PHYSICAL MEDICINE AND REHABILITATION BOARD REVIEW

PHYSICAL MEDICINE AND REHABILITATION BOARD REVIEW

Sara Cuccurullo, M.D.
Editor

Clinical Assistant Professor and Residency Program Director
Director, JFK Medical Center Consult Service
Department of Physical Medicine and Rehabilitation
University of Medicine and Dentistry of New Jersey
Robert Wood Johnson Medical School
JFK Johnson Rehabilitation Institute, Edison, New Jersey

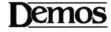

Demos Medical Publishing, 386 Park Avenue South, New York, New York 10016

Library of Congress Cataloging-in-Publication data
Physical medicine and rehabilitation board review / by Sara J.
   Cuccurullo, editor.
      p. ; cm.
   Includes bibliographical references and index.
   ISBN 1-888799-45-5
   1. Medicine, Physical—Examinations, questions, etc.   2. Medical
   rehabilitation—Examinations, questions, etc.
[DNLM: 1. Physical Medicine—Examination Questions. 2.
Rehabilitation—Examination Questions. WB 18.2 P4776 2002] I.
Cuccurullo, Sara J., 1960-
RM701.6.P48 2002
615.8'2'076—dc21
2002000889
Manufactured in the United States of America

Great care has been taken to maintain the accuracy of the information contained in this volume. However, Demos Medical Publishing cannot be held responsible for errors or for any consequences arising from the use of the information contained herein.

■

DEDICATION

I dedicate this book to my dear friend Kathy Wong, M.D. The spirit, integrity and grace she brought to her patients and the field of Physical Medicine and Rehabilitation is greatly missed since she died of breast cancer at the young age of 36.

This book is also dedicated to:
>   my husband Alec (my loving partner in life);
>   my four children, Michelle, Alexander, Amanda, and Nicholas (who are the joys of my life);
>   my parents, Connie and Pat Cuccurullo, (my support system throughout my entire life);
>   my mentors and teachers, especially my chairman Dr. Thomas E. Strax (my inspiration and supporter in all aspects of medicine both clinical and academic), and Dr. Ernest W. Johnson (my encouragement to take on a challenge);
>   and the residents of the UMDNJ, Robert Wood Johnson Medical School, JFK Johnson Rehabilitation Institute Residency Program (whose hunger for knowledge inspired the concept of this review book).

It is only because of the support and encouragement of these people that this project could be completed.

PRODUCTION STAFF

JFK Johnson Rehabilitation Institute
Project Manager: Heather Platt, B.S.

DM Cradle Associates, Publishing Services
Project Manager: Carol Henderson

We gratefully acknowledge the contributions made by the artists involved in this project. We sincerely thank them for their dedication, expertise, creativity and professionalism. Special thanks to Bob Silvestri and the JFK Johnson Rehabilitation Institute Prosthetic and Orthotic Laboratory.

Al Garcia Photography
Photographs

4.28	4.55	4.81	4.105	4.164	6.35
4.37	4.57	4.82	4.106	6.10	6.36
4.38	4.77	4.100	4.117	6.16	6.37
4.44	4.78	4.101	4.159	6.17	
4.45	4.79	4.102	4.160	6.24	
4.49	4.80	4.103	4.163	6.34	

Andrew F. Pecoraro
Illustrations

4.8	6.11	6.27	7.24	10.3	10.12
4.11	6.13	6.38	7.25	10.4	10.17
6.5	6.14	7.4	7.36	10.5	10.18
6.6	6.15	7.13	7.37	10.6	11.7
6.7	6.23	7.14	9.6	10.7	11.11
6.8	6.25	7.16	9.9	10.8	11.12
				10.11	11.13

Ethan F. Geehr, CMI
Illustrations

5.4	5.21	5.38	5.77	5.97	5.113
5.6	5.22	5.39	5.78	5.98	5.114
5.8	5.25	5.43	5.79	5.99	5.115
5.10	5.26	5.44	5.81	5.103	5.116
5.11	5.27	5.46	5.83	5.106	5.117
5.12	5.28	5.47	5.84	5.108	5.125
5.13	5.31	5.48	5.88	5.109	8.2
5.14	5.35	5.65	5.91	5.110	8.3
5.15	5.36	5.71	5.94	5.111	9.1
5.20	5.37	5.72	5.95	5.112	9.5

Table 5.4

George Higgins
Photographs

4.16	4.22	4.107
4.17	4.53	4.118
4.21	4.67	4.156

Heather L. Platt
Illustrations

4.9	4.54	4.93	4.121	4.157	7.9
4.13	4.58	4.94	4.123	4.161	7.10
4.15	4.59	4.95	4.124	4.162	7.11
4.25	4.60	4.96	4.125	4.165	7.18
4.32	4.63	4.97	4.127	4.172	7.19
4.33	4.70	4.98	4.128	4.173	7.20
4.34	4.71	4.99	4.129	4.174	7.21
4.35	4.72	4.108	4.130	4.180	7.22
4.36	4.73	4.109	4.131	4.185	7.30
4.39	4.74	4.110	4.132	4.186	7.34
4.40	4.75	4.111	4.134	4.187	7.35
4.41	4.76	4.112	4.136	4.188	8.1
4.46	4.88	4.116	4.137	7.3	10.1
4.47	4.91	4.119	4.138	7.5	10.2
4.52	4.92	4.120	4.146	7.6	10.9
			4.147	7.7	10.16
			4.154	7.8	10.19

Acknowledgment

I've had the pleasure of helping residents learn what they need to know for their PM&R Boards at JFK Johnson Rehabilitation Institute, UMDNJ Robert Wood Johnson Medical School for more than ten years. Over these years, I have had many requests for my yearly revised notes from former residents and from residents outside our program. For this reason I gathered together an expert group of knowledgeable physicians to put together a comprehensive PM&R board review text.

The *Physical Medicine and Rehabilitation Board Review* reflects the commitment of the authors and the faculty in the Department of Physical Medicine and Rehabilitation at UMDNJ Robert Wood Johnson Medical School, based at JFK Johnson Rehabilitation Institute, to produce a text that would be used as a guide containing selected topics considered important for physicians preparing for either the certifying or the recertifying examination offered by the American Board of Physical Medicine and Rehabilitation. This text presents clear practical information for both residents studying for the boards of PM&R and for practicing physicians. This text should be of great value in not only preparing for the American Board of PM&R board exam, but also for caring for patients.

The credit for this textbook coming to print must be given to Thomas Strax, M.D., Chairman of the Department of Physical Medicine and Rehabilitation. His constant encouragement and willingness to support this project has been a true inspiration in seeing this textbook come to realization. Special thanks have to be given to the administration of JFK Johnson Rehabilitation Institute and JFK Medical Center for their encouragement and financial support without which this book would not have been possible. Specifically, I would like to sincerely thank J. Scott Gebhard, Anthony Cuzzola, Marci Gietter and John P. McGee.

I will also be eternally grateful to three of my former students, Edgardo Baerga, Eric Freeman, and Priscila Gonzalez. It was their stamina and perseverance that enabled this text to come to fruition. Their energy and enthusiasm were truly inspirational. I am grateful to all the authors for their completion of the manuscripts. I greatly acknowledge the support of Demos Medical Publishing and DM Cradle Associates, Publishing Services.

Special thanks must also be given to Heather Platt, project manager of the book. Heather was there from the day the idea of this book was conceived and has been truly dedicated and committed to seeing that the text realizes publication. Her countless hours of commitment to this project and her dedication are things for which I will always be grateful.

I would also like to thank Ernie Johnson who has been very inspirational in any educational project I have undertaken. He is truly one of the giants in the field of PM&R. His interest in reading the book, writing the foreword, and giving his input prior to its publication is greatly appreciated. I would like to acknowledge the enormous support and understanding I have received from my husband, four children, and parents during the formulation of this text. I hope that the *Physical Medicine and Rehabilitation Board Review* will receive a warm reception. My coauthors and I look forward to receiving comments and suggestions from the readers.

Sara Cuccurullo, M.D.

FOREWORD

Over the years many residents have confronted the problem of "what to study for the Boards."

This is a serious problem that had a few, generally unsatisfactory, solutions:

1. Attend one of the review courses. Can't cover everything but makes a 5-day effort. Costs!!!!
2. Have weekly conferences with senior residents to argue about vague recollections by former residents of previous Part I of the Boards. Some of the more enterprising programs usually had files of old exams to generate discussion.
3. Home perusal of the two major PM&R texts and electrodiagnostic medicine. This is a stupendous (one could say—outrageous) task, hardly possible for a busy fourth year resident to manage.
4. Review all of the literature. One of our former residents made the mistake of trying to review the last 10 years of the *Archives of PM&R*, and the *Am J PM&R, Muscle & Nerve*. He obviously believed he had learned everything. He only later discovered this time-consuming preparation interfered with his performance rating in the residency program, severely compromised his "moonlighting," and almost broke up his marriage.

In the old days when we had only one skinny journal, one of my resident colleagues decided to review three textbooks—neurology, orthopedics, and internal medicine, with pediatrics in reserve (if time was available). He discovered too late he could not cover the key subjects—even if he only read the boldface type. (**N.B.** Textbooks are five years old when published.)

However, this elegant volume will finally fulfill this critical void and will supply reasonable and current PM&R diagnostic and management facts for the prospective Board candidate.

It can be studied in a reasonable time without speed reading *and* it is up-to-date with valuable and relevant information. With over 500 pages of nuggets, I predict the next Elkins award winner will have read this study guide.

Thank you, Dr. Sara Cuccurullo!

Ernest W. Johnson, M.D.

CONTRIBUTORS

AUTHORS

Michael Alexander, M.D.
Clinical Professor, Department of Pediatric Rehabilitation, Jefferson Medical College of Thomas Jefferson University, A.I. duPont Hospital for Children, Wilmington, Delaware

Edgardo Baerga, M.D.
Attending Physiatrist, Department of Physical Medicine and Rehabilitation, Shore Rehabilitation Institute, Diplomate, American Board of Physical Medicine and Rehabilitation, Point Pleasant, New Jersey

David Brown, D.O.
Clinical Assistant Professor, Department of Physical Medicine and Rehabilitation, University of Medicine and Dentistry of New Jersey—Robert Wood Johnson Medical School, Director, Outpatient Services, JFK Johnson Rehabilitation Institute, Edison, New Jersey

Sara Cuccurullo, M.D.
Clinical Assistant Professor and Residency Program Director, Department of Physical Medicine and Rehabilitation, University of Medicine and Dentistry of New Jersey—Robert Wood Johnson Medical School, JFK Johnson Rehabilitation Institute, Director, JFK Medical Center Consult Service, Edison, New Jersey

Elie Elovic, M.D.
Associate Professor Kessler Institute for Rehabilitation, University of Medicine and Dentistry of New Jersey—New Jersey Medical School, Co-Director TBI Research, Kessler Medical Rehabilitation Research Education Corporation, Newark, New Jersey

Eric D. Freeman, D.O., F.A.A.P.M.R.
Physiatrist, New Jersey Orthopaedic Sports and Spine Institute, Edison, New Jersey

Ted L. Freeman, D.O., F.A.A.P.M.R., F.A.A.E.M.
Medical Director, Freeman Spine and Sports Medicine Institute, Laurelton Medical Center, Brick, New Jersey, Medical Director, Freeman Occupational Healthcare, Oakhurst, New Jersey

Priscila Gonzalez, M.D.
Attending Physiatrist, Private Practice, Oakhurst, New Jersey

Barbara Hoffer, D.O.
Attending Physiatrist, Healthsouth Reading Rehabilitation Hospital, Director, Oncology Services, Reading, Pennsylvania

Iqbal Jafri, M.D.
Clinical Assistant Professor, Department of Physical Medicine and Rehabilitation, University of Medicine and Dentistry of New Jersey—Robert Wood Johnson Medical School, Director, Pain Management Program, JFK Johnson Rehabilitation Institute, Edison, New Jersey

Ernest W. Johnson, M.D.
Clinical Professor, Department of Physical Medicine and Rehabilitation, Associate Dean for External Affairs, College of Medicine and Public Health, Ohio State University, Columbus, Ohio

Steven Kirshblum, M.D.
Associate Professor, University of Medicine and Dentistry of New Jersey—New Jersey Medical School, Associate Medical Director, Director of Spinal Cord Injury Services, Kessler Institute for Rehabilitation, Newark, New Jersey

Leslie Lazaroff, D.O.
Attending Physiatrist, Department of Physical Medicine and Rehabilitation, Somerset Medical Center, Somerset, New Jersey

Lisa Luciano, D.O.
Clinical Assistant Professor, Department of Physical Medicine and Rehabilitation, University of Medicine and Dentistry of New Jersey—Robert Wood Johnson Medical School, Medical Director, Independent Health Systems, Attending Physiatrist, JFK Johnson Rehabilitation Institute, Edison, New Jersey

Thomas Nucatola, M.D.
Arthritis, Allergy, Immunology Center, Edison, New Jersey

David S. Rosenblum, M.D.
Diplomate, American Board of Physical Medicine and Rehabilitation, and Medical Director, SCI & Neuro-Orthopaedic Division, Gaylord Hospital, Wallingford, Connecticut

Roger Rossi, D.O.
Clinical Assistant Professor, Department of Physical Medicine and Rehabilitation, University of Medicine and Dentistry of New Jersey—Robert Wood Johnson Medical School, Director, Rehabilitation Services Hartwyck, Edison Estates, Director, Graduate Medical Student Education Program, JFK Johnson Rehabilitation Institute, Edison, New Jersey

Thomas E. Strax, M.D., Assistant Editor
Clinical Professor and Chair, Department of Physical Medicine and Rehabilitation, University of Medicine and Dentistry of New Jersey—Robert Wood Johnson Medical School, Medical Director, JFK Johnson Rehabilitation Institute, Edison, New Jersey

Heikki Uustal, M.D.
Clinical Assistant Professor, Department of Physical Medicine and Rehabilitation, University of Medicine and Dentistry of New Jersey—Robert Wood Johnson Medical School, Medical Director, Prosthetics and Orthotics Team, JFK Johnson Rehabilitation Institute, Edison, New Jersey

Alan W. Young, D.O.
Physician, Department of Rehabilitation Medicine, Rehabilitation Institute of San Antonio, President, Alamo Regional Alternative Rehabilitation Center, San Antonio, Texas

Richard D. Zorowitz, M.D.
Assistant Professor, Department of Rehabilitation Medicine, University of Pennsylvania School of Medicine, Director, Stroke Rehabilitation, Medical Director, Piersol Rehabilitation Unit, Philadelphia, Pennsylvania

REVIEWERS

Steven Escaldi, D.O.
Clinical Assistant Professor, Department of Physical Medicine and Rehabilitation, University of Medicine and Dentistry of New Jersey—Robert Wood Johnson Medical School, Medical Director, Day Hospital Rehabilitation Program, JFK Johnson Rehabilitation Institute, Edison, New Jersey

Ernest W. Johnson, M.D.
Clinical Professor, Department of Physical Medicine and Rehabilitation, Associate Dean for External Affairs, College of Medicine and Public Health, Ohio State University, Columbus, Ohio

Lei Lin, Ph.D., M.D., Assistant Editor
Clinical Assistant Professor, Department of Physical Medicine and Rehabilitation, University of Medicine and Dentistry of New Jersey—Robert Wood Johnson Medical School, Attending Physiatrist, JFK Johnson Rehabilitation Institute, Edison, New Jersey

Ian Maitin, M.D.
Assistant Professor, Temple University School of Medicine, and Director, NeuroRehabilitation Services, Residency Program Director, Department of Physical Medicine and Rehabilitation, Philadelphia, Pennslyvania

Caroline McCagg, M.D.
Clinical Associate Professor, Department of Physical Medicine and Rehabilitation, University of Medicine and Dentistry of New Jersey—Robert Wood Johnson Medical School, Associate Medical Director, Director of Inpatient Services, Medical Director, Center for Head Injury, JFK Johnson Rehabilitation Institute, Edison, New Jersey

Matthew Raymond, D.O.
Diplomate, American Board of Physical Medicine and Rehabilitation; Attending Physiatrist, Musculoskeletal Medicine, Gaylord Hospital, Wallingford, Connecticut

Thomas E. Strax, M.D., Assistant Editor
Clinical Professor and Chair, Department of Physical Medicine and Rehabilitation, University of Medicine and Dentistry of New Jersey—Robert Wood Johnson Medical School; Medical Director, JFK Johnson Rehabilitation Institute, Edison, New Jersey

CONTENTS

PREFACE

The Physical Medicine and Board Review Book will appeal to medical students, residents, and practicing physiatrists. The book concentrates on board-related concepts in the field of Rehabilitation Medicine. Residents will find the book essential in preparing for Part I and Part II of the Physical Medicine and Rehabilitation Board Certification because it is one of the only books of its kind with major focus on board-related material giving a synopsis of up-to-date PM&R orthopedic, neurologic, and general medical information all in one place. Over 500 diagrams simplify material that is board pertinent. In this way, important concepts are clarified and reinforced through illustration. All of the major texts of this specialty have been referenced to give the board examinee the most timely and relevant information and recommended reading.

This book is clearly different than most texts. It is written in outline form and is about one-third the size of most textbooks. The topics are divided into major subspecialty areas and are authored by physicians with special interests and clinical expertise in the respective subjects. Board pearls are highlighted with an open-book icon in the margins of many of the paragraphs. These pearls are aimed at stressing the clinical and board-eligible aspects of the topics. This format was used to assist with last minute preparation for the board examination and was inspired by the *Mayo Clinic Internal Medicine Board Review*. The contents are modeled after the topic selection of the *American Academy of Physical Medicine and Rehabilitation (AAPMR) Self-Directed Medical Knowledge Program* [which is used by residents nationwide to prepare for the Self-Assessment Examination (SAE)]. This was done specifically to help all residents, Post Graduate Year 2, 3, 4, in yearly preparation and carryover from the SAE preparation to board exam preparation.

Two key points need to be addressed prior to using this text. This book is not a comprehensive textbook of PM&R. All chapters are prepared under the assumption that readers will have studied at length one or more of the standard textbooks of PM&R before studying this review.

My hope is that this text is a valuable tool to all physicians preparing for both the written and oral board exams, and also in managing issues of patient care. Practicing physiatrists should also find this book helpful in preparation for the recertifying exam. Because this is one of the first textbooks designed specifically for PM&R board preparation, the authors welcome any ideas for improvement from any of the readers. We wish you all the best in your studies.

Sara Cuccurullo, M.D.

INTRODUCTION:
BOARD CERTIFICATION

The discussion in this chapter is aimed primarily at candidates preparing for the American Board of Physical Medicine and Rehabilitation (ABPM&R) certifying or recertifying examinations in Physical Medicine and Rehabilitation.

The following information was collected and calculated by the ABPM&R and published in the *Diplomate News* July 2003.

In May 2003, the ABPM&R administered the 56th certification examinations to 806 candidates. With 266 candidates achieving Board certification, the total number of Diplomates rose to 7,460. The table and graph below summarize the results for both the written exam (Part I) and the oral exam (Part II).

	PART I			PART II	
All Candidates					
Passed	361	79%		266	76%
Failed	97	21%		82	24%
First Time	366			314	
Passed	328	89.6%		245	78%
Failed	38	10.4%		69	22%
Repeat	92			34	
Passed	33	36%		21	62%
Failed	59	64%		13	38%

As the data in the table suggest, the pass rate for first-time candidates on both exams continues to be high, with pass rates of 89.6% and 78% for Part I and Part II respectively.

In 1998, the Board began analyzing results based on the content areas in the examination outline for Part I. The Part I exam outline consists of two independent dimensions or content domains, and all test questions are classified into each of these domains. The major content domains appear below.

I. Type of Problem/Organ System
    A. Neurologic Disorders
    B. Musculoskeletal Medicine
    C. Amputation
    D. Cardiovascular and Other Systems
    E. Rehabilitation Problems and Outcomes
    F. Basic Sciences
II. Focus of Question/Patient Management
    A. Patient Evaluation and Diagnosis
    B. Electrodiagnosis
    C. Patient Management
    D. Rehabilitation Technology
    E. Applied Sciences

All Part 1 candidates received performance feedback in the form of scaled scores for each of these content domains. To allow performance in one section to be compared to performance in other sections, the section scores were scaled to fall between 1 and 10. A score of 1 would indicate that a candidate performed no better than chance, while a score of 10 indicates that a candidate answered all questions correctly in that section.

According to psychometric data available to the Board following each examination, it is apparent that this year, as in previous years, the sections are not equally difficult for the group as a whole. Candidates in 2003 performed better in the Musculoskeletal Medicine section, while lower scores were recorded in Amputation and Rehabilitation Technology.

THE PURPOSE OF CERTIFICATION

The intent of the certification process as defined by Member Boards of the ABMS (American Board of Medical Specialties) is to provide assurance to the public that a certified medical specialist has successfully completed an accredited residency training program and an evaluation, including an examination process, designed to assess the knowledge, experience and skills requisite to the provision of high quality patient care in that specialty. Diplomates of the ABPM&R possess particular qualifications in this specialty.

THE EXAMINATION

As part of the requirements for certification by the ABPMR, candidates must demonstrate satisfactory performance in an examination conducted by the Board covering the field of PM&R. The examination for certification is given in two parts, computer based (Part I) and oral (Part II).

EXAMINATION ADMISSIBILITY REQUIREMENTS

Part I

Part I of the ABPMR's certification examination is administered as computer-based testing (CBT). To be admissible to Part I of the Board certification examination, candidates are required to complete at least 48 months of ACGME-accredited postgraduate residency training, of which at least 36 months should be spent in supervised education and clinical practice in an ACGME-accredited PM&R residency training program.

Part II

Part II of the ABPMR's certification examination is administered as an oral examination. At least one full-time or equivalent year of PM&R clinical practice, PM&R-related clinical fellowship, or a combination of these activities is required after satisfactory completion of an accredited PM&R residency training program.

The clinical practice must provide evidence of acceptable professional, ethical, and humanistic conduct attested to by two Board-certified physiatrists in the candidate's local or regional area. In rare instances in which a physiatrist is not geographically available, two licensed physicians in the area may support the candidate's application for Part II.

Additional information about the certification and re-certification examinations are provided in several brochures published by the ABPMR. The brochures are titled *Preparing for the Computer-Based ABPMR Examination, Computer-Based Testing Fact Sheet*, and *Preparing for the ABPMR Oral Examination*. These brochures can be obtained from the Board office.

Part I Examination

The Board made the decision to implement computerized testing for the Part I certification exam because they felt it offered many advantages to examinees. These include access and conveniences, enhanced security, and cutting-edge technology (e.g., graphics, simulation). Computer-based testing (CBT) is the administering of an exam using an electronic multiple-choice question format.

The ABPMR transitioned from paper-and-pencil exams to CBTs with the May 2002 certification exam. The Part I exam is administered on an electronic testing system that eliminates the use of paper and pencil exam booklets and answer sheets. Candidates use a keyboard or mouse to select answers to exam questions presented on the computer screen. The computer stores responses and automatically time the exam. The time remaining and the number of the question currently being answered are visible on the computer screen throughout the exam. Answers can be changed, skipped, and marked for review. Computer based testing provides simple, easy-to-follow instructions via a tutorial to complete the exam. The ABPMR uses a simple, proven computer interface that will require only routine mouse or cursor movements, and the use of the mouse or enter-key on the keyboard to record the option chosen to answer the question. Examinees have the option of using a brief tutorial on the computer prior to beginning the actual exam. Time spent with the tutorial does not reduce your testing time, so they recommend that examinees take advantage of it. The tutorial is available at the beginning of each section of the exam. It includes detailed instructions on taking the computerized exam and provides an opportunity to respond to practice questions. You also become familiar with placement of information on the computer screen.

The ABPMR's computer-based exam is offered at over three hundred and fifty (350) technology centers located in most of the major cities throughout the United States and Canada through an arrangement with Prometric. Candidates should call to schedule their exam as soon as possible after they receive their admissibility letter from the Board. Candidates who wait too long to call may not be able to test at the location they prefer. Candidates will be able to indicate preference for sites. However, in some regions due to large numbers of candidates, it will be first-come, first-served based on site capacity and numbers of sites in the area. Once you have received admissibility and authorization from the ABPMR, you may arrange for a test site location by calling Prometric Candidate Services Call Center. Contact information will be provided by the ABPMR. Prometric Technology Centers typically consist of a waiting area, check-in area, and testing room with six to fifteen individual computer testing stations. One or more Prometric staff members will be on hand to check-in candidates and supervise the testing session. Prometric monitors exam sessions by several wall-mounted video cameras, as is noted by signage in each center.

The exam is administered on one day annually at selected Prometric Technology Center sites throughout the United States and Canada. The exam is a 400-item test that is divided into a morning section consisting of 200 questions and an afternoon section composed of the remaining 200 questions. The question format is the same as it has been on the pencil-paper exam. There are four options for each question with one best answer. Examinees are allowed eight hours to take the full exam. Each section of the exam (morning, afternoon) is allotted four hours for completion.

Exam content outline remains the same as previous ABPMR certifying exams. The questions used for the computerized exam are selected from the same item pool as the paper and pencil exams. The ABPMR introduces several hundred new items to the pool every year. This continues with computer-based testing. The software allows examinees to skip and/or mark items for later review within each four-hour section. Once a section is completed, however, the examinee is not able to go back and review or change answers.

Each test center is staffed with Prometric personnel to assist examinees in the event of a computer malfunction. If the problem is not resolved in a reasonable time-frame, examinees will be notified of how to proceed. If you require wheelchair seating, it is crucial that you indicate your needs during the application process, as such accommodations are limited at the various sites. The Board will make reasonable accommodations for candidates with dis-

xxiv ■ BOARD CERTIFICATION

abilities, provided appropriate medical documentation is submitted with the request for special testing accommodations. Contact the ABPMR for a copy of the *Request for Special Examination Accommodations* form. The form must be returned to the Board office by January 1 of the exam year.

Exam results and score reports are mailed to examinees from the Board office within six weeks after the testing day. No results are given via telephone, fax, or e-mail. Prometric is not able to provide exam results. Although the exam only requires eight hours to administer, there is significant post-exam activity done by the ABPMR. Only after this statistical analysis is carefully completed can the results be reported to the examinees. The examinee score report includes the examinee's scaled score and the scaled score required to pass the exam. In addition, scaled sub-scores for the specific content areas (based on the exam outline) are reported.

The ABPMR has prepared a document that describes the computer testing process. The brochure, titled *Preparing for the ABPMR's Computer-Based Certification Exam,* will be mailed with your admissibility information. Candidates should arrive at the testing center thirty minutes before the beginning of the scheduled exam session. Candidates who arrive more than fifteen minutes late for either section of the exam will forfeit their reservations and will be excluded from taking the exam. The following items will be required at the test center when reporting to the exam:

- Two forms of government-issued identification, one that includes your photo and signature, and the other that bears your signature.
- The admissibility letter from the Board office.

To ensure that all candidates are tested under equally favorable conditions, the following regulations and procedures are observed at each test center:

- Candidates are not permitted to take personal belongings into the testing room. Items that candidates bring to the room must be placed in a small, square locker; you will keep the locker key for the duration of the exam. Prometric Technology Centers are not responsible for lost or misplaced items.
- Candidates are not permitted to eat, drink, or smoke during the test.
- Under no circumstances will candidates be permitted to work beyond the time allotted for the exam. Time limits are generous; candidates should have ample time to answer all questions and check all work.
- Candidates may not leave the room during an exam without notifying the on-site manager. Candidates will be required to sign-out when leaving and sign-in upon returning to the testing room. Candidates who need to leave the exam room for any reason will not be allowed additional time for the exam.
- Candidates causing any disturbance or engaging in any kind of misconduct—such as giving or receiving help, using notes, books, or other aids, taking part in an act of impersonation, or removing notes from the testing room—may be summarily dismissed from the exam.
- No visitors, guests, or children are allowed at the test center.

The test center manager will escort you to your assigned seat and log you on to your computer. At the end of the time allotted for each section of the exam, the screen will indicate that time has expired and further access will be denied. For candidates who complete either section of the exam early, clicking the "end" button will close down their access to that section of the exam. Notify the test center manager if you complete either section of the exam early. You will sign out upon leaving the facility.

The ABPMR web site will be updated periodically. Each issue of the *Diplomate News* also includes reports from the Electronic Exam Committee, and other news.

CONTENT OF THE EXAMINATION

The examination questions are designed to test the candidate's knowledge of basic sciences and clinical management as related to PM&R and will be in the form of objective testing.

PART I (COMPUTER-BASED) EXAMINATION OUTLINE

Examination Outline for the Written Examination

Class 1: Type of Problem/Organ System

A. Neurologic Disorders
1. Stroke
2. Spinal Cord Injury
3. Traumatic Brain Injury
4. Neuropathies
   a. Mononeuropathies
   b. Polyneuropathies
   c. Carpal Tunnel Syndrome
   d. Other Entrapment Neuropathies
5. Other Neurologic Disorders
   a. Multiple Sclerosis
   b. Motor Neuron Disease
   c. Poliomyelitis
   d. Guillain-Barré Syndrome
   e. Cerebral Palsy
   f. Spina Bifida
   g. Duchenne Muscular Dystrophy
   h. Myotonic Muscular Dystrophy
   i. Inflammatory Myopathies
   j. Other Myopathies
   k. Thoracic Outlet Syndrome
   l. Plexopathy
   m. Radiculopathy
   n. Parkinson's Disease
   o. Other Neuromuscular Disorders
B. Musculoskeletal Medicine
1. Arthritis
   a. Rheumatoid Arthritis
   b. Osteoarthritis
   c. Collagen Disease
   d. Other Arthritis
2. Soft Tissue & Orthopedic Problems
   a. Acute Trauma
   b. Chronic Trauma/Overuse
   c. Complex Regional Pain Syndrome Type 1 (Reflex Sympathetic Dystrophy)
   d. Fibrositis/Myofascial Pain/Soreness
   e. Burns
   f. Fractures
   g. Osteoporosis
   h. Back and Spine Disorders
   i. Strain/Sprains
   j. Tendonitis/Bursitis
   k. Orthopedic/Rheumatology
   l. Heterotopic Ossification
   m. Other Soft Tissue Disease
C. Amputation
1. Upper Extremity
2. Lower Extremity
D. Cardiovascular & Other Systems
1. Cardiovascular
   a. Ischemic Heart Disease
   b. Other Heart Disease
   c. Peripheral Artery Disease
   d. Venous Disease
   e. Vascular Disorders
   f. Lymphedema
   g. Hypertension
   h. Other Cardiovascular
2. Pulmonary Disease
   a. Asthma
   b. COPD
   c. Pneumonia
   d. Impaired Ventilation
   e. Other Pulmonary Problems
3. GU/GI Disorders
   a. Neurogenic Bladder
   b. Renal Impairment/Failure
   c. Neurogenic Bowel
   d. Sexuality and Reproductive Issues
   e. Other GU/GI Disorders
4. Cancer
5. Infectious Disease
E. Rehabilitation Problems & Outcomes
1. Physical Complications
   a. Spasticity
   b. Contracture
   c. Hydrocephalus
   d. Seizures
   e. Pressure Ulcer
   f. Posture/Balance Disorders
   g. Abnormal Gait
   h. Dysphagia/Aspiration

i. Bed Rest/Deconditioning
j. Paralysis/Weakness
k. Heterotopic Ossification
l. Other Physical Complications
2. Cognitive/Sensory Dysfunction
   a. Speech and Language Disorders
   b. Hearing Impairment
   c. Visual Dysfunction
   d. Cognitive Disorders
   e. Sleep Disorders

f. Other Cognitive/Sensory Dysfunctions
3. Psychiatric/Psychological Problems
   a. Depression
   b. Substance Abuse
   c. Dementia/Pseudodementia
   d. Vegetative State
   e. Other Psychiatric Problems
4. Pain
F. Basic Sciences

Class 2: Focus of Question/Patient Management

A. Patient Evaluation & Diagnosis
   1. Physical Exam, Signs & Symptoms
   2. Diagnosis & Etiology
   3. Diagnostic Procedures
      a. Cardiopulmonary Assess/Stress Test
      b. Gait Analysis
      c. Urodynamics
      d. Lab Studies
      e. Synovial Fluid Analysis
      f. Medical Imaging
      g. Neuropsychological Evaluations
      h. Other Diagnostic Procedures
   4. Functional Evaluation
   5. Prognosis
B. Electrodiagnosis
   1. General Electrodiagnosis
   2. Instrumentation
   3. Nerve Conduction
   4. Electromyography
   5. Somatosensory Evoked Potential
   6. Neuromuscular Transmission
   7. H Reflex/F Wave
   8. Special Studies
C. Patient Management
   1. Clinical Decision-Making (incl. Ethics)
   2. Physical Agents
      a. Heat/Cryotherapy
      b. Hydrotherapy
      c. Electrostimulation
      d. Ultrasound
      e. Biofeedback
   3. Therapeutic Exercise and Manipulation
      a. Motor Control
      b. Mobility and Range of Motion
      c. Strength and Endurance
      d. Manipulation and Massage
      e. Traction/Immobilization
   4. Pharmacologic Interventions
      a. Analgesics

b. Antiseizure and Antispasmodics
c. Antibiotics
d. Psychopharmacologies
e. Anti-Inflammatory
f. Other medications
5. Procedural/Interventional
   a. Nerve Blocks
   b. Anesthetic Injections
   c. Surgery
   d. Other Procedural/Interventional
6. Behavioral/Psychological Modalities
   a. Relaxation Therapy
   b. Behavior Modification
   c. Psychotherapy/Counseling
   d. Education
D. Rehabilitation Technology
   1. Prosthetics
   2. Orthotics
   3. Other Rehabilitation Technology
      a. Shoes
      b. Functional Electrical Stimulation
      c. Transcutaneous Electrical Nerve Stimulation
      d. Augmentation Communication
      e. Ventilation
      f. Wheelchair/Seating
      g. Other Devices
E. Applied Sciences
   1. Anatomy
      a. Central Nervous System
      b. Peripheral Nerves
      c. Head/Neck
      d. Shoulder
      e. Arm
      f. Wrist
      g. Hand
      h. Hip
      i. Knee
      j. Leg

k. Ankle
l. Foot
m. Muscle
n. Bone
o. Back/Spine: General
p. Spine: Cervical
q. Spine: Thoracic
r. Spine: Lumbosacral
s. Other Anatomy
2. Physiology
   a. Neurophysiology
   b. Neuromuscular
   c. Cardiovascular
   d. Pulmonary
   e. Genitourinary

f. Gastrointestinal
g. Skin and Connective Tissue
h. Bone and Joints
i. Autonomic Nervous System
j. Endocrine
3. Pathology/Pathophysiology
4. Kinesiology/Biomechanics
5. Histology
6. Epidemiology/Risk Factors
7. Nutrition
8. Biochemistry
9. Pharmacology
10. Research and Statistics
11. Growth and Development
12. Other Basic Science (e.g., Physics)

QUESTION FORMAT

The 1998 ABPMR Booklet gave an idea of how the exam looks. These items are *not* from previous ABPM&R exams, nor will they appear on future tests. They are given by ABPM&R as a sample for your use. All items are of the "best single choice answer multiple choice" type.

1. Post-acute recovery and community reintegration of the traumatically brain-injured patient are most often hampered by
   A. Language impairment
   B. Memory impairment
   C. Physical impairment
   D. Financial disincentives
   E. Personality and behavioral impairment
2. Which best describes a feature of short-wave diathermy?
   A. It is used to heat the hip joint
   B. It produces both direct and reflex blood flow increase
   C. It is used around the thigh to improve circulation in an ischemic limb
   D. The dose is regulated by measuring the flow of the high-frequency current through the patient
   E. Commercially available machines operate at a frequency of 950 MHz
3. The single most reliable clinical sign for the detection of inflammatory arthritis is
   A. Local tenderness
   B. Painful, limited range of motion
   C. Synovial swelling
   D. Joint effusion
   E. Skin color change
4. Which condition is most likely a contraindication for intra-articular corticosteroid injection therapy?
   A. Crystal-induced synovitis
   B. Diabetes mellitus
   C. Peptic ulcer
   D. Bacteremia
   E. Osteoarthritis

Answers for the above examples are as follows; 1. E, 2. B, 3. C, 4. D. Attempts have been made to avoid ambiguity and typographical or spelling errors, but occasionally they occur. They are not intended to "trip you up" or confuse you. Further details regarding the examination, training requirements, eligibility requirements and other related information can be obtained from the ABPM&R.

PREPARATION FOR THE TEST

Training during medical school forms the foundation on which advanced clinical knowledge is accumulated during residency training. However, the serious preparation for the examination actually starts at the beginning of the residency training in PM&R. Most candidates will require a minimum of 6-8 months of intense preparation for the examination. Cramming just before the examination is counterproductive. Some of the methods for preparation for the Board examination are described below. Additionally, each candidate may develop his or her own system.

It is essential that each candidate study a standard textbook of PM&R from beginning to end. Any of the standard textbooks of PM&R should provide a good basic knowledge base in all areas of PM&R. Ideally, the candidate should read one good textbook and not jump from one to another, except for reading certain chapters that are outstanding in a particular textbook. This book and similar board review syllabi are excellent tools for brushing up on important Board-relevant information several weeks to months before the examination. They, however, cannot take the place of comprehensive textbooks of PM&R. This book is designed as a study guide rather than a comprehensive textbook of PM&R. Therefore, it should not be used as the sole source of medical information for the examination.

HELPFUL RESOURCES

Use past Self-Assessment Examinations-for Residents (SAE-R). These are extremely valuable for obtaining practice in answering multiple choice questions. These annual exam questions are available in print-format from the Academy of Physical Medicine and Rehabilitation. These questions are not used on the Board exams, but serve as a means to assess your knowledge on a range of PM&R topics. For a nominal fee, the AAPM&R will send requestors an exam booklet with answers and references for one exam.

Formation of study groups, three to five candidates per group, permits study of different textbooks and review articles in journals. It is important that the group meet regularly and that each candidate be assigned reading materials. Selected review papers and state-of-the-art articles on common and important topics in PM&R should be included in the study materials. Indiscriminate reading of articles from many journals should be avoided. In any case, most candidates who begin preparation 6 to 8 months before the examination will not find time for extensive study of journal materials. Notes and other materials the candidates have gathered during their residency training are also good sources of information. These clinical "pearls" gathered from mentors will be of help in remembering certain important points.

Certain diseases, many peculiar and uncommon, are eminently "Board-eligible," meaning that they may appear in the Board examinations more frequently than in clinical practice. Most of these are covered in this book. Several formulas and points should be memorized (such as Target Heart Rate). Most significantly, the clinical training obtained and the regular study habits formed during residency training are the most important aspects of preparation for the examination. Review courses are also available if desired.

DAY OF THE EXAMINATION

Adequate time is allowed to read and answer all the questions; therefore, there is no need to rush or become anxious. You should watch the time to ensure that you are at least halfway through the examination when half of the time has elapsed. Start by answering the first question and continue sequentially (do not skip too many). Do not be alarmed by lengthy questions; look for the question's salient points. When faced with a confusing question, do not become distracted by that question. Mark it so you can find it later, then go to the next question and come back to the unanswered ones at the end. Extremely lengthy stem statements or case presentations are apparently intended to test the candidate's ability to separate the essential from the unnecessary or unimportant information.

Some candidates may fail the examination despite the possession of an immense amount of knowledge and the clinical competence necessary to pass the examination. Their failure to pass the examination may be caused by the lack of ability to understand or interpret the questions properly. The ability to understand the nuances of the question format is sometimes referred to as "boardsmanship." Intelligent interpretation of the questions is very important for candidates who are not well versed in the format of multiple-choice questions. It is very important to read the final sentence (that appears just before the multiple answers) several times to understand how an answer should be selected. For example, the question may ask you to select the *correct* or *incorrect* answer. Nevertheless, it is advisable to recheck the question format before selecting the correct answer. It is important to read each answer option thoroughly through to the end. Occasionally a response may be only partially correct. Watch for qualifiers such as "next," "immediately," or "initially." Another hint for selecting the correct answer is to avoid answers that contain absolute or very restrictive words such as "always," "never," or "must." Another means to ensure that you know the correct answer is to cover the answers before tackling the question; read each question and then try to think of the answer before looking at the list of potential answers. Assume you have been given all the necessary information to answer the question. If the answer you had formulated is not among the list of answers provided, you may have interpreted the question incorrectly. When a patient's case is presented, write down the diagnosis before looking at the list of answers. It will be reassuring to realize (particularly if your diagnosis is supported by the answers) that you are on the "right track." If you do not know the answer to the question, very often you are able to rule out one or several answer options and improve your odds at guessing.

Candidates are well advised to use the basic fund of knowledge accumulated from clinical experience and reading to solve the questions. Approaching the questions as "real-life" encounters with patients is far better than trying to second-guess the examiners or trying to analyze whether the question is tricky. There is no reason for the ABPM&R to trick the candidates into choosing the wrong answers.

It is better not to discuss the questions or answers (after the examination) with other candidates. Such discussions usually cause more consternation, although some candidates may derive a false sense of having performed well in the examination. In any case the candidates are bound by their oath to the ABPM&R not to discuss or disseminate the questions.

PART II EXAMINATION

The Directors of the Board give the oral examinations, with the assistance of selected guest examiners. Three examiners examine the candidate, each examiner conducting a 40-minute segment of the total 120-minute examination. Two 5-minute breaks divide the three portions of the oral examination.

Candidates will be expected to present in a concise, orderly fashion evidence of the proficiency in the management of various clinical conditions that come within the field of PM&R. During the oral examination, the examiner will ask questions about diagnostic procedures, therapeutic procedures, and patient management.

The candidate should be prepared to demonstrate familiarity with the literature of basic and clinical research, as well as recent significant literature pertinent to PM&R. Conciseness and clarity of statements are expected. Evidence of the professional maturity of the candidate in clinical procedures and factual knowledge will be sought.

In addition to clinical PM&R, the oral portion of the examination may cover certain aspects of the basic sciences. The basic science components of the examinations may include anatomy, physics, physiology, pathology, and other fundamental clinical sciences and competencies as listed under Residency Training Requirements.

In the event a candidate taking both Parts I and II examinations in the same year fails Part I of the examination, results of Part II will not be counted or be recognized in any way. Both Parts I and II would need to be retaken for certification.

RECERTIFICATION

Please note: This information is taken directly from the ABPM&R Informational Booklet.

The content of the Booklet of Information is subject to change from year to year. For the most current information, please obtain the Booklet of Information for the present year, or call the ABPM&R office.

It is the applicant's responsibility to seek information concerning the current requirements of recertification in PM&R. The most current requirements supercede any prior requirements and are applicable to each candidate for recertification.

Beginning in 1993, the Board issued time-limited certificates that are valid for 10 years. To maintain certification beyond the 10-year period, Diplomates certified since 1993 must participate in the recertification program.

The guiding principle of the recertification program of the ABPMR is to foster the continuing development of excellence in patient care and all aspects of the practice of PM&R by its Diplomates. Through its recertification program, the ABPMR seeks to encourage, stimulate, and support its Diplomates in a program of self-directed, life-long learning through the pursuit of continuing medical education.

The recertification process permits Diplomates to demonstrate that they continue to meet the requirements of the ABPMR. Recertification also provides patients and their families, funding agencies, and the public in general with assurance of the continuing up-to-date knowledge of PM&R Diplomates.

To participate in the recertification program, an ABPMR Diplomate must:

- Hold a current, valid, unrestricted license to practice medicine or osteopathy in a United States licensing jurisdiction or Puerto Rico, or licensure in Canada. Evidence of unrestricted licensure in all states where a license is held will be required;
- Pay an annual fee;
- Provide evidence of an average of 50 continuing medical education (CME) credits annually, for a total of 500 CME hours over the 10-year period (with all such CME credits being recognized by the AMA or AOA); and
- Successfully complete a written or computer-based examination. Beginning in 2005, this will be a proctored examination. The recertification exam given in 2005 and beyond will be computer-based testing administered at selected locations.

Diplomates are automatically enrolled in the recertification program upon issuance of their time-limited ABPMR certificates. Holders of certificates that are not time-limited may participate in the program and may request, in writing, to be enrolled.

The recertification examination is an open-book, take-home test consisting of 200 multiple-choice questions. Diplomates have 10 weeks to complete the examination and return it to the ABPMR. The examination content is organized into modules. All participants complete a core module. The participants then select two additional modules from specific subspecialty areas in PM&R. For complete information on the recertification process and the requirements, please request a copy of the current *Recertification Booklet of Information* from the ABPMR Office. It can also be downloaded from their website at http://www.abpmr.org.

CONTENT

Examination content is organized into modules. A core module, which must be completed by all participants, contains 100 question on topics pertinent to the broad practice of PM&R. Two additional modules, with 50 questions each, will be selected by the participant from four available content areas: neuro-rehabilitation and related topics, musculoskeletal rehabilitation and related topics, electrodiagnosis and related topics, and general PM&R topics.

Examination Content	Number of Questions
PM&R Core Module (mandatory)	100
Modules (select 2)	100
1. Neuro-rehabilitation and Related Topics	
2. Musculoskeletal Rehabilitation and Related Topics	
3. Electrodiagnosis and Related Topics	
4. General PM&R Topics	
Total questions on the examination	200

EXAMINATION APPLICATION PROCESS AND FEES

Beginning in June 2000, recertification examination application forms became available to program participants wishing to take the recertification examination that year. To apply for the examination, a program participant must complete the form and mail it to the ABPM&R office with the examination fee.

ADMINISTRATION AND SCORING

Each November applicants are notified of their admissibility status. In early December, eligible participants receive the examination booklet(s), answer sheet(s), and instructions for completing the examination. Participants are allowed 10 weeks from the date of mailing to complete the examination. The date by which the completed examination must be returned to the ABPMR office is printed on the examination booklet(s).

The passing score for each module is determined by the Board. Participants will also receive statistical information on their performance on each test module.

NOTIFICATION OF RESULTS

Approximately six weeks after the examination is returned to the ABPMR office, participants will receive their examination score reports and notification of their pass/fail status.

Most Diplomates who participate in the recertification program will likely be successful. Those who do not fulfill the basic requirements and/or the CME requirements, or do not pass the examination, are encouraged to continue to seek recertification. These Diplomates will need to submit a new examination application and an examination fee each time they apply to the take the recertification examination. There is no limit to the number of times Diplomates may take the recertification examination, so long as such individuals continue to meet the annual program requirements expected of all active participants.

REPORTING CME CREDITS

To maintain their status as active participants in the recertification program, Diplomates must annually report their progress toward completing the required CME credits. The

ABPMR requires completion of 500 CME credits over the 10-year recertification program, at least 300 of which must be recognized by the ACCME or the AOA as Category 1 credits. The remaining 200 credits may be ACCME or AOA Category 2 credits.

Diplomates enrolled in the recertification program receive a form for reporting CME credits. The completed form must be returned to the ABPMR office by August 15 of each year. Typically, the active participant accumulates an average of 50 CME credits each year. Diplomates may accumulate more credits in some years and fewer in other years, but must accumulate 500 CME credits before being recertified.

RECERTIFICATION EXAMINATION PRIOR TO CERTIFICATE EXPIRATION

Diplomates may take the recertification examination before their certificate expires, beginning with the seventh year of the 10-year period of the certificate, if they meet these criteria:

- They have been active participants in the recertification program for at least four years prior to the date they wish to take the examination.
- They have completed an average of 50 CME credits per year during the time they have participated in the program and there are no outstanding fees to be paid.
- They hold a current, valid, and unrestricted license to practice medicine.

Although a Diplomate may take and pass the examination before his or her certificate expires, the CME credits and annual fee for each of the remaining years of the 10-year program are still required. If all requirements have been met, a certificate will be issued in the same year that the original certificate expires. The new time-limited certificate is in effect for 10 years from the date the previous certificate expires, not from the date the recertification exam is taken.

THE CERTIFICATE

The Board will issue a time-limited certificate to each Diplomate who successfully completes the recertification process. This certificate will be dated from the year the Diplomate's original certificate was due to expire.

Participants must submit their CME statement and pay the annual fee for the 10th year of the recertification program before the certificate will be issued.

Participants earn certificates if all requirements of the recertification program are met, including:

1. All fees paid;
2. Total of 500 CME credits accumulated and reported in the 10-year period prior to issuing the certificate;
3. Examination passed.

The Board will issue the new certificate after the expiration date on the original certificate.

Further details and current information for the certification and recertification programs can be obtained by writing to the ABPMR or by visiting their website.

ABPMR
21 Southwest 1st St.
Suite 674
Rochester, MN 55902-3092
Telephone: (507) 282-1776
ABPMR E-mail: office@abpmr.org
ABPMR website: http://www.abpmr.org
Prometric website: www.prometric.com *or* www.2test.com

1

STROKE

Richard Zorowitz, M.D., Edgardo Baerga, M.D., and Sara Cuccurullo, M.D.

INTRODUCTION

📖 DEFINITION OF STROKE

- Sudden focal (sometimes global) neurologic deficit secondary to occlusion or rupture of blood vessels supplying the brain
- Symptoms > 24 hours = stroke
- Symptoms < 24 hours = transient ischemic attack (TIA)
- Reversible ischemic neurologic deficit (RIND) = (this term is no longer used)

EPIDEMIOLOGY

- Stroke, after heart disease and cancer, is the third leading cause of death in the United States.
- The American Heart Association (AHA) estimates 600,000 strokes annually; 500,000 new cases, and 100,000 recurrent cases. (2000 AHA Heart and Stroke Statistical Update)
- Nearly four million stroke survivors in the United States
- 46% decline in cerebral infarcts and hemorrhages from 1950–1954 period to 1975–1979 period (Broderick, 1993)
  - Decline attributed to better management of blood pressure (BP), heart disease, decrease in cigarette smoking, etc.
- Incidence increases 17% from 1975–1979 period to 1980–1984 period (attributed to increased use of CT scan)
- There has been no change in the incidence of aneurysmal rupture
- Mortality from strokes has been steadily declining since 1950s
  - A sharp decline noted in the 1970s, possibly related to improved diagnosis (Dx) and treatment (Tx) of hypertension (HTN)
  - Improved Dx by modern diagnostic imaging tools (CT and MRI), may also have created a statistical decline in calculated mortality as smaller (less severe) strokes were identified (Sacco, 1995).

📖 RISK FACTORS (Stewart, 1999)

Nonmodifiable:

- Age—single most important risk factor for stroke worldwide; after age 55, incidence increases for both males and females
- Risk more than doubles each decade after age 55
- Sex (male > female)
- Race (African Americans 2× > whites > Asians)
- Family history (Hx) of stroke

1

Modifiable (treatable) risk factors:

- Hypertension—probably the most important modifiable risk factor for both ischemic and hemorrhagic stroke; increases risk by sevenfold
- History of TIA/prior stroke (~ 5% of patients with TIA will develop a completed stroke within 1 month if untreated)
- Heart disease (Dz.)
  - Congestive heart failure (CHF) and coronary artery disease (CAD): increases risk by twofold
  - Valvular heart Dz. and arrhythmias atrial fibrillation (A. Fib.)—increases risk of embolic stroke
    - A. Fib.: fivefold increase risk (Ryder, 1999)
- Diabetes—twofold increase in risk; unfortunately, good blood sugar control has not been shown to alter the risk of stroke
- Cigarette smoking
- Carotid stenosis (and carotid bruit); risk of stroke decreases with carotid endarterectomy (CEA) on selected symptomatic patients (> 70% stenosis)
- ETOH abuse/cocaine use
- High-dose estrogens (birth control pills)—considerable increase in risk when linked to cigarette smoking
- Systemic diseases associated with *hypercoagulable states*
  - Elevated RBC count, hematocrit, fibrinogen
  - Protein S and C deficiency
  - Sickle-cell anemia
  - Cancer
- Hyperlipidemia—several clinical trials have shown a reduction in stroke with use of cholesterol reducing agents (~ 30% reduction risk of stroke with use of HMG-CoA reductase inhibitors)
- Migraine headaches
- Sleep apnea
- Patent Foramen Ovale

[Obesity/sedentary life style (no clear relationship with increased risk of stroke)]

■

BASIC NEUROANATOMICAL REVIEW OF THE MAJOR VESSELS INVOLVED IN STROKE

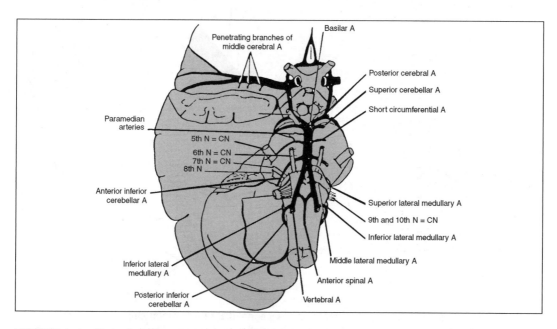

FIGURE 1–1   The principle vessels of the vertebrobasilar system in relation to the brainstem. A = artery; CN = cranial nerve

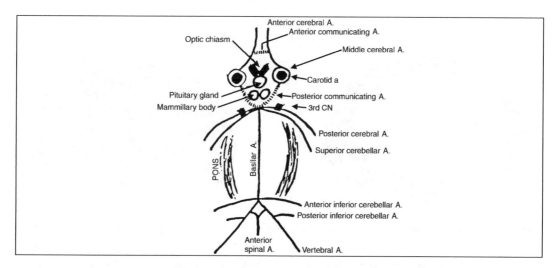

FIGURE 1–2   The Circle of Willis is a ferocious spider that lives in the brain. His name is Willis! Note that he has a nose, angry eyebrows, two suckers, eyes that look outward, a crew cut, antennae, a fuzzy beard, 8 legs, a belly that, according to your point of view, is either thin (basilar artery) or fat (the pons, which lies from one end of the basilar artery to the other), two feelers on his rear legs, and male genitalia. In Fig. 1–2 the brain is seen from below, so the carotid arteries are seen in cross section. (Reprinted with permission from Goldberg S. Clinical Neuroanatomy Made Ridiculously Simple. Miami: Medmaster Inc.; 1997.)

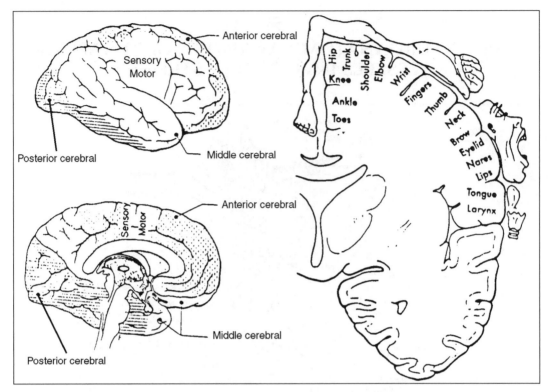

FIGURE 1–3   Major vascular supply to brain and functional diagram of motor strip. It is evident that lower-limb motor strip is in anterior cerebral artery distribution while upper-extremity motor strip is supplied by middle cerebral artery. (Reprinted with permission from Rosen P. Emergency Medicine–Stroke 3rd ed. St. Louis: Mosby; 1992.)

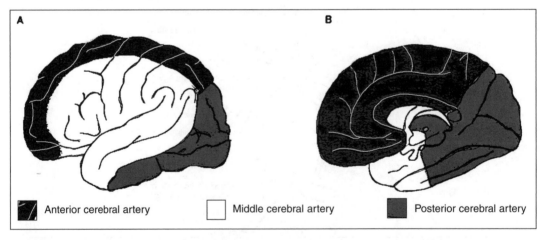

FIGURE 1–4   The three cerebral arteries' cortical territories. **A.** Lateral aspect of the hemisphere. **B.** Medial and inferior aspects of the hemisphere.

1. Most of the lateral aspect of the hemisphere is mainly supplied by the middle cerebral artery.
2. The anterior cerebral artery supplies the medial aspect of the hemisphere from the lamina terminalis to the cuneus.
3. The posterior cerebral artery supplies the posterior inferior surface of the temporal lobe and the visual cortex.

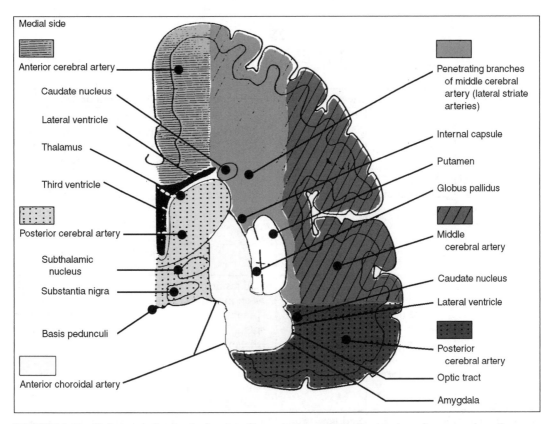

FIGURE 1–5 Major vascular territories are shown in this schematic drawing of a coronal section through the cerebral hemisphere at the level of the thalamus and the internal capsule.

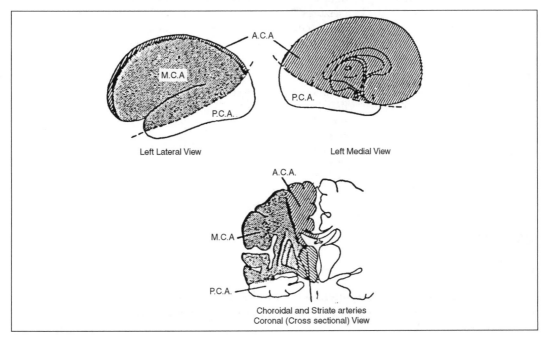

FIGURE 1–6 The cerebral blood circulation. MCA, middle cerebral artery; ACA, anterior cerebral artery; PCA, posterior cerebral artery. (Reprinted with permission from Goldberg S. Clinical Neuroanatomy Made Ridiculously Simple. Miami: Medmaster Inc.; 1997.)

▪

📖 TYPES OF STROKE

TABLE 1–1

	Ischemic 85%			Hemorrhagic 15%	
Type	Thrombotic	Embolic	Lacunar	Intracerebral (hypertensive) hemorrhage	Subarachnoid hemorrhage (ruptured aneurysms)
Frequency (%)	35	30	20	10	5
Factors associated with onset	Occurs during sleep	Occurs while awake		In 90% of cases occurs when the patient is calm and unstressed Blacks > whites	Occurs during activity (often strenuous activity)
Major causes/ etiology	Perfusion failure distal to site of severe stenosis or occlusion of major vessels	Due mainly to cardiac source	Small lesions seen mainly: −putamen −pons −thalamus −caudate −internal capsule/corona radiata	Hypertension	From ruptured aneurysms and vascular malformations
Presentation	Slowly (gradually) progressive deficit	Sudden, immediate deficit (seizures may occur)	Abrupt or gradual onset	Gradual onset (over minutes to days) or sudden onset of local neurologic deficits	Sudden onset
Link with TIA	50% with preceding TIA (50% occurring same vascular territory of preceding TIA)	TIA less common than in thrombotic 11% with preceding TIA	23% with preceding TIA	8% with preceding TIA	7% with preceding TIA

ISCHEMIC STROKES

Thrombotic (large artery thrombosis): 35% of all strokes

- Usually occurs during sleep (patient often awakens unaware of deficits)
- May have "stuttering," intermittent progression of neurologic deficits or be slowly progressive (over 24–48 hours)
- Profound loss of consciousness rare, except when area of infarction is large or when brainstem involved

- Neurologic deficit varies according to cerebral territory affected
- Perfusion failure distal to site of severe stenosis or occlusion of major vessels
- Emboli from incompletely thrombosed artery may precipitate an abrupt deficit. May have embolism from extracranial arteries affected by stenosis or ulcer

Embolic: 30% of all strokes

- Usually occurs during waking hours
- Deficit is immediate
- Seizures may occur at onset of stroke
- Cortical signs more frequent
- Most often embolus plugs one of the branches of the middle cerebral artery. An embolus may cause severe neurologic deficits that are temporary; symptoms resolve as the embolus fragments
- Presence of atrial fibrillation, history of recent myocardial infarction (MI) and occurrence of emboli to other regions of the body support Dx of cerebral embolism
- Suggested by history and by hemorrhagic infarction on CT (seen in 30% of patients with embolism) also by large low-density zone on CT encompassing entire territory of major cerebral artery or its main divisions
- Most commonly due to cardiac source: mural thrombi and platelet aggregates
- Chronic atrial fibrillation is the most common cause. Seen with myocardial infarction, cardiac aneurysm, cardiomyopathy, atrial myxoma, valvular heart disease (rheumatic, bacterial endocarditis, calcific aortic stenosis, mitral valve prolapse), sick sinus syndrome
- 75% of cardiogenic emboli go to brain

Lacunar infarction: 20% of all strokes

📖 Lacunes are small (less than 15 mm) infarcts seen in the putamen, pons, thalamus, caudate, and internal capsule
- Due to occlusive arteriolar or small artery disease (occlusion of deep penetrating branches of large vessels)
- Occlusion occurs in small arteries of 50—200 μm in diameter
- Strong correlation with hypertension (up to 81%); also associated with micro-atheroma, microembolism or rarely arteritis
- Onset may be abrupt or gradual; up to 30% develop slowly over or up to 36 hours
- CT shows lesion in about 2/3 of cases (MRI may be more sensitive)
- Relatively pure syndromes often (motor, sensory)—discussed below
- Absence of higher cortical function involvement (language, praxis, non-dominant hemisphere syndrome, vision)

Neuroanatomic Location of Ischemic Stroke (Adams, 1997)

1. Anterior Circulation

INTERNAL CAROTID ARTERY (ICA): (most variable syndrome): Occlusion occurs most frequently in the first part of the ICA immediately beyond the carotid bifurcation. ICA occlusions often asymptomatic (30–40% of cases) (Fig. 1–7)

- Ocular infarction: (embolic occlusion of either retinal branch or central retinal artery)
- Transient monocular blindness *(amaurosis fugax):* the ICA nourishes the optic nerve and retina as well as the brain; transient monocular blindness occurs prior to onset of stroke in approximately 25% of cases of internal carotid occlusion. Central retinal artery ischemia is very rare because of collateral supply

- Cerebral infarction: Presentation of complete ICA occlusion variable, from no symptoms (if good collateral circulation exists) to severe, massive infarction on ACA and MCA distribution. Failure of distal perfusion of internal carotid artery may involve all or part of the middle cerebral territory and, when the anterior communicating artery is small, the ipsilateral anterior cerebral artery. Contralateral motor and/or sensory symptoms present.

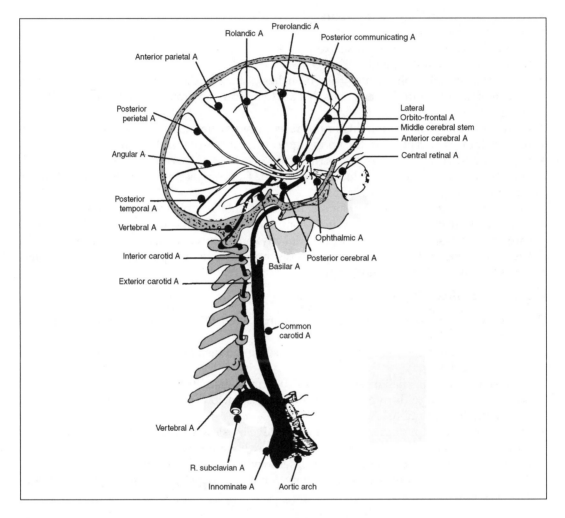

FIGURE 1–7 Arterial anatomy of major vessels on the right side carrying blood from the heart to the brain. Note location and course of the internal carotid artery.

MIDDLE CEREBRAL ARTERY (MCA): Occlusion occurs at stem of middle cerebral or at one of the two divisions of the artery in the sylvian sulcus. (Figure 1–8)

Superior Division

📖 Most common cause of occlusion of superior division of MCA is an embolus (superior division of MCA supplies rolandic and prerolandic areas)

Presentation:
- Sensory and motor deficits on contralateral face and arm > leg
- Head and eyes deviated toward side of infarct
- With left-side lesion (dominant hemisphere)—global aphasia initially, then turns into Broca's aphasia (motor speech disorder)

- Right side lesion (nondominant hemisphere)—deficits on spatial perception, hemineglect, constructional apraxia, dressing apraxia
- Muscle tone usually decreased initially and gradually increases over days or weeks to spasticity
- Transient loss of consciousness is uncommon

Inferior division (lateral temporal and inferior parietal lobes)

Presentation:
- With lesion on either side—superior quadrantanopia or homonymous hemianopsia
- Left side lesion—Wernicke's aphasia
- Right side lesion—left visual neglect

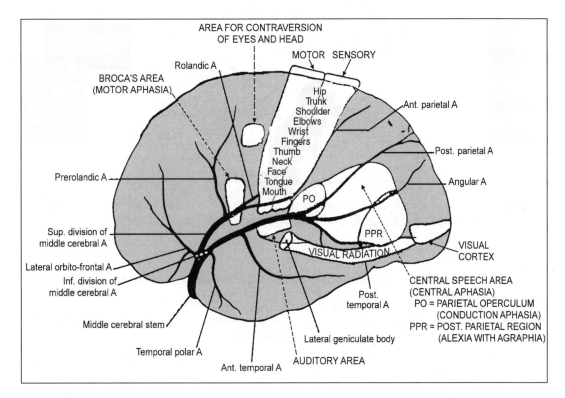

FIGURE 1–8 The distribution of the middle cerebral artery on the lateral aspect of the cerebral hemisphere. Principal regions of cerebral localization are noted.

ANTERIOR CEREBRAL ARTERY (ACA) (Figure 1–9):

- If occlusion is at the stem of the anterior cerebral artery proximal to its connection with the anterior communicating artery ⇒ it is usually well tolerated because adequate collateral circulation comes from the artery of the opposite side
- 📖 If both anterior cerebral arteries arise from one stem ⇒ major disturbances occur with infarction occurring at the medial aspects of both cerebral hemispheres resulting in aphasia, paraplegia, incontinence and frontal lobe/personality dysfunction
- Occlusion of one anterior cerebral artery distal to anterior communicating artery results in:
  - 📖 Contralateral weakness and sensory loss, affecting mainly distal contralateral leg (foot/leg more affected than thigh)
  - Mild or no involvement of upper extremity

- Head and eyes may be deviated toward side of lesion acutely
- Urinary incontinence with contralateral grasp reflex and paratonic rigidity may be present
- May produce transcortical motor aphasia if left side is affected
- 📖 Disturbances in gait and stance = gait apraxia

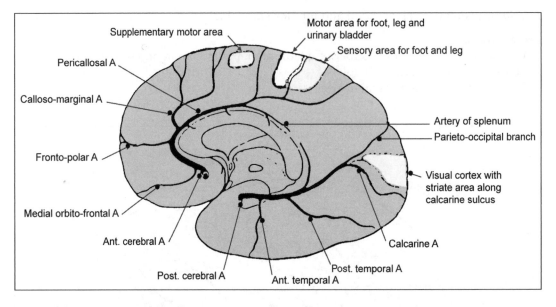

FIGURE 1–9 The distribution of the anterior cerebral artery on the medial aspect of the cerebral hemisphere, showing principal regions of cerebral localization.

2. Posterior Circulation: Vertebrobasilar Arteries & Posterior Cerebral Arteries

POSTERIOR CEREBRAL ARTERY (PCA):
Occlusion of PCA can produce a variety of clinical effects because both the upper brainstem and the inferior parts of the temporal lobe and the medial parts of the occipital lobe are supplied by it.

Particular area of occlusion varies for PCA because anatomy varies

- 70% of times both PCAs arise from basilar artery; connected to internal carotids through posterior communicating artery
- 20%–25%: one PCA comes from basilar; one PCA comes from ICA
- 5%—10%: both PCA arise from carotids

Clinical presentation includes:

- Visual field cuts (including cortical blindness when bilateral)
- May have prosopagnosia (can't read faces)
- palinopsia (abnormal recurring visual imagery)
- alexia (can't read)
- transcortical sensory aphasia (loss of power to comprehend written or spoken words; patient can repeat)
- 📖 Structures supplied by the interpeduncular branches of the PCA include the oculomotor cranial nerve (CN 3) and trochlear (CN 4) nuclei and nerves

- 📖 Clinical syndromes caused by the occlusion of these branches include oculomotor palsy with contralateral hemiplegia = Weber's syndrome (discussed below) and palsies of vertical gaze (trochlear nerve palsy)

VERTEBROBASILAR SYSTEM:
- Vertebral and basilar arteries: supply midbrain, pons, medulla, cerebellum, and posterior and ventral aspects of the cerebral hemispheres (through the PCAs.)
- Vertebral arteries: branches of the subclavian; are the main arteries of the medulla. At the pontomedullary junction, the two vertebral arteries join to form the basilar artery, which supplies branches to the pons and midbrain. Cerebellum is supplied by posterior-inferior cerebellar artery (PICA) from vertebral arteries, and by anterior-inferior cerebellar artery (AICA) and superior cerebellar artery, from basilar artery
- Vertebrobasilar system involvement may present any combination of the following signs/symptoms: vertigo, nystagmus, abnormalities of motor function often bilateral. usually ipsilateral cranial nerve dysfunction
- Crossed signs: motor or sensory deficit on ipsilateral side of face and opposite side of body; ataxia, dysphagia, dysarthria

📖 **Important:** There is *absence* of *cortical signs* (such as aphasias or cognitive deficits) that are characteristic of anterior circulation involvement

Syndromes of the Vertebrobasilar System

I. 📖 Lateral Medullary (Wallenberg's) Syndrome

This syndrome is one of the most striking in neurology. It occurs due to occlusion of the following:

1. vertebral arteries (involved in 8 out of 10 cases)
2. posterior inferior cerebellar artery (PICA)
3. superior lateral medullary artery
4. middle lateral medullary artery
5. inferior lateral medullary artery

- **Wallenberg's syndrome** also known as lateral medullary syndrome, PICA syndrome, and vertebral artery syndrome.
  Signs and symptoms include the following:
  – Ipsilateral side
    ▪ Horner's syndrome (ptosis, anhydrosis, and miosis)
    ▪ decrease in pain and temperature sensation on the ipsilateral face
    ▪ cerebellar signs such as ataxia on ipsilateral extremities (patient falls to side of lesion)
  – Contralateral side
    ▪ Decreased pain and temperature on contralateral body
  – Dysphagia, dysarthria, hoarseness, paralysis of vocal cord
  – Vertigo; nausea and vomiting
  – Hiccups
  – Nystagmus, diplopia
    Note: No facial or extremity muscle weakness seen in this syndrome

II. Benedikt's Syndrome (Red Nucleus/Tegmentum of Midbrain):

- Obstruction of interpeduncular branches of basilar or posterior cerebral artery or both
- Ipsilateral III nerve paralysis with mydriasis, contralateral hypesthesia (medial lemniscus), contralateral hyperkinesia (ataxia, tremor, chorea, athetosis) due to damage to red nucleus

III. Syndromes of the ParamedianArea (Medial Brainstem):

Paramedian area contains:
- Motor nuclei of CNs
- Cortico-spinal tract
- Medial lemniscus
- Cortico-bulbar tract

Signs/symptoms include:
- contralateral hemiparalysis
- ipsilateral CN paralysis

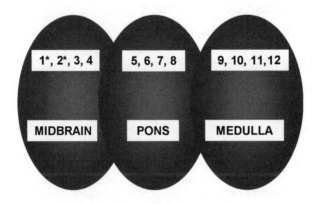

Location (grossly) of cranial nerve nuclei on brainstem
⬚ NOTE: nucleus of CN 1 and CN 2 located in forebrain. Spinal division of CN 11 arises from ventral horn of cervical segments C1–C6.

TABLE 1–2 Syndromes of the Paramedian Area (Medial Brainstem)

Weber Syndrome	Millard-Gubler Syndrome	Medial Medullary Syndrome "Another Lesion"
• Ipsilateral CN 3 palsy	• Ipsilateral CN 6 paralysis (often CN 7 also involved)	• Ipsilateral CN 12 palsy
• Contralateral hemiplegia	• Contralateral hemiplegia (extension into medial lemniscus is Foville's Syndrome with gaze palsy to side of lesion).	• Contralateral hemiplegia
	• Contralateral lemniscal (tactile sensation) sensory loss secondary to damage to medial lemniscus	• Contralateral lemniscal sensory loss

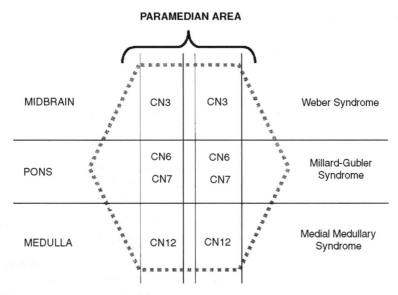

Gross depiction of the paramedian area of the brainstem and associated syndromes.

Weber Syndrome

(Base of midbrain): Obstruction of interpeduncular branches of posterior cerebral artery or posterior choroidal artery or both. Ipsilateral CN 3 cranial nerve paralysis, contralateral hemiplegia, contralateral Parkinson's signs, contralateral dystaxia (mild degree of ataxia).

Millard-Gubler Syndrome

(Base of pons): Obstruction of circumferential branches of basilar artery. Ipsilateral facial (CN 7) and abducens (CN 6) palsy, contralateral hemiplegia, analgesia, hypoesthesia.

- Extension to medial lemniscus = Raymond-Foville's Syndrome (with gaze palsy to side of lesion)

📖 Medial Medullary Syndrome

Caused by an infarction of the medial medulla due to occlusion (usually atherothrombotic) of penetrating branches of the vertebral arteries (upper medulla) or anterior spinal artery (lower medulla and medullo-cervical junction).

- Rare; ratio of medial medullary infarct to lateral medullary infarct ~ 1–2 : 10
- Typical syndrome:
  - Ipsilateral hypoglossal palsy (with deviation toward the side of the lesion)
  - Contralateral hemiparesis
  - Contralateral lemniscal sensory loss (proprioception and position sense)

TABLE 1–3 Syndromes of the Brainstem

	Main Arteries	Medial Brain Stem Lesions (Paramedian area syndromes)	Lateral Brain Stem Lesions
Midbrain	PCA	Weber syndrome	
Pons	Basilar	Millard-Gubler syndrome	
Medulla	Vertebral (or anterior spinal artery)	Medial medullary syndrome	Wallenberg syndrome

IV. Basilar Artery Occlusion Syndrome

Occlusion may arise in several ways:

- atherosclerotic plaque in the basilar artery itself (usually lower third)
- occlusion of both vertebral arteries
- occlusion of one vertebral artery when it is the only one of adequate size

Note:

- Thrombosis usually only obstructs a branch of basilar artery rather than the trunk
- Emboli, if they get through the vertebral arteries, usually lodge in one of the posterior cerebral arteries or at the upper bifurcation of the basilar artery

May cause internuclear ophthalmoplegia, conjugate horizontal gaze palsy, ocular bobbing. Ptosis, nystagmus common but variable. May see palatal myoclonus, coma.

📖 *Locked-in syndrome:* tetraparesis with patients only able to move eyes vertically or blink; patient remains fully conscious secondary to sparing of the reticular activating system; caused by bilateral lesions of the ventral pons (basilar artery occlusion). Some degree of paresis accompanies nearly all cases of basilar artery occlusion.

Neuroanatomic Location of Lacunar Infarction Syndromes

TABLE 1–4

Lacunar Syndrome	Anatomical Location
1. Pure motor hemiplegia –Weakness involves face, arm, and leg; no sensory deficits, aphasia or parietal signs	Posterior limb of internal capsule Corona radiata Pons
2. Pure sensory stroke	Thalamus (ventro-lateral) Parietal white matter Thalamocortical projections
3. 📖 Dysarthria—clumsy hand syndrome	Basis pontis Internal capsule (anterior limb)
4. Sensorimotor stroke	Junction of internal capsule and thalamus
5. Ataxia and leg paralysis	Pons Midbrain Internal capsule Cerebellum Parietal white matter Coronal Radiata
6. Hemichorea-hemiballismus	Head of the caudate Thalamus Subthalamic nucleus

HEMORRHAGIC STROKES (see Table 1–1)

15% of all strokes may be secondary to hypertension, ruptured aneurysm, arteriovenous malformation (AVM), blood dyscrasias/bleeding disorders, anticoagulants, bleeding into tumors, angiopathies.

I. Hypertensive Intracerebral Hemorrhage

- Linked to chronic HTN (> one-third occur in normotensives)
- Sudden onset of headache, and/or loss of consciousness
- Vomiting at onset in 22%–44%
- Seizures occur in 10% of cases (first few days after onset)
- Nuchal rigidity common
- Sites: putamen, thalamus, pons, cerebellum; some from white matter
- Frequently extends to ventricular subarachnoid space
- Preceded by formation of "false" aneurysms (microaneurysms) of Charcot & Bouchard = arterial wall dilations 2° to HTN

Locations

1. **Putamen:** Most common; hemiplegia 2° to compression of adjacent internal capsule. Vomiting in ~ 50%; headache frequent but not invariable
   - Large hemorrhage: Stupor/coma + hemiplegia with deterioration in hours.
   - With smaller hemorrhages: Headache (HA) leading to aphasia, hemiplegia, eyes deviate away from paretic limbs
   - These symptoms, occurring over few minutes to one-half hour, are strongly suggestive of progressive intracerebral bleeding
2. **Thalamus:** Hemiplegia by compression of adjacent internal capsule; contralateral sensory deficits; aphasia present with lesions of the dominant side; contralateral hemineglect with involvement on the nondominant side. Ocular disturbances with extension of hemorrhage into subthalamus
3. **Pontine:** Deep coma results in a few minutes; total paralysis, small pupils (1 mm) that react to light; decerebrate rigidity → death occurs in few hours. Patient may survive if hemorrhage is small (smaller than 1 cm)
4. **Cerebellum:** Develops over several hours. Coma/loss of consciousness (LOC) unusual vomiting, occipital HA, vertigo, inability to sit, stand or walk, eyes deviate to opposite side (ipsilateral CN 6 palsy); dysarthria, dysphagia
5. **Lobar hemorrhage:** HA and vomiting. A study of 26 patients revealed:
   - 11 occipital: Dense homonymous hemianopsia and pain ipsilateral eye
   - 7 temporal: Partial hemianopsia/fluent aphasia/pain ear
   - 4 frontal: Contralateral hemiplegia (mainly the arm) and frontal headache
   - 3 parietal: Hemisensory deficit (contralateral)/anterior temporal HA

II. Subarachnoid Hemorrhage (SAH) (Ruptured Saccular Arterial Aneurysm)

- Saccular aneurysms = Berry aneurysms
- Arterial dilations found at bifurcations of larger arteries at base of brain (circle of Willis or major branches). (Fig. 1–10)

  📖 90%–95% of saccular aneurysms occur on the anterior part of the circle of Willis. Presumed to result from congenital medial and elastica defects vs hemodynamic forces causing focal destruction of internal elastic membrane at bifurcations. (Adams, 1997)
- Multiple in 20% of patients (either unilateral or bilateral)
- Other types of aneurysms: arteriosclerotic, mycotic, dissecting aneurysms, traumatic, neoplastic
- More likely to rupture if 10mm or larger (rupture may occur in smaller aneurysms)
- Rupture occurs usually when patient is active rather than during sleep (e.g., straining, coitus)
- Peak age for rupture = fifth and sixth decade

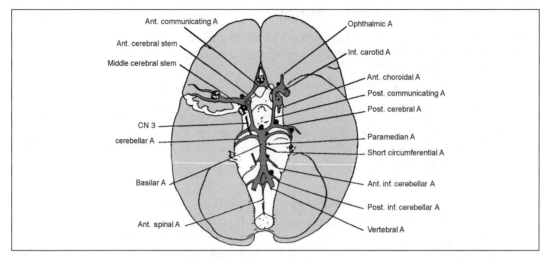

FIGURE 1–10 The principle sites of saccular aneurysms. The majority (approximately 90%) of aneurysms occur on the anterior half of the Circle of Willis.

Clinical Presentation of Saccular Aneurysms/SAH:
Symptoms due to aneurysms; presentation can be either:
1. None, usually asymptomatic prior to rupture. (intracranial aneurysms are common, found during 3%–5% of routine autopsies)
2. Compression of adjacent structures
   📖 (e.g., Compression of oculomotor nerve (CN 3) with posterior communicating— internal carotid junction aneurysm or posterior communicating—posterior cerebral artery aneurysm)

   Signs of CN 3 involvement:
   • Deviation of ipsilateral eye to lateral side (lateral or divergent strabismus) because of unopposed action of lateral rectus muscle
   • Ptosis
   • Mydriasis (dilated pupil) and paralysis of accommodation due to interruption of parasympathetic fibers in the CN 3
3. Rupture of aneurysm producing subarachnoid hemorrhage with or without intracerebral hematoma
   • "Sentinel" HA prior to rupture in ~ 50% of patients
   • With subarachnoid hemorrhage, blood is irritating to the dura causing severe HA classically described as "worst headache of my life"
   • Sudden, transient loss of consciousness in 20%–45% at onset
   • May have CN 3 or CN 6 palsy (from direct pressure from the aneurysm vs. accumulation of an intracerebral hematoma vs early development of arterial spasm), hemiparesis, aphasia (dominant hemisphere), memory loss
   • Seizures: 4% at onset/25% overall
   • Mortality 25% during first 24 hours
   • Risk of rebleeding within one month 30%; 2.2% per year during first decade
   • Mortality from rebleeding in the early weeks after initial event: 50% to 60%
   • Vasospasm: common complication occurring in ~ 25% of cases; caused by the presence of blood breakdown products (vasoactive amines) on the subarachnoid space, acting in the adventitia of the arteries. Occurs 3–12 days after rupture (frequently ~ 7 days after rupture)

- Meds: nimodipine, a calcium channel blocker, is useful in the treatment of cerebral blood vessel spasm after subarachnoid hemorrhage (see Treatment section below)

III. Vascular Malformations/AVMs

- Consists of a tangle of dilated vessels that form an abnormal communication between the arterial and venous systems: an arteriovenous (AV) fistula
- Congenital lesions originating early in fetal life
- AVM composed of coiled mass of arteries and veins with displacement rather than invasion of normal brain tissue
- 📖 AVMs are usually low-pressure systems; the larger the shunt, the lower the interior pressure. Thus, with these large dilated vessels there needs to be an occlusion distally to raise luminal pressures to cause hemorrhage
- Hemorrhage appears to be more common in smaller malformations, which is probably due to higher resistance and pressure within these lesions
- Patients are believed to have a 40%–50% risk of hemorrhage from AVM in life span
- Natural history of AVMs: bleeding rate per year = 2%–4%
- Rebleeding rate 6% first year post-hemorrhage
- Annual mortality rate: 1% (per year)
- First hemorrhage fatal in ~10% of these patients
- Bleeding commonly occurs between the ages of 20–40 years

Clinical Presentation of AVM Rupture:

- Hemorrhage: Majority of symptomatic patients present with hemorrhage. Cerebral hemorrhage first clinical manifestation in ~ 50% of cases; may be parenchymal (41%), subarachnoid (23%), or intraventricular (17%) (Brown et al., 1996)
- Seizures: presenting feature in 30% of cases
- Headaches: presenting complaint in 20% of cases; 10% (overall) with migraine-like headache

▪

DIAGNOSTIC STUDIES

TABLE 1–5   Diagnostic Studies

	Infarct	Hemorrhage
CT	Focally decreases density (hypodense) = darker than normal **BLACK** Not seen immediately (unless there is a mass effect) May be seen after 24 hrs. (due to increase in edema); seen best within 3 to 4 days	Blood Hyperdense (radio-opaque) **WHITE** Seen immediately
MRI	Edema Fluid: high density **WHITE** Can be seen immediately as bright area on T_2	Blood Low signal density **BLACK** (on either T1 or T2)

1. **CT Scan:**

   Major role in evaluating presence of blood (cerebral hemorrhage or hemorrhagic infarction), especially when anticoagulation is under consideration.

   If intracranial (IC) hemorrhage suspected, *CT scan without contrast* is the study of choice Why?: To avoid confusing blood with contrast, as both appear white on CT scan.

   Cerebral Infarction:
   - Regardless of stroke location or size, CT is often normal during the first few hours after brain infarction
   - Infarcted area appears as hypodense (black) lesion usually after 24–48 hours after the stroke (occasionally positive scans at 3–6 hours ↔ subtle CT changes may be seen early with large infarcts, such as obscuration of gray-white matter junction, sulcal effacement, or early hypodensity)
   - Hypodensity initially mild and poorly defined; edema better seen third or fourth day as a well-defined hypodense area
   - CT with contrast: IV contrast provides no brain enhancement in day 1 or 2, as it must await enough damage to blood brain barrier; more evident in 1–2 weeks. Changes disappear in 2 to 3 months
   - Some studies suggest worse prognosis for patients receiving IV contrast early
   - Hemorrhage can occur within an infarcted area, where it will appear as a hyperdense mass within the hypodense edema of the infarct

   Hemorrhagic Infarct:
   - High density (white) lesion seen immediately in ~100% cases. Proved totally reliable in hemorrhages 1.0 cm or more. Demonstration of clot rupture into the ventricular system (32% in one series) not as ominous as once thought

   Subarachnoid Hemorrhage:
   - Positive scan in 90% when CT performed within 4–5 days (may be demonstrated for only 8–10 days). SAH can really be visualized only in the acute stage, when blood is denser (whiter) than the cerebrospinal fluid (CSF)
   - Appears as hyperdense (or isodense) area on CT scan—look for blood in the basal cisterns or increase density in the region around the brainstem. May sometimes localize aneurysm based upon hematoma or uneven distribution of blood in cisterns.
   - Once diagnosis of SAH has been established, angiography is generally performed to localize and define the anatomic details of the aneurysm and to determine if others aneurysms exist

2. **MRI Scan:**

   More sensitive than CT scan in detecting small infarcts (including lacunar) and posterior cranial fossa infarcts (because images are not degraded by bone artifacts); ischemic edema detected earlier than with CT—within a few hours of onset of infarct.

   Cerebral Infarction:
   - Early, increased (white) signal intensity on T2 weighted images, more pronounced at 24 hours to 7 days (Tl may show mildly decreased signal)
   - Chronically (21 days or more), decreased Tl and T2 weighted signals

   Intracerebral Hemorrhage:
   - Acute hemorrhage: decreased (black) signal or isointense on Tl and T2 weighted images
   - Edema surrounding hemorrhage appears as decreased intensity on Tl weighted image; increased (white) signal on T2 images
   - As hemorrhage ages, it develops increased signal on Tl and T2 images

   Subarachnoid or Intraventricular Hemorrhage:
   - Acutely, low signal (black) on Tl and T2 images

MRI/MRA:
Detects most aneurysms on the basal vessels; insufficient sensitivity to replace conventional angiography

Lacunes:
CT scan documents most supratentorial lacunar infarctions, and MRI successfully documents both supratentorial and infratentorial infarctions when lacunes are 0.5 cm or greater

3. **Carotid Ultrasound:**
   Real time B-mode imaging; direct doppler examination. Screening test for carotid stenosis; identification of ulcerative plaques less certain. Useful in following patients for progression of stenosis.

4. **Angiography:**
   Conventional angiography, intravenous digital subtraction angiography (DSA), and intra-arterial digital subtraction angiography
   - DSA studies: safer, may be performed as outpatient
   - Evaluation of extracranial and intracranial circulation
   - Valuable tool for diagnosis of aneurysms, vascular malformations, arterial dissections, narrowed or occluded vessels, and angiitis
   - Complications: occur in 2% to 12%; complications include aortic or carotid artery dissection, embolic stroke, vascular spasm, and occlusion
   - Morbidity associated with procedure: 2.5%
   - Carotid and vertebral angiography—only certain means of demonstrating an aneurysm—positive in 85% of patients with "clinical" SAH

   MRA:
   Can reliably detect extracranial carotid artery stenosis; may be useful in evaluating patency of large cervical and basal vessels

5. **Lumbar Puncture:**
   Used to detect blood in CSF; primarily in subarachnoid hemorrhage when CT not available or, occasionally, when CT is negative and there is high clinical suspicion

6. **Transesophageal Echo:**
   Transesophageal echocardiographic findings can be helpful for detecting potential cardiac sources of embolism in patients with clinical risks for cardioembolism or unexplained stroke.

■

TREATMENT

IMMEDIATE MANAGEMENT (Ferri, 1998; Rosen, 1992; Stewart, 1999)

- **Respiratory support**/ABCs of critical care
- **Airway obstruction** can occur with paralysis of throat, tongue, or mouth muscles and pooling of saliva. Stroke patients with recurrent seizures are at increased risk of airway obstruction. Aspiration of vomiting is a concern in hemorrhagic strokes (increased association of vomiting at onset). Breathing abnormalities (central) occasionally seen in patients with severe strokes
- **Control of blood pressure** (see following)

- **Indications for emergent CT scan**
  - Because the clinical picture of hemorrhagic and ischemic stroke may overlap, CT scan without contrast is needed in most cases to definitively differentiate between the two
  - Determine if patient is a candidate for emergent thrombolytic therapy
  - Impaired level of consciousness/coma: If there is acute deterioration of level of consciousness, evaluate for hematoma/acute hydrocephalus; treatment: emergency surgery
  - Coagulopathy present (i.e., rule out (R/O) hemorrhage)
  - Fever and concern regarding brain ulcers or meningitis
- **Seizure management (see below)**
- **Obtain blood sugar levels** immediately
  - Hypoglycemia → bolus 50% dextrose
  - Hyperglycemia: shown to potentiate severity of brain ischemia in animal studies.
  - Insulin if blood sugar > 300 mg/dl
- **Control of Intracranial Pressure (ICP) (see below)**
- **Fever**: potentially damaging to the ischemic brain.
  - Antipyretics (acetaminophen) should be given early while the source of fever is being ascertained
- **Intravenous Fluid**: Normal Saline Solution (NSS) or Ringer's lactate; avoid hypotonic solutions or excessive loading because they may worsen brain edema
- **Keep patient NPO** if at risk of aspiration

Blood Pressure Management:

Management of blood pressure after acute ischemic and hemorrhagic stroke is controversial. Many patients have HTN after ischemic or hemorrhagic strokes but few require emergency treatment. Elevations in blood pressure usually resolve without antihypertensive medications during the first few days after stroke. (Biller and Bruno, 1997)

Antihypertensive treatment can lower cerebral perfusion and lead to worsening of stroke. The response of stroke patients to antihypertensive medications can be exaggerated.

Current treatment recommendations are based on the type of stroke, ischemic vs. hemorrhagic

Ischemic Stroke:

TABLE 1–6   American Heart Association Recommendations for HTN Management in *Ischemic Stroke*

Nonthrombolytic candidates	Treat if :	SBP >220
		DBP >120
		or MAP >120
Thrombolytic candidates	Treat if :	SBP >185
(before thrombolytic treatment give)		DBP >110

- IV labetalol and enalapril are favored antihypertensive agents.

Hemorrhagic Strokes:

Treatment of increased BP during hemorrhagic strokes is controversial. Usual recommendation is to treat at lower levels of blood pressure than for ischemic strokes because of concerns of rebleeding and extension of bleeding.

- Frequent practice is to treat BP if: SBP > 180, DBP > 105
- Agent of choice: IV labetalol (labetalol does not cause cerebral vasodilation, which could worsen increased ICP)

Seizure Management:

- Recurrent seizures: potentially life-threatening complication of stroke (see Stroke Rehabilitation)
- Seizures can substantially worsen elevated ICP
- Benzodiazepines = first-line agents for treating seizures
- IV lorazepam or diazepam
- If seizures don't respond to IV benzodiazepines, treat with long acting anticonvulsants:
  Phenytoin – 18 mg/kg
  Also fosphenytoin – 17 mg/kg
        Phenobarbital – 1000 mg or 20 mg/kg

Intracranial Pressure Management:

- Increased ICP reduces cerebral blood perfusion
- Cerebral perfusion calculated by subtracting ICP from mean arterial pressure (MAP). It should remain > 60 mm Hg to ensure cerebral blood flow
- Fever, hyperglycemia, hyponatremia, and seizures can worsen cerebral edema by increasing ICP

> **Keep ICP <20 mmHg**

Management of ICP:
- **Correction of factors exacerbating increased ICP**
  - Hypercarbia
  - Hypoxia
  - Hyperthermia
  - Acidosis
  - Hypotension
  - Hypovolemia

- **Positional**
  - Avoid flat, supine position; elevate head of bed 30°
  - Avoid head and neck positions compressing jugular veins

- **Medical Therapy**
  - Intubation and hyperventilation: reduction of $PaCO_2$ through hyperventilation is the most rapid means of lowering ICP. Keep ICP < 20 mmHg
  - Hyperventilation should be used with caution because it reduces brain tissue PO_2 ($PbrO_2$); hypoxia may lead to ischemia of brain tissue, causing further damage in the CNS after stroke
  - Optimal $PaCO_2$ ~ 25–30 mmHg
  - Hyperosmolar therapy with mannitol improves ischemic brain swelling (by diuresis and intravascular fluid shifts)
  - Furosemide/acetazolamide may also be used
  - High doses of barbiturates (e.g., thiopental) rapidly lower ICP and suppress electrical brain activity

- **Fluid Restriction**
  - Avoid glucose solutions; use normal saline; maintain euvolemia
  - Replace urinary losses with normal saline in patients receiving mannitol

- **Surgical Therapy**
  - Neurosurgical decompression

THROMBOLYTIC THERAPY

IV tissue – plasminogen activator (t-PA)

First FDA approved Tx for ischemic strokes in selected patients
- In National Institute of Neurologic Disorders (1995) trial, patients given t-PA within three hours of onset of stroke were 30% more likely to have minimal or no disability at three months compared to patrents treated with placebo
- There was a tenfold increase in hemorrhage (overall) with t-PA compared to placebo (6.4% vs. 0.6%) and in fatal ICH (3% vs. 0.3%)
- However, mortality was higher in placebo group than in t-PA groups; overall mortality: 17% t-PA (including hemorrhage cases) vs. 21% placebo

Inclusion criteria

- Age 18 yrs or older
- Time of onset of symptoms well established to be < three hours before treatment would begin
- Patients with measurable neurologic deficits (moderate to severe stroke symptoms)
- CT negative for blood

Exclusion criteria

- Minor stroke symptoms/TIA (symptoms rapidly improving)
- CT positive for blood
- Blood Pressure > 185/100 despite moderate Tx
- Increased PT/PTT
- Decreased PLTs
- Blood Sugar < 50, > 400
- Hx stroke past 3 month
- Hx of ICH, AVM or aneurysm
- Seizure at onset of stroke

Streptokinase

Three recent large randomized trials of streptokinase in stroke suspended because of increase in hemorrhage and mortality in treatment group

ANTICOAGULANT THERAPY

Heparin
- Frequently used in patients with acute ischemic stroke, but its value is unproven
- There is no unanimity on when heparin should be started, desired level of anticoagulation or if bolus dose should be given or not

Low molecular-weight heparin
- has more selective antithrombotic action than heparin (may be safer)
- Kay et al. (1995) study reporting improvement in survival and decrease in eventual rate of dependency (rated by Barthel Index) in patients treated with low molecular-weight heparin (LMWH) within 48 hours of onset of stroke compared to placebo

Aspirin, warfarin, ticlopidine (Ticlid®), clopidogrel, Plavix® (Creager, 1998)
- All have been shown to decrease the risk of subsequent stroke in patients with TIA.
- Usefulness in Tx of acute stroke unknown
- Anticoagulant therapy with warfarin: Stroke incidence and mortality in patients at high risk reduced; might be the best option for patients with a history of atrial fibrillation, prior stroke (or TIA), HTN, diabetes and CHF (Ryder, 1999)

Indications for Anticoagulation (Controversial)

- **Stroke in evolution:**

Neurologic deficit developing in stepwise progression (over 18 to 24 hours in carotid circulation; up to 72 hours in vertebrobasilar circulation). IV heparin efficacy unproven as previously mentioned. Generally, IV heparin given for at least several days to increase PTT to 1.5 to 2.5 times control. Coumadin® may be used for longer period (e.g, 6-month trial)

- **Cardiac emboli** (best reason to anticoagulate):
  - Primarily from nonvalvular atrial fibrillation and mural thrombus from myocardial infarction (MI)
  - Anticoagulation reported to reduce incidence of cerebral emboli in patients with MI by 75%
  - Timing of anticoagulation in patients with cardiac emboli controversial; probable risk of inducing cerebral hemorrhage or hemorrhagic infarction within large infarcts if anticoagulated in first 24–32 hours
  - If neurologic deficit is mild (and CT shows no hemorrhage) may begin anticoagulation immediately
  - If deficit severe (clinically and/or CT), wait 3–5 days before starting anticoagulation
  - 15% of cardiogenic emboli lodge in the brain. The most common cause is chronic atrial fibrillation

- **Transient Ischemic Attacks:**
  - Some studies suggest that a cluster of recent, frequent ("crescendo") TIAs is an indication for anticoagulation therapy. Use of anticoagulants (heparin, Coumadin®) in TIA is empirical
  - May consider use of Coumadin® when antiplatelet drugs fail to reduce attacks

- **Completed Stroke:**
  - Anticoagulation not considered beneficial after major infarction and usually not of great value once stroke is fully developed
  - Empirically, some will utilize anticoagulation (initially with IV heparin) in setting of mild infarct to theoretically prevent further progression in same vascular territory Coumadin® may be continued for several weeks to 3 to 6 months
  - Anticoagulation generally not employed for lacunar infarction

CORTICOSTEROIDS:

- No value in ischemic strokes
- Some studies suggest worsening in prognosis of stroke patients due to hyperglycemia

CAROTID ENDARTERECTOMY (CEA)

Symptomatic carotid stenosis

CEA for symptomatic lesions with > 70% stenosis (70%–99%) is effective in reducing the incidence of ipsilateral hemisphere stroke. (North American Symptomatic Carotid Endarterectomy Trial Collaborators, 1991), (Endarterectomy for moderate symptomatic carotid stenosis: Interim results from the MRC European Carotid Surgery Trial, 1996) (Executive Committee for Asymptomatic Carotid Artherosclerosis Study, 1995)

American Heart Association (AHA) guidelines for CEA (Moore, 1995)

1. CEA is proven beneficial in:
   - Symptomatic patients with one or more TIAs (or mild stroke) within the past 6 months and carotid stenosis ≥ 70%

2. CEA is "Acceptable but not proven":
   - TIAs or mild and moderate strokes within the last 6 months and stenosis 50% to 69%
   - Progressive stroke and stenosis ≥ 70%

CEA for Asymptomatic Carotid Stenosis

- Indications—Controversial
- AHA guidelines (Moore, 1995)

"Acceptable but not proven": in stenosis > 75% by linear diameter (asymptomatic cases)

Note: recent studies present opposing views on indications for surgery in asymptomatic carotid stenosis

---

Asymptomatic Carotid Atherosclerosis Study (ACAS) (Executive Committee for the Asymptomatic Carotid Artherosclerosis Study, 1995) (Young et al., 1996)

- Study showed a significant reduction (53%) in risk of ipsilateral stroke in a five-year period in asymptomatic patients with > 60% carotid stenosis (and < 3% rate perioperative morbidity/mortality); risk was 5.1% on patients treated surgically vs. 11.0% in patients treated medically.
- ACAS study not evaluated for AHA guidelines on 1995

ECST (Endarterectomy for moderate symptomatic carotid stenosis: Interim results from the MRC European Carotid Surgery Trial, 1996). This 3 year study showed:

- In patients with asymptomatic carotid stenosis < 70%, risk of stroke is low, 2%. In patients with stenosis > 70%, risk also is low, 5.7%
- Conclusion of study was that CEA is not justified in asymptomatic carotid stenosis.

TREATMENT OF SUBARACHNOID HEMORRHAGE (see also Tx of ICP)

- Bed rest in a quiet, dark room with cardiac monitoring (cardiac arrhythmias are common)
- Control of headaches with acetaminophen and codeine
- Mannitol to reduce cerebral edema
- Control of blood pressure—have the patient avoid all forms of straining (give stool softeners and mild laxatives)
- Early surgery (with clipping of aneurysm) better; reduces risk of rebleeding; does not prevent vasospasm or cerebral ischemia
- Nimodipine (calcium channel blocker) shown to improve outcome after SAH (decreased vasospasms). It is useful in the treatment of cerebral blood vessel spasm after SAH. It decreases the incidence of permanent neurologic damage and death. Therapy should be initiated within 96 hours of the onset of hemorrhage

TREATMENT OF INTRACRANIAL HEMORRHAGE

- Management of increased ICP and blood pressure (see previous)
- Large intracranial or cerebellar hematomas often require surgical intervention

TREATMENT OF ARTERIOVENOUS MALFORMATION (AVM) (Hamilton and Septzler, 1994; Schaller, Scramm, and Haun, 1998)

- Treatment advised in both *symptomatic* and *asymptomatic* AVMs
- Surgical excision if size and location feasible (and depending on perioperative risk)
- Embolization
- Proton Beam Therapy (via stereotaxic procedure)
- Small asymptomatic AVMs: radiosurgery/microsurgical resection recommended

▪
STROKE REHABILITATION

INTRODUCTION

The primary goal of stroke rehabilitation is functional enhancement by maximizing the independence, life style, and dignity of the patient.

This approach implies rehabilitative efforts from a physical, behavioral, cognitive, social, vocational, adaptive, and re-educational point of view. The multidimensional nature of stroke and its consequences make coordinated and combined interdisciplinary team care the most appropriate strategy to treat the stroke patient.

Recovery from impairments

Hemiparesis and motor recovery have been the most studied of all stroke impairments. Up to 88% of acute stroke patients have hemiparesis

The process of recovery from stroke usually follows a relatively predictable, stereotyped series of events in patients with stroke-induced hemiplegia. These sequence of events have been systematically described by several clinical researchers.

Twitchell (1951) published a highly detailed report describing the pattern of motor recovery following a stroke (pattern most consistent in patients with cerebral infarction in the MCA distribution)
- His sample included 121 patients, all except three having suffered either thrombosis or embolism of one of the cerebral vessels
- Immediately following onset of hemiplegia there is total loss of voluntary movement and loss or decrease of the tendon reflexes
- This is followed (within 48 hours) by increased deep tendon reflexes on the involved side, and then (within a short time) by increased resistance to passive movement (tone returns → spasticity), especially in flexors and adductors in the upper extremity (UE) and extensors and adductors in the lower extremity (LE)
- As spasticity increased, clonus (in ankle plantar flexors) appeared in 1–38 days post- onset of hemiplegia
- Recovery of movement:
  - 6 to 33 days after the onset of hemiplegia, the first "intentional" movements (shoulder flexion) appears
  - In the UE, a flexor synergy pattern develops (with shoulder, elbow, wrist and finger flexion) followed by development of an extensor synergy pattern. Voluntary movement in the lower limb also begins with flexor synergy (also proximal—hip) followed by extensor synergy pattern
- With increase of voluntary movement, there is a decrease in the spasticity of the muscles involved
- Tendon reflexes remain increased despite complete recovery of movement
- At onset of hemiplegia, the arm is more involved than the leg, and eventual motor recovery in the leg occurs earlier, and is more complete, than in the arm
- Most recovery takes place in the first three months and only minor additional recovery occurs after six months post onset

Predictors of motor recovery:
- Severity of arm weakness at onset:
  - With complete arm paralysis at onset, there is a poor prognosis of recovery of useful hand function (only 9% gain good recovery of hand function)

- Timing of return of hand movement:
  - If the patient shows some motor recovery of the hand by four weeks, there is up to 70% chance of making a full or good recovery
  - Poor prognosis with no measurable grasp strength by four weeks
- Poor prognosis associated also with:
  - Severe proximal spasticity
  - Prolonged "flaccidity" period
  - Late return of proprioceptive facilitation (tapping) response > nine days
  - Late return of proximal traction response (shoulder flexors/adductors) > 13 days

Brunnstrom (1966, 1970) and Sawner (1992) also described the process of recovery following stroke-induced hemiplegia. The process was divided into a number of stages:

1. Flaccidity (immediately after the onset)
   No "voluntary" movements on the affected side can be initiated

2. Spasticity appears
   Basic synergy patterns appear
   Minimal voluntary movements may be present

3. Patient gains voluntary control over synergies
   Increase in spasticity

4. Some movement patterns out of synergy are mastered (synergy patterns still predominate)
   Decrease in spasticity

5. If progress continues, more complex movement combinations are learned as the basic synergies lose their dominance over motor acts
   Further decrease in spasticity

6. Disappearance of spasticity
   Individual joint movements become possible and coordination approaches normal

7. Normal function is restored

REHABILITATION METHODS FOR MOTOR DEFICITS: Major theories of rehabilitation training

Traditional Therapy:

Traditional therapeutic exercise program consists of positioning, ROM exercises, strengthening, mobilization, compensatory techniques, endurance training (e.g., aerobics). Traditional approaches for improving motor control and coordination: emphasize need of repetition of specific movements for learning, the importance of sensation to the control of movement, and the need to develop basic movements and postures. (Kirsteins, Black, Schaffer, and Harvey, 1999)

Proprioceptive (or peripheral) Neuromuscular Facilitation (PNF) (Knott and Voss, 1968)
- *Uses spiral and diagonal components of movement rather than the traditional movements in cardinal planes of motion with the goal of facilitating movement patterns that will have more functional relevance than the traditional technique of strengthening individual group muscles*
- Theory of spiral and diagonal movement patterns arose from observation that the body will use muscle groups synergistically related (e.g., extensors vs. flexors) when performing a maximal physical activity

- Stimulation of nerve/muscle/sensory receptors to evoke responses through manual stimuli to increase ease of movement-promotion function
- It uses resistance during the spiral and diagonal movement patterns with the goal of facilitating "irradiation" of impulses to other parts of the body associated with the primary movement (through increased membrane potentials of surrounding alpha motoneurons, rendering them more excitable to additional stimuli and thus affecting the weaker components of a given part)
- Mass-movement patterns keep Beevor's axiom: Brain knows nothing of individual muscle action but only movement

Bobath approach / neurodevelopmental technique (NDT) (Bobath, 1978)
- *The goal of NDT is to normalize tone, to inhibit primitive patterns of movement, and to facilitate automatic, voluntary reactions and subsequent normal movement patterns.*
- Based on the concept that pathologic movement patterns (limb synergies and primitive reflexes) must not be used for training because continuous use of the pathologic pathways may make it too readily available to use at expense of the normal pathways
- Probably the most commonly used approach
- Suppress abnormal muscle patterns before normal patterns introduced
- Mass synergies avoided, although they may strengthen weak, unresponsive muscles, because these reinforce abnormally increased tonic reflexes, spasticity
- Abnormal patterns modified at *proximal* key points of control (e.g., shoulder and pelvic girdle)
- *Opposite to Brunnstrom approach* (which encourages the use of abnormal movements); see the following

Brunstrom approach/Movement therapy (Brunnstrom, 1970)
- *Uses primitive synergistic patterns in training in attempting to improve motor control through central facilitation*
- Based on concept that damaged CNS regressed to phylogenetically older patterns of movements (limb synergies and primitive reflexes); thus, synergies, primitive reflexes, and other abnormal movements are considered normal processes of recovery before normal patterns of movements are attained
- Patients are taught to use and voluntarily control the motor patterns available to them at a particular point during their recovery process (e.g., limb synergies)
- Enhances specific synergies through use of cutaneous/proprioceptive stimuli, central facilitation using Twitchell's recovery
- *Opposite to Bobath* (which inhibits abnormal patterns of movement)

Sensorimotor approach/Rood approach (Noll, Bender, and Nelson, 1996)
- Modification of muscle tone and voluntary motor activity using cutaneous sensorimotor stimulation
- Facilitatory or inhibitory inputs through the use of sensorimotor stimuli, including, quick stretch, icing, fast brushing, slow stroking, tendon tapping, vibration, and joint compression to promote contraction of proximal muscles

Motor relearning program/Carr and Shepard approach (Carr et al., 1985)
- Based on cognitive motor relearning theory and influenced by Bobath's approach
- Goal is for the patient to relearn how to move functionally and how to problem solve during attempts at new tasks
- Instead of emphasizing repetitive performance of a specific movement for improving skill, it teaches general strategies for solving motor problems.
- Emphasizes functional training of specific tasks, such as standing and walking, and carry-over of those tasks

Behavioral approaches (Noll, Bender, and Nelson, 1996) include:
- Kinesthetic or positional biofeedback and forced-use exercises
- Electromyographic biofeedback EMGBF: makes patient aware of muscle activity or lack of it by using external representation (e.g., auditory or visual cues) of internal activity as a way to assist in the modification of voluntary control
  - In addition to trying to modify autonomic function, EMGBF also attempts to modify pain and motor disturbances by using volitional control and auditory, visual, and sensory clues
  - Electrodes placed over agonists/antagonists for facilitation/inhibition
  - Accurate sensory information reaches brain through systems unaffected by brain → via visual and auditory for proprioception

UPPER EXTREMITY MANAGEMENT (Black-Shaffer, Kirsteins, and Harvey, 1999)

- Shoulder pain: 70%–84% of stroke patients with hemiplegia have shoulder pain with varying degrees of severity
- Of the patients with shoulder pain, the majority (85%) will develop it during the spastic phase of recovery
- It is generally accepted that the most common causes of hemiplegic shoulder pain are the shoulder-hand syndrome/reflex sympathetic dystrophy (RSD) and soft-tissue lesions (including plexus lesions)

Complex Regional Pain Syndrome Type I (CRPS, Type I)/Reflex Sympathetic Dystrophy (RSD)

- Disorder characterized by sympathetic-maintained pain and related sensory abnormalities, abnormal blood flow, abnormalities in the motor system, and changes in both superficial and deep structures with trophic changes
- Has been reported in 12% to 25% of hemiplegic stroke patients
- CRPS Type I = RSD
  (CRPS type II = causalgia—pain limited to a peripheral nerve distribution)
- Most common subtype of RSD in stroke is shoulder-hand syndrome

Stages:
- **Stage 1—acute:** burning pain, diffuse swelling/edema, exquisite tenderness, vasomotor changes in hand/fingers (with increased nail and hair growth, hyperthermia or hypothermia, sweating). Lasts three to six months
- **Stage 2—dystrophic:** pain becomes more intense and spreads proximally, skin/muscle atrophy, brawny edema, cold insensitivity, brittle nails/nail atrophy, decrease ROM, mottled skin, early atrophy and osteopenia (late). Lasts three to six months
- **Stage 3—atrophic:** pain decreases, trophic changes, hand skin pale and cyanotic, with a smooth, shiny appearance and feels cool and dry, bone demineralization progresses with muscular weakness/atrophy, contractures/flexion deformities of shoulder/hand, tapering digits, no vasomotor changes

Pathogenesis
- Multiple theories postulated including:
  - Abnormal adrenergic sensitivity develops in injured nociceptors, and circulating or locally secreted sympathetic neurotransmitters trigger the painful afferent activity
  - Cutaneous injury activates nociceptor fibers → central pain-signaling system → pain
  - Central sensitization of pain-signaling system
  - Low-threshold mechanoreceptor input develops capacity to evoke pain
  - With time, efferent sympathetic fibers develop capacity to activate nociceptor fibers

Diagnosis

- **X rays**—in initial stages, X rays normal; periarticular osteopenia may be seen in later stages; use is questionable, given that bone mineral density starts to decrease in the paralytic arm one month after stroke
  - Need 30%–50% demineralization for detection

- **Bone Scan**—30 stroke survivors < 3 months onset, evaluated for CRPS Type I using triple phase bone scan (Kozin, 1981; Simon and Carlson, 1980; Habert, Eckelman, and Neuman, 1996)
  - Sensitivity ~ 92%
  - Specificity ~ 56%
  - Positive predictive value (PPV) ~ 58%
  - Negative predictive value (NPV) ~ 91% (Holder and Mackinnon, 1984)
  - Diffusely increased juxta-articular tracer activity on delayed images is the most sensitive indicator for RSD (sensitivity 96%, specificity 97%, and PPV 88%)

- **EMG**—as predictor for RSD (Cheng and Hong, 1995)
  - Association between spontaneous activity and eventual development of RSD (vs no spontaneous activity on EMG)

- **Clinical** (Wang et al., 1998)
  - Clinical diagnosis difficult, presentation fairly incomplete
  - Most consistent early diagnostic signs: shoulder pain with ROM (flexion/abduction/external rotation), absence of pain in elbow and with forearm pronation/supination; wrist dorsiflexion pain with dorsal edema; pain MCP/PIP flexion with fusiform PIP edema
  - Pain out of proportion to injury and clinical findings
  - Shoulder/hand pain preceded by rapid ROM loss
  - Tepperman et al. (1984) Greyson and Tepperman (1984)
  - Studied 85 consecutive post-CVA hemiplegic patients
  - 25% had radionuclide evidence for RSD: positive diagnosis was evident when delayed image showed increased uptake in wrist, MCP and IP joints
  - In this study, the most valuable clinical sign was MCP tenderness to compression with 100% predictive value, sensitivity 85%, and specificity 100%

- **Stellate ganglion block**
  - Alleviation of pain following sympathetic blockade of the stellate ganglion using local anesthetic: is the gold standard Dx of sympathetically mediated CRPS Type I

Treatment (Arlet and Mazieres, 1997)

- ROM exercises involved joint-pain free within three weeks, most < four to six days with passive stretch of involved joints
- Corticosteroids (systemic): a large majority of patients respond to systemic steroids instituted in the acute phase of the disease. Usually prednisone in doses up to 100–200 mg/day or 1 mg/kg, and tapered over two weeks
  - More effective in RSD confirmed by bone scan than on "clinical" RSD with negative bone scan. Bone scan may be useful not only in establishing the Dx of RSD, but also in identifying patients likely to respond to oral steroid therapy. In a study, 90% of the patients. with positive bone scan findings for RSD treated with corticosteroids had good or excellent response, whereas 64% of the patients, without bone scan abnormalities had poor or fair response.

    – In recent study, 31/34 MCA stroke patients with RSD became pain free by 14 days after starting methylprednisolone 8 mg PO QID (patients treated for two weeks, followed by two-week taper)
- Intra-articular injections with corticosteroids
- Analgesics (NSAIDs)
- Tricyclic antidepressants
- Diphosphonates
- Calcitonin
- Anticonvulsants (as Neurontin® or Tegretol®)
- Alpha-adrenergic blockers (clonidine, prazosin)
- Beta-blockers (propranolol and pindolol)
- Calcium channel blockers (nifedipine)
- Topical capsaicin
- TENS
- Contrast baths
- Edema control measures
- Desensitization techniques
- Ultrasound (U/S)
- Sympathetic ganglion blocks (i.e., stellate ganglion) may be diagnostic as well as therapeutic
- Local injections (procaine, corticosteroid)
- Sympathectomy

Shoulder Subluxation

Characterized by the presence of a palpable gap between the acromion and the humeral head

Etiology is unknown, but may be due to changes in the mechanical integrity of the gleno-humeral joint

Pathogenesis: factors that are thought to be related to shoulder subluxation include: angulation of the glenoid fossa, the influence of the supraspinatus muscle on the humeral head sitting, the support of the scapula on the rib cage, the contraction of the deltoid and rotator cuff muscles on the abducted humerus
- A number of recent studies have failed to show any correlation between shoulder subluxation and pain
- There might be a correlation with between-shoulder pain and decrease in arm external rotation
- *Basmajian Principle:* Decreased trapezius tone—the scapula rotates and humeral head subluxates from glenoid fossa

Treatment
Shoulder slings: use is controversial
Routine use of sling for the subluxed shoulder (or for shoulder pain) is not indicated
- 📖 **Friedland**—sling does not prevent/correct subluxation, not necessary to support pain-free shoulder (Friedland, 1975)
- 📖 **Hurd**—no appreciable difference in shoulder ROM, subluxation, or shoulder pain in patients wearing slings or not (Hurd et al., 1974)

Pros: May be used when patient ambulates to support extremity (may prevent upper extremity trauma, which in turn may cause increase pain or predispose to development of RSD)

Cons: May encourage contractures in shoulder adduction/internal rotation, elbow flexion (flexor synergy pattern)

Other widely used treatments for shoulder subluxation:
• Functional Electrical Stimulation (FES)
• Armboard, arm trough, lapboard—used in poor upper-extremity recovery, primary wheelchair users
    – Arm board may overcorrect subluxation
• Overhead slings—prevents hand edema (may use foam wedge on armboard)

Prevention:
• Subluxation may be prevented by combining the early reactivation of shoulder muscula- ture (specifically supraspinatus and post- and mid-deltoid) with the provision of FES or a passive support of the soft-tissue structures of the glenohumeral joint (e.g., arm trough)

📖 Brachial Plexus/Peripheral Nerve Injury

Etiology: "Traction" neuropathy

Diagnosis:
• Clinical: atypical functional return, segmental muscle atrophy, finger extensor contracture, delayed onset of spasticity
• Electrodiagnostic studies (EMG)—lower motor neuron findings

Treatment:
• Proper bed positioning to prevent patient from rolling onto his paretic arm, trapping it behind his back or through the bed rails and place a traction stress on it.
• ROM to prevent contracture while traction avoided
• 45-degree shoulder-abduction sling for nighttime positioning
• Sling for ambulation to prevent traction by gravity
• Armrest in wheelchair as needed

Prognosis—may require 8 to 12 months for reinnervation

Bicipital Tendinitis

• Chronic pain anterolateral shoulder, pain in abduction/external rotation, painful over bicipital groove
• Positive Yergason test: with arm on side and elbow flexed, external rotation of the arm is exerted by the examiner (while pulling downward on the elbow) as the patient resists the movement. If the biceps tendon is unstable on the bicipital groove, it will pop-out and the patient will experience pain
• Greatest excursion of long head biceps from flexion/internal rotation, to elevation/abduc- tion, depression/external rotation/extension
• May progress to adhesive capsulitis (frozen shoulder)

Diagnosis may be confirmed with decreased pain after injection of tendon sheath with lido- caine; bicipital tendinitis may respond to steroid injection of the tendon sheath.

Rotator Cuff Tear, Impingement Syndrome, Adhesive Capsulitis (frozen shoulder):

All are causes of poststroke shoulder pain—see Table 1.7; see Musculoskeletal chapter

TABLE 1–7 Post-Stroke Shoulder Pain

	Inferior Subluxation	Rotator Cuff Tear	CRPS Type 1 (RSD)	Frozen Shoulder	Impingement Syndrome	Biceps Tendinitis
EXAM	• Acromio-humeral separation • Flaccid	• Positive abduction test • Positive drop arm test • Flaccid or spastic	• MCP compress-ion test • Skin changes color • Flaccid or spastic	• External rotation less than 15° • Early decrease in scapular motion • Spastic	• Pain with abduc-tion of 70°–90° • End-range pain with forward flexion • Usually spastic	• Positive Yergason's test • Flaccid or spastic
DIGNOSTIC TEST	• X ray in stand-ing position • Scapular plane view	• X ray • Arthrogram • Subacromial injection of lidocaine • MRI	• Triple phase bone scan • Stellate ganglion block	• Arthrogram	• Subacromial injection of lidocaine	• Tendon sheath injection of lidocaine
THERAPY	• Sling when upright • FES	• Steroid injection • PT/ROM • Possible surgical repair • Reduction of internal rotator cuff tone	• Oral corticosteroids • Stellate ganglion block	• PT/ROM • Debridement manipulation • Subacromial steroids • Intra-articular steroids • Reduction of internal rotator cuff tone	• PT/ROM • Scapular mobilization • Subacromial steroids • Reduction of internal rotator cuff tone	• Tendon sheath injection of steroids

Abbreviations: CRPS1: Complex/regional Pain Syndrome type 1
FES: Functional electrical stimulation
MCP: metacarpophalangeal
PT/ROM: Physical Therapy/Range of Motion

MRI: magnetic resonance imaging
RSD: Reflex Sympathetic Dystrophy
(Black-Schaffer, 1999)

Heterotopic Ossification

- Infrequent (in stroke), but may be seen in elbow, shoulder
- Occurs only on extensor side of elbow
- No problems in pronation/supination since proximal radioulnar joint not involved
- Treatment: joint mobilization/ROM, etidronate disodium

Dependent Edema

May be treated with use of compression glove, foam wedge, pneumatic compression, retrograde massage, arm elevation

OTHER ASPECTS OF STROKE REHABILITATION

Spasticity Management

For a detailed discussion of spasticity, see the Spasticity chapter

Spasticity in stroke:
- Usually seen days to weeks after ischemic strokes
- Usually follows classic upper-extremity flexor and lower-extremity extensor patterns
- Clinical features include velocity-dependent resistance to passive movement of affected muscles at rest, and posturing in the patterns previously mentioned during ambulation and with irritative/noxious stimuli

Treatment:
- Noninvasive Tx: stretching program, splints/orthosis, serial casting, electrical stimulation, local application of cold

- Medications:
  - The use of benzodiazepines, baclofen, dantrolene, and the alpha agonists clonidine and tizanidine, in stroke patients, remains controversial
  - These drugs have modest effects on the hypertonicity and posturing associated with stroke and their side-effects limit their usefulness

- Injection of chemical agents:
  - Botulinum toxin: may be particularly useful in control of increased tone in smaller muscles of the forearm and leg (e.g., brachioradialis, finger, wrist, and thumb flexors, in the upper extremity, and long and short toe flexors, extensor hallucis injury (EHL), and ankle invertors in the lower extremity)
  - Phenol: may remain the agent of choice for injection of large muscle groups (e.g., hip adductors and extensors, the pectorals, lats, and biceps)

- Intrathecal baclofen: limited experience of its use in stroke patients; usefulness remains to be determined in this population

- Surgical procedures:
  - Uncommonly used in stroke, probably because of expected decrease in survival and increase in rate of medical co-morbidities
  - May be useful in selected cases when specific goals are pursued (e.g., increase in function, improve hygiene, decrease in pain)

Deep Vein Thrombosis (DVT)

- Common medical complication after stroke; occurring in 20%–75% of untreated stroke survivors (60%–75% in affected extremity, 25% proximal DVT; PE, 1%–2%)

- **Diagnosis**: Usually can be made using noninvasive techniques:
  - Ultrasonography
  - Impedance plethysmography
  - Contrast venography reserved for cases with inconclusive results.
  - D-dimer assays (a cross-linked fibrin degradation product): may be useful as screening tool for DVT in stroke patients

- **Prophylaxis**:
  Currently, recommended prophylaxis regimens include:
  - Low dose subcutaneous (SQ) heparin/low molecular weight heparin
  - Intermittent pneumatic compression (IPC) of the lower extremity (LE) (for patients with a contraindication to heparin)
  - Gradient compression stockings in combination with SQ heparin or IPC

Bladder Dysfunction

- Incidence of urinary incontinence is 50%–70% during the first month after stroke and 15% after 6 months (similar to general population—incidence ≈ 17%.)
- Incontinence may be caused by CNS damage itself, UTI, impaired ability to transfer to toilet or impaired mobility, confusion, communication disorder/aphasia, and cognitive-perceptual deficits that result in lack of awareness of bladder fullness
- Types of voiding disorders: areflexia, uninhibited spastic bladder (with complete/incomplete emptying), outlet obstruction
- Treatment: implementation of timed bladder-emptying program
  - Treat possible underlying causes (e.g., UTI)
  - Regulation of fluid intake
  - Transfer and dressing-skill training
  - Patient and family education
  - Medications (if no improvement with conservative measures)
- Remove indwelling catheter—perform postvoid residuals, intermittent catheterization—perform urodynamics evaluation

Bowel Dysfunction

Patient unable to inhibit urge to defecate → incontinence
- Incidence of bowel incontinence in stroke patients 31%
- Incontinence usually resolves within the first two weeks; persistence may reflect severe brain damage
- Decrease in bowel continence may be associated with infection resulting in diarrhea, inability to transfer to toilet or to manage clothing, and communication impairment/inability to express toileting needs
- Tx: treat underlying causes (e.g., bowel infection, diarrhea), timed-toileting schedule, training in toilet transfers and communication skills
Impairment of intestinal peristalsis—constipation
- Management: adequate fluid intake/hydration, modify diet (e.g., increase in dietary fiber), bowel management (stool softeners, stool stimulants, suppositories), allow commode/bathroom privileges

Dysphagia

Dysphagia (difficulty swallowing), in stroke, has an incidence of 30% to 45% (overall)
- 67% of brainstem strokes
- 28% of all left hemispheric strokes
- 21% of all right hemispheric strokes
- More common in bilateral hemisphere lesions than in unilateral hemisphere lesions
- More common in large-vessel than in small-vessel strokes

Predictors on bed-side swallowing exam of aspiration include:
- Abnormal cough
- Cough after swallow
- Dysphonia
- Dysarthria
- Abnormal gag reflex
- Voice change after swallow (wet voice) (Aronson, 1990)

SWALLOWING

Three phases:
1. Oral
2. Pharyngeal
3. Esophageal

TABLE 1–8   Oral Phase

Voluntary vs. reflex	• Voluntary
Phase duration	• Variable; voluntary phase with duration influenced by consistency of material ingested, number of times person chews, etc.
Hallmarks of this phase	• Preparation of bolus • Tongue elevates and occludes the anterior oral cavity and compresses the bolus toward the oropharynx • Contraction of the palatopharyngeal folds • Elevation of the soft palate
Phase requires:	• Intact lip closure • Mobile tongue • Functional muscles of mastication
Problems seen in this phase:	• Drooling, pocketing, head tilt

TABLE 1–9   Pharyngeal Phase

Voluntary vs. reflex	• Reflex
Phase duration	• Lasts ~ 0.6 to 1 sec
Hallmarks of this phase	• Bolus propelled from mouth to esophagus • Aspiration most likely to occur during this phase • With initiation of pharyngeal phase, inhibition of breathing occurs to prevent aspiration.
▥ Phase requires:	• Tongue elevation • Soft palate elevation (also seen in the oral phase) and velopharyngeal port closure—to close off the nasal cavity and prevent regurgitation into the nasopharynx • Laryngeal elevation, with folding of epiglottis and vocal cord adduction to prevent aspiration • Coordinated pharyngeal constriction and cricopharyngeal (upper esophageal sphincter) relaxation—to facilitate bolus transport into the esophagus
Problems seen in this phase:	• Food sticking, choking and coughing, aspiration, wet/gurgling voice, nasal regurgitation

TABLE 1–10   Esophageal Phase

Voluntary vs. reflex	• Reflex
Phase duration	• Longest phase—lasts 6–10 sec
Hallmarks of this phase	• Bolus passed from pharynx → esophagus → stomach • Esophageal clearance is assisted by gravity but requires relaxation of the gastroesophageal sphincter
Phase requires:	• Cricopharyngeal muscle contraction • Coordinated peristalsis and LES relaxation
Problems seen in this phase:	• Heartburn, food sticking

Important Definitions

- ▥ **Chin tuck**—compensatory technique to provide airway protection by preventing entry of liquid into the larynx (probably by facilitating forward motion of the larynx). Also, chin tuck decreases the space between the base of the tongue and the posterior pharyngeal wall, and so creates increased pharyngeal pressure to move the bolus through the pharyngeal region

- ▥ **Aspiration**
  - Aspiration, by definition, is the penetration of a substance into the laryngeal vestibule and below the vocal folds (true vocal cords) into the trachea
  - Aspiration is missed on bedside swallowing evaluations in 40% to 60% of patients (i.e., silent aspiration)
  - It can be reliably diagnosed on videofluoroscopic swallowing study (penetration of contrast material below the true vocal cords)
  - Using videofluoroscopic swallowing study, aspiration has been found to occur in 40% to 70% of stroke patients.
  - Predictors of aspiration on videofluoroscopic swallowing study include:
    - Delayed initiation of the swallow reflex
    - Decreased pharyngeal peristalsis

- **Aspiration pneumonia**
  Risk factors for development of pneumonia secondary to aspiration include:
  - Decreased level of consciousness
  - Tracheostomy
  - Emesis
  - Reflux
  - Nasogastric tube (NGT) feeding
  - Dysphagia
  - Prolonged pharyngeal transit time

As dysphagia is a frequent and potentially serious (because of aspiration) complication of stroke, careful bedside swallowing evaluation should be performed in all patients before oral feeding is started. If a patient is believed to be at high risk of recurrent aspiration after bedside and/or videofluoroscopic evaluation, he/she should be kept NPO and enterally fed, initially via NGT, and then via G-tube or J-tube if long-term enteral feeding is required.

- **Non-oral feeding:**
  - Clear contraindication for oral feeding is pulmonary pathology due to aspiration in the presence of documented airway contamination
  - NPO also indicated in patients at high risk of aspiration because of reduced alertness, reduced responsiveness to stimulation, absent swallow, absent protective cough, and difficulty handling secretions, or when there is significant reduction of oral pharyngeal and laryngeal movements
  - NPO is disadvantageous in treating dysphagia because swallowing itself is the best treatment

Treatment of dysphagia/prevention of aspiration:
- Changes in posture and head position
- Elevation of the head of the bed
- Feeding in the upright position
- Chin tuck
- Turning the head to the paretic side
- Diet modifications (e.g., thickened fluids, pureed or soft foods in smaller boluses)

Inconclusive evidence of long-term efficacy in dysphagia:
- Thermal stimulation (to sensitize the swallowing reflex)
- Oral/motor exercises (to improve tongue and lip strength, ROM, velocity, and precision, and vocal-fold adduction)

Other complications of dysphagia include dehydration and malnutrition:
- Malnutrition found in 49% of patients admitted to rehabilitation in recent study and was associated with a prolonged length of stay and slower rate of functional gains
- Malnourished patients—higher stress reaction, frequency of infection and decubiti

Recovery of dysphagia in stroke:
Few studies available on recovery of dysphagia in stroke:
- Gresham (1990) reports his findings regarding 53 patients in a swallowing program post-stroke
  - 85% (45/53) on full oral nutrition at discharge
  - 17% (9/53) could not drink thin liquids safely
  - 8% (4/53) could not adequately maintain cohesive bolus of varied texture
- Gordon (1987)
  - 41 of 91 (45%) stroke patients + dysphagia
  - 90% hemispheric lesions (17% bilateral)

- Swallowing function regained within 14 days in 86% (of patients who survived unilateral stroke)
- 📖 Logemann (1991)
  - Recovery of swallowing function in most brainstem strokes occurs in the first three weeks poststroke

📖 **Nasal speech**: hypernasality caused by partial or complete failure of soft palate to close-off the nasal cavity from the oral cavity or by incomplete closure of the hard palate. Uplifting the soft palate prevents nasal speech (speech abnormally resonated in the nasal cavities).

APHASIA

- Aphasia is an impairment of the ability to utilize language due to brain damage. Characterized by paraphasias, word-finding difficulties, and impaired comprehension. Also common, but not obligatory, features are disturbances in reading and writing, non-verbal constructional and problem-solving difficulty and impairment of gesture

TABLE 1–11 Aphasias

Fluent				Nonfluent			
+ COMPREHENSION		– COMPREHENSION		+ COMPREHENSION		– COMPREHENSION	
REPETITION ⇓		*REPETITION* ⇓		*REPETITION* ⇓		*REPETITION* ⇓	
+	–	+	–	+	–	+	–
NAMING	conduction	Transcortical sensory	Wernicke's	Transcortical motor	Broca's	Mixed transcortical	Global

NAMING	
+	–
normal	anomia

Fluent	Non-fluent
Wernicke's	Broca's
Transcortical sensory	Transcortical motor
Conduction	Global
Anomia	Mixed transcortical

ANATOMIC LOCATION OF MAJOR SPEECH AREAS

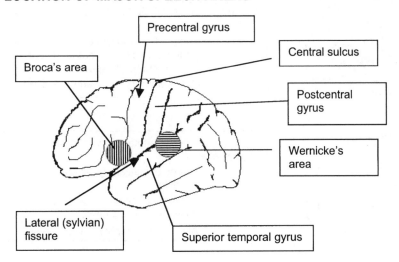

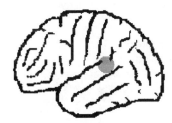

Wernicke's aphasia

📖 Location: posterior part of superior (first) temporal gyrus of the dominant (usually left) hemisphere
Characteristics:
- Fluent speech (normal rate/speed)
- Impaired comprehension
- Word deafness, difficulty in reading (alexia) and writing (agraphia)
- Marked paraphasias & neologisms

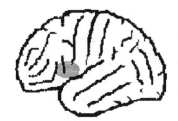

Broca's aphasia (remember "broken" speech)

Location: posterior-inferior frontal lobe (third frontal convolution) of dominant (usually left) hemisphere → anterior to motor cortex areas that supply the tongue, lips and larynx
Characteristics:
- Nonfluent speech (telegraphic)
- Impaired repetition
- Preserved comprehension
- Paraphasias & articulatory errors or struggle

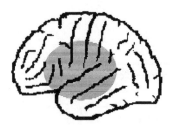

Global aphasia

Location: vary in size and location but usually involve distribution of the left MCA (entire perisylvian region)
Characteristics:
- Ranges from mutism (non-fluent) to total repetitive jargon or neologistic output (fluent but incomprehensible speech)
- Poor comprehension and repetition

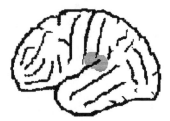

Anomic aphasia

Location: temporo-parietal injury, angular gyrus
Characteristics:
- Fluent, essentially good comprehension and repetition
- Decreased output of nouns
- Word-finding difficulties
- Alexia and agraphia may be present

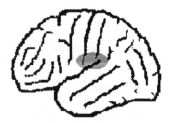

Conduction aphasia

Location: lesion of the parietal operculum (arcuate fasciculus) or insula or deep to the supramarginal gyrus (usually left side)
Characteristics:
- Normal rate of speech (fluent)
- Preserved comprehension
- Impaired repetition
- Literal paraphasias with "targeting" of words (until getting the right one)

Note: **arcuate fasciculus** is a band of white matter running deep to the supramarginal gyrus and insula that joins Broca's and Wernicke's areas

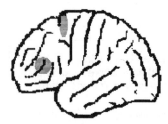

Transcortical motor aphasia

Location: frontal lobe, anterior or superior to Broca's area or in the subcortical region deep to Broca's area
Characteristics:
- Reduced rate of speech, limited language output (with some fluent utterances)
- Reduced initiation & organization of speech good comprehension
- Preserved repetition

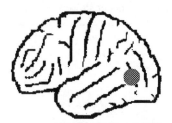

Transcortical sensory aphasia

Location: watershed lesion isolating perisylvian speech structures (Broca's and Wernicke's areas) from the posterior brain; angular gyrus or posterio-inferior temporal lobe
Characteristics:
- Poor comprehension
- Fluent speech (neologisms)
- Preserved repetition (possibly echolalia)

Transcortical mixed aphasia: Lesions in border zone of frontal, parietal, and temporal areas

Characteristics:
• Poor comprehension
• Nonfluent (decrease rate and initiation of speech)
• Preserved repetition (echolalia)
📖 Note: Language areas are anatomically clustered around the sylvian fissure of the dominant hemisphere—left hemisphere in 95% of people.

Paraphasias: Incorrect substitutions of words or part of words

• Literal or phonemic paraphasias: similar sounds (e.g., "sound" for "found")
• Verbal or semantic paraphasias: word substituted for another from same semantic class (e.g., "fork" for "spoon")

📖 **Recovery Language Deficits/Aphasia Post Stroke:**

The greatest amount of improvement in patients with aphasia occurs in the first two to three months after the onset; after six months, there is a significant drop in the rate of recovery.

In the majority of cases of patients with aphasia spontaneous recovery does not seem to occur after a year. However, there are reports of improvements many years after their stroke in patients undergoing therapy.

MEDICAL MANAGEMENT PROBLEMS

Poststroke Depression

• **Etiology:**
  – Organic: May be related to catecholamine depletion through lesion-induced damage to the frontal nonadrenergic, dopaminergic and serotonergic projections (Heilman and Valenstein, 1993)
  – Reactive: Grief/psychological responses for physical and personal losses associated with stroke, loss of control that often accompany severe disability, etc.
• Prevalence of depression in stroke patients reported ≈ 40% (25% to 79%); occur in similar proportion in their caregivers. (Flick, 1999)
• Most prevalent six months to two years
• A psychiatric evaluation for DSM-IV criteria and vegetative signs may be a clinically useful diagnostic tool in stroke patients
• There may be higher risk for major depression in left frontal lesions (relationship still controversial)
• Risk factors: prior psychiatric Hx, significant impairment in ADLs, high severity of deficits, female gender, nonfluent aphasia, cognitive impairment, and lack of social supports
• Persistent depression correlates with delayed recovery and poorer outcome
• Treatment: Active Tx should be considered for all patients with significant clinical depression
• Psychosocial interventional program: psychotherapy
• Medications: SSRIs preferred because of fewer side effects (compared to TCAs); methylphenidate has also been shown to be effective in poststroke depression
• SSRIs and TCAs also been shown to be effective in poststroke emotional lability

Sexual Dysfunction

- Well documented that the majority of elderly people continue to enjoy active and satisfying sexual relationships
- No significant changes in sexual interest or desire, but marked decline in behavior in both sexes (after stroke)
- There is a marked decline in sexual activity poststroke
- Fugl-Meyer (1980)—67 patients sexually active prestroke (Fugl-Meyer and Jaaski, 1980)
  - 36% remained active poststroke
  - 33% men resumed unaltered intercourse
  - 43% women resumed unaltered intercourse
  - Decreased frequency due to altered sensation, custodial attitudes taken by spouse

  Other factors related to decrease in sexual activity poststroke:
  Emotional factors—fear, anxiety and guilt; low self esteem; and fear of rejection by partner
  Treatment: supportive psychotherapy, counseling.

Seizures

- Can be classified as occurring:
  - At stroke onset
  - Early after stroke (1–2 weeks)
  - Late after stroke (> 2 weeks)

- In prospective study after first time stroke, 27 of 1099 (2.5%) of patients had seizures within 48 hours postictus.
- Seizures associated with older age, confusion, and large parietal or temporal hemorrhages
- Majority of seizures were generalized tonic-clonic
- In-hospital mortality higher in patients with seizures
- Early seizures tend not to recur; these are associated with acute metabolic derangement associated with ischemia or hemorrhage.
- Stroke patients requiring inpatient rehabilitation have higher probability of developing seizures than the general stroke population
- Seizures occurring > 2 weeks after stroke have higher probability of recurrence
- In study with 77 ischemic stroke victims followed two to four years
  - 6%–9% develop seizures
  - 6/23 (26%) patients with cortical lesions develop seizures
  - 1/54 (2%) patients with subcortical lesions develop seizures
- Risk Factors: Cortical lesions, persistent paresis (6/12 = 50%)
- Treatment: choice of anticonvulsant drugs for patients with cerebral injury discussed in the TBI chapter.

FACTORS THAT PREDICT MORTALITY AND FUNCTIONAL RECOVERY IN STROKE PATIENTS

Mortality Factors

- Mortality of ischemic strokes in the first 30 days ranges from 17%–34%
- Hemorrhagic strokes are more likely to present as severe strokes and with mortality rate reported to be up to 48%

- Mortality in the first year after stroke 25% to 40%
- The risk of another stroke within the first year 12% to 25%

RISK FACTORS FOR ACUTE STROKE MORTALITY — 30 DAY MORTALITY

- Stroke severity
- Low level of consciousness
- Diabetes mellitus
- Cardiac disease
- Electrocardiograph abnormalities
- Old age
- Delay in medical care
- Elevated blood sugar in non-diabetic
- Brainstem involvement
- Hemorrhagic stroke
- Admission from nursing home

Functional Recovery and Disability Factors

- As stroke mortality has declined in the last few decades, the number of stroke survivors with impairments and disabilities has increased
- There are 300,000 to 400,000 stroke survivors annually
- 78% to 85% of stroke patients regain ability to walk (with or without assistive device)
- 48% to 58% regain independence with their self-care skills
- 10% to 29% are admitted to nursing homes

RISK FACTORS FOR DISABILITY AFTER STROKE

- Severe stroke (minimal motor recovery at 4 weeks)
- Low level of consciousness
- Diabetes mellitus
- Cardiac disease
- Electrocardiograph abnormalities
- Old age
- Delay in medical care
- Delay in rehabilitation
- Bilateral lesions
- Previous stroke
- Previous functional disability
- Poor sitting balance
- Global aphasia
- Severe neglect
- Sensory and visual deficits
- Impaired cognition
- Incontinence (>1–2 weeks)

Negative Factors of Return to Work (Black-Shaffer and Osberg, 1990)
- Low score on Barthel Index at time of rehabilitation discharge
- Prolonged rehabilitation length of stay
- Aphasia
- Prior alcohol abuse

(Barthel Index is a functional assessment tool that measures independence in ADLs on 0–100 scale)

REFERENCES

Adams RD, Victor M, Ropper AH. *Principles of Neurology 6th ed*. New York: McGraw-Hill; 1997.

American Heart Association. 2000 Heart and Stroke Statistical Update. Dallas: American Heart Association, 1999.

Arlet J, Mazieres B. Medical Treatment of RSD. *Hand Clinics* 1997;13:477–483.

Aronson AE. *Clinical Voice Disorders 3rd ed*. New York: Thieme Medical Publishers, 1990.

Biller J, Bruno A. "Acute Ischemic Stroke" in *Current Therapy in Neurologic Disease 5th ed*. St. Louis: Mosby, 1997.

Black-Schaffer RM, Kirsteins AE, Harvey RL. Stroke rehabilitation. 2. Co-morbidities and complications. *Arch Phys Med Rehabil*. 1999;80(suppl):S8–16.

Black-Schaffer RM, Osberg JS. Return to work after stroke: development of a predictive model. *Arch Phys Med Rehabil*. 1990;71:285–90.

Bobath B. *Adult hemiplegia: Evaluation and treatment*. London: Spottiswood Ballintype, 1978.

Broderick JP. Stroke trends in Rochester, Minnesota, during 1945 to 1984. *Ann Epidemiol*. 1993;3:476–9.

Brown RD, Whisnant JP, Sicks JD, O'Fallon WM, Wiebers DO. Stroke incidence, prevalence, and survival: secular trends in Rochester, Minnesota, through 1989. *Stroke*. 1996;27:373–80.

Brunnstrom S. Motor testing procedures in hemiplegia: based on sequential recovery stages. *Phys Ther*. 1966;46:357–75.

Brunnstrom S. *Movement Therapy in Hemiplegia: A Neurophysiological Approach*. New York: Medical Dept., Harper & Row, 1970.

Carr JH, Shepherd RB, Nordholm L, Lynne D. Investigation of a new motor assessment scale for stroke patients. *Phys Ther*. 1985;65:175–80.

Cheng PT, Hong CZ. Prediction of reflex sympathetic dystrophy in hemiplegic patients by electromyographic study. *Stroke*. 1995;26:2277–80.

Creager MA. Results of the CAPRIE trial: efficacy and safety of clopidogrel. Clopidogrel versus aspirin in patients at risk of ischemic events. *Vasc Med* 1998;3:257–60.

Endarterectomy for moderate symptomatic carotid stenosis: Interim results from the MRC European Carotid Surgery Trial. *Lancet*. 1996;347:1591–3.

Executive Committee for the Asymptomatic Carotid Atherosclerosis Study. Endarterectomy for asymptomatic carotid artery stenosis. *JAMA*. 1995;273:1421–8.

Ferri, FF. *Practical Guide to the Care of the Medical Patient 4th ed*. St. Louis: Mosby, 1998.

Fix JD. HighYield Neuroanatomy. Baltimore: Williams & Wilkins, 1995.

Flick CL. Stroke Rehabilitation: 4. Stroke outcome and psychosocial consequences. *Arch Phys Med Rehabil*. 1999;80(suppl):21–26

Friedland E. Physical Therapy. In Licht S. ed. Stroke and its Rehabilitation. New Haven, CT: E. Licht, 1975.

Fugl-Meyer AR, Jaaski L. Post-stroke hemiplegia and sexual intercourse. *Scand J Rehabil Med*. 1980;7:158–66.

Goldberg S. *Clinical Neuroanatomy Made Ridiculously Simple*. Miami: Medmaster Inc., 1997.

Gordon C, Hewer RL, Wade DT. Dysphagia in acute stroke. *Br Med J (Clin Res Ed)*. 1987;295:411–4.

Gresham SL. Clinical assessment and management of swallowing difficulties after stroke. *Med J Aust* 1990;153:397–99.

Greyson ND, Tepperman PS. Three-phase bone studies in hemiplegia with reflex sympathetic dystrophy and the effect of disuse. *J Nucl Med*. 1984;25:423–9.

Habert JC, Eckelman WC, Neumann RD. *Nuclear Medicine, Diagnosis and Therapy*. Thieme Medical Publishers, 1996.

Hamilton MG, Spetzler RF: The Prospective Application of a Grading System for Arteriovenous Malformations. *Neurosurgery*. 1994;34:2–7.

Heilman KM, Valenstein E. *Clinical Neuropsychology*. New York: Oxford University Press, 1993.

Holder Le, Mackinnon SE. Reflex sympathetic dystrophy in the hands: clinical and scintographic criteria. *Radiology*. 1984;152:517–22.

Hurd MM, Farrell KH, Waylonis GW. Shoulder Sling for hemiplegia: Friend or foe? *Arch Phys Med Rehabil*. 1974; 55:519–22.

Kay R, Wong KS, Yu YL, Chan YW, Tsoi TH, Ahuja AT, et al. Low-molecular-weight heparin for the treatment of acute ischemic stroke. *N Engl J Med*. 1995;333:1588–93.

Kirsteins AE, Black-Schaffer RM, Harvey RL. Stroke rehabilitation: 3. Rehabilitation management. *Arch Phys Med Rehabil*. 1999;80(suppl):17–20.

Knott M, Voss DE. *Proprioceptive Neuromuscular Facilitation: Patterns and Techniques, 2nd ed*. Hagerstown: Harper and Row, 1968.

Kozin F. Bone Scintigraphy in the RSD Syndrome. *Radiol*. 1981;138:437.

Logemann JA. Approaches to management of disordered swallowing. *Baillieres Clin Gastroenterol*. 1991;5:269–80.

National Institute of Neurologic Disorders and Stroke rt-PA Stroke Study Group. Tissue plasminogen acticator for acute ischemic stroke. *N Engl J Med* 1995;333:1581–7.

Moore WS. The American Heart Association Consensus Statement on guidelines for carotid endarterectomy. *Semin Vasc Surg*. 1995;8:77–81.

Noll SF, Bender CE, Nelson MC. Rehabilitation of Patients With Swallowing Disorders. In Braddom RL. *Physical Medicine and Rehabilitation*. Philadelphia: W.B. Saunders Co., 1996.

North American Symptomatic Carotid Endarterectomy Trial Collaborators. Beneficial effect of carotid endarterectomy in symptomatic patients with high-grade carotid stenosis. *N Engl J Med*. 1991;325:445–53.

Rosen P, ed. *Emergency Medicine—Stroke 3rd ed*. St. Louis: Mosby, 1992.

Ryder KM, Benjamin EJ. Epidemiology and significance of atrial fibrillation. *Am J Cardiol*. 1999;84(9A):131R-138R.

Sacco RL. *Merrit's Textbook of Neurology, 9th ed.—Pathogenesis, Classification, and Epidemiology of Cerebrovascular Disease*. Baltimore: Williams & Wilkins, 1995.

Sawner KA, LaVigne JM. *Brunnstrom's Movement Therapy in Hemiplegia: A Neurophysiological Approach, 2nd ed*. Philadelphia: J.B. Lippincott, 1992.

Schaller C, Scramm J, Haun D. Significance of Factors Contributing to Surgical Complications and to Late Outcome After Elective Surgery of Cerebral Arteriovenous Malformations. *J Neurol Neurosurg Psychiatry* 1998;65:547–54.

Simon H, Carlson DH. The use of bone scanning in diagnosis of RSD. *Clin Nucl Med*. 1980;3:116.

Stewart DG. Stroke rehabilitation: 1. Epidemiologic aspects and acute management. *Arch Phys Med Rehabil*. 1999;80(suppl);4–7.

Tepperman PS, Greyson ND, Hilbert L, Jimenez J, Williams JI. Reflex sympathetic dystrophy in hemiplegia. *Arch Phys Med Rehabil*. 1984;65:442–7.

Twitchell TE. The restoration of motor function following hemiplegia in man. *Brain* 1951;74:443–80.

Wang YL, Tsau JC, Huang MH, Lee BF, Li CH. Reflex sympathetic dystrophy syndrome in stroke patients with hemilegia—three-phase bone scintography and clinical characteristics. *Kaohsiung J Med Sci*. 1998:14:40–7.

Young B, Moore WS, Robertson JT, Toole JF, Ernst CB, Cohen SN, et al. An analysis of perioperative surgical mortality and morbidity in the asymptomatic carotid atherosclerosis study. *Stroke*. 1996;27:2216–24.

RECOMMENDED READING

DeLisa JA. Rehabilitation Medicine: Principles and Practice, 3rd ed. Philadelphia: JB Lippincott, 1998; 253–256.

Logemann JA. Evaluation and Treatment of Swallowing Disorders 2nd ed. Austin, TX: PRO-ED, 1998.

Miller J, Fountain N. Neurology Recall. Baltimore: Williams & Wilkins, 1997.

Mohr JP, Caplan LR, Melski JW, et al. The Harvard Cooperative Stroke Registry: A prospective registry. *Neurology*. 1978;28:754–762.

O'Young B, Young MA, Stiens SA. PM&R Secrets. Philadelphia: Hanley and Belfus Inc.;1997.

Stroke: Hope Through Research. Bethesda, MD; National Institute of Neurologic Disorders and Stroke, National Institutes of Health, 1999. NIH Publication No. 99–2222.

Tan JC. *Practical Manual of Physical Medicine and Rehabilitation*. New York: Mosby, 1998.

Zorowitz R. Stroke Rehabilitation. Grand rounds clinical lecture presented at: JFK Johnson Rehabilitation Institute August 1999; presented at Kessler Rehabilitation Institute Board Review Course 2000.

2

TRAUMATIC BRAIN INJURY

Elie Elovic, M.D., Edgardo Baerga, M.D., and Sara Cuccurullo, M.D.

■

INTRODUCTION

EPIDEMIOLOGY

- Trauma is the leading cause of death in ages 1–44 and more than half of these deaths are due to head trauma. Traumatic brain injury (TBI) is arguably the primary cause of neurologic mortality and morbidity in the United States
- About 500,000 per year traumatic brain injuries (requiring hospitalization) in the United States
- National Health Interview Survey (1985) provided the only national estimate of incidence of nonfatal TBI (hospitalized and non-hospitalized cases) for 1985–1987:
  - 1.975 million head injuries per year
  - Estimate probably includes head injuries in which no brain injury occurred
  - Fife (1987) concluded that only 16% of these injuries resulted in admission to a hospital
  - As a result of TBI Act, CDC is now sponsoring State Registries
- Overall incidence of traumatic brain injury 200 per 100,000 (150,000–235,000) per year (TBI cases requiring hospitalization)
  - Incidence is higher in males than in females (148–270 per 100,000 vs. 70–116 per 100,000)
- There is some evidence that TBI incidence is decreasing in the United States, comparing numbers from the 1970s and 1980s with more recent data (1990s) (Sosin, 1991)
- Peak ages 15–18 to 25 years
  - Age distribution is bimodal, with second peak in the elderly (ages 65–75); this group has a higher mortality rate
- Male to female ratio ⇒ 2.5 : 1
  - Mortality in males is 3–4 times higher than in females
- Motor vehicle accident (MVA) is the most common cause (overall) of head injury in adolescents and adults (~ 50% of cases)
  - 📖 The single most common cause of death and injury in automobile accidents is ejection of the occupant from the vehicle. (Spitz, 1991)
- Violence/assault is the second most common cause of TBI in young adults
- ETOH use clearly related to TBI
  - Alcohol detected in blood in up to 86% of TBI patients
  - ETOH blood levels 0.10% or higher in 51% to 72% of patients at the time of the injury (Gordon, Mann, a nd Wilier, 1993)

TBI Model Systems Program from 1989 to 1998

Data collected from the 17 model system centers in the United States between March 1989 and Sept 1998, on 1,086 TBI cases: (U.S. Dept. of Ed., 1999)
- 58% MVA-related injuries
- 26% violence-related injuries
- 53% positive blood alcohol level at injury

Mortality in TBI

- There has been a change in trends from 1980s to 1990s in TBI mortality with success in decreasing deaths secondary to MVA, but failure to prevent injuries (and deaths) due to firearms/violence
- Study in TBI deaths from 1979 to 1992 (Sosin, Snizek, and Waxweiler, 1995)
  - Average 52,000 deaths per year in the United States secondary to TBI
  - There was a decline in overall TBI-related deaths of 22% from 1979 to 1992 (reasons not known, but may include more vehicles with air bags, increase in use of seat belts and other improvements in vehicle safety features, roadway safety improvements, etc.)
  - 25% decline in MVA-related deaths
  - 13% increase in firearm-related deaths
  - Firearms surpassed MVA as the largest single cause of death in TBI in 1990
- Mortality rate TBI : 14–30 per 100,000 per year
- Gunshot wound (GSW) to head—mortality risk 75%–80%
- The majority of GSW-related TBI are self-inflicted

Geriatrics

- The risk of TBI increases sharply after age 65
- TBI among the elderly are more frequently due to falls
- Severity of TBI among the elderly tends to be higher than that observed in other age groups; mortality is also higher in the elderly compared to other groups
- Predominant sex: none; male = female (grossly) (1.2 : 1 ratio)
  (National Institute on Disability and Rehabilitation Research, Traumatic Brain Injury Model Systems Program, 1999)

Pediatrics

- As mentioned above, TBI is the leading cause of death in children > 1 year of age
- 10 in every 100,000 children die each year secondary to head injuries
- Annual incidence of TBI in children—185 per 100,000
- Causes:
  - Transportation related (39%)
  - Falls (28%)
  - Sports and recreational activities (17%)
  - Assault (7%)

■

MECHANISM AND RECOVERY OF HEAD INJURY

MECHANISMS OF INJURY

Primary
Occurs at the moment of the impact and as a direct result of trauma
    A. Contusions and lacerations of the brain surfaces—(Figure 2–1)
    B. Diffuse axonal injury (DAI)—(Figure 2–2)
    C. Diffuse vascular injury/multiple petechial hemorrhages
    D. Cranial nerve injury

Secondary
Damage that occurs after the initial trauma and as a result of the injuring event. Most secondary injury occurs during the first 12 to 24 hours after trauma, but may occur up to 5 to 10 days postinjury in very severe brain injury. Because of the delayed presentation, secondary injury may be preventable.
  A. Intracranial hemorrhage (epidural, subdural, subarachnoid and intracerebral hematoma)
  B. Brain swelling/brain edema (see below)
  C. Elevated Intracranial Pressure (ICP)
    – ↑ ICP ⇒ ↓ perfusion ⇒ ischemic brain damage
  D. Brain damage secondary to hypoxia
  E. Intracranial infection
  F. Hydrocephalus
  G. ↑ release of excitatory neurotransmitters secondary to diffuse axonal injury (DAI) = excitotoxicity
    – This will increase the activity of certain brain areas and overall metabolic demand in the already injured brain
  H. Production of free-radical molecules

Other secondary causes of brain injury include:
• Hypotension
• Electrolyte imbalances
• Anemia
• Hyperthermia
• Hyperglycemia
• Hypercarbia
• Hypoglycemia
• Hyperemia
• Hyponatremia
• Infection
• Carotid dissection
• Epilepsy/seizures
• Vasospasm/ischemia

Primary Head Injury

Contusion—bruising of cerebral (cortical) tissue
• Occurs on the undersurface of the frontal lobe (inferior frontal or orbitofrontal area) and anterior temporal lobe, regardless of the site of impact (Figure 2–1)
• May produce focal, cognitive, and sensory-motor deficits
• Is not directly responsible for loss of consciousness following trauma
• May occur from relatively low velocity impact, such as blows and falls

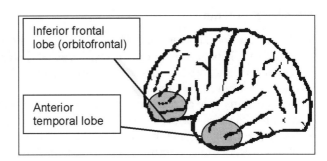

FIGURE 2–1. Location of Contusions

Diffuse axonal injury (DAI):
• DAI is seen exclusively in TBI
• Damage seen most often in the corpus callosum and other midline structures involving the parasagittal white matter, the interventricular septum, the walls of the third ventricle and the brain stem (midbrain and pons) (Figure 2–2)

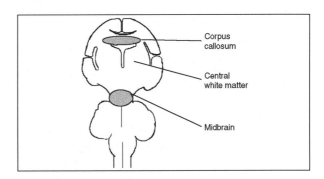

FIGURE 2–2. Locations of Diffuse Axonal Injury

- Responsible for the initial loss of consciousness seen in acute TBI
- Results from acceleration-deceleration and rotational forces associated with high-velocity impact (MVAs)
- The axonal injury seen in severe TBI is thought to be secondary to damage to the axoplasmic transport in axons (with $\uparrow$ Ca^{++} influx) leading to axonal swelling and detachment

Secondary Head Injury

Brain Swelling
- Occurs after acute head injury within 24 hours.
- Identified in CT as collapse of ventricular system and loss of cerebral spinal fluid (CSF) cisterns around the midbrain
- Is due to an increase in cerebral blood volume (intravascular blood)

Brain Edema
- Occurs later after head injury (in comparison to brain swelling)
- Is due to an increase in brain volume secondary to $\uparrow$ brain water content $\Rightarrow$ extravascular fluid
- Two types:
  1. **Vasogenic** edema:
     - Due to outpouring of protein rich fluid through damaged vessels
     - *Extracellular* edema
     - Related to cerebral contusion
  2. **Cytogenic** edema:
     - Found in relation to hypoxic and ischemic brain damage
     - Due to failing of the cells' energy supply system $\Rightarrow$ $\uparrow$ cell-wall pumping system $\Rightarrow$ *intracellular* edema in the dying cells

PENETRATING HEAD INJURIES

Missile/Fragments

- Deficits are focal corresponding to location of lesions caused by bullet/fragment
- If the brain is penetrated at the lower levels of the brain stem, death is instantaneous from respiratory and cardiac arrest. 80% of patients with through-and-through injuries die at once or within a few minutes
- The mortality rate of patients who are initially comatose from gunshot wounds to head is 88%; this is more than twice the mortality from closed-head injury (CHI)
- Focal or focal and generalized seizures occur in the early phase of the injury in 15% to 20% of cases. Risk of long-term posttraumatic epilepsy is higher in penetrating head injuries compared to nonpenetrating injuries

RECOVERY MECHANISMS

📖 Plasticity

- Brain plasticity is when the damaged brain has the capabilities to repair itself by means of morphologic and physiologic responses
- Plasticity is influenced by the environment, complexity of stimulation, repetition of tasks, and motivation

  It occurs via 2 mechanisms:
  1) Neuronal regeneration/neuronal (collateral) sprouting
  2) Unmasking neural reorganization

Neuronal Regeneration

Intact axons establish synaptic connections through dendritic and axonal sprouting in areas where damage has occurred

- May enhance recovery of function, may contribute to unwanted symptoms, or may be neutral (with no increase or decrease of function)
- Thought to occur weeks to months post-injury

Functional Reorganization/Unmasking

Healthy neural structures not formerly used for a given purpose are developed (or reassigned) to do functions formerly subserved by the lesioned area.

> Brain plasticity—remember "PUN"
> Plasticity = Unmasking + Neuronal sprouting

OTHER RELATED PHENOMENA ASSOCIATED WITH HEAD INJURY RECOVERY

Synaptic Alterations

Includes diaschisis and increased sensitivity to neurotransmitter levels

📖 **Diaschisis**: Mechanism to explain spontaneous return of function (Figure 2–3)

1. Lesions/damage to one central nervous system (CNS) region can produce altered function in other areas of the brain (at a distance from the original site of injury) that were not severed if there is connection between the two sites (through fiber tracts). Function is lost in both injured and in morphologically intact brain tissue.

2. There is some initial loss of function secondary to depression of areas of the brain connected to the primary injury site, and resolution of this functional deafferenation parallels recovery of the focal lesion (Feeney, 1991).

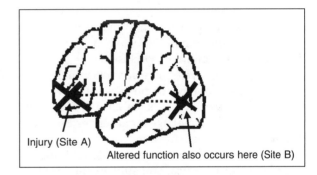

FIGURE 2–3. Example of Diaschisis: Injury to site A will produce inhibition on function at site B, which was not severed by the initial injury and is distant from the original site of injury (site A). Recovery of functions controlled by site B will parallel recovery of site A

Functional Substitution/Behavioral Substitution

Techniques/new strategies learned to compensate for deficits and achieve a particular task

Other Theories of Recovery Include

- **Redundancy**: Recovery of function based on activity of uninjured brain areas (latent areas) that normally would contribute to that function (and are capable of subserving that function)
- **Vicariation**: Functions taken over by brain areas not originally managing that function. These areas alter their properties in order to subserve that function.

■

DISORDERS OF CONSCIOUSNESS

LOCATION OF CONTROL OF CONSCIOUSNESS

📖 Consciousness

Consciousness is a function of ascending reticular activating system (RAS) and the cerebral cortex

RAS is composed of cell bodies in the central reticular core of the upper brain stem (mainly midbrain) and their projections to widespread areas of the cerebral cortex via both the thalamic and the extrathalamic pathways.

Lesions that interrupt the metabolic or structural integrity of the RAS or enough of the cortical neurons receiving RAS projections can cause coma.

DISORDERS OF CONSCIOUSNESS

Coma

- It is a state of unconsciousness from which the patient cannot be aroused; there is no evidence of self- or environmental-awareness
- Coma is essentially universal in severe TBI
- Up to 50% of patients in coma > 6 hours die without ever regaining consciousness. Survivors who remain unresponsive for > 2–4 weeks evolve into vegetative state
- Eyes remain continuously closed
- No sleep-wake cycles on electroencephalogram (EEG)
- There is *no* spontaneous purposeful movement (e.g., patient will not scratch himself, will not grab bedrail); there is inability to discretely localize noxious stimuli
- No evidence of language comprehension or expression
- It is believed that transition from coma to vegetative state signals the return of brain stem arousal mechanisms and that persistent unconsciousness reflects damage to the thalamus and/or global cortical and subcortical damage

Vegetative State (VS)

- **Definition:** Loss of capacity to interact with the environment despite the preserved potential for spontaneous or stimulus-induced arousal (due to absence of cortical activity)
- **Characteristics:**
  - Patient opens eyes (either spontaneously or with noxious stimuli)
  - VS is characterized by the presence of intermittent wakefulness evidenced by sleep-wake cycles (these may be demonstrated on EEG)
  - In VS there is no perceivable evidence of purposeful behavior
  - There is no evidence of intelligible verbal or gestural communication
  - This condition may persist for years following TBI, but this is very rare
  - Coma and VS are characterized by the absence of function in the cerebral cortex as judged behaviorally
- The term persistent vegetative state (redefined by The Multi-Society Task Force on PVS, 1994) is used for vegetative state that is present ≥ one month after a traumatic or nontraumatic brain injury

The Task Force also introduced the term *permanent vegetative state* to denote irreversibility after 3 months following nontraumatic brain injury and 12 months following traumatic brain injury (Howsepian, 1996).

Persistent VS	VS present ≥ 1 month after TBI or Nontraumatic brain injury
Permanent VS	VS present > 3 months after Nontraumatic brain injury or VS present > 12 months after TBI, in both children and adults

- American Congress of Rehabilitation Medicine (1995)—advocates to simply use the term vegetative state (VS) followed by the length of time it persists instead of the terms persistent and permanent. The Aspen Neurobehavioral Conference (1996), supported the ACRM recommendations to use the term VS + specify cause of injury + specify length of time since onset.
- Neuropathology of VS ⇒
  - Related to diffuse cortical injury
  - Bilateral thalamic lesions are prominent findings in VS
- Transition to VS, when preceded by coma, is signaled by re-emergence of eye opening and spontaneous control of autonomic functions.
  - Vegetative or autonomic functions include respiration, cardiovascular, thermoregulatory and neuroendocrine functions
- Visual tracking is considered a signal of transition out of VS

Minimally Conscious State (MCS)

- Severely altered consciousness with minimal but definite behavioral evidence of self- or environmental-awareness.
- Patients in MCS demonstrate inconsistent but definite reproducible behavioral evidence of self-awareness or awareness of the environment
- There is evidence that the following behaviors are reproducible (or sustained), but inconsistent:
  - Simple command following
  - Object manipulation
  - Intelligible verbalization
  - Gestural or verbal yes/no responses
- Patient may also show:
  - Visual fixation
  - Smooth pursuit tracking
  - Emotional or motor behaviors that are contingent upon the presence of specific eliciting stimuli [e.g., patient will cry or get agitated (and behavior is reproducible) only after hearing voices of family members but not with voices of hospital staff]
- Emergence from MCS is signaled by:
  - Consistent command following
  - Functional object use
  - Reliable use of a communication system
- Prognosis is better for MCS than for VS

Treatment
- There is no evidence to support that any kind of therapy-based program (e.g., coma stimulation/sensory-stimulation program) will induce or accelerate the cessation of coma or VS

- Nevertheless, an organized treatment approach to low-functioning patients permits a quantifiable assessment of responses to stimulation and early recognition of changes or improvements in response to therapeutic interventions or through spontaneous recovery

Management/Therapy Program for Patients with Disorders of Consciousness
- Neuromedical stabilization
- Preventive therapeutic interventions may be implemented:
  - Manage bowel and bladder (B/B) function
  - Maintain nutrition
  - Maintain skin integrity
  - Control spasticity
  - Prevent contractures
- Pharmacologic treatment/intervention
  A. Elimination of unnecessary medicines (e.g., histamine-2 blockers, metoclopramide, pain meds, etc.) and selection of agents with fewest adverse effects on cognitive and neurologic recovery
  B. Addition of agents to enhance specific cognitive and physical functions
     - In patients emerging out of coma or VS, the recovery process may be (theoretically) hastened through the use of pharmacotherapy
     - Agents frequently used include:
       - Methylphenidate
       - Dextroamphetamine
       - Dopamine agonists (levocarbidopa and carbidopa)
       - Amantadine
       - Bromocriptine
       - Antidepressants—tricyclic antidepressants (TCA's) & selective serotonin reuptake inhibitors (SSRIs)
     - The efficacy of pharmacologic therapy to enhance cognitive function has not been proven
- Sensory stimulation—widely used despite little evidence of efficacy as previously mentioned.
  - Sensory stimulation should include all five senses, addressed one at a time, in specific therapy sessions and/or in the environmental state and developed in the room
  - Avoid overstimulation (educate family)
  - Patient may have adverse responses due to overstimulation, as ↑ confusion or agitation, ↑ reflex responses or avoidance reactions, which may interfere with performance

■

POSTURING SECONDARY TO HEAD INJURY

📖 DECEREBRATE POSTURING

- This postural pattern was first described by Sherrington, who produced it in cats and monkeys by transecting the brain stem
- There is extension of the upper and lower extremities (hallmark: elbows extended) (Figure 2–4 A)

- Seen with midbrain lesions/compression; also with cerebellar and posteria fossa lesions
- In its fully developed form it consists of opisthotonus, clenched jaws, and stiff, extended limbs with internal rotation of arms and ankle plantar flexion (Feldman, 1971)

DECORTICATE POSTURING

- Posturing due to lesions at a higher level (than in decerebrate posture)—seen in cerebral hemisphere/white matter, internal capsule and thalamic lesions
- Flexion of the upper limbs (elbows bent) and extension of the lower limbs (Figure 2–4 B)

> **Hint:**
> Remember, deCORticate → "COR" = heart = ♥
> ⇒ Patient brings hands close to his heart by flexing the elbows

- Arms are in flexion and adduction and leg(s) extended

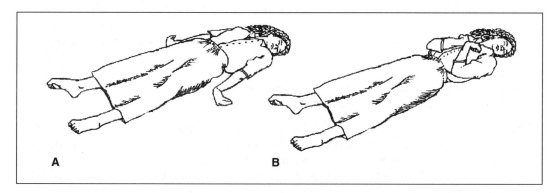

FIGURE 2–4. **A** Decerebrate Posture: There is extension of the upper and lower extremities.
B Decorticate Posture: There is flexion of the upper extremities and extension of the lower limbs.

▪

PREDICTORS OF OUTCOME AFTER TBI

📖 WIDELY USED INDICATORS OF SEVERITY IN ACUTE TBI

- The best Glasgow Coma Scale (GCS) score within 24 hours of injury
- Length of coma
- Duration of posttraumatic amnesia (PTA)
  - Note: The *initial* GCS and the *worst* GCS (within the first 24 hours) have also been proposed as acute indicators of severity in TBI

Glasgow Coma Scale

TABLE 2–1   📖 Glasgow Coma Scale: (Teasdate and Jennett, 1974)

Score	Best Motor Response 6	Best Verbal Response 5	Eye Opening 4
1	None	None	None
2	Decerebrate posturing (extension) to pain	Mutters unintelligible sounds	Opens eyes to pain
3	Decorticate posturing (flexion) to pain	Says inappropriate words	Opens eyes to loud voice (verbal commands)
4	Withdraws limb from painful stimulus	Able to converse— confused	Opens eyes spontaneously
5	Localizes pain/pushes away noxious stimulus (examiner)	Able to converse—alert and oriented	
6	Obeys verbal commands		

- Total GCS score is obtained from adding the scores of all three categories.
- Highest score = 15
- Lowest score = 3
- With GCS score < 8: patient is said to be comatose
- The lower the score, the deeper the coma

📖 The GCS is a simple scoring for assessing the depth of coma
- Highest GCS score within the first few hours after the injury preferred as this reduces the likelihood of using excessively low, very early scores (often before cardiopulmonary resuscitation (CPR)) and of confounding factors such as decreased arousal due to use of sedatives or paralytic agents
- Severity of injury:
  GCS score of 3 to 8 = severe injury
           9 to 12 = moderate injury
           13 to 15 = mild injury

- 📖 Of the three items in GCS, *best motor response* is the best acute predictor of outcome
- Jennet (1979): Relationship between best GCS score (within the first 24 hours) and outcome:
  - GCS scores of 3–4 resulted in death or VS in 87% of patients
  - Scores 5–7 = death or VS in 53% and moderate or good recovery in 34%
  - Scores 8–10 = moderate or good recovery in 68%
  - Score of 11 = moderate or good recovery in 87%
- Glasgow-Liege scale: Born (1985) proposed the addition of the brain stem reflex scale to the Glasgow Coma Scale—Glasgow-Liege Scale
    The Glasgow-Liege Scale has been tested for reliability and prognostic power and has been shown to amplify the information provided by the standard GCS in comatose patients
    Brain stem reflexes included in this scale:
  - Fronto-orbicular reflex (orbicularis oculi): Orbicularis oculi contraction on percussion of the glabella
  - Vertical oculocephalic and horizontal oculocephalic or oculovestibular reflex: "Doll's eye" maneuver (horizontal—moving head forward from side to side; vertical—moving head up and down)
  - The pupillary light reflex
  - The oculocardiac reflex: Bradycardia induced by increasing pressure on the eyeball

Duration of Posttraumatic Amnesia (PTA)

- PTA is one of the most commonly used predictors of outcome
- PTA is the interval of permanently lost memory that occurs following the injury
- 📖 Resolution of PTA clinically corresponds to the period when incorporation of ongoing daily events occurs in the working memory
- Duration of PTA has a proportional relationship to coma duration. Katz and Alexander (1994)—PTA correlates with Glasgow Outcome Scale (GOS) score at 6 and 12 months—predictor of outcome
- PTA correlates strongly with length of coma (and with GOS—see below) in patients with DAI but poorly in patients with primarily focal brain injuries (contusions)
- 📖 Galveston Orientation and Amnesia Test (GOAT)—developed by Harvey Levin and colleagues, is a standard technique for assessing PTA. It is a brief, structured interview that quantifies the patient's orientation and recall of recent events
  - The GOAT includes assessment of orientation to person, place, and time, recall of the circumstances of the hospitalization, and the last preinjury and first postinjury memories
  - The GOAT score can range from 0 to 100, with a score of 75 or better defined as normal
  - The end of PTA can be defined as the date when the patient scores 75 or higher in the GOAT for two consecutive days. The period of PTA is defined as the number of days beginning at the end of the coma to the time the patient attains the first of two successive GOAT scores ≥ 75 (Ellenberg, 1996)
- Categories of PTA: Duration of PTA is often used to categorize severity of injury according to the following criteria:

TABLE 2–2. Posttraumatic Amnesia

Duration of PTA	Severity of Injury Category
Less than 5 minutes	Very mild
5–60 minutes	Mild
1–24 hours	Moderate
1–7 days	Severe
1–4 weeks	Very severe
Greater than 4 weeks	Extremely severe

TABLE 2–3. Classification of Posttraumatic Amnesia

Length of PTA	Likely Outcome
1 day or less	Expect quick and full recovery with appropriate management (a few may show persisting disability)
More than 1 day, less than 1 week	Recovery period more prolonged—now a matter of weeks or months. Full recovery possible, for most of these cases, with good management.
1–2 weeks	Recovery a matter of many months. Many patients are left with residual problems even after the recovery process has ended, but one can be reasonably optimistic about functional recovery with good management.
2–4 weeks	Process of recovery is very prolonged—1 year or longer is not unusual. Permanent deficits are likely. There must be increasing pessimism about functional recovery when PTA reaches these lengths.
More than 4 weeks	Permanent deficits, indeed significant disability, now certain. It is not just a matter of recovery but of long-term retraining and management.

From Brooks DN and McKinlay WW, Evidence and Quantification in Head Injury: Seminar notes. Unpublished material, 1989, with permission.

Duration of Coma

- Katz and Alexander (1994): defined as the date when the patient shows the first unequivocal sign of responsiveness. In this study, the sign of responsiveness used was evidence of the patient following commands

Other Indicators of Outcome after TBI Include:

- **Age**
  - Children and young adults tend to have a generally more positive prognosis than older adults. However, young children (< 5 yrs) and older adults (> 65 yrs) have greater mortality
  - Katz and Alexander (1994): Age ≥ 40 correlates with worse functional outcome when compared with patients < 40
- **Rate of early recovery** reflected in serial disability rating scales (DRS): found to be predictive of final outcome
- **Pupillary reaction** to light:
  - 50% of patients with reactive pupils after TBI achieve moderate disability to good recovery (in DRS scale) vs 4% with nonreactive pupils
- **Time**
  - Most recovery usually occurs within the first 6 months postinjury
- **Postcoma use of phenytoin:**
  - Long-term use of phenytoin has been reported to have adverse cognitive effects (neurobehavioral effects in severe TBI patients compared to placebo group)

HEAD INJURY PREDICTOR SCALES AND TESTING

📖 Prognosis in Severe Head Injury

TABLE 2–4

Predicative Indicator	Poorer	Better
Glasgow Coma Scale score	< 7	> 7
CT scan	Large blood clot; massive bihemispheric swelling	Normal
Age	Old age	Youth
Pupillary light reflex	Pupils remain dilated	Pupil contracts
Doll's eye sign	Impaired	Intact
Caloric testing with ice water	Eyes do not deviate	Eyes deviate to irrigated side
Motor response to noxious stimuli	Decerebrate rigidity	Localizes defensive gestures
Somatosensory evoked potentials	Deficient	Normal
Posttraumatic amnesia length	> 2 wks	< 2 wks

(Reprinted with permission from Braddom, RL. Physical Medicine and Rehabilitation. Philadelphia: W.B. Saunders Company; 1996: p. 1033, table 49-4.)

📖 Glasgow Outcome Scale (GOS)

TABLE 2–5

	Category	Description
1	Death	Self-evident criteria
2	Persistent vegetative state	Prolonged unconsciousness with no verbalization, no following of commands. Absent awareness of self and environment; patient may open eyes; absence of cortical function as judged behaviorally; characterized by the presence of sleep-wake cycles
3	Severe disability	Patient unable to be independent for any 24-hour period by reason of residual mental and/or physical disability
4	Moderate disability	Patient with residual deficits that do not prevent independent daily life; patient can travel by public transport and work in a sheltered environment
5	Good recovery	Return to normal life; there may be minor or no residual deficits

- Widely used scale; documented correlation between acute predictors of outcome and GOS score at 6 months and 12 months
- Cons:
  - In the GOS, categories are broad; scale not sensitive enough
  - Not real indicator of functional abilities

(Continued)

📖 Disability Rating Scale (DRS)

TABLE 2–6

1. Eye Opening	2. Communication	3. Motor Response
0 Spontaneous	0 Oriented	0 Obeying
1 To Speech	1 Confused	1 Localizing
2 To Pain	2 Inappropriate	2 Withdrawing
3 None	3 Incomprehensible	3 Flexing
	4 None	4 Extending
		5 None
4. Feeding	**5. Toileting**	**6. Grooming**
0.0 Complete	0.0 Complete	0.0 Complete
0.5	0.5	0.5
1.0 Partial	1.0 Partial	1.0 Partial
1.5	1.5	1.5
2.0 Minimal	2.0 Minimal	2.0 Minimal
2.5	2.5	2.5
3.0 None	3.0 None	3.0 None

7. Level of functioning (physical and cognitive disability)	8. "Employability" (as full-time worker, homemaker, or student)
0.0 Completely independent	0.0 Not restricted
0.5	0.5
1.0 Dependent in special environment	1.0 Selected jobs, competitive
1.5	1.5
2.0 Mildly dependent—limited assistance (nonresident helper)	2.0 Sheltered workshop, noncompetitive
2.5	2.5
3.0 Moderately dependent—moderate assistance (person in home)	3.0 Not employable
3.5	
4.0 Markedly dependent—assist all major activities, all times	
4.5	
5.0 Totally dependent—24-hr nursing care	

(Rappaport et al., 1982)

This is a 30-point scale covering the following eight dimensions:
1. Eye opening
2. Verbalization/communication
3. Motor responsiveness
4. Feeding*
5. Toileting*
6. Grooming*
7. Overall level of functioning/dependence
8. Employability

*Note: measuring cognitive skills only in these categories.

- The DRS was developed specifically for brain injury
- It provides a quantitative index of disability
- It is more sensitive to clinical changes than GOS

Rancho Los Amigos Levels of Cognitive Function Scale (LCFS)

TABLE 2–7

Level	Description
I	No response
II	Generalized response to stimulation
III	Localized response to stimuli
IV	Confused and agitated behavior
V	Confused with inappropriate behavior (nonagitated)
VI	Confused but appropriate behavior
VII	Automatic and appropriate behavior
VIII	Purposeful and appropriate behavior

(Reprinted with Permission from Rancho Los Amigos National Rehabilitation Center.)

- Eight-level global scale that focuses on cognitive recovery and behavior after TBI
- (Gouvier et al., 1987)—LCFS has lower validity and reliability than the Disability Rating Scale (DRS)

Functional Independence Measure (FIM)

- Ordinal scale with 18 items and 7 levels to assess physical and cognitive function
- Documented validity and reliability

TABLE 2–8 FIM

L E V E L S	7 Complete Independence (Timely, Safely) 6 Modified Independence (Device)	NO HELPER

	Modified Dependence
	  5 Supervision
	  4 Minimal Assist (Subject = 75% +)
	  3 Moderate Assist (Subject = 50% +)
	
	Complete Dependence
	  2 Maximal Assist (Subject = 25% +)
	  1 Total Assist (Subject = 0% +)
		HELPER

	ADMIT	DISCHG	FOL-UP
Self-Care A. Eating B. Grooming C. Bathing D. Dressing - Upper Body E. Dressing - Lower Body F. Toileting	☐	☐	☐
Sphincter Control G. Bladder Management H. Bowel Management	☐	☐	☐
Transfers I. Bed, Chair, Wheelchair J. Toilet K. Tub, Shower	☐	☐	☐
Locomotion L. Walk/Wheelchair Walk/Wheelchair/Both M. Stairs	☐	☐	☐
Motor Subtotal Score	☐	☐	☐
Communication N. Comprehension Auditory/Visual/Both O. Expression Vocal/Non-vocal/Both	☐	☐	☐
Social Cognition P. Social Interaction Q. Problem Solving R. Memory	☐	☐	☐
Cognitive Subtotal Score	☐	☐	☐
Total FIM	☐	☐	☐

NOTE: Leave no blanks; enter 1 if patient not testable due to risk

(FIM™ Guide for Uniform Data Set for Medical Rehabilitation, SUNY-Buffalo, 1996.)

Coma Recovery Scale (CRS)

- Theorizes hierarchical responses (from generalized to cognitively mediated) for 25 items in 6 areas: auditory, visual, motor, oromotor/verbal, communication, and arousal
- Giacino et al. (1991) found that changes in CRS scores showed stronger correlations with outcome (as measured by the Disability Rating Scale) than initial, one-time scores. The change as a percentage of total score was greater for the CRS than for the GCS or DRS (Horn and Zasler 1996)

📖 Neuropsychological Testing

Prior to the development of the CT Scan, neuropsychological assessment was targeted at determining whether a brain lesion was or was not present, and, if present, discerning its location and type

This diagnostic approach supported the development of the *Halstead-Reitan Neuropsychological Battery (HRNB)*. This battery was initially designed to assess frontal-lobe disorders by W.C. Halstead (1947) and subsequently used by Reitan (1970 1974), who added some tests and recommended its use as a diagnostic test for all kinds of brain damage. Most examiners administer this battery in conjunction with the WAIS-R (Wechsler Adult Intelligence Scale—Revised) and WMS (Wechsler Memory Scale) or the Minnesota Multiphasic Personality Inventory (MMPI)

- *Wechsler Adult Intelligence Scale—Revised (WAIS-R):* eleven subtests (6 determine verbal IQ and 5 determine performance IQ), WAIS-R is the most frequently used measure of general intellectual ability.
- *Minnesota Multiphasic Personality Inventory (MMPI)* consists of 550 true/false questions that yield information about aspects of personality. It is the most widely and thoroughly researched objective measure of personality.

▪

MEDICAL COMPLICATIONS AFTER TBI

Posttraumatic Hydrocephalus (PTH)

- Ventriculomegaly (ventricular dilation) is common after TBI , reported in 40%–72% of patients after severe TBI. However, true hydrocephalus is relatively rare; incidence is 3.9 to 8%
- Ventriculomegaly is usually due to cerebral atrophy and focal infarction of brain tissue (*ex vacuo* changes)
- Hydrocephalus in TBI is most often of the communicating or normal-pressure type
- Unfortunately, the classic triad of incontinence, ataxia/gait disturbance and dementia is of little help in severe TBI cases
- Radiographic evaluation (CT Scan) and further work-up (to rule out hydrocephalus) should be considered if there is failure to improve or deterioration of cognitive or behavioral function
- CT-Scan—periventricular lucency, lack of sulci, and uniformity in ventricular dilation favors PTH
- Initial manifestations of hydrocephalus can be intermittent HA, vomiting, confusion, and drowsiness
- Tx: Lumbar puncture, shunt placement

Elevated Intracranial Pressure (ICP)

- In a normal adult, reclining with the head and the trunk elevated to 45°, the ICP is between 2 to 5 mmHg
- ICP levels up to 15 mmHg are considered harmless
- Raised ICP: defined as ICP > 20 mmHg for more than 5 minutes
- Common after severe TBI (53% reported in a recent series)
- When ICP > 40 mmHg, there is neurologic dysfunction and impairment of the brain's electrical activity
- An ICP > 60 mmHg is invariably fatal; pressures in 20–40 mmHg area associated with increased morbidity
- 75% of the patients post severe TBI die due to deformation of tissue, shift, the development of internal hernias and secondary damage to the CNS
- If unchecked an increased ICP may cause death mainly because of deformation of tissue, brain shifts, herniation, and cerebral ischemia
- A unilateral mass lesion causes distortion of the brain, a reduction of the CSF volume, and, in the closed skull, the formation of internal hernias (including tentorial/uncal herniation—see below)
- Increased ICP reduces cerebral blood perfusion
- It is more important to maintain an adequate cerebral perfusion pressure (CPP) than controlling only the ICP
- Cerebral perfusion is calculated by subtracting ICP from mean arterial pressure (MAP). It should remain > 60 mmHg to ensure cerebral blood flow
- CPP = MAP—ICP
- Fever, hyperglycemia, hyponatremia, and seizures can worsen cerebral edema by ↑ ICP

Indications for Continuous Monitoring of Intracranial Pressure and for Artificial Ventilation

1. Patient in coma (GCS < 8) and with CT findings of ↑ ICP (absence of third ventricle and CSF cisterns)
2. Deep coma (GCS < 6) without hematoma
3. Severe chest and facial injuries and moderate/severe head injury (GCS < 12)
4. After evacuation of IC hemorrhage if patient is in coma (GCS < 8) beforehand

---

Factors that May Increase ICP
- Turning head, especially to left side if patient is completely horizontal or head down
- Loud noise
- Vigorous physical therapy
- Chest PT
- Suctioning
- Elevated blood pressure

Methods Used to Monitor ICP
- Papilledema: papilledema is rare in the acute stage after brain injury, despite the fact that ↑ ICP is frequent
  - Usually occurs bilaterally
  - May indicate presence of intracranial mass lesion
  - Develops within 12 to 24 hours in cases of brain trauma and hemorrhage, but, if pronounced, it usually signifies brain tumor or abscess, i.e., a lesion of longer duration
- CT Scan (see earlier)—if CT-Scan equivocal, cysternography may be done

- Lumbar puncture (LP) if no papilledema (must rule out mass lesion first)
  - LP carries a certain risk of causing fatal shift of brain tissue (i.e., herniation)

Management of ICP
- Elevate head of bed 30°
- Intubation and hyperventilation: reduction of $PaCO_2$ through hyperventilation is the most rapid mean of lowering ICP. However, it may negatively impact outcome
  - Hyperventilation should be used with caution as it reduces brain tissue PO_2 this may cause brain tissue hypoxia $\Rightarrow$ this may lead to ischemia $\Rightarrow$ ischemia may cause further damage in the CNS tissue of the head injury (HI) patient
  - Optimal $PaCO_2 \sim 30$ mmHg
- Osmotic agents (e.g., mannitol)—improves ischemic brain swelling (by diuresis and intravascular fluid shifts)
- Furosemide/acetazolamide may also be used
- Avoid HTN: can increase brain blood volume and increase ICP
- High doses of barbiturates (e.g., thiopental) rapidly lower ICP and suppress electrical brain activity
- Neurosurgical decompression
- Hypothermia may be used to $\downarrow$ ICP and it may protect brain tissue by lowering cerebral metabolism. Marion (1997)—treatment with hypothermia for 24 hours in severe TBI patients (GCS 5–7) associated with improved outcome
- Steroids—not proven to be beneficial management of ICP

Temporal Lobe—Tentorial (UNCAL) Herniation

- Uncal herniation results when the medial part of one temporal lobe (uncus and parahippocampal gyrus) is displaced over the edge of the ipsilateral tentorium so as to compress the third cranial nerve, midbrain, cerebral cortex, and subthalamus
- Occurs as a result of increased supratentorial pressure. It is commonly associated with hematoma (subdural or epidural) secondary to trauma or to a brain tumor
- Uncal herniation of the medial temporal lobe produces:
  1. Stretching of the third cranial nerve (oculomotor nerve) causes ipsilateral pupillary dilation; this may lead to complete ipsilateral third nerve palsy (with fixed pupil dilation, ptosis, and later, ophthalmoplegia)
  2. Ipsilateral hemiparesis results due to pressure on the corticospinal tract located in the contralateral crus cerebri
  3. Contralateral hemiparesis may result due to pressure (from edema or mass effect) on the precentral motor cortex or the internal capsule
- In uncal herniation, reduced consciousness and bilateral motor signs appear relatively late. Central hyperventilation may also occur late in uncal herniation

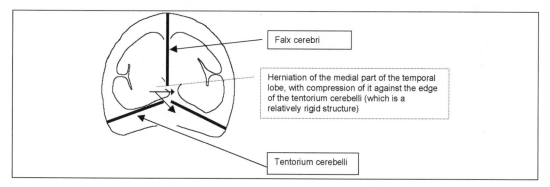

FIGURE 2–5. Temporal Lobe—Tentorial (Uncal) Herniation

Heterotopic Ossification (HO)

- HO is the formation of mature lamellar bone in soft tissue
- Common in TBI, with an incidence of 11%–76% (incidence of clinically significant cases is 10%–20%)

📖 **Risk factors:**
- Prolonged coma (> 2 weeks)
  - Immobility
  - Limb spasticity/↑ tone (in the involved extremity)
  - Associated long-bone fracture
  - Pressure ulcers
  - Edema
- Period of greater risk to develop HO: 3 to 4 months post injury

Signs/Symptoms
- Most common: pain and ↓ range of motion (ROM)
- Also: local swelling, erythema, warmth joint, muscle guarding, low-grade fever
- In addition to pain and ↓ ROM, complications of HO include bony ankylosis, peripheral nerve compression, vascular compression, and lymphedema
- Joints most commonly involved:
  1. Hips (most common)
  2. Elbows/shoulders
  3. Knees

Differential Dx: DVT, tumor, septic joint, hematoma, cellulitis, and fracture

Diagnostic Tests/Labs

Serum Alkaline Phosphatase (SAP)
- SAP elevation may be the earliest and least expensive method of detection of HO
- It has poor specificity (may be elevated for multiple reasons, such as fractures, hepatic dysfunction, etc.)

Bone Scan
- Is a sensitive method for early detection of HO
- HO can be seen within the first 2–4 weeks after injury in Phase I (blood-flow phase) and Phase II (blood-pool phase) of a triple phase bone scan, and in Phase III (static phase/delayed images) in 4–8 weeks with normalization by 7 to 12 months

Plain X-rays
- Require 3 weeks to 2 months post injury to reveal HO. Useful to confirm maturity of HO

Prophylaxis
- ROM exercises
- Control of muscle tone
- Non Steroidal Anti-inflammatory Drugs (NSAIDs)
- Radiation—used perioperatively to inhibit HO in total hip replacement patients; concerns about ↑ risk of neoplasia limit its use in younger patient populations (e.g., TBI patients). Also, as radiation is used prophylactically to prevent HO formation of a particular joint, to use it in TBI patients would require essentially irradiation of the whole body (as HO can develop practically at any joint), which is not practical

Treatment

- Diphosphonates and NSAIDs (particularly indomethacin) have been used on patients to arrest early HO and to prevent postop recurrence, but their efficacy has not been clearly proven (TBI population)
- ROM exercises—used prophylactically to prevent HO and also used as a treatment for developing HO (to prevent ankylosis)
- Surgery—surgical removal of HO indicated only if ↑ in function is a goal (to ↑ hygiene, sitting, etc.)
- Surgical resection usually postponed 12 to 18 months to allow maturation of HO

Hypertension (HTN)

- Frequently observed post-TBI
- Estimated incidence 11%–25% post head injury
- Posttraumatic hypertension usually resolves spontaneously—long-term use of antihypertensive agents is rarely necessary
- Post TBI hypertension related to sympathetic hyperactivity usually seen in severe TBI—demonstrated by ↑ plasma and urine catecholamines levels
- Cases of HTN have been reported secondary to hydrocephalus several years after TBI
- If medication needed, propanolol recommended because:
  - ↓ plasma catecholamines levels
  - ↓ cardiac index
  - ↓ myocardial oxygen demand
  - ↓ heart rate
  - Improves pulmonary ventilation-perfusion inequality

Venous Thromboembolic Disease

- Venous thromboembolic disease (VTE), including deep vein thrombosis (DVT) and pulmonary embolus (PE), are among the most significant complications of TBI as they are related to ↑ mortality in the rehabilitation setting
- The incidence of DVT in TBI rehabilitation admissions is approximately 10%–18% (Cifu, 1996)
- VTE/DVT often clinically silent in the TBI population, with sudden death from PE being the first clinical sign in 70%–80%
- DVT occurs most commonly in the lower limbs and is traditionally associated with immobility, paresis, fracture, soft-tissue injuries, and ages > 40
- Remember Virchow's triad: venous stasis, vessel-wall damage, and hypercoagulable state

Prophylactic Regimens for DVT

- Low-dose unfractionated heparin (5000 U q 8 to 12 hours) and low-molecular-weight heparin—adequate anticoagulation generally achieved with these treatments
- Intermittent pneumatic compression—provide effective DVT prophylaxis in patients at risk of bleeding complications
- Warfarin (Coumadin®)
- Inferior vena cava (IVC) filter

Diagnostic tests

Doppler ultrasonography, impedance plethysmography (IPG), ^{125}I-fibrinogen scanning and contrast venography

TABLE 2–9

Diagnostic Test	Pros	Cons
Doppler ultrasonography	• 95% sensitivity and 99% specificity for symptomatic proximal thrombi	• Limited ability to detect calf thrombi
Impedance plethysmography	• 90%–93% sensitivity and 94% specificity for proximal thrombi	• Limited ability to detect calf thrombi
^{125}I-fibrinogen scanning	• 60%–80% sensitive in proximal thrombi	• Invasive • Involves injection of radioactive agent
Contrast venography	• Remains the gold standard for diagnosis of clinically suspected DVT	• Invasive • Contrast-induced thrombosis • Contrast allergy

Treatment of DVT

• Anticoagulation is first initiated with IV heparin or adjusted-dose subcutaneous heparin followed by oral anticoagulation; anticoagulation continued for 3–6 months. IVC filter used when anticoagulation is contraindicated

Posttraumatic Epilepsy/Posttraumatic Seizures (PTS)

Posttraumatic epilepsy is classified as:
1. Generalized (grand mal and tonic-clonic)
2. Partial (*simple*, if consciousness is maintained, or *complex*, if not)

The majority of PTS are of the partial type

Posttraumatic seizures are further classified as:
• Immediate PTS—occur within the first 24 hours post injury
• Early PTS—occur within the first week (24 hours to 7 days)
• Late PTS—occur after the first week
  – Immediate PTS has better prognosis than early epilepsy; early PTS associated with increased risk of late PTS

Incidence

Varies greatly according to the severity of the injury, the time since the injury, and the presence of risk factors (see below)
• 5% of hospitalized TBI patients (overall, closed-head injury) have late *PTS*
• 4%–5% of hospitalized TBI patients have one or more seizures in the first week after the injury (early PTS) (Rosenthal et al., 1990)

Study to evaluate association between different characteristics (severity) of TBI and development of seizures post injury. A group of 4541 patients with TBI {characterized by loss of consciousness (LOC), posttraumatic amnesia (PTA), SDH or skull fracture}, were divided into three categories:

Mild TBI—LOC or amnesia < 30 minutes
Moderate TBI—LOC for 30 minutes to 24 hours or skull fractures
Severe TBI—LOC or amnesia > 24 hours, SDH or brain contusion

Incidence of seizures in the different categories:

Mild TBI—1.5%
Moderate TBI -2.9%
Severe TBI -17%
Overall incidence (all patients)—3.1%

(Annegers et al., 1998)

📖 Risk Factors Associated with Late Posttraumatic Seizures:

- Penetrating head injury—33%–50%
- Intracranial hematoma—25%–30%
- Early seizure (> 24 hours to 7 days)—25%
- Depressed skull fracture—3%–70%
- Prolonged coma or posttraumatic amnesia (> 24 hours)—35%

Other Risk Factors
- Dural tearing
- Presence of foreign bodies
- Focal signs such as aphasia and hemiplegia
- Age
- Alcohol abuse
- Use of tricyclic anti-depressants (TCAs)

Risk Factors Associated with Late Posttraumatic Seizures

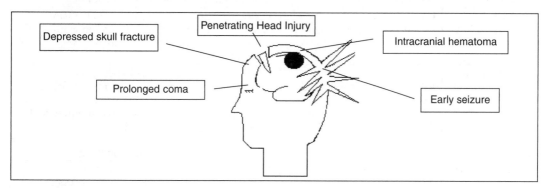

FIGURE 2–6.

- 50%–66% of PTS occur within one year; 75%–80% occur within two years; most PTS occur 1–3 months after injury
- 50% of patients with PTS will have only one seizure, and 25% have no more than three episodes

Diagnosis
- Clinical
- EEG
  - Standard
  - Sleep-deprived
  - 24 hour
- Prolactin level: ↑ prolactin level confirms true seizure activity (but normal prolactin levels will not exclude seizure activity)

Prophylactic Anticonvulsants
- Greater risk of development of PTS: within the first 2 years post injury
- Prophylactic use of anticonvulsants has not been proven effective in prospective, randomized, controlled studies
- Phenytoin—proven to be effective only during the first week post injury (with no benefit thereafter) at preventing early PTS. There is no proof of change in outcome with prophylactic use of phenytoin (Temkin et al., 1990)

Treatment

It has been suggested that carbamazepine and valproic acid are the drugs of choice (DOC) for the treatment of partial and generalized PTS, respectively.

TABLE 2–10 Anticonvulsant Medications: Uses and Adverse Reactions

Medication	Uses	Adverse Reactions
Carbamazepine	• Partial seizures • Tonic-clonic; generalized seizures • Stabilization of agitation and psychotic behavior • Bipolar affective disorder • Neuralgia	• Acute: stupor or coma, hyperirritability, convulsions, respiratory depression • Chronic: drowsiness, vertigo, ataxia, diplopia, blurred vision, nausea, vomiting, aplastic anemia, agranulocytosis, hypersensitivity reactions (dermatitis, eosinophilia, splenomegaly, lymphadenopathy), transient mild leukopenia, transient thrombocytopenia, water retention with decreased serum osmolality and sodium, transient elevation of hepatic enzymes
Gabapentin	• Partial seizures	• Somnolence, dizziness, ataxia, fatigue
Lamotrigine	• Partial seizures • Tonic-clonic; generalized seizures	• Dizziness, ataxia, blurred or double vision, nausea, vomiting, rash, Stevens-Johnson syndrome, disseminated intravascular coagulation
Phenobarbital	• Partial seizures • Tonic-clonic; generalized seizures	• Sedation, irritability, and hyperactivity in children, agitation, confusion, rash, exfoliative dermatitis, hypothrombinemia with hemorrhage in newborns whose mothers took phenobarbital, megaloblastic anemia, osteomalacia • Nystagmus and ataxia at toxic doses
Phenytoin	• Partial seizures • Tonic-clonic; generalized seizures • Neuralgia	• Intravenous administration: cardiac arrhythmias, hypotension, CNS depression • Oral administration: disorders of the cerebellar and vestibular systems (such as nystagmus, ataxia, and vertigo), cerebellar atrophy, blurred vision, mydriasis, diplopia, ophthalmoplegia, behavioral changes (such as hyperactivity, confusion, dullness, drowsiness, and hallucination), increased seizure frequency, gastrointestinal symptoms, gingival hyperplasia, osteomalacia, megaloblastic anemia, hirsutism, transient liver enzyme elevation, decreased antidiuretic hormone secretion leading to hypernatremia, hyperglycemia, glycosuria, hypocalcemia, Stevens-Johnson syndrome, systemic lupus erythematosus, neutropenia, leukopenia, red cell aplasia, agranulocytosis, thrombocytopenia, lymphadenopathy, hypothrombinemia in newborns whose mothers received phenytoin, reactions indicative of drug allergy (skin, bone marrow, liver function)
Valproic Acid	• Partial seizures • Tonic-clonic; generalized seizures • Myoclonic seizures • Absence seizures • Stabilization of agitation and psychotic behavior	• Transient gastrointestinal symptoms such as anorexia, nausea, and vomiting; increased appetite; sedation; ataxia; tremor; rash; alopecia; hepatic enzyme elevation, fulminant hepatitis (rare, but fatal); acute pancreatitis; hyperammoniemia

From Rosenthal M, Griffith ER, Kreutzer JS, Pentland B. Rehabilitation of the Adult and Child with Traumatic Brain Injury 3rd ed. Philadelphia: F.A. Davis; 1999, p. 67, table 4–2, with permission

- Anticonvulsant medications are usually started once *late* seizures occur
- ▢ In the TBI population, carbamazepine (for partial seizures) and valproic acid (for generalized seizures) are often preferred to medications that are more sedating or associated with cognitive impairment (such as phenobarbital and phenytoin). Their superiority over phenytoin has been debated (differences among these three agents are probably minimal); carbamazepine may be as sedating as phenytoin. (Brain Injury Special Interest Group of the American Academy of Physical Medicine and Rehabilitation, 1998)
- Important to remember that all anticonvulsants may cause some degree of sedation and cognitive deficits (usually psychomotor slowing)
- Phenobarbital is clearly associated with greater cognitive impairment; this medication should not be used as first choice of anticonvulsant therapy in the TBI patient
- Long-term use of phenytoin has been associated with adverse cognitive effects. Animal and clinical (extrapolated from strokes) studies suggest that phenytoin may impede recovery from brain injury (Dikmen, 1991)
- Second generation anticonvulsants, such as gabapentin and lamotrigine, may also be used for treatment of PTS as adjuvant agents (not approved yet for monotherapy). These agents appear to have fewer cognitive side effects, but are still under investigation in the TBI population.

▢ *Drug Interactions*

TABLE 2–11. **Anticonvulsant Medications: Common Drug Interactions**

Medication	Drug Interaction
Carbamazepine	• Increased metabolism of carbamazepine (decreased levels) with phenobarbital, phenytoin, and valproic acid • Enhances metabolism of phenobarbital • Enhances metabolism of primidone into phenobarbital • Reduces concentration and effectiveness of haloperidol • Carbamazepine metabolism inhibited by propoxyphene and erythromycin
Lamotrigine	• When used concurrently with carbamazepine, may increase levels of 10,11–epoxide (an active metabolic of carbamazepine) • Half-life of lamotrigine is reduced to 15 hours when used concurrently with carbamazepine, phenobarbital, or primidone • Reduces valproic acid concentration
Phenobarbital	• Increased levels (as much as 40%) of phenobarbital when valproic acid administered concurrently • Phenobarbital levels may be increased when concurrently administering phenytoin • Phenobarbital has a variable reaction with phenytoin levels
Phenytoin	• Phenytoin levels may increase with concurrent use of chloramphenicol, cimetidine, dicumarol, disulfiram, isoniazid, and sulfonamides • Free phenytoin levels may increase with concurrent use of valproic acid and phenylbutazone • Decreased total levels of phenytoin may occur with sulfisoxazole, salicylates, and tolbutamide • Decreased phenytoin levels with concurrent use of carbamazepine • Decreased carbamazepine levels with concurrent use of phenytoin • Increased or decreased levels of phenytoin when concurrently administered with phenobarbital • When concurrently used with theophylline, phenytoin levels may be lowered and theophylline metabolized more rapidly • May decrease effectiveness of oral contraceptives • Enhances metabolism of corticosteroids
Valproic Acid	• Increases level of phenobarbital • Inhibits metabolism of phenytoin • Rare development of absence status epilepticus associated with concurrent use of clonazepam

(Reprinted with permission from Rosenthal et al., 1999, p. 68, table 4–3)

Withdrawal of Anticonvulsants (For Patients with Posttraumatic Seizures):
- 📖 No clear indications. It has been suggested to withdraw anticonvulsant medications after a seizure-free interval of 3 months to 6 months up to 1–2 years. (One to two year seizure-free interval is used more often as time frame for withdrawal of anticonvulsant therapy.)
- Spontaneous resolution of PTS can occur

Posttraumatic Agitation

- Posttraumatic agitation is usually a self-limiting problem lasting 1–4 weeks
- Reported to occur in 33%–50% of patients with TBI in the acute care setting
- Posttraumatic agitation has been described as
  - A subtype of delirium unique to TBI survivors, in which the survivor is in a state of posttraumatic amnesia, and there are excesses of behavior, including a combination of aggression, disinhibition and/or emotional lability
    - Delirium is related to, but not sufficient for, a diagnosis of agitation.
- Often no pharmacologic intervention is required

First-line Intervention
- Patient should be maintained in a safe, structured, low-stimulus environment, which is frequently adequate to manage short-term behavior problems. Agitation may be controlled with alterations in environment and staff or family behavior
- Floor beds can eliminate need for restraints
- Use physical restraints only if patient is a danger to self or others; should be applied only to minimal degree and not as a substitute for floor bed or one-to-one or other environmental interventions

TABLE 2–12.   Environmental Management of Agitation

1. Reduce the level of stimulation in the environment Place patient in quiet private room Remove noxious stimuli if possible, tubes, catheters, restraints, traction Limit unnecessary sounds, TV, radio, background conversations Limit number of visitors Staff to behave in a calm and reassuring manner Limit number and length of therapy sessions Provide therapies in patient room
2. Protect patient from harming self or others Place patient in a floor bed with padded side panels (Craig bed) Assign 1:1 or 1:2 sitter to observe patient and ensure safety Avoid taking patient off unit Place patient in locked ward
3. Reduce patient's cognitive confusion One person speaking to patient at a time Maintain staff to work with patient Minimize contact with unfamiliar staff Communicate to patient briefly and simple, one idea at a time
4. Tolerate restlessness when possible Allow patient to thrash about in floor bed Allow patient to pace around unit with 1:1 supervision Allow confused patient to be verbally inappropriate

(Reprinted with permission from Braddom RL. Physical Medicine and Rehabilitation, Philadelphia: W.B. saunders Company; 1996: Table 49-8.)

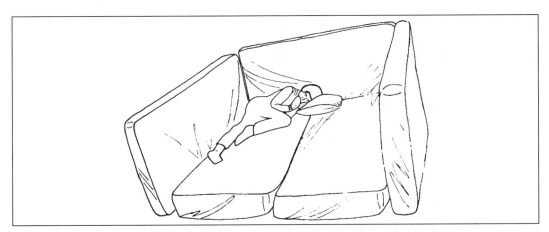

FIGURE 2–7   Agitated non-ambulatory patients often benefit from the use of a floor (Craig) bed. Mattresses can be laid on the floor and 3–4 ft. padded walls on four sides allow the patient to roll around. The use of a floor bed with one-to-one supervision and with the use of mitts and a helmet (if necessary) often eliminates the need for restraints. (Reprinted with permission from Braddom, R.L. Physical Medicine and Rehabilitation. Philadelphia: W.B. Saunders; 1996: p. 1038, figure 49-7.)

Medications for Treatment of Posttraumatic Agitation

- Pharmacologic treatment for agitation is controversial but it includes carbamazepine (Tegretol®) (most commonly used agent for posttraumatic agitation), TCAs, trazodone (Desyrel®), beta-blockers, SSRIs, valproic acid (Depakote®), lithium, amantadine (Symmetrel®), buspirone (BuSpar®)
- Avoid haloperidol (Haldol®), which is shown to decrease recovery in the injured brain tissue in animals (Feeny et al., 1982)

Urinary Dysfunction

- Neurogenic bladder with uninhibited detrusor reflex (contraction)
- TBI patients are frequently incontinent, usually presenting a disinhibited type of neurogenic bladder, in which the bladder volume is reduced but empties completely with normal postvoiding intravesicular volumes ⇒ Small voids with normal residuals
- 📖 For this type of dysfunction, a time-void program is usually helpful, in which the patient is offered the urinal or commode at a regular scheduled interval
- Anticholinergic meds (to ↑ bladder capacity) may also be used
- (Note—For a more detailed description of bladder function, types of neurogenic bladder and treatments, see SCI section) (Rosenthal, 1999)

Cranial Neuropathies

Most frequently affected cranial nerves in blunt head trauma:
- Olfactory nerve (CN I)
- Facial nerve (CN VII)
- Audiovestibular/vestibulocochlear nerve (CN VIII)
- CN affected with intermediate frequency
  - optic nerve (CNII)
  - ocular motor nerves (CN IV > CN III > CN VI)
- Trigeminal nerve (CN V) and the lower cranial nerves are rarely involved

CN I (Olfactory)

- 📖 Cranial nerve most often damaged by blunt head trauma
- Overall incidence ~ 7%, rising to 30% with severe head injuries or anterior fossa fractures

- Anosmia (loss of the ability to smell) is more common with occipital than with frontal blows and can result from trauma to any part of the head
- Anosmia and an apparent loss of taste result from CN I disruption thought to be secondary to a displacement of the brain with tearing of the olfactory nerve filaments in or near the cribriform plate through which they course
- Often associated with ↓ appetite/altered feeding behavior
- Associated with CSF rhinorrhea
- Recovery occurs in > one-third of cases, usually during the first 3 months

CN VII (Facial)
- Especially vulnerable to penetrating or blunt trauma to head because of its long, tortuous course through the temporal bone

CN VIII (Vestibulocochlear)
- Damage to the vestibulocochlear nerve results in loss of hearing or in postural vertigo and nystagmus coming on immediately after the trauma

CN II (Optic Nerve)
- Partial damage may result in scotomas and a troublesome blurring of vision or as homonymous hemianopsia. If nerve is completely involved or transected, patient will develop complete blindness (pupil dilated, unreactive to direct light but reactive to light stimulus to the opposite eye (consensual light reflex)

Endocrine Complications

Syndrome of Inappropriate Antidiuretic Hormone Secretion (SIADH)
- Water retention resulting from excessive antidiuretic hormone (ADH) secretion from the neurohypophysis secondary to multiple causes including head trauma
- In SIADH, ADH excess considered to be inappropriate because it occurs in the presence of plasma hypo-osmolality
- In SIADH, Na^+ excretion in the urine is maintained by hypervolemia, suppression of the renin-angiotensin-aldosterone system, and ↑ in the plasma concentration atrial natriuretic peptide (usually > 20 mmol/L)

Common Causes of SIADH

- CNS Diseases
  - Thrombotic or hemorrhagic events
  - Infection
    - Meningitis
    - Encephalitis
    - Brain abscess
- Head Trauma
- Lung Disease
  - Pneumonia
  - Lung abscess
  - Positive pressure ventilation
- Malignancy
  - CA of the lung (especially small cell CA)
  - GI malignancy (e.g., pancreatic cancer)
  - Prostate CA
  - Thymoma
  - Lymphoma
- Drugs
  - 📖 Carbamazepine
  - Vincristine
  - Clofibrate
  - Chlorpropamide
  - Phenotiazines
  - Amtriptyline
  - Morphine
  - Nicotine

Signs and Symptoms in SIADH:
- In mild SIADH (with Na^+ 130–135), or in gradually developing SIADH, symptoms may be absent or limited to anorexia and nausea/vomiting

- In severe SIADH (with significant hyponatremia) or in acute onset SIADH, there might be an increase in body weight and symptoms of cerebral edema—restlessness, irritability, confusion, coma, convulsions
- Edema (peripheral/soft tissue) almost always absent

Treatment
- Fluid restriction to ~ 1.0 L/day (800 ml to 1.2 L/day) (either alone or with a loop diuretic)
- Careful daily monitoring of weight changes and serum Na^+ until sodium level > 135 mmol/L
- Hypertonic saline (e.g., 5% NaCl solution), 200–300 ml, should be infused IV over 3–4 hours in patients with severe symptoms as confusion, convulsions, or coma
- It is important not to raise Na^+ concentration too rapidly to avoid development of serious neurological damage, pontine myelinolysis, or congestive heart failure (CHF); sodium may be corrected not more than 10 mEq/L over 24 hours until sodium reaches 125 mEq/L
- Chronic SIADH may be treated with demeclocycline, which normalizes serum Na^+ by inhibiting ADH action in the kidney; lithium carbonate acts similarly but is rarely used because it is more toxic

Cerebral Salt-Wasting (CSW) Syndrome
- CSW is another common cause of hyponatremia in TBI; may probably be a more common cause of hyponatremia in TBI patients than SIADH
- Hyponatremia in TBI is generally present in a hypotonic setting with either normal extracellular volume (isovolemia = SIADH) or reduced extracellular volume (hypovolemia = CSW).
- CSW is thought to occur because of direct neural effect on renal tubular function
- In CSW, hyponatremia is not dilutional (as in SIADH)—CSW patients are, in fact, volume depleted

- *Hallmark of CSW*
  - Decreased blood volume (↓ extracellular volume = hypovolemia) secondary to sodium loss (in urine) ⇒ this triggers ↑ in ADH secretion that is appropriate rather than inappropriate (differentiating this condition from SIADH)
  - Signs of dehydration

- *Treatment*
- Hydration/fluid replacement and electrolyte (Na+) correction
- It is important to differentiate CSW from SIADH and to recognize that there is water depletion in this condition, because treating it with fluid restriction (adequate Tx for SIADH) may further ↓ the extracellular fluid with disastrous results to the patient

Diabetes Insipidus (DI)
- Hallmark: Deficiency of ADH (vasopressin)
- May occur in severe head injuries; often associated with fractures of the skull
- 📖 A fracture in or near the sella turcica may tear the stalk of the pituitary gland, with resulting DI (due to disruption of ADH secretion from the posterior lobe of the pituitary) in addition to other clinical syndromes depending on the extent of the lesion
- Spontaneous remissions of traumatic DI may occur even after 6 month, presumably because of regeneration of disrupted axons within the pituitary stalk

Clinical Manifestations
- Polyuria, excessive thirst and polydipsia
- Urinary concentration (osm < 290 mmol/kg, SG 1.010) is below that of the serum in severe cases but may be higher than that of serum (290–600 mmol/kg) in mild DI

- Normal function of the thirst center ensures that polydipsia closely matches polyuria, so dehydration is seldom detectable except by a mild elevation of serum Na^+
- However, when replenishment of excreted water is inadequate, dehydration may become severe, causing weakness, fever, psychic disturbances, prostration, and death
- These features are associated with a rising serum osmolality and serum Na^+ concentration, the latter is sometimes > 175 mmol/L

Treatment
- Hormone replacement
  - DDAVP® (desmopressin acetate)—analog of antidiuretic hormone (ADH) with prolonged antidiuretic effect and no significant pressor activity
  - May be given intranasally or intramuscular (IM)
- Chlorpropamide potentiates the effects of ADH on the renal tubules—used in partial ADH deficiency

TABLE 2–13.   Comparison of SIADH, CSW and DI

	SIADH	DI	CSW syndrome
Serum ADH (rarely done as routine lab work)	↑ (inappropriately elevated)	↓	↑ (appropriately elevated)
Diagnostic Labs			
Serum Na^+	↓	↑	↓
Serum osmolality	↓	↑	↓
Extracellular volume	Normal (isovolemic)	Normal (isovolemic)	Reduced (hypovolemic)
Urine osmolality and SG	↑ (concentrated urine with osmolality usually > 300 mmol/kg)	↓	Normal

Spasticity

- Disorders of motor tone (e.g., spasticity, rigidity) are common after TBI
- Please refer to the Spasticity section for a full discussion on definition, clinical assessment/grading and treatment options for spasticity

■

MILD TRAUMATIC BRAIN INJURY AND POSTCONCUSSIVE SYNDROME

- Mild TBI constitutes 80% to 90% of TBI cases in the United States
- ~ 2.3 million cases in the United States
- Multiple terms, definitions, and diagnostic criteria available for mild or minor traumatic brain injury
- The American Congress of Rehabilitation (1995) has defined mild TBI as a traumatically induced physiologic disruption of brain function with at least one of four manifestations:
  - Any loss of consciousness (LOC)
  - Any loss of memory for events immediately before or after the injury
  - Any alteration in mental status at the time of the accident
  - Focal neurological deficits that may or may not be transient
- Usually, mild TBI has negative radiological findings (CT/MRI)

- The injury cannot exceed the following severity criteria:
  - LOC greater than 30 minutes
  - Posttraumatic amnesia (PTA) > 24 hours
  - Initial GCS ≤ 12 (13 to 15)
- Signs and symptoms after mild TBI include:
  - Headache (most common)
  - Dizziness
  - Tinnitus
  - Hearing loss
  - Blurred vision
  - Altered taste and smell
  - Sleep disturbances/insomnia
  - Fatigue
  - Sensory impairments
  - Attention and concentration deficits
  - Slowed mental processing (slowed reaction and information processing time)
  - Memory impairment (mostly recent memory)
  - Lability
  - Irritability
  - Depression
  - Anxiety
- Most mild TBI patients have a good recovery with symptoms clearing within the first few weeks or months postinjury (usually within 1 to 3 months)
- In some patients the symptoms (previously mentioned) persist and are associated with social and vocational difficulties that appear to be out of proportion to the severity of the neurologic insult. This condition has been termed postconcussive syndrome (PCS)
- In a recent study, 14 mild TBI patients with unusually persistent deficits evaluated with single photon emission computed tomography (SPECT) showed significant anterior mesial temporal (lobe) hypoperfusion and less striking dominant (left) orbitofrontal abnormalities
- Memory and learning deficits have been associated with lesions at the hippocampus and related structures in the medial temporal lobes or with injuries to structures that control attention, concentration, and information processing in the frontal and temporal lobe
- Pharmacologic intervention may be used including antidepressants and psychostimulants

Concussion/Sports Related Head Injuries

- Classification of concussion is controversial
- The most widely used grading systems for concussion/mild head injury are the Colorado and the Cantu guidelines

TABLE 2–14. Cantu and Colorado Head Injury Grading Systems

Grade	Cantu	Colorado
Grade I—mild	• No LOC • PTA < 30 min	• No LOC • Confusion w/o amnesia
Grade 2—moderate	• LOC < 5 min • PTA > 30 min	• No LOC • Confusion with amnesia
Grade 3—severe	•LOC > 5 min • PTA > 24 hrs	• LOC

LOC = loss of consciousness
PTA = posttraumatic amnesia
(Cantu, 1992) (Report of the Quality Standards Subcommittee, 1997)

Return to Play Guidelines
- Return to play criteria have been similarly controversial
- Colorado Medical Society and Cantu Guidelines are among the most widely used.

TABLE 2–15. Cantu's Guidelines for Return to Play after Concussion

Grade	First Concussion	Second Concussion	Third Concussion
Grade I— mild	May return to play if asymptomatic for 1 week	May return to play in 2 weeks if asymptomatic for 1 week	Terminate season, although patient may return to play next season if asymptomatic
Grade 2— moderate	May return to play after asymptomatic for 1 week	Minimum of 1 month out of competition, may return to play then if asymptomatic for 1 week and consider termination of season dependent on symptoms	Same as above
Grade 3— severe	Minimum of 1 month, may return to play if asymptomatic for 1 week	Terminate season, although may return to play next season if asymptomatic	

(Cantu , 1998)

The American Academy of Neurology endorsed the Colorado Medical Society Guidelines for classification and management of concussion in sports in its Report of the Quality Standards Subcommittee Practice Parameter published in Neurology, 1997.

TABLE 2–16. When to Return to Play—Colorado Medical Society Guidelines

Grade of Concussion:	Return to play only after being asymptomatic with normal neurologic assessment at rest with exercise:
Grade 1 concussion	15 minutes or less
Multiple Grade 1 concussions	1 week
Grade 2 concussion	1 week
Multiple Grade 2 concussions	2 weeks
Grade 3—brief loss of consciousness (seconds)	1 week
Grade 3—prolonged loss of consciousness (minutes)	2 weeks
Multiple Grade 3 concussions	1 month or longer, based on decision of evaluating physician

(Report of the Quality Standards Subcommittee, 1997)

REFERENCES

American Congress of Rehabilitation Medicine. Recommendations for use of uniform nomenclature pertinent to patients with severe alterations in consciousness. *Arch Phys Med Rehabil.* 1995 Feb;76:205-9.

Annegers JF, Hauser WA, Coan SP, Rocca WA. A population-based study of seizures after traumatic brain injuries. *N Engl J Med.* 1998 Jan 1; 338(1):20-4.

Aspen Neurobehavioral Conference: Draft Consensus Statement. 1996.

Born JD, Born JD, Albert A, Hans P, Bonnal J. Relative prognostic value of best motor response and brain stem reflexes in patients with severe brain injury. *Neurosurgery* 16: 595, 1985.

Braddom RL. Physical Medicine and Rehabilitation. Philadelphia: W.B. Saunders Company; 1996.

Brain Injury Special Interest Group of the American Academy of Physical Medicine and Rehabilitation. Practice Parameter: Antiepileptic drug treatment of posttraumatic seizures. *Arch Phys Med Rehabil* 1998;79(suppl)594-7.

Cantu RC. Cerebral concussion in sport. Management and prevention. *Sports Med.* 1992;14:64–74.

Cantu RC. Return to play guidelines after a head injury. *Clin Sports Med.* 1998;17:45–60.

Cifu DX, Kaelin DL, Wall BE. Deep venous thrombosis: Incidence on admission to a brain injury rehabilitation program. *Arch Phys Med Rehabil.* 1996; 77:118–25.

Dikmen SS, Temkin NR, Miller B, Machamer J, Winn HR. Neurobehavioral effects of phenytoin in prophylaxis in post-traumatic seizures. *JAMA* 1991; 265:1271-1277.

Ellenberg JH, Levin HS, Saydjari C. Posttraumatic amnesia as a predictor of outcome after severe closed head injury. Prospective assessment. *Arch Neurol.* 1996 ;53:782–91.

Feeney DM, Gonzalez A, Law WA. Amphetamine, haloperidol, and experience interact to affect rate of recovery after motor cortex injury. *Science.* 1982; 217:855–7.

Feeney DM. Pharamcologic modulation of recovery after brain injury: A reconsideration of diaschisis. *J Neurol Rehabil.* 1991; 5:113–28.

Feldman MH. The decerebrate state in the primate. I. Studies in monkeys. *Arch Neurol.* 1971, 25:501–16.

Fife D.Head injury with and without hospital admission: comparisons of incidence and short-term disability. *Am J Public Health.* 1987; 77:810–2.

Functional Indepence Measure. (Guide for the Uniform Data Set for Medical Rehabilitation, 1996) FIM(TM) is a trademark of the Uniform Data System for Medical Rehabilitation, a division of UB Foundation Activities, Inc.

Giacino JT, Kezmarsky MA, DeLuca J, Cicerone KD. Monitoring rate of recovery to predict outcome in minimally responsive patients. *Arch Phys Med Rehabil.* 1991; 72:897–901.

Gordon WA, Mann N, Wilier B. Demographic and social characteristics of the traumatic brain injury model system database. *J Head Trauma Rehabil* 1993; 8(2):26–33.

Gouvier WD, Blanton PD, LaPorte KK, Nepomuceno C. Reliability and validity of the Disability Rating Scale and the Levels of Cognitive Functioning Scale in monitoring recovery from severe head injury. *Arch Phys Med Rehabil.* 1987; 68:94–7.

Gouvier WD. Assessment and treatment of cognitive deficits in brain-damaged individuals. *Behav Modif.* 1987; 11:312–28.

Halstead, WC. Brain and intelligence; a quantitative study of the frontal lobes. Chicago, University of Chicago Press; 1947.

Horn LJ, Zasler ND. Medical Rehabilitation of Traumatic Brain Injury. Philadelphia: Hanley and Belfus; 1996.

Howsepian AA.The 1994 Multi-Society Task Force consensus statement on the Persistent Vegetative State: a critical analysis. *Issues Law Med.* 1996 Summer; 12:3–29.

Jennett B. Defining brain damage after head injury. *J R Coll Physicians Lond.* 1979 Oct;13(4):197–200.

Katz DI, Alexander MP. Traumatic brain injury. Predicting course of recovery and outcome for patients admitted to rehabilitation. *Arch Neurol.* 1994 Jul; 51:661–70.

Marion DW, Penrod LE, Kelsey SF, et al. Treatment of traumatic brain injury with moderated hypothermia. *N Engl J Med.* 1997; 336:540–6.

National Health Interview Survey 1985. Hyattsville, MD; U.S. Dept. of Health and Human Services, National Center for Health Statistics. 1987.

National Institute on Disability and Rehabilitation Research, Traumatic Brain Injury Model Systems Program. TBI model system grants. *J Head Trauma Rehabil.* 1999; 14:189–200.

Rancho Los Amigos National Rehabilitation Center. Levels of Cognitive Function Scale. Downey, CA.

Rappaport M, Hall KM, Hopkins K, Belleza T, Cope DN. Disability rating scale for severe head trauma: coma to community. *Arch Phys Med Rehabil*. 1982; 63:118–123.

Reitan RM. Sensorimotor functions, intelligence and cognition, and emotional status in subjects with cerebral lesions. *Percept Mot Skills*. 1970; 31:275–84.

Reitan, RM, Davison LA, eds. Clinical neuropsychology: current status and applications. Washington, D.C.: Hemisphere Pub. Corp.; 1974.

Report of the Quality Standards Subcommittee. Practice parameter: the management of concussion in sports (summary statement). Neurology. 1997; 48:581–5.

Rosenthal M, Griffith ER, Bond MR, Miller JD, eds. Rehabilitation of the Adult and Child with Traumatic Brain Injury, 2nd ed. Philadelphia: F.A. Davis; 1990.

Rosenthal M, Griffith ER, Kreutzer JS, Pentland B. Rehabilitation of the Adult and Child with Traumatic Brain Injury, 3rd edition. Philadelphia, PA: F.A. Davis Company; 1999.

Sosin DM, Sniezek JE, Thurman DJ. Incidence of mild and moderate brain injury in the United States, 1991. *Brain Inj*. 1996; 10:47–54.

Sosin DM, Sniezek JE, Waxweiler RJ, Trends in death associated with TBI, 1979 through 1992. *JAMA*. 1995; 273:1778–1780.

Spitz WE, Fisher RS. Medicolegal Investigation of Death: Guidelines for the application of pathology to crime investigation, 2nd edition. Springfield, IL; Charles C. Thomas Publisher; 1991.

Teasdate G, Jennett B. Assessment of Coma and impaired consciousness. Lancet 1974; 2:81–84.

Temkin NR, Dikmen SS, Wilensky AJ, et al. A randomized, double-blind study of phenytoin for the prevention of post-traumatic seizures. *N Engl J Med*. 1990; 23; 323:497–502.

The Multi-Society Task Force on PVS. Medical aspects of the persistent vegetative state (1). *N Engl J Med*. 1994;330:1499–508.

United States Department of Education, National Institute on Disability and Rehabilitation Research, Traumatic Brain Injury Model Systems National Data Center; Traumatic Brain Injury Facts and Figures. 1999;4(1).

RECOMMENDED READING

Adams RD, Victor M, Ropper AH. Principles of Neurology, 6th ed. New York: McGraw-Hill; 1997.

Whyte J, Hart T, Laborde A, Rosenthal M. Rehabilitation of the Patient with Traumatic Brain Injury. In Delisa JA, ed-in-chief; Gans B, ed. Rehabilitation Medicine: Principles and Practice, 3rd ed. Philadelphia: Lippincott-Raven; 1998.

Molnar G, Alexander M. Pediatric Rehabilitation, 3rd ed. Philadelphia: Hanley & Belfus; 1999.

3

RHEUMATOLOGY

Thomas R. Nucatola, M.D., Eric Freeman, D.O., and David P. Brown, D.O.

■

RHEUMATOID ARTHRITIS (RA)

DEFINITION (Klippel, 1997; Kelly et al, 1997)

Systemic autoimmune inflammatory disord of unknown etiology that primarily affects the synovial lining of the diarthrodial joints. Th chronic, symmetric erosive synovitis develops in the joints and leads to destruction. These erosions are pathognomonic of RA.

> **Diarthrodial Joint**
> - Type II Hyaline Cartilage
> - Subchondral Bone
> - Synovial Membrane
> - Synovial Fluid
> - Joint Capsule

Results of Joint Destruction in RA

- Injury to synovial microvasculature
- Synoviocytes are activated via class III HLA Ag (cellular process): Synovial cells proliferate
- Leads to congestion, edema, and fibrin exudation
- T Lymphocytes infiltrate
- Synovium is hypertrophied (cartilage is destroyed)
- Pannus formation

📖 Pannus Formation is the Most Important Destructive Element in RA

Pannus:
- Membrane of granulation tissue that covers the articular cartilage at joint margins
- Fibroblast-like cells invade and destroy the periarticular bone and cartilage at joint margins
- Vascular granulation tissue is composed of:
  - Proliferating fibroblasts
  - Numerous small blood vessels
  - Various number of inflammatory cells mainly T lymphocytes (Polymorphic Neutrophil PMN are in fluid)
  - Occasionally collagen fibers are seen within phagolysosomes of cells at the leading edge of pannus
- Joint ankylosis may occur in later stages

EPIDEMIOLOGY

- Female to male ratio is 2:1
- Prevalence: approximately 1% of the population
- Genetic
- Major Histocompatability Complex (MHC) on chromosome #6
- Class II MHC allele HLA-DR4 (HLA-DR4 haplotype)
- Age range from 20 to 60 years, prevalence rises with age, peak incidence between 4th and 5th decade

ETIOLOGY

Two major theories:
1. Infectious agents
2. Immunogenetic→ Class II surface antigens-presenting cells

PATTERN OF ONSET

📖 Insidious → 50%–70%

- Initial symptoms can be systemic or articular
- Slow onset from weeks to months
- Constitutional symptoms: fatigue, malaise
- Diffuse musculoskeletal pain may be the first nonspecific complaint with joint involvement later
- Most commonly symmetric involvement although asymmetric involvement may be seen early
- Morning stiffness in the involved joints lasting one hour or more
- Swelling, erythema
- Muscle atrophy around the affected joints
- Low grade fever without chills

Acute Onset → 10%–20%

- Onset over several days
- Less symmetric in presentation
- Severe muscle pain

Intermediate Onset→ 20%–30%

- Onset over several days to weeks
- Systemic complaints more noticeable

📖 DIAGNOSIS OF RA: 1988 American Rheumatologic Association Criteria (Arnett et al., 1988)

- **Must satisfy 4–7 criteria**
- **Criteria 1 through 4 must be present for at least six weeks**

ARA Criteria:
1. Morning Stiffness
   - In and around the joint
   - Must last at least one hour before maximal improvement
2. Arthritis of Three or More Joints
   - Three or more joint areas simultaneously affected with soft tissue swelling or fluid
   - Observed by a physician
   - 14 possible joint areas are bilateral proximal interphalangeal (PIP), metacarpal phalangeal (MCP), wrist, elbow, knee, ankle and metatarsal phalangeal (MTP)

3. **Arthritis of the Hand Joints**
   - At least one joint area swollen in the wrist, MCP and/or PIP
4. **Symmetric Arthritis**
   - Simultaneous involvement at the same joint area on both sides of the body
   - Absolute symmetry is not needed
5. **Rheumatoid Nodules**
   - Subcutaneous nodules over extensor surfaces, bony prominence or in juxta-articular regions
   - Observed by a physician
6. **Serum Rheumatoid Factor (RF [+]).**
7. **Radiographic Changes (Hand and Wrist)**
   - Erosions, bony decalcification, and symmetric joint-space narrowing

---

📖 **Duration and Location in the Major Arthritides of Morning Stiffness**
- Rheumatoid Arthritis → PIP, MCP, MTP Joints
  Duration > 1–2 hours
- Osteoarthritis (OA) → Distal Interphalangeal Joint (DIP)
  Duration < 30 minutes
- Ankylosing Spondylosis → Lumbosacral Spine
  Duration ~ 3 hours

LAB TESTS

Although no single test is definitive in diagnosing RA, typical laboratory findings in active disease include:
- Rheumatoid factor
- Acute phase reactants: ESR and C-reactive protein
- CBC: thrombocytosis, hypochromic microcytic anemia, eosinophilia
- Synovial fluid analysis

📖 **Synovial Fluid In RA**
- Low viscosity
- WBC → 1,000–75,000 mm^3
- > 70% PMNs
- Transparent - cloudy

- Hypergammaglobulinemia
- Hypocomplementemia

Rheumatoid Factor (+)

- 📖 85% of the patients with RA have a (+) Rheumatoid Factor (RF [+])
- Associated with severe active disease with increased systemic manifestations (nodules)
- Serial titers are of no value
- Can still be RF (–) and have RA because (+) diagnosis needs four to seven diagnostic criteria
- + RF can be seen in other diseases: Rheumatic (SLE, scleroderma, Sjögren's), viral, parasitic, bacterial, neoplasms, hyperglobulinemic

Increased ESR and C Reactive Protein

- Acute phase reactants
- Nonspecific, not used in diagnosis

📖 RADIOGRAPHIC FINDINGS IN RA

- Marginal bone erosions (near attachment of joint capsule)
- (+) Juxta-articular osteopenia (bone wash-out)
- Predilection of swelling of joints in wrists, MCP, PIP, MTP not DIP
- Erosion of the ulnar styloid
- Erosion of the metatarsal head of the MTP joint
- Disease may be asymmetric at first then progress to symmetric
- Cervical spine involvement may lead to cervical atlantoaxial (A-A) subluxation (> 2.5–3 mm) (Martel, 1961; Park et al. 1979)
- Ulnar deviation and volar subluxation seen at the MCP joint of the phalanges
- Radial deviation of the radiocarpal joint
- Hallux valgus
- Early findings
  - Soft tissue swelling
  - ↑ joint space
- Late findings
  - Uniform joint space narrowing due to loss of articular cartilage (hips, knees, etc.)
  - Axial migration of the hip (Protrusio Acetabulum)
  - Malalignment and fusion of joints

JOINT DEFORMITIES OF RHEUMATOID ARTHRITIS

> **The joints commonly involved in RA**
> - Hands and wrist
> - Cervical spine—C1 to C2
> - Feet and ankles
> - Hips and knees

Disease Progression
1. **Morning stiffness** → universal feature of synovial inflammation > one hour
2. **Structural inflammation** → warm swollen tender joints seen superficially
3. **Structural damage** → cartilage loss and erosion of the periarticular bone

Hand and Wrist Deformities

📖 **Boutonnière Deformity** (Calliet, 1982) (Figure 3–1)

Mechanism
- Weakness or rupture of the terminal portion of the extensor hood (tendon or central slip), which holds the lateral bands in place
- The lateral bands slip downward (or sublux) to the axis of the PIP joint turning them into flexors
- The PIP then protrudes through the split tendon as if it were a button hole (boutonnière = button hole)
- The distal phalanx hyperextends

Result
- Flexion of the PIP
- Hyperextension of the DIP
- Hyperextension of the MCP

Note: Positioning of the finger as if you were buttoning a button

Orthotic
- Tripoint finger splint

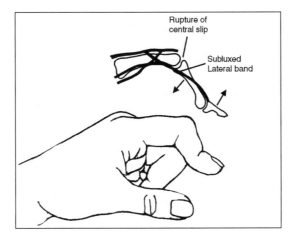

FIGURE 3–1. Boutonnière Deformity

Swan Neck Deformity (Calliet, 1982) (Figure 3–2)

Mechanism
- Contracture of the intrinsic and deep flexor muscles and tendons of the fingers

Result
- Flexion contracture of the MCP
- Hyperextension of the PIP
- Flexion of the DIP

Orthotic
- Swan neck ring splint

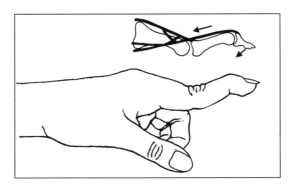

FIGURE 3–2. Swan Neck Deformity

Ulnar Deviation of the Fingers (Calliet, 1982)

Mechanism
- Weakening of the extensor carpi ulnaris (ECU), ulnar and radial collateral ligament
- Wrist deviates radially
- Increases the torque of the stronger ulnar finger flexors
- Flexor/extensor mismatch deviates the fingers in the ulnar direction as the patient tries to extend the joint

Result
- Ulnar deviation is due to the pull of the long finger flexors

Orthotic
- Ulnar deviation splint

Tenosynovitis of the Flexor Tendon Sheath

- One of the most common manifestation of the hands in RA
- Can be a major cause of hand weakness

Result
- Diffuse swelling of the volar surfaces of the phalanges between the joints with palpable grating of the flexor tendon sheath
- May be confused with deQuervain's disease

DeQuervain's disease
- Tenosynovitis of the extensor pollicis brevis (EPB) and abductor pollicis longus tendon (APL)
- Thickening of the tendon sheath results in tenosynovitis and inflammation
- Pain over the tendons on the radial wrist EPB and APL
- Test: Finkelstein Test (Figure 3–3)

Full flexion of the thumb into the palm followed by ulnar deviation of the wrist will produce pain and is diagnostic for deQuervain's tenosynovitis

---

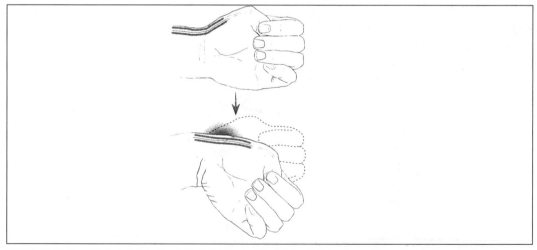

FIGURE 3–3. Finkelstein's Test: Full flexion of the thumb into the palm will produce pain when the wrist is deviated in the ulnar direction. From Snider RK. Essentials of Musculoskeletal Care. Rosemont, Illinois: American Academy of Orthopaedic Surgeons, 1997, with permission.

Carpal Bones Rotate in Zig-Zag Pattern

Mechanism
- Ligament laxity
- Radial deviation of the wrist
- Ulnar styloid rotates dorsally
- Carpal bones rotate
  - Proximal row: volarly
  - Distal row: dorsally

Result
- Zig-zag pattern

Floating Ulnar Head (Piano-Key Sign, Think of the Black Keys)

Mechanism
- Proliferating synovium leads to rupture or destruction of the ulnar collateral ligament

Result
- The ulnar head raises up to the dorsal wrist
- Easily compressible elevated ulnar styloid
- Ulnar head floats

Resorptive Arthropathy

Mechanism
- Digits are shortened and phalanges appear retracted with skin folds

Result
- Telescoping appearance of the digits
- Most serious arthritic involvement

Pseudobenediction Sign

Mechanism
- Stretched radioulnar ligaments allow the ulna to drift upward
- Extensor tendons of the fourth and fifth digit are subject to abrasion from rubbing on the sharp elevated ulnar styloid

Result
- Extensor tendon rupture
- Inability to fully extend the fourth and fifth digit

Cervical Spine

Atlantoaxial Joint Subluxations → Most Common are Anterior Subluxations
- **Instability**
  - Odontoid or Atlas can erode
  - With flexion, the Atlantoaxial (AA) space should not increase significantly: any space larger than 2.5 or 3 mm is considered abnormal (Martel, 1961; Park et al., 1979)
  - Tenosynovitis of the transverse ligament of C1
  - Cervical myelopathy → erosion of the odontoid process, ligament laxity or rupture

Foot and Ankle Deformities

Foot

- Hammer Toe Deformities
  - Hyperextension of the MTP and DIP with flexion of the PIP
- Claw Toe Deformities
  - Hyperextension at the MTP joint and flexion of the PIP and DIP joints
  - Pain on the metatarsal heads on weight bearing
- Hallux Valgus Deformity
- Lateral Deviation of the Toes

Ankle

- Ligament weakness leading to pronation of the hindfoot
- Tarsal tunnel syndrome
  - Synovial inflammation leads to compression of the posterior tibial nerve

Hip Deformities

- Occurs in about 50% of patients with RA (Duthie and Harris, 1969)
- Symmetric involvement
- Protrusio acetabulum can occur

What is a Protrusio?: Inward bulging of the acetabulum into the pelvic cavity
- Accompanied by arthritis of the hip joint, usually due to RA

Shoulders

- Glenohumeral arthritis
  - Limitation of Internal rotation is an early finding
- Effusions can occur; decreased range of motion (ROM) may lead to frozen shoulder
- Rotator cuff injuries which include:
  - Superior subluxations, tears, fragmenting of tendons secondary to erosion of the greater tuberosity

Elbow

- Subcutaneous nodules
- Olecranon bursitis
- Loss of full elbow extension is an early problem and may lead to flexion deformities
- Ulnar Neuropathies

Knee Deformities

- Common symmetric joint involvement
- Loss of full knee extension which may lead to flexion contractures
- Quadriceps atrophy leading to increased amount of force though the patella
- Force leads to increased intra-articular pressure in the knee joint causing the synovial fluid to drip into the popliteal space called a popliteal (Baker's) cyst

EXTRA-ARTICULAR MANIFESTATIONS OF RA

More common in patients that are:
- RF (+)
- With rheumatoid nodules

- Severe articular disease
- MHC class HLA DRB1 Alleles

General

- Malaise or fatigue

Skin

- **Subcutaneous Nodules**
  - Present in 50% of RA patients
  - Form subcutaneously, in bursae, and along tendon sheaths
  - Typically located over pressure points
  - Extensor surface of the forearm
  - Can occur singly or aggregate in clusters
  - Methotrexate may enhance the development or accelerate the development of rheumatoid nodules

> 📖 **Subcutaneous nodules are seen in**:
> - RA
> - Gout

- **Vasculitic Lesions**
  - Leukocytoclastic vasculitis and palpable purpura

Ocular

- Keratoconjunctivitis sicca (dry-eye syndrome)
- Episcleritis → benign, self-limited
- Scleritis → severe inflammation may erode through the sclera into the choroid causing scleromalacia perforans

Pulmonary

- Interstitial lung disease
  - Interstitial fibrosis
  - Rheumatoid nodules
- Pulmonary fibrosis
- Pleurisy
- Inflammation of the cricoarytenoid joint → dysphagia, dysphonia
- Bronchiolitis obliterans

> **Caplan's Syndrome**
> - Intrapulmonary nodules—histologically similar to rheumatoid nodules
> - (+) rheumatoid factor
> - Associated with rheumatoid arthritis and pneumoconiosis in coal workers
> - Granulomatous response to silica dust

Cardiac

- Pericarditis
  - May lead to constrictive pericarditis with right-sided heart failure
  - May be found in about half of RA patients
  - Rarely symptomatic
- Valvular heart disease

Gastrointestinal:

- Xerostomia—dryness of the mouth secondary to decreased salivary secretion
- Gastritis and Peptic Ulcer Disease (PUD) associated with non-steroidal anti-inflammatory drugs (NSAIDs) (not directly linked to disease)

Renal

- Rare glomerular disease usually related to drug (gold)
- May see renal involvement if amyloidosis develops

Neurologic

- Cervical spine
  - Most common at C1-C2, destruction of the transverse ligament or the dens itself
  - 📖 Cervical myelopathy
  - Gradual onset of bilateral sensory paraesthesia of the hands and motor weakness
  - Neurologic exam findings may include → Babinski, Hoffman's, hyperactive Deep Tendon Reflexes (DTRs)
- Entrapment neuropathies
  - This is secondary to fluctuation in synovial inflammation and joint postures
- Mononeuritis multiplex —inflammatory—not due to compression

Hematologic

- Hypochromic-microcytic anemia
- Felty's syndrome

Felty's Syndrome
"She felt her spleen"
- Classic triad of RA, splenomegaly, leukopenia
- Seen in seropositive RA, usually with nodules
- Occurs in the fifth to seventh decades with RA > 10 years
- Women comprise two-thirds of cases
- Often associated with leg ulcers

TREATMENT OF RHEUMATOID ARTHRITIS (Hicks, Sutin, 1988; Berkow, Elliot 1995)

Education

- Joint protection
- Home exercise program

Relative Rest

- Required for the acutely inflamed joint

Exercise

- Acute disease: with severely inflamed joints, actual splinting to produce immobilization with twice daily full and slow passive range of motion to prevent soft tissue contracture
- 📖 Mild disease: (moderate synovitis) requires isometric program

Isometric Exercise
- Causes least amount of periarticular bone destruction and joint inflammation
- Restores and maintains strength
- Generates maximal muscle tension with minimal work, fatigue and stress
- Isotonics and isokinetic may exacerbate the flare and should be avoided

Modalities

- Superficial moist heat
  - Should not be used in acutely inflamed joints
  - Depth of 1 cm
  - Decreases pain and increases collagen extensibility
  - Increases collagenase enzyme activity which causes increased joint destruction
- Other superficial heating/modalities: paraffin, fluidotherapy
- Cryotherapy
  - Pain relief in an acutely inflamed joint
  - Decreases the pain indicators of inflammation

ORTHOTICS

Indications
- Decrease pain and inflammation
- Reduce weight through joint
- Decrease joint motion—stabilization
- Joint rest

- Splinting of the wrist in RA will most likely help to:
  - Decrease pain and inflammation (Stenger et al., 1998)
  - May help with disease progression, but is not proven
- The major function of an orthosis used to combat early deformity in RA is to prevent MCP flexion
  Remember: There is no evidence that splinting will stop these deformities, but stabilizing the MCP joint accompanied with exercise may help prevent or slow the progression. The MCP is thought to be the primary site of RA and inflammation can lead to weakening of joint supporting structures.
- Wrist-hand orthosis contributes to decrease in pain and is used mainly for strength maneuvers rather than dexterity
- Does not deter the progression of the disease

Medications

- Early diagnosis should be done within the first month to prevent joint pathology
- Poor prognostic factors
- Help with assessing treatment

> **Poor Prognosis in RA**
> 1. Rheumatoid Nodules
> 2. RF (+)
> 3. Xray consistent with Erosive Disease
> 4. Persistent Synovitis
> 5. Insidious Onset

Surgical Options

- Synovectomy
- Arthroplasty
- Arthrodesis
- Tendon repairs

TABLE 3–1. Treatment Options for Rheumatoid Arthritis (Verhoeven, 1998)

Disease Stage	Poor Prognostic Features	Treatment	Medications
Mild	(–)	1. Education 2. PT/OT 3. Compliance	1. NSAID, salicylates 2. Disease-modifying antirheumatic drug (DMARD) • Hydroxychloroquine • Sulfasalazine • Oral gold
Moderately severe	(+)	1. Education 2. PT/OT 3. Compliance	1. NSAID, salicylates 2. DMARD • Parental gold, methotrexate—weekly 3. Short course of corticosteroids • 3–5 day taper
Severe	(+)	Mandatory 1. Education 2. PT/OT 3. Compliance	1. NSAID, salicylates 2. DMARD-chronic use • IM gold • Weekly oral or parental methotrexate • May add a second DMARD 3. Corticosteroids

PT = Physical Therapy
OT = Occupational Therapy
NSAID = non-steroidal anti-inflammatory drugs
DMARD = disease modifying anti-rheumatic drug

TABLE 3–2. Drugs Used in Rheumatoid Arthritis and Common Side Effects (Gerber, Hicks, 1995)

DMARDs (Disease Modifying Anti-rheumatic Drugs)	Toxic Profile	General Degree of Toxicity
Hydroxychloroquine	Macular damage	Safer
Sulfasalazine	Myelosuppression, gastrointestional (GI) distrubances	Safer
Auranofin	GI disturbances, diarrhea, nausea, vomiting, anorexia, rash pruritus, conjunctivitis, stomatitis, anemia, thrombocytopenia, proteinuria, elevated liver enzymes	Safer
Methotrexate	Stomatitis, myelosuppression, hepatic fibrosis, cirrhosis, pulmonary involvement, worsens rheumatoid nodules	More toxic
Cyclosporine	Renal dysfunction, tremor, hirsutism, hypertension, gum dysplasia	More toxic
Gold, Intramuscular, Oral	Myelosuppression, renal → proteinuria Diarrhea (#1, oral), Rash (#1, Intramuscular)	More toxic
Azathioprine	Myelosuppression, hepatotoxicity, lymphoproliferative disorders	More toxic
D-Penicillamine	Oral ulcers, bone marrow suppression induction of autoimmune disease, proteinuria	More toxic
Chlorambucil	Bone marrow suppression, GI disturbances, nausea, vomiting, diarrhea, oral ulceration, central nervous system (CNS) disturbances, tremors, confusion, seizures, skin hypersensitivity, pulmonary fibrosis, hepatotoxicity, drug fever peripheral neuropathy, infertility, leukemia and 2° malignancies	Very toxic
Cyclophosphamide	Carcinogenesis, impairment of fertility, mutagenesis, GI disturbances, nausea, vomiting, anorexia, alopecia, leukopenia, thrombocytopenia, anemia, cystitis, urinary bladder fibrosis, interstitial pulmonary fibrosis, anaphylactic reaction	Very toxic

Other Drugs for the Treatment of Rheumatoid Arthritis	Toxic Profile
ASA, NSAID	GI ulceration and bleeding Therapeutic levels for ASA 15 mg/dl–25 mg/dl Toxic > 30 mg/dl
Corticosteroids	Hyperglycemia, inhibits immune response, osteoporosis, peptic ulcer disease, emotional liability

■

OSTEOARTHRITIS (OA)

DEFINITION

A noninflammatory progressive disorder of the joints leading to deterioration of the articular cartilage and new bone formation at the joint surfaces and margins
- Disease of the cartilage initially, not bone

PREVALENCE

Most common form of arthritis and the second most common form of disability in the United States
- Prevalence increases with age: approximately 70% population > 65 years old have radiographic evidence of osteoarthritis (Lane, 1997)
- Increase in occupations with repetitive trauma
- Male:female ratio is equal between the ages of 45–55. After 55 years old, it is more common in women.
- Obesity → OA of the knee is most common

PATHOLOGY

- Microscopically
  - Early → Hypercellularity of chondrocytes
    Cartilage breakdown
    Minimal inflammation
  - Later → Cartilage fissuring, pitting, and erosions
    Hypocelluarity of chondrocytes
    Inflammation 2° synovitis
    Osteophytes spur formation—seen at the joint margins
    Subcondral bone sclerosis (eburnation)
    Cyst formation in the juxta-articular bone
- Increased water content of OA cartilage leads to damage of the collagen network
- Loss of proteoglycans

CLASSIFICATION

- Primary OA → Idiopathic
  - Knees, MTP, DIP, carpal metacarpal joint (CMC), hips and spine
- Secondary → Follows a recognizable underlying cause
  - Elbows and shoulder involvement
  - Chronic or acute trauma, connective tissue disease, endocrine or metabolic, infectious, neuropathic and crystal deposition, bone dysplasias
- Erosive inflammatory OA
- DISH → Diffuse Idiopathic Skeletal Hyperostosis (Snider, 1997)

> **OA Affected Joints**
> - Primary OA: Knees, MTP, DIP, CMC, Hips, Spine
> - Secondary OA: Elbows and Shoulders

SIGNS & SYMPTOMS

Signs

- Dull aching pain increased with activity, relieved by rest
- Later pain occurs at rest
- Joint stiffness < 30 minutes, becomes worse as the day goes on
- Joint giving away
- Articular gelling → stiffness lasting short periods and dissipates after initial ROM
- Crepitus on ROM

Symptoms

- Monoarticular, shows no obvious joint pattern
- Localized tenderness of joints
- Pain and crepitus of involved joints
- Enlargement of the joint → changes in the cartilage and bone secondary to proliferation of synovial fluid and synovitis

SPECIFIC JOINT INVOLVEMENT

- Heberden's Nodes → Spur formation at the DIP joints
- Bouchard's Nodes → PIP
- First CMC
- Knee Joint—Narrowing of medial compartment
- Hips—Narrowing of superior lateral compartment, loss of ROM
- Acromioclavicular Joint
- First MTP Joint
- Spine
- Spondylosis
- Involvement of the intervertebral fibrocartilaginous disc and vertebrae
- Diffuse Idiopathic Skeletal Hyperostosis (DISH) (Snider, 1997)

> **DISH**
> - Variant form of primary OA
> - Osteophytes extending to the length of the spine leading to spinal fusion
> - Hallmark → ossification spanning three or more intervertebral discs
> - Common in the thoracic, thoracolumbar spine
> - More prevalent in white males > 60 years old
> - Multisystem disorder, associated with:
>   - diabetes mellitus (DM), obesity, hypertension (HTN), coronary artery disease (CAD)
>   - Stiffness in the morning or evening
>   - Dysphagia if cervical involvement

RADIOGRAPHIC FINDINGS:

- Asymmetric narrowing of the joint space
  - Knee—medial joint space narrowing
  - Hip—superior lateral joint space narrowing
- Subchondral bony sclerosis—new bone formation (white appearance, eburnation)
- Osteophyte formation
- Osseous cysts—microfractures may cause bony collapse
- Loose bodies
- No osteoporosis/osteopenia (no bone washout)
- Joint involvement
  - First CMC
  - DIP—Heberden's
  - Large joints—knee and hip
  - Luschka joint's—uncinate process on the superior/lateral aspect of the cervical vertebral bodies (C3-C5) making them concave

TREATMENT

- Patient education
  - Weight loss
- PT/OT
  - ROM, strengthening exercises
  - Assistive devices
  - Joint protection and energy conservation
- Pharmacologic
  - NSAIDs
  - Acetaminophen
  - Narcotics—rare
  - Steroids
    - Intra-articular may be beneficial in acute flares
    - Oral steroids are contraindicated—not proven

📖 **Erosive X-Ray Changes**

Osteoarthritis
- No erosive changes seen on X-ray

Rheumatoid Arthritis
- Marginal or central erosions seen on X-ray

TABLE 3–3. Summary RA Compared to OA

RADIOGRAPHIC FINDINGS IN RA	RADIOGRAPHIC FINDING IN OA

• Uniform joint space narrowing—hips, knees, etc.
• Symmetrical joint involvement
• Marginal bone erosions
• Juxta-articular osteopenia—bone wash-out
• Ulnar deviation of phalanges
• Radial deviation of the radiocarpal joint
• Erosion of the ulnar styloid
• Atlantoaxial separation (> 2.5–3 mm) → subluxation
• Small joint involvement—MCP, PIP, carpal
	• Asymmetric narrowing of the joint space
	  – Knee—medial joint space narrowing;
	  – Hip—superior lateral joint space narrowing
	• Joint involvement does not have to be symmetric
	• No erosive changes seen on x-ray
	• No osteoporosis/osteopenia (bone wash-out)
	• Subchondral bony sclerosis—new bone formation with white appearance
	• Osteophyte formation
	• Osseous cysts—microfractures may cause bony collapse
	• Loose bodies
	• Joint involvement; first CMC, DIP, large joints—knee and hip

EXTREMITY INVOLVEMENT	EXTREMITY INVOLVEMENT
• Wrist • MCP • PIP • Ankle Joint • Talonavicular joint • MTP	• First CMC • PIP • DIP • MTP

■

JUVENILE RHEUMATOID ARTHRITIS (JRA)

- The most common form of childhood arthritis
- Cause → unknown
- ARA diagnostic criteria → JRA
  Chronic arthritic disease in children
  General criteria of diagnosis of JRA
- Three clinical subtypes: systemic, polyarticular, pauciarticular

---

ARA Diagnostic Criteria for JRA
- Onset less than 16 years of age
- Persistent arthritis in one or more joints at least six weeks
- Exclusion of other types of childhood arthritis—rheumatic fever, infection, systemic lupus erythematosus(SLE), vasculitis, etc.
- Type of onset of disease during the 1st six months classified as polyarthritis, oligoarthritis, or systemic arthritis with intermittent fever

---

THREE CLINICAL SUBTYPES OF JUVENILE RHEUMATOID ARTHRITIS

Systemic "Still's Disease" (approximately 10% of JRA)

- JRA- Poly or Oligoarthritis (Oligo—few)
- Onset peak—1 to 6 years old, male:female equal
- Persistent intermittent fever daily > 101° spikes daily or twice daily
- Rash—transient, non-pruritic seen on the trunk
- Clinically—multisystemic involvement
  - Growth delay
  - Osteoporosis, osteopenia
  - Diffuse lymphadenopathy
  - Hepatosplenomegaly
  - Pericarditis
  - Pleuritis
  - Anemia
  - Leukocytosis
  - ↑ acute phase reactants
- RF) (+): < 2%
- Uveitis rare

Polyarticular

- JRA—mild systemic manifestations
- Females >> males, onset usually > 8 years old
- Gradual onset of swelling, stiffness involving the cervical spine and hips
- Growth retardation—early closure of the epiphyseal plates
- Five or more joints involved during the first 6 months
- RF (+): 5–10%

RF (+) Polyarticular (only 5–10%)

- Females > 10 years old
- Erosive and chronic
- Unremitting: This group has the worst prognosis if disease is unremitting
- Uveitis does not occur
- Subcutaneous nodules

RF (–) Polyarticular (90–95%)

- 25% males < 6 years old

Pauciarticular

- JRA—oligoarticular
- Fewer than 4 joints during the first 6 months
- ⬚ Knee is the most common joint involved, followed by ankle, wrist, elbows
- Hips usually spared, (–) Sacroilitis
- Two distinct types
- Early onset—females, < 5 years old
- Late onset—males
- (+) HLA B27
- RF positive (+) < 2% (Klippel, 1997)
- Antinuclear antibody (+) (ANA) have greater risk of eye involvement
- Chronic iridocyclitis—leads to cataracts, glaucoma, blindness

---

Key Points

- (+) ANA, RF (-)
- (+) HLA B27
- Iridocyclitis
- No erosions

⬚ **When diagnosed with Pauciarticular Rheumatoid Arthritis**
- Ophthalmology referral is mandatory
- Slit lamp exam is required four times per year, for four years

---

TREATMENT

- Therapeutic Goals
  - Relieving symptoms
  - Maintaining ROM—two to three times per day
  - Joint protection
  - Family training
- Pharmacologic
  - Manifestations:
    - NSAIDs with food and gastrointestinal (GI) protection
    - Methotrexate—more commonly in systemic and polyarticular types
- 70% of children with JRA improve without serious disability (worst prognosis if polyarticular with unremitting disease)
- 10% of children suffer severe functional disability
- Poor prognosis indicators
  - RF (+)
  - Nodules
  - Bone erosions on x-ray
  - Polyarticular group with unremitting disease

- Treatment (Rapoff, Purviance, and Lindsley, 1988)
  - Salicylates
  - NSAIDs: tolmetin, naprosyn, ibuprofen (approved for kids)
  - Corticosteroids (preferably intra-articular)
  - Orthosurgery (if severe)
  - Dz modifying agents: methotrexate, injectable gold, sulfasalazine (Stenger et al., 1998)

■

JUVENILE SPONDYLOARTHROPATHIES

DIAGNOSIS

- Many years to diagnose
- Symptoms before age of 16

CLASSIFICATION

- Spondyloarthropathies in childhood encompass four discrete clinical entities
  - Juvenile Ankylosing Spondylosis (RF +, ANA +)
  - Reiter's Syndrome
  - Psoriatic Arthritis
  - Enteropathic Arthropathy
- Since these diseases take many years to fully evolve and satisfy existing diagnostic criteria, it is not uncommon for children to have symptoms but not satisfy full criteria for diagnosis. Because of this, it is suggested that spondyloarthropathies in children include another syndrome, Seronegative Enthesopathy and Arthropathy (SEA)
- SEA Syndrome
  - (–) RF
  - (–) ANA
  - Enthesitis and either arthritis or arthralgia

TABLE 3–4. Key Points of Juvenile Arthritides

JUVENILE RHEUMATOID ARTHRITIS			JUVENILE SPONDYLO-ARTHROPATHIES
SYSTEMIC Multisystemic Involvement	**POLYARTICULAR** Many joints	**PAUCIARTICULAR**	
RF(–) (~98%) Still's Disease High fever Rheum. rash Lymphadenopathy Hepatosplenomegaly Anemia	RF(–) (90–95%) No extraarticular manifestations of systemic onset dz. Gradual onset of: Swelling Stiffness + cervical spine, + hip Growth retardation Early closure of epiphyseal plates *This group has the worst progress when disease is unremitting	RF(–) (> 98%) 1–4 joint involvement Few systemic effects Chronic Iridocyclitis: < 6 yrs. occurs in 20–40%; more frequently with Females. w/+ANA Must have ophthamology exam four times/year (+) HLA B27 (–) Bony erosions on X-ray	• Ankylosing Spondylosis (AS) • Reiter's • Psoriatic arthritis • Arthritis of inflammatory bowel disease Presents like adult spondylo-arthropathies (see below) SEA Syndrome – RF (–) – ANA (–) – Enthesitis/Arthritis/ Arthralgia

INFLAMMATORY ARTHRITIS	NONINFLAMMATORY ARTHRITIS
Increase in WBC and ESR Acute painful onset Erythema, warmth and tenderness Connective Tissue Disease (CTD) – SLE, polymyositis/dermatomyositis, Progressive Systemic Sclerosis (PSS), RA Crystal – Gout and pseudogout Infectious Seronegative spondyloarthropathies	Degenerative joint disease – OA, Avascular Necrosis (AVN) Traumatic Joint tumors Hemophilia Metabolic – hemochromatosis, alkaptonuria, rheumatic fever, Wilson's disease

TABLE 3–5. Crystal Induced Synovitis

	GOUT	PSEUDOGOUT
🔲 **Crystal**	• Monosodium Urate • Sodium urate • Acute synovitis in the synovial membrane and joint cavity	• "Articular chondrocalcinosis" • Calcium pyrophosphate dihydrate (CPPD) • Hyaline cartilage and fibrocartilage joints
Aspirate: Microscopic	Negative Birefringence 🔲 (Moderate-severe inflammation WBC 15–20,000—Neutrophils)	Positive Birefringence 🔲
Epidemiology	Male >> Female Age—30–50 yrs	Male > Female Age—30–50 yrs
Sequelae	• Gouty arthritis • Acute recurrent attacks • Chronic tophaceous arthritis • Uric acid calculi • Urate nephropathy	Acute Pseudogout • Inflammatory host response to CPPD crystals shed from the cartilaginous tissues to the synovial cavity 🔲 Pseudogout may have associations with: hypothyroidism amyloidosis hyperparathyroidism hypomagnesemia hemochromatosis hypophosphatasia

Clinical Presentation	• Asymptomatic hyperuricemia
	• Acute intermittent → Acute gouty arthritis
	🔲 Exquisite pain, warm tender swelling—first MTP joint (Podagra)
	  • Monoarticular
	  • Other sites: midfoot, ankles, heels, knees
	  • Fever, chills, malaise, cutaneous erythema
	  • May last days to weeks with a mean time of 11 months between attacks
	  • Chronic Tophaceous Gout
	  • Tophi form after several years of attacks
	  • Cause structural damage to the articular cartilage and adjacent bone
	  • Polyarticular Gout
	  • Sites of involvement: Olecranon bursae, wrists, hands, renal parenchyma with uric acid nephrolithiasis
		• Inflammation in one or more of the large joints
		🔲 • Most common—knee
		  • Others: first MTP, wrist, MCP, hips, shoulder, elbow, crowded dens syndrome
		• Symmetric
		• Flexion contracture of the knee is common
		• Less painful than gout, self-limiting, lasts two days—weeks
		• Fever, chills, malaise

Provocative Factors	Acute gout attacks • Trauma—Influx of synovial fluid urate production • Alcohol—Increase uric acid production • Drugs—Thiazides • Hereditary	• Hereditary • Idiopathic • Metabolic disease • Trauma • Surgery, illness (MI, CVA)
Labs	Hyperuricemia	Uric acid normal
Radiologic	Acute gouty arthritis • Soft tissue swelling around the affected joint • Asymmetric • MTP most frequent joint involved • Others: fingers, wrists, elbows Chronic tophaceous • Tophi appear as nodules in lobulated soft tissue masses • Bone erosions develop near the tophi just slightly removed from the periarticular surface, develop overhanging margins Joint space is preserved No osteopenia	Chondrocalcinosis • Punctate fine line of crystals in the articular hyaline or fibrocartilage tissues • #1—Menisci of the knee: resulting in narrowing of the femoral tibial joint • Other large joint: acetabulum labrum, pubic symphysis, articular disc of the wrist, annulus fibrosis of the disc Joint effusions
Treatment	Goals → Pain relief, prevent attacks, tophi, and joint destruction Acute attack • Colchicine—inhibits phagocytosis of the urate crystals • NSAIDs—Indocin • Corticosteroids Chronic • Allopurinol—decrease synthesis of urate • Probenecid—uricosuric increases the renal excretion of urate	NSAIDs Corticosteroids Colchicine

■

SERONEGATIVE SPONDYLOARTHROPATHIES

DEFINITION

- Group of multisystem inflammatory disorders affecting various joints, including the spine, peripheral joints and periarticular structures
- Associated with extraarticular manifestations
- Majority are HLA B27 (+) and RF (–)
- There are four major seronegative spondyloarthropathies:
  - Ankylosing Spondylitis (AS)
  - Reiter's Syndrome
  - Psoriatic Arthritis
  - Arthritis of Inflammatory Bowel Disease

📖 ANKYLOSING SPONDYLITIS

Definition

- Chronic inflammatory disorder of the axial skeleton affecting the sacroiliac joint and the spine
- The hallmark is bilateral sacroiliitis

Epidemiology

- Onset → late adolescent and early adulthood
- Males >> Females
- More common in whites
- Genetic marker → (+) HLA-B27~ 90%

> 📖 **HLA B27 Positive Diseases**
> - Ankylosing Spondylitis
> - Reiter's Syndrome
> - Psoriatic Arthritis—HLA Cw6
> - Enteropathic Arthropathy
> - Pauciarticular JRA

Mechanism

- Exact mechanism is unknown
- Synovitis and inflammation with intimal cell hyperplasia—lymphocyte and plasma cell infiltrate

---

AS vs. RA

Both have synovial inflammation that can lead to destruction of articular cartilage and ankylosis of the joint

Ankylosing Spondylitis	Rheumatoid Arthritis
More common in males	More common in females
Absence of rheumatoid nodules	Presence of rheumatoid nodules
RF (–)	RF (+) in 85% of cases
Prespinous calcification	

Clinical Manifestations

Skeletal Involvement

- Insidious onset, back pain or tenderness in the bilateral SI joint
  - First site of involvement is SI joint
  - Initially asymmetric
- Persistent symptoms of at least three months
- Lumbar morning stiffness that improves with exercise
- Lumbar lordosis—decreased and thoracic kyphosis—increased
- Cervical ankylosis develops in 75% of the patients who have AS for 16 years or more
- Lumbar spine or lower cervical is the most common site of fracture
- Enthesitis (An inflammatory process ocurring at the site of insertion of muscle.)
  - Tenderness over the ischial tuberosity, greater trochanter, ASIS, iliac crests.
- Hip and shoulder involvement more common in the juvenile onset, < 16 years old
- Respiratory restriction with limited chest expansion
  (Normal is 7–8 cm, if < 7–8 cm, then risk of restrictive lung disease pattern)
  Once restrictive lung disease pattern ensues:
  - Chest expansion decreases
  - Patient develops diaphragmatic breathing
  - Thoracic spine involvement—costovertebral, costosternal, manubriosternal, sternoclavicular

> **📖 Sites of Involvement in AS**
> - 1 → SI joint
> - 2 → Lumbar Vertebrae
> - 3 → Thoracic Vertebrae
> - 4 → Cervical Vertebrae

Extraskeletal Involvement

- Other complaints include—fatigue, weight loss, low-grade fever
- Acute iritis/iridocyclitis → most common extraskeletal manifestation of AS
  More progressive in Reiter's syndrome:
  - Unilateral, recurrent
  - Pain, photophobia, blurred vision
- Cardiac
  - Aortitis leading to fibrosis
  - Conduction defects
- Apical pulmonary fibrosis
  - May experience dyspnea and cough
- Amyloidosis
- Neurologic
  - Cauda equina syndrome
  - C1 to C2 subluxation

Lab Findings

- (+) HLA-B27, 90%—(clinically: test to find HLA-B27 factor is expensive)
- ↑ ESR and C-Reactive Protein
- Anemia—normochromic/normocytic
- RF (–) and ANA (–)

Radiographic Findings:

- SI Joint narrowing—Symmetric, may lead to fusion
- Pseudo-widening of the joint space
  - Subchondral bone resorption—blurring
  - Erosion sclerosis
  - Calcification leading to ankylosis
- Bamboo spine
  - Ossification of the anterior spinal ligament and ankylosis of the apophyseal joint leading to complete fusion
- Syndesmophyte formation—Squaring of lumbar vertebrae's anterior concavity
  - Reactive bone sclerosis
  - Squaring and fusion of the vertebral bodies and ossification of the annulus fibrosis at the dorsolumbar and lumbosacral area
- Osteopenia—Bone wash-out
- Straightening of the C-spine
- Hip and shoulder involved to a lesser extent

Other Tests

- **Schober Test**
  - Used for detecting limitation of forward flexion and hyperextension of the lumbar spine (Figure 3–4)
  - While standing erect, place a landmark midline at a point 5 cm below the iliac crest line and 10 cm above on the spinous processes. On forward flexion, the line should increase by greater than 5 cm to a total of 20 cm or more (from 15 cm)
  - Any increase less than 5 cm is considered a restriction

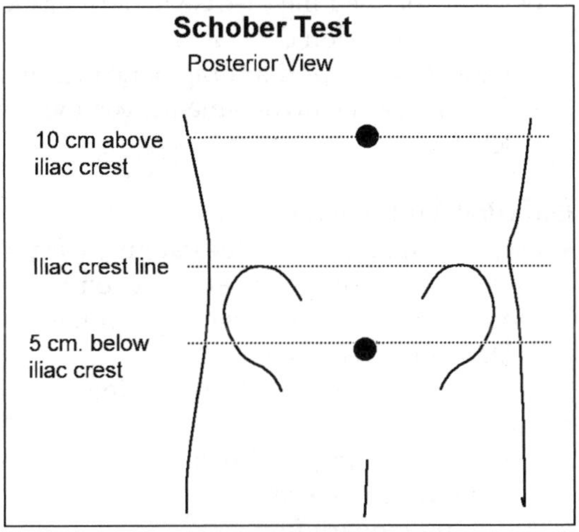

Schober Test
Posterior View

10 cm above iliac crest

Iliac crest line

5 cm. below iliac crest

FIGURE 3–4

Treatment

- Education
  - Good posture
  - Firm mattress, sleep straight—Supine or prone
  - Prevent flexion contractures
- Physical Therapy
  - Spine mobility—Extension exercises
  - Swimming is ideal
  - Joint protection
- Pulmonary—Maintain chest expansion
  - Deep breathing exercises
  - Cessation of smoking
- Medications
  - NSAIDs—Indocin
    - Control pain and inflammation
    - Allow for physical therapy

- Corticosteroids—Tapering dose, PO and Injections
- Sulfasalazine
  - Improves peripheral joint symptoms
  - Modify disease process
- Methotrexate
- Topical corticosteroid drops—Uveitis

REITER'S SYNDROME

Triad of Reiter's Syndrome

1. Conjunctivitis
2. Arthritis
3. Nongonococcal urethritis

> ~ 3%–10% of Reiter's progress to AS

Epidemiology

- Males >> females
- Organisms → Chlamydia, Campylobacter, Yersinia, Shigella, Salmonella
- More common in whites
- Associated with HIV

Clinical Manifestations

Arthritis
- Arthritis appears 2 to 4 weeks after initiating infectious event—GU or GI
- Asymmetric
- Oligoarticular—average of four joints
  - LE involvement >> UE
  - More common in the knees, ankles, and small joints of the feet
  - Rare hip involvement
  - UE → Wrist, elbows, and small joints of the hand
- Sausage digits (dactylitis)
  - Swollen tender digits with a dusklike blue discoloration
  - Pain on ROM
- Enthesopathies—Achilles tendon
  - Swelling at the insertion of tendons, ligaments, and fascia attachments
- Low back pain—Sacroilitis

Ocular
- Conjunctivitis, iritis, uveitis, episcleritis, corneal ulceration

Genitourinary
- Urethritis, meatal erythema, edema
- Balanitis Circinata—small painless ulcers on the glans penis, urethritis

Skin and Nails
- Keratoderma blennorrhagica—hypertrophic skin lesions on palms and soles of feet
- Reiter's Nails—thickened and opacified, crumbling, nonpitting

Cardiac
- Conduction defects

General
- Weight loss, fever
- Amyloidosis

Lab Findings

- Synovial fluid—inflammatory changes

> **Reiter's Syndrome: Synovial Fluid**
> - Turbid
> - Poor viscosity
> - WBC 5-50,000-PMN
> - ↑ protein, normal glucose

- Increased ESR
- RF (–) and ANA (–)
- Anemia–normochromic/normocytic
- **(+)** HLA B27

📖 Radiographic Findings

- "Lover's Heel"—erosion and periosteal changes at the insertion of the plantar fascia and Achilles tendons
- Ischial tuberosities and greater trochanter
- Asymmetric sacroiliac joint involvement
- Syndesmophytes
- Pencil in cup deformities of the hands and feet—more common in psoriatic arthritis

PSORIATIC ARTHRITIS

Prevalence

- ~5% to 7% of persons with psoriasis will develop some form of inflammatory joint disease
- Affects 0.1 % of the population
- Male: Female ratio is equal
- Age of onset ranges between 30–55 years
- More common in whites
- Associated with HIV ⟶

> **📖 Psoriatic arthritis and HIV**
> - Foot and ankle involvement is most common and severe
> - Treatment—Same as psoriatic.
>   - NO oral corticosteroids
>   - First line-NSAIDs
>   - NO methotrexate

Pathogenesis

- Unknown
- Genetic—(+) HLA-B27
- Environmental—infectious, trauma
- Immunologic

Clinical Manifestations

Skin and Nails:
- Psoriatic skin lesions—erythematous, silvery scales
- Auspitz sign—gentle scraping of the lesions results in pinpoint bleeding

- Located over the extensor surfaces
- Nail pitting

Arthritis

- Stiffness of the spine lasting ~ 30 min
- Asymmetric
- Oligoarticular and monoarticular
  - Large joints → knee
  - DIP involvement
    - Arthritis mutilans—osteolysis of the phalanges and metacarpals of the hand resulting in "Telescoping of the finger"
- Enthesopathy: Inflammation of the enthesis (insertion of ligament, tendon, joint capsule and bone)
- Spondylitis, sacroiliitis

Others
- Conjunctivitis—one-third
- Aortic insufficiency

Lab Findings

- Nonspecific—increased incidence in patients with +HLA-B27

Radiographic

- "Pencil in Cup" appearance of the DIP
- Asymmetric sacroiliitis → fusion
- "Fluffy Periostitis"—hands, feet, spine, and SI joint
- Syndesmophytes—see AS Radiology
- Bone erosion

📖 Treatment

- ROM to all joints
- Do not abuse an inflamed joint → exacerbation
- Meds—similar to RA, PUVA (long wave ultraviolet A light)
- Steroids—oral steroids not proven, injection may help

ENTEROPATHIC ARTHROPATHY

Definition

- Arthritis secondary to inflammatory bowel disease (Crohn's disease and ulcerative colitis)
- Bacterial etiology

Epidemiology

- Males >> female
- Peripheral arthritis occurs in ~ 10% to 20% of the patients with Crohn's disease and ulcerative colitis

Clinical Manifestations

- Asymmetric joint involvement
- Synovitis affecting the peripheral joints
- Monoarticular or polyarticular
- ⌨ Large joints—knees, ankles, feet
- Two types of arthropathies can occur
  - Enteropathic arthritis
  - AS
- Sacroilitis
- Peripheral arthritis will subside with remission of bowel disease

Extra-articular Manifestations

- Erythema nodosa—Crohn's
- Pyoderma gangraenosa—ulcerative colitis
- Painful deep oral ulcers
- Uveitis
- Fever and weight loss during bowel episodes

Lab Test

- Anemia
- ↑ ESR, C-reactive protein
- RF (–), ANA (–)
- (+) anti neutrophil cytoplasmic antibodies ~60% (antimyeloperoxidase)
- Increase incidence of HLA-B27

TABLE 3–6. Seronegative Spondyloarthropathy Fact Sheet

The following are all Seronegative Spondyloarthropathies. 1. Anklyosing Spondyloarthropathy 2. Reiter's Syndrome 3. Psoriatic Arthropathy 4. Arthritis of Inflammatory Bowel Disease				
All have the following characteristics:	Ankylosing Spondyloarthropathy	Reiter's Syndrome	Psoriatic Arthropathy	Arthritis of Inflammatory Bowel Disease
1. Increased incidence in patients with (+) HLA-B27	✔	✔	✔	✔
2. Mucocutaneous lesions	✔	✔	✔	✔
3. Frequent inflammation of the enthesis	✔	✔	✔	✔
4. Spondylitis with SI joint involvement	✔	✔	✔	✔
5. RF (–) ✔	✔	✔	✔	

■
CTD (CONNECTIVE TISSUE DISORDERS) AND SYSTEMIC ARTHRITIC DISORDERS

MCTD: MIXED CONNECTIVE TISSUE DISORDERS

- Combination
  1. SLE
  2. Scleroderma
  3. Polymyositis

SYSTEMIC LUPUS ERYTHEMATOSUS

- Multisystemic disease, autoimmune
- Females > > > males

> **Diagnosis of SLE**
> - Any 4 of 11 criteria present
> - Serially and simultaneously

Criteria—American Rheumatologic Association (ARA)

1. Malar Butterfly rash—Malar eminences spares nasolabial folds
2. Discoid rash—Raised erythematous patches with keratotic scaling
3. Photosensitivity
4. Oral ulcers—painless ulcers
5. Arthritis—Nonerosive arthritis involving two or more peripheral joints with tenderness, swelling and effusion
6. Serositis—Pleuritis or pericarditis (most common cardiac event)
7. Renal disorder—Proteinuria, red cell casts
8. Neurologic disorder—Seizure, psychosis
9. Hematologic disorder—Hemolytic anemia, leukopenia, thrombocytopenia, lymphopenia
10. Immunologic—(+)LE cell preparation or Anti-DNA antibody, or Anti-SM, false positive test for syphilis
11. ANA

Clinical

- Fatigue, fever, weight loss, GI complaints
- Alopecia
- Vasculitis
- Arthritis
  - Small joints of the hands, wrist, and knees
  - Symmetric
  - Migratory, chronic, nonerosive
  - Soft tissue swelling
  - Subcutaneous nodules
  - Synovial analysis—ANA (+)
  - Jaccoud's arthritis
- Arthralgias
- Muscle pain and weakness

> **Jaccoud's Arthritis**
> - Nonerosive deforming arthritis
> - Ulnar deviations of the fingers and subluxations which are reversible early
> - May become fixed

Labs

- Depressed complement—C3 and C4
- Ds-DNA
- Anti-SM

Treatment

- NSAIDs, corticosteroids, antimalarials, methotrexate, cyclophosphamide, azathioprine, cyclosporine A

PROGRESSIVE SYSTEMIC SCLEROSIS (SCLERODERMA)

Progressive Chronic Multisystem Disease

- Classified by the degree of skin thickening
- Fibrosis-like changes in the skin and epithelial tissues of affected organs
- Subsets:
  - Diffuse Cutaneous Scleroderma
    - Heart, lung, GI, kidney
    - ANA(+)
    - Anticentromere Antibody (–)
    - Rapid onset after Raynaud's phenomenon
    - Variable course—poor prognosis
  - Limited cutaneous Scleroderma—CREST Syndrome
    - Progression after Raynaud's phenomenon
    - Anticentromere Antibody (+)
    - Good prognosis
  - Overlap syndromes
    - Combinations of connective tissue disease
  - Undefined CTD
    - No clinical or laboratory findings
  - Localized scleroderma
    - Morphea, linear scleroderma

> **Crest Syndrome**
> - Calcinosis
> - Raynaud's phenomenon
> - Esophageal dysmotility
> - Sclerodactyly
> - Telangiectasia

Clinical

- Skin thickening—face, trunk, neck
- Symmetric arthritis with involvement of the fingers, hands, arm, legs
- Initial symptoms—Raynaud's phenomenon with fatigue, and musculoskeletal complaints

📖 **Raynaud's Phenomenon**

- Vasospasm of the muscular digital arteries can lead to ischemia, ulceration of the fingertips
- Triggered by cold and emotional stresses
- Reversal of episode occurs after stimulus has ended—and digits rewarmed
- Present in 90% of patients with scleroderma
- Treatment
  - Education against triggers—cold, smoking
  - Rewarming
  - Calcium channel blockers—nifedipine
  - EMG and biofeedback—self-regulation

> **Causes of Raynaud's**
> - Collagen vascular disease—PSS, SLE, RA, Dematomyositis/Polymyositis
> - Arterial occlusive disease
> - Pulmonary HTN
> - Neurologic—SCI, CVA
> - Blood dyscrasia
> - Trauma
> - Drugs—ergots, beta blockers, cisplatin
>
> (Braunwald, et al., 2001)

Treatment

- Rehabilitation
- Maintain ROM—twice per day
- ↑ skin elasticity
- Strengthening exercises

📖 Eosinophilic Fascitis
- Variant of PSS
- Precipitated by strenuous exercise
- Exercise should be done in a noninflammatory state
- Pain and swelling
- Tx—Steroids

POLYMYOSITIS/DERMATOMYOSITIS

Striated muscle involvement with profound symmetrical weakness of the proximal muscles:
- Shoulder and hip girdle
- Anterior neck flexors
- Pharyngeal involvement; dysphagia results

Five Types

- TYPE 1—Primary idiopathic polymyositis; insidious onset
  - Weakness starts at the pelvic girdle → shoulder girdle → neck
  - Dysphagia/dysphonia
  - Remission and exacerbation common
  - Moderate-severe arthritis
  - Atrophic skin over knuckles
- TYPE II—Primary idiopathic dermatomyositis; acute onset
  - Proximal muscle weakness, tenderness
  - Heliotrope rash with periorbital edema
  - Malaise, fever and weight loss
- 📖 TYPE III—Dermatomyositis or polymyositis; associated with malignancy—5% to 8%
  - Male > 40 years old
  - Poor prognosis
- TYPE IV—Childhood dermatomyositis or polymyositis
  - Rapid progressive weakness
  - Respiratory weakness
  - 📖 Severe joint contractures—more disabling in a child
- TYPE V—Polymyositis or dermatomyositis; associated with collagen vascular disease

📖 Clinical Features of Polymyositis/Dermatomyositis-Modified ARA Criteria

- Symmetric proximal muscle weakness
  - Hips first then the shoulders
  - (+/–) respiratory muscle involvement
  - Dysphagia
- 📖 Muscle biopsy
  - Perifascicular atrophy
  - Evidence of necrosis of type I and II fibers
  - Variation in fiber size
  - Large nuclei
- Elevation of muscle enzymes
  - Increased aldolase creatinine kinase (CK), transaminases, LDH
- 📖 EMG—Myopathic changes—positive sharp waves, fibrillation potentials and complex repetitive discharges (CRD)
  - Small, short polyphasic motor units, with early recruitment

  - Decreased amplitude
  - Decreased duration
- Dermatologic features—Dermatomyositis
  - Lilac heliotrope rash with periorbital edema
  - Gottron's papules—scaly dermatitis over the dorsum of the hand—MCP, PIP

Poor Prognostic Factors

- Old age
- Malignancy
- Cardiac involvement
- Delayed initiation of corticosteroid therapy
- Respiratory muscle weakness—aspiration pneumonia
- Joint contractures

Treatment

- Corticosteroids, second line—azathioprine or MTX
- ROM, isometric exercises
- Follow—serum enzymes and manual muscle strength

📖 Juvenile Dermatomyositis

- Seen more commonly than polymyositis in children
- Slight female preponderance
- Heliotrope rash is a predominant feature
- Presence of clumsiness is often unrecognized
- Clinically—transient arthritis, elevated rash
- 80% to 90% respond well to corticosteroids

KEY POINTS OF ARTHRIDITIES

The following tables indicate in what circumstances ANA, RF and HLA-B27 are positive or negative.

📖 ANA AND RF

	ANA	RF
MCTD	+	+
RA	+	+
SLE	+	−
Scleroderma (PSS)	+	−
Polymyositis	+	−
Sjögren's	+	+

📖 (+) HLA-B27

- AS
- Reiter's
- Psoriatic arthritis
- Enteropathy arthropathy
- Pauciarticular JRA

▪
VASCULITIS

POLYARTERITIS NODOSA

- Systemic necrotizing vasculitis
- Male:female ratio is 2:1
- Small, medium artery involvement
- Glomerulonephritis—#1 cause of death
- Lungs spared
- Skin—palpable purpura
- Mononeuritis multiplex, arthritis

Also seen in:
• RA
• SLE
• Sjögren's

GIANT CELL ARTERITIS: ALSO KNOWN AS TEMPORAL ARTERITIS (TA)

- More common in females > 50 years old
- Large arteries
- Tenderness of the scalp and in the muscle of mastication
- Headaches, abrupt visual loss in 15% of patients
- Diagnosis: Elevated ESR, temporal artery biopsy
- Treatment: High dose steroids imperative to prevent permanent visual loss

📖 Polymyalgia Rheumatica (PMR)

In view of clinical similarities between PMR patients with and without signs of arteritis in a temporal artery biopsy, many authors believe that PMR is an expression of giant cell arteritis
- Fever, weight loss, malaise
- Proximal muscles—neck, pelvic
- Shoulder
- Morning stiffness—muscle tenderness
- Abrupt myalgias/arthralgia
- Diagnosis: ↑ ESR > 50
- Treatment: steroids

WEGENER'S GRANULOMATOSIS

- Small artery involvement
- Male, middle aged
- Necrotizing granulomatous vasculitis involving
  - Upper/lower respiratory tract
  - Focal segmental glomerulonephritis
- "Saddle-nose" deformity
- Pulmonary, tracheal, ocular, and cutaneous manifestation

TAKAYASU

- Elastic large arteries—Aorta
- Asian females, 40 years old
- Erythema nodosum on the legs
- Pulselessness, arm claudication

BEHÇET'S

- Small vessels
- Oral and genital skin ulcers
- 20% experience venous thrombosis

GOODPASTURE'S

- Pulmonary and kidney involvement

■

SJÖGREN'S SYNDROME

Autoimmune-mediated disorder of the exocrine glands

📖 CLINICAL PRESENTATION: (sicca symptoms)

- Dry eyes
- Dry mouth
- Skin lesions
- Parotid involvement

LABS: ANA (+), RF (+)

Classification: Primary and secondary forms
- Primary—Dry eyes and mouth with ANA (+) , RF (+)
- Secondary—sicca symptoms
  - Sjögren's syndrome plus evidence of SLE, RA, PSS, Polymyositis

EXTRAGLANDULAR MANIFESTATIONS

- Arthralgias
- Raynaud's phenomenon

ARTHRITIS AND INFECTIOUS DISORDERS

SEPTIC ARTHRITIS

Clinical Picture: Septic Arthritis

- Rapid onset of moderate to severe joint pain, erythema, and decreased ROM
- Monoarticular, leukocytosis
- Knee is the most common joint
- Risk factors—age, prosthetic joints, comorbidities such as anemia, chronic diseases, hemophilia.
- 📖 N. gonorrhea → most common in adults
- 📖 Staph. aureus → most common in children

Children

Causes
- Otitis, infected IV lines

Presentation
- Large joints, monoarticular
- Polyarticular infections
- Neonates and greater than two years: Staph. aureus and group B strep
- Six months to two years: H. influenza

Adults/Elderly

Causes
- In adults ≤ 60 years of age, main cause is STD (sexually transmitted disease)
- > 60 years of age—source is commonly from another focus

Presentation
- N. gonorrhea—Most common form of acute bacterial arthritis

Rheumatoid Arthritis
- Staph. aureus

Most Common Organisms That Cause Septic Arthritis (by Age category)

Neonates	6 Mo–2 Yrs of Age	Children > 2 Yrs	Adults	RA
Staph. aureus Group B Strep	H. influenza	Staph. aureus Group B strep	N. gonorrhea	Staph. aureus

Diagnostic Approach

- Synovial fluid analysis—most important test
- Inflammatory
- Radiologic exam
- Plain films
  Early: soft tissue swelling
  Later: joint space narrowing, erosions, gas formation (E. Coli)
- Bone scans

Treatment

- Antibiotic coverage
- Frequent needle aspirations with arthroscopic lavage

📖 **TABLE 3–7.** Joint Fluid Analysis

Property	Normal	Noninflammatory	Inflammatory	Septic
Viscosity	High	High	Low	Variable
Color	Colorless	Straw	Yellow	Turbid-Yellow
Clarity	Transluscent	Transluscent	Transluscent	Opaque
WBC	< 200	< 5000	1000–75000	> 100,000
PMN%	< 25	< 25	> 50	> 85
Culture	Negative	Negative	Negative	Positive
Mucin clot	Good	Good	Fair	Poor
Glucose	Equal to blood	Equal to blood	< 50 mg/dl lower than blood	> 50 mg/dl lower than blood

OTHER INFECTIOUS CAUSES OF ARTHRITIS

- **Viral Infections**—Rubella, infectious hepatitis
- **Fungi**—Seen in Immunocompromised adults
- **Mycobacterium**—tuberculosis of the spine (Pott's disease)
  - Thoracic involvement
  - 📖 TB arthritis—Hips and knees
    - Monoarticular
    - Radiologic findings—Phemister's triad
      - ♦ Juxta-articular osteoporosis
      - ♦ Marginal erosions
      - ♦ Joint space narrowing
- **Lyme Disease**
  - Tick borne—Borrelia burgdorferi
  - Classic presentation
    - Erythema migrans—bull's eye rash
    - Cardiac, neurologic, articular manifestations
  - 📖 Intermittent migratory episodes of polyarthritis
  - Commonly affects the knee
  - Synovial fluid—Inflammatory
  - Diagnosis—ELISA, Western blot analysis
  - Management—First-line antibiotics:
    - Adults: Doxycycline
    - Children: Amoxicillin
  - Pattern of Onset:
    - Bite
    - Rash
    - Systemic dz.
    - Neurologic involvement

▪
DEPOSITION AND STORAGE DISEASE

HEMOCHROMATOSIS

- Organ damage and tissue dysfunction secondary to excessive iron stores and the deposition of hemosiderin
- Organs → Hepatic cirrhosis, cardiomyopathy, DM, pituitary dysfunction
- Skin pigmentation
- Chronic progressive arthritis
  - Occurs commonly in second and third MCP, PIP joints. It may also affect the hip joints
- Males ~40–50 years old
- Treatment: Phlebotomy, NSAIDs

ALKAPTONURIA (OCHRONOSIS)

- Autosomal recessive
- Deficiency in the enzyme homogentisic acid oxidase leads to its increase
- Alkalinization and oxidation causes darkening of tissue parts termed 🕮 ochronosis
  - Blueish discoloration of the urine, cartilage, skin, sclera secondary to the accumulation of homogentisic acid
- Progressive degenerative arthropathy
  - Onset—in the fourth decade
  - Spinal column involvement
  - Arthritis of the large joints, chondrocalcinosis, effusions, osteochrondral bodies

WILSON'S DISEASE

- Autosomal recessive
- Deposition of copper leads to destruction:
  - Liver leading to cirrhosis
  - Brain
  - Kidneys
  - Ocular—Kayser-Fleischer rings
- OA—wrists, MCP, knees, spine
- Osteoporosis
- Treatment: Copper chelation with penicillamine, dietary restriction

GAUCHER'S DISEASE

- Autosomal recessive—Ashkenazi Jews
- Glucocerebroside accumulates in the reticuloendothelial cells of the spleen, liver, and bone marrow
- Monoarticular hip and knee degeneration

■

OTHER SYSTEMIC DISEASES

SARCOIDOSIS

- Systemic chronic granulomatous disease—can affect any organ system
- Pathogenesis: disseminated noncaseating granulomatous
- Eight times more common in blacks, females > males
- Clinical features:
  - Pulmonary
  - Hilar adenopathy
  - Fever, weight loss, fatigue
  - Arthritis: polyarthritis, 4-6 joints
    - Knees, PIP, MCP, wrists
  - Skin—Lofgren's Syndrome
  - Arthritis, Hilar adenopathy, Erythema nodosum

AMYLOIDOSIS

- Homogeneous eosinophilic material seen with Congo red dye
- Deposition of amyloid in the kidneys, liver and spleen
- Clinical features:
  - Renal disease is primary clinical feature
  - Cardiomyopathy
  - Median neuropathy
  - Pseudoarthritis—periarticular joint inflammation
  - Effusions: Arthrocentesis—"Shoulder-pad" sign

HEMOPHILIA ARTHROPATHY

- X-linked recessive disorder, predominately in males—associated with HIV 2° to transfusions of factor and blood
- Blood coagulation disorder caused by Factor VIII deficiency (classic hemophilia A) and Factor IX deficiency (Christmas disease, hemophilia B)
- Bleeding into bones and soft tissue causes hemarthrosis, necrosis and compartment syndrome
- Elbow, knee, wrist are common
- 📖 Arthritis is caused by the remaining blood in the joint depositing hemosiderin into the synovial lining → proliferation of the synovium and pannus formation
- Radiologic: Joint space narrowing, subchondral sclerosis and cyst formation
- 📖 Treatment: Conservative care (immobilization, rest, ice), Factor VIII replacement, rehabilitation, joint aspiration as a last resort

SICKLE-CELL DISEASE

- Biconcave RBC changes to an elongated crescent sickle-shape causing obstruction of the microvasculature
- Musculoskeletal complications:
  - Painful crisis—Most common event
    - Abdomen, chest, back
    - Pain in the large joints from juxta-articular bone infarcts with synovial ischemia

– Dactylitis—"Hand-Foot" Syndrome
  ▪ Painful non-pitting swelling of the hands and feet
– Osteonecrosis
  ▪ Local hypoxia with occlusion to the venous system by the sickled cells
  ▪ 1/3 femoral heads and 1/4 humeral heads go on to osteonecrosis
– Osteomyelitis—most commonly caused by Salmonella

■

NEUROPATHIC ARTHROPATHY (CHARCOT'S JOINT)

DEFINITION

Chronic progressive degenerative arthropathy, secondary to a sensory neuropathy with loss of proprioception and pain sensation, leading to instability and joint destruction

CAUSES → "STD" "SKA" → SHOULDER, KNEE, ANKLE

- Syringomyelia → Shoulder
- Tabes dorsalis # 2 → Syphilis → Knee
- Diabetic Neuropathy → # 1 cause → Ankle

CLINICAL

- Early findings: Painless swelling, effusion and joint destruction
- Late findings: Crepitation, destruction of cartilage and bones, intra-articular loose bodies
- Subtle fractures

RADIOLOGIC

- Joint destruction
- Hypertrophic osteophytes
- Loose bodies caused by micro fractures
- Disorganization of the joint—Subluxation and dislocation

TREATMENT

- Immobilization
- Restriction of weight bearing

📖 **Charcot Joint vs. Osteoarthritis**

May mimic OA early in the disease—
Both have:
- Soft tissue swelling
- Osteophytes
- Joint effusion

Charcot joints have:
- Bony fragments
- Subluxation
- Periarticular debris

TABLE 3–8. Hip Pain in Children (Janig and Stanton-Hicks 1996; Kaggs and Tolo 1996; Koop Quanbeck 1996; Jensen et al. 1990)

	Congenital Hip Dislocation	Slipped Capital Femoral Epiphysis (SCFE)	Legg-Calve-Perthes Disease (LCPD)
Definition	Dislocated hip at birth	Femoral head may slip, displacing it medially and posteriorly in relation to the shaft of the femur at the level of the proximal femoral epiphysis	Idiopathic AVN of the femoral head
Present	Birth	2:1 males: females 13–16 yrs males 11–13 yrs females Bilateral involvement: 30–40%	Onset: 2–12 yrs old; if onset is > 12 yrs old it is considered AVN not LCPD Boys >> girls Majority—unilateral
Etiologic Factors	First born—tight uterine and abdominal musculature of mother Inhibits fetal movement Breech position Left hip > right Hormonal factors More common in white	Strain on the growth plate During its growth spurt secondary to increased weight 📖 Endocrinopathies linked w/SCFE Hypothyroidism—most common Growth hormone abnormalities Down Syndrome	Bone age low for age results in short stature Etiology unknown Linked w/hypothyroid abnormality
Physical Exam/ Signs and Symptoms	*Barlow's Test—dislocation* Start with hip in flexion and abduction, then the femoral head is dislocated on hip flexion and adduction *Ortolani's Test—relocation* Hip is relocated on hip flexion and abduction	Pain and altered gait Pain in the groin, medial thigh and knee *Chronic Slip*-most common Loss of internal rotation—when the hip is flexed it rolls into external rotation *Acute Slip* Trauma, sudden onset of pain on weight bearing Acute or Chronic Chondrolysis Erosion and degeneration of the cartilage inflaming the synovial membrane on activity	Mild to intermittent or no pain Stiffness Painless limp→ antalgic gait Hip flexion contracture—use Thomas test Limitations in abduction and internal rotation Disuse atrophy Short stature
Radiologic Findings	Not useful until 6 weeks Negative finding on x-ray does not rule out a dislocation Proximal and lateral migration of the femoral head from the acetabulum Acetabular dysplasia Delayed ossification	Must obtain AP and frog leg position Grading based on degree of displacement of the epiphysis Grade I: < 33% Grade II: 33–50% Grade III: > 50%	Plain films and frog-leg views of the pelvis Chronological Sequence 1. Growth arrest—avascular stage 2. Subchondral fracture—"Crescent sign" 3. Resorption 4. Reossification 5. Healed

TABLE 3-8   *(Continued)*

	Congenital Hip Dislocation	Slipped Capital Femoral Epiphysis (SCFE)	Legg-Calve-Perthes Disease (LCPD)
Treatment	• Goal—return the hip into its normal position until there is resolution of the pathologic changes • Closed Reduction— < 6 mo • Position devices Triple diapers Frejka pillows Splints: Craig, Von Rosen-Pavlik harness: allows hip motion within the safe zone while maintaining abduction • Traction, casting, surgical	• Bed rest—weight relief • Prevention of further displacement • Surgery is the preferred method of treatment— Knowles pinning • Nonsurgical—traction, body casts, hormonal therapy	1. Eliminate hip pain 2. Restoration of motion 3. Prevent femoral head collapse Containment techniques • Permit weight bearing of the femoral head to assist healing and remodeling • Greater than 6 years old • Abduction braces Petrie casts, Toronto brace, Salter stirrup • Surgical— Epiphysiodesis Valgus Osteotomy
Complication	1. AVN	1. Chondrolysis 2. AVN 3. OA	1. AVN

Thomas Test:
To detect flexion contractures of the hip and evaluate range of hip flexion
1. Patient Supine, hand under lumbar region to stabilize—Flex hip
2. Notice where patient back touches hand
3. Flex one hip, then other as far as possible
4. Have patient hold one leg on chest, lower other leg flat

Indicators of fixed flexion contracture/deformity:
1. Hip does not extend fully
2. Pt. rocks forward, lifts thoracic region, or arches back to reform lordosis

---

Acute Transient Synovitis
• Most common cause of hip pain in kids
• Self-limiting, preadolescent
• Good outcome

Cause of Avascular Necrosis
"Plastic Rags"

P—pancreatitis	R—radiation
L—lupus	A—amyloid
A—alcohol	G—Gaucher's disease
S—steroids	S—sickle cell
T—trauma	
I—idiopathic, infection	
C—caisson disease, collagen vascular disease	

■
FIBROMYALGIA SYNDROME (FMS)

CLINICAL FEATURES

- Diffuse aching stiffness and fatigue with multiple tender points in specific areas
  - Headaches
  - Neck and upper trapezius discomfort
  - Upper extremity paraesthesias
  - Fatigue—lack of sleep
- Females—20–60 years old
- May experience morning stiffness but it varies throughout the day
- Triggers may exacerbate symptoms:
  1. Physical activity
  2. Inactivity
  3. Sleep disturbance
  4. Emotional stress
- May be associated with Irritable Bowel Syndrome, RA, Lyme, hyperthyroidism

ARA CLASSIFICATION:

1. Widespread pain—pain in the left and right side of the body above and below the waist.
   Axial involvement—Cervical, anterior chest, thoracic, and low back
2. Pain in 11–18 tender points (Figure 3-5)
   Bilateral involvement
   Occipital, lower cervical, trapezius, supraspinatus, second rib, lateral epicondyle, gluteal, greater trochanter, knee

> **Classification**
> - Need to have satisfied both criteria
> - Present at least three months

FMS SHOULD BE DIFFERENTIATED FROM MYOFASCIAL PAIN SYNDROME AND CHRONIC FATIGUE SYNDROME

Myofascial Pain Syndrome

- Local pain and tender points that resolves with local treatment, but may recur
- Fatigue, morning stiffness uncommon

Chronic Fatigue Syndrome

- Disabling fatigue at least six months
- Preceded by a viral syndrome

TREATMENT OF FMS

- Patient education and reassurance
- Nortriptyline—sleep disturbance

- NSAIDs and corticosteroids
- Combination therapy is effective
- Biofeedback, tender point injection
- Acupuncture, aerobic exercise

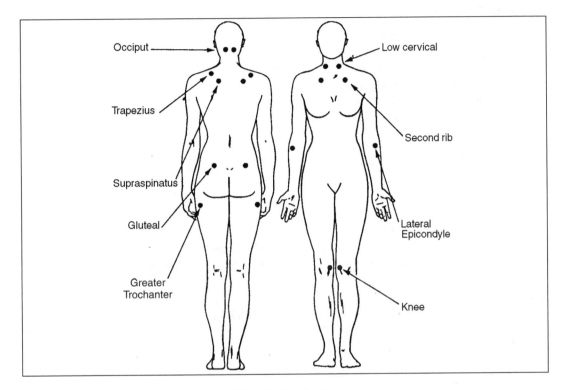

FIGURE 3–5. Fibromyalgia: Location of Specific Tender Points

■

COMPLEX REGIONAL PAIN DISORDER (CRPD)

OTHER NAMES

- Sudeck's atrophy
- Algodystrophy
- Shoulder hand syndrome
- RSD: Reflex Sympathetic Dystrophy

CHARACTERISTICS

- Limb pain, swelling, and autonomic dysfunction
- Most commonly caused by minor or major trauma

CLINICAL FEATURE

- Pain, deep burning exacerbated by movement
  - Allodynia—pain induced by a nonnoxious stimulus
  - Hyperalgesia—lower pain threshold and enhanced pain perception
- Local edema and vasomotor changes
  - Extremity is warm, red, and dry initially
  - Later becomes cool, mottled, and cyanotic
- Muscle weakness
- Dystrophic changes
  - Thin, shiny skin, brittle nails

CLINICAL STAGES

1. Acute—few weeks–6 months
   - Pain, hypersensitivity, swelling, and vasomotor changes
   - Increased blood flow creating temperature and skin-color changes
   - Hyperhidrosis
2. Dystrophic—3–6 months
   - Persistent pain, disability, and atrophic skin changes
   - Decreased blood flow, decreased temperature
   - Hyperhidrosis
3. Atrophic
   - Atrophy and contractures
   - Skin glossy, cool, and dry

RADIOGRAPHIC FINDINGS

1. Plain radiographs
   - Sudeck's atrophy—patchy osteopenia, ground-glass appearance
2. Three-phase bone scan
   - First two phases are nonspecific, osteoporosis
   - Third phase—abnormal, with enhanced uptake in the peri-articular structures

TREATMENT

1. Immediate mobilization—Passive and active ROM, massage, contrast baths, TENS
2. Pain control—NSAIDs, narcotic
3. Inflammation—Corticosteroids, initial dose 60–80 mg/day qid dosing for two weeks then gradual tapering the next two weeks
4. Cervical sympathetic ganglia block for the upper extremities, lumbar ganglion block for the lower extremities
5. Surgical sympathectomy—if block is beneficial but transient

TABLE 3–9. 📖 CRPD: Complex Regional Pain Disorder Children and Adolescents vs. Adults (Janig and Stanton Hicks, 1995)

	Children	Adults
Site	Lower extremity	Upper extremity
Spontaneous pain	Common	Common
Allodynia	Most patients	Most patients
Sex ratio	Female:male 4:1	Mixed
Three-phase bone scan	• Mixed results: Used to rule out other pathology • See decreased uptake of the extremity—decreased atrophic changes • Occasionally normal • Will have increased uptake normally secondary to bone growth	Increased uptake in the third phase of the affected extremity
Treatment	• Physical therapy alone • Noninvasive—TENS, Biofeedback • Meds—Tricyclic antidepressant • Blocks more common in the upper extremity	Sympathetic blocks
Prognosis	Good	Poor

📖 SYMPATHETIC AND NONSYMPATHETIC CRPD

Four tests used to determine if pain is sympathetically mediated; the first two are used more commonly.

1. Symptomatic block with local anesthetic:
   Local anesthetic is injected at the stellate ganglion (upper extremity) or the lumbar paravertebral ganglion (lower extremity). If relief, then suspect sympathetic etiology
2. Guanethidine test:
   Injection of guanethidine into the extremity distal to a suprasystolic cuff. The test is positive if the pain is reproduced after injection and is immediately relieved after cuff is released
3. Pentolamine test:
   IV pentolamine will reproduce the pain
4. Ischemia test:
   Inflation of the suprasystolic cuff decreases the pain

▪

TENDON DISORDERS

📖 DUPUYTREN'S CONTRACTURE: (Snider, 1997) (Figure 3–6)

- Fibrous contracture of the palmar fascia creating a flexion contracture at the MCP and PIP joints
- More common in white men ~50–70 years of age
- Associated with → epilepsy, pulmonary TB, alcoholism, diabetes mellitus

Mechanism

- The palmar fascia is a continuation of the palmaris longus tendon attaching to the sides of the PIP and middle phalanges
- The fascia is connected to the skin, as it contracts and fibroses, the skin dimples
- Contraction of the fibrous bands into nodules and the fingers develop a flexion contracture

Clinically

- Painless thickening of the palmar surface and underlying fascia
- Most commonly at the fourth and fifth digits

Treatment

- Nonoperative—Trypsin, chymotrypsin, lidocaine injection follow by forceful extension rupturing the skin and fascia improving ROM
- Modalities—heating, stretching, ultrasound
- Surgical—fasciotomy, amputation

- Flexion contracture at the PIP and MCP joints of fourth and fifth digit
- Palmar surface
- Painless

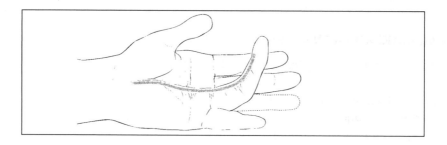

FIGURE 3–6. Dupuytren's Contracture. From Snider RK. Essentials of Musculoskeletal Care. Rosemont, Illinois: American Academy of Orthopaedic Surgeons, 1997, with permission.

TRIGGER FINGER: "SNAPPING FINGER SENSATION" (Figure 3–7)

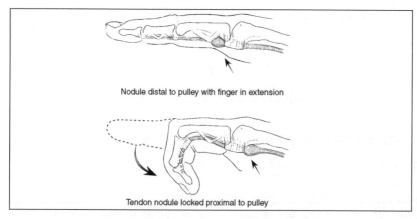

Nodule distal to pulley with finger in extension

Tendon nodule locked proximal to pulley

FIGURE 3–7. Trigger Finger: With finger in extension, nodule is distal to the pulley. When finger is flexed, the tendon locks proximal to the pulley. (Reprinted with permission of American Society for Surgery of the Hand, from Snider RK. Essentials of Musculoskeletal Care. Rosemont, Illinois: American Academy of Orthopaedic Surgeons, 1997, with permission.

- Trauma to the flexor portion of the fingers pinching the flexor tendon within its synovial sheath
- Ligamentous sheath thickens and a nodule is formed within it
- When the finger is flexed, the nodule moves proximally, re-extension is prevented
- A locking sensation is felt or clicking when the nodule passes though the tendon sheath

📖 MALLET FINGER

- Most common extensor tendon injury (Snider, 1997)
- Rupture of the extensor tendon into the distal phalanx secondary to forceful flexion
- The DIP drops remains in a flexed position and cannot be extended actively
- Treatment: Splinting to immobilize the distal phalanx in hyperextension
  Acute—6 week
  Chronic—12 weeks
- Surgical: poor healing, volar subluxation, avulsion > one third of bone

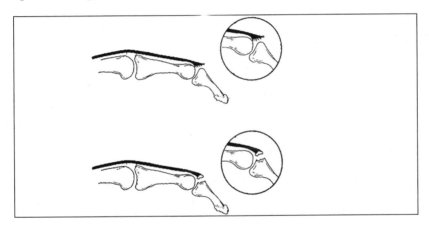

FIGURE 3–8. Mallet finger caused by: Top: Rupture of the extensor tendon at its insertion. Bottom: Avulsion of a portion of the distal phalanx.

REFERENCES

Arnett FC, Edworthy SM, Bloch DA, et al: The American Rheumatism Association 1987 reviied criteria for the classification of rheumatoid arthritis. Arthritis Rheum. 1988; 31:315–324.

Berkow R, Elliott L. Rheumatoid Arthritis: New Approaches for Its Evaluation and Management. *Arch Phys Med Rehabil* 1995; 76:190–201.

Braunwald E, Fauci AS, Kaspar DL, et al, eds. Harrisons Principles of Internal Medicine 15th ed. New York: McGraw-Hill, 2001.

Cailliet, R, *Hand Pain and Impairment 3rd ed*. Philadelphia: F.A. Davis Company, 1982.

Gerber LH, Hicks JE, Surgical and Rehabilitation Options in the Treatment of the Rheumatoid Arthritis Patient Resistant to Pharmacologic Agents. *Rheum Dis Clin North Am*. 1995; 21:19–39

Hicks JE, Sutin J, Rehabilitation in Joint and Connective Tissue Diseases: Approach to the Diagnosis of Rheumatoid Diseases. *Arch Phys Med Rehabil*. 1988; 69:(suppl):S78–83.

Janig W, Stanton-Hicks M, eds. *Progress in Pain Research and Management vol 6. Reflex Sympathetic Dystrophy in Children and Adolescents: Differences from Adults. Reflex Sympathetic Dystrophy: A Reappraisal.* Seattle: IASP Press, 1996.

Jensen HP, Steinke MS, Mikkelsen SS, et al., Hip physiolysis. Bilaterally in 62 cases followed for 20 years. Acta Orthop Scand. 1990, 61(5):419–420.

Kelly WN, Harris ED Jr., Ruddy S, Sledge CB, *Textbook of Rheumatology 5th ed. vol 1,2*. Philadelphia: W.B. Saunders Co., 1997.

Klippel, JH, *Primer on the Rheumatic Diseases 11th ed*. Atlanta: Arthritis Foundation, 1997.

Koop S, Quanbeck D. Three common causes of childhood hip pain. Pediatr Clin North Am. 1996, 43(5):1053–1066.

Lane NE, Pain Management in Osteoarthritis: The Role of Cox-2 Inhibitors. *J Rheumatol.* 1997, 24:20–24.

Martel W. The occipito-atlanto-axial joints in rheumatoid arthritis and ankylosing spondylitis. AJR. 1961, 86(2):223–239.

Park WM, O'Neill M, McCall IW. The radiology of rheumatoid involvement of the cervical spine. Skeletal Radiol. 1979, 4:1–7.

Rapoff MA, Purviance MR, Lindsley CB, Educational and Behavioral Strategies for Improving Medication Compliance in Juvenile Rheumatoid Arthritis. *Arch Phys Med Rehabil.* 1988; 69: 439–41.

Skaggs DL, Tolo VT. Legg-Calve-Perthes Disease. *J Am Acad Orthop Surg.* 1996, 4(1):9–16.

Snider RK, Essentials of Musculoskeletal Care. Rosemont, Illinois: American Academy of Orthopaedic Surgeons, 1997.

Stenger AA, vanLeeuwen MA, Houtman PM, et al., Early Effective Suppression of Inflammation in Rheumatoid Arthritis Reduces Radiologic Progression. *Br J Radiol.* 1998; 37: 1157–1163.

Verhoeven AC. Combination Therapy in Rheumatoid Arthritis: Updated Systematic Review. *Br J Radiol.* 1998; 37:612–619.

RECOMMENDED READING

Cailliet, R. *Neck and Arm Pain 3rd ed.* Philadelphia: F.A. Davis Company, 1991.

DeLisa JA, *Rehabilitation Medicine: Principles and Practice.* Philadelphia: JB Lippincott, 1988.

Duthie RB, Harris CM, A Radiographic and Clinical Survey of the Hip Joint in Sero-positive Arthritis. *Acta Orthop Scand.* 1969;40:346–64.

Nicholas JJ. *Rehabilitation of Patients with Rehsumatic Disorders.* In Braddom RL. Physical Medicine and Rehabilitation. Philadelphia: W.B. Saunders Co.; 1996.

Sponsellar PD, and Stevens HM, *Handbook of Pediatric Orthopedics.* Boston: Little, Brown and Company, 1996.

Wall PD, Melzack R, *Textbook of Pain 3rd ed.* New York: Churchhill Livingstone, 1994: 685–691.

4

MUSCULOSKELETAL MEDICINE

UPPER EXTREMITIES—David P. Brown, D.O., Eric D. Freeman, D.O.,
and Sara Cuccurullo, M.D.
LOWER EXTREMITIES—David P. Brown, D.O., Eric D. Freeman, D.O.,
and Sara Cuccurullo, M.D.
SPINE—Ted L. Freeman, D.O. and Eric D. Freeman D.O.

■

UPPER EXTREMITIES—SHOULDER REGION

FUNCTIONAL ANATOMY

Range of Motion (Figure 4–1)

- Flexion: 180°
- Extension: 60°
- Abduction: 180°
  - Abduction of 120° is seen in normals with the thumb pointed down.
- Adduction: 60°
- Internal rotation: 90° (with arm abducted)
- External rotation: 90° (with arm abducted)

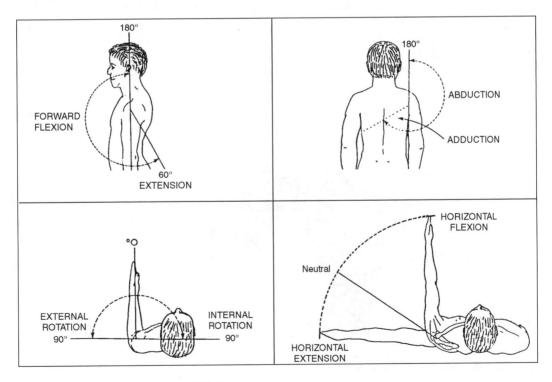

FIGURE 4–1. Shoulder Range of Motion.

Shoulder Motion

Flexion (Figure 4–2)

- Deltoid, anterior portion (axillary nerve from posterior cord, C5, C6)
- Pectoralis major, clavicular portion (medial and lateral pectoral nerve, C5, C6, C7, C8, T1)
- Biceps brachii (musculocutaneous nerve from lateral cord, C5, C6)
- Coracobrachialis (musculocutaneous nerve from lateral cord, C5, C6)

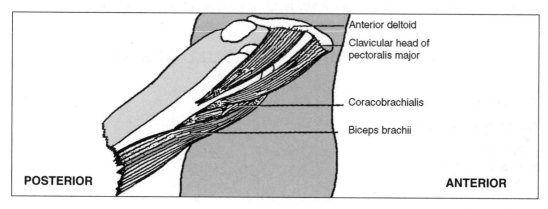

FIGURE 4–2. Arm Flexors (lateral view).

Extension (Figure 4–3)

- Deltoid, posterior portion (axillary nerve from posterior cord, C5, C6)
- Latissimus dorsi (thoracodorsal nerve from posterior cord, C6, C7, C8)
- Teres major (lower subscapular nerve from posterior cord, C5, C6)
- Triceps long head (radial, C6, C7, C8)
- Sternocostal portion of pectoralis major (medial and lateral pectoral nerve, C5, C6, C7, C8, T1)

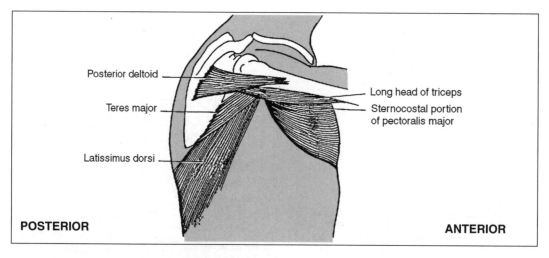

FIGURE 4–3. Arm Extensors (lateral view).

Abduction (Figure 4–4)

- Deltoid, middle portion (axillary nerve from posterior cord, C5, C6)
- Supraspinatus (suprascapular nerve from upper trunk, C5, C6)

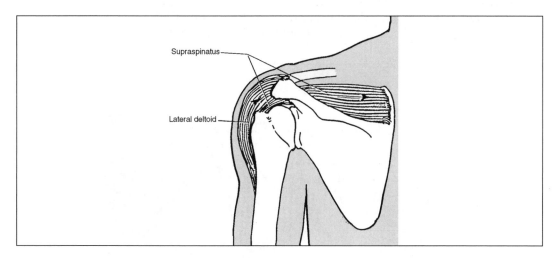

FIGURE 4–4. Arm Abductors (posterior view).

Adduction (Figure 4–5)

- Pectoralis major (medial and lateral pectoral nerve, C5, C6, C7, C8, T1)
- Latissimus dorsi (thoracodorsal nerve from posterior cord, C6, C7, C8)
- Teres major (lower subscapular nerve from posterior cord, C5, C6)
- Coracobrachialis (musculocutaneous nerve from lateral cord, C5, C6, C7)
- Infraspinatus (suprascapular nerve from upper trunk, C4, C5, C6)
- Long head of triceps (radial nerve from posterior cord, C6, C7, C8)
- Anterior and posterior deltoid (axillary nerve from posterior cord, C5, C6)

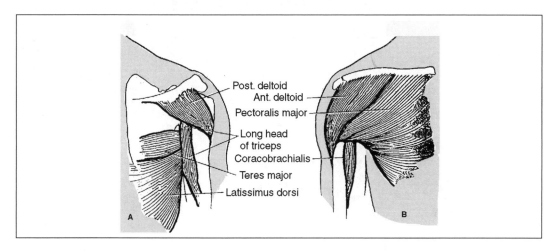

FIGURE 4–5. Arm Adductors. **A.** Posterior View. **B.** Anterior View.

Internal (Medial) Rotation (Figure 4–6)

- Subscapularis (upper and lower subscapular nerve from the posterior cord, C5, C6)
- Pectoralis major (medial and lateral pectoral nerve, C5, C6, C7, C8, T1)
- Latissimus dorsi (thoracodorsal nerve from posterior cord, C5, C6)
- Deltoid, anterior portion (axillary nerve from posterior cord, C5, C6)
- Teres major (lower subscapular nerve from posterior cord C5, C6)

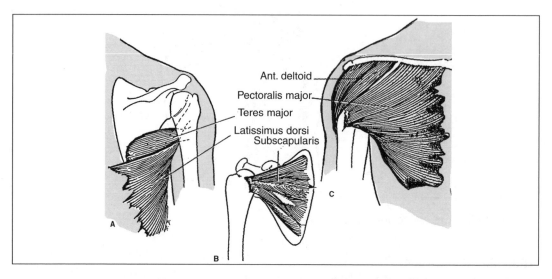

FIGURE 4–6. Major Medial Rotators of the Arm. **A.** Posterior View. **B.** and **C.** Anterior View.

External (Lateral) Rotation (Figure 4–7)

- Infraspinatus (suprascapular nerve from upper trunk, C5, C6)
- Teres minor (axillary nerve from posterior cord, C5, C6)
- Deltoid, posterior portion (axillary nerve from posterior cord, C5, C6)
- Supraspinatus (suprascapular nerve from upper trunk, C4, C5, C6)

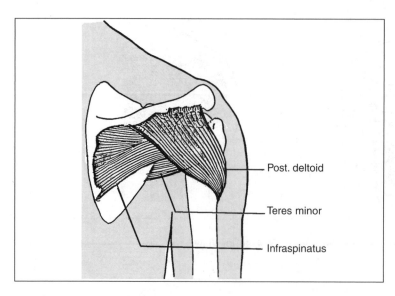

FIGURE 4–7. Major Lateral Rotators of the Arm (posterior view).

Shoulder Girdle Complex: Glenohumeral Joint

Glenoid Fossa
Articulates with 30% of the humeral head

Labrum (Figure 4–8)
- The labrum is a redundant fibrocartilaginous fold of capsular tissue surrounding the glenoid fossa
- This tissue deepens the fossa increasing the contact between the humeral head and glenoid by roughly 70%
- It serves as an attachment for the glenohumeral ligaments and tendons, and prevents anterior and posterior humeral head dislocation

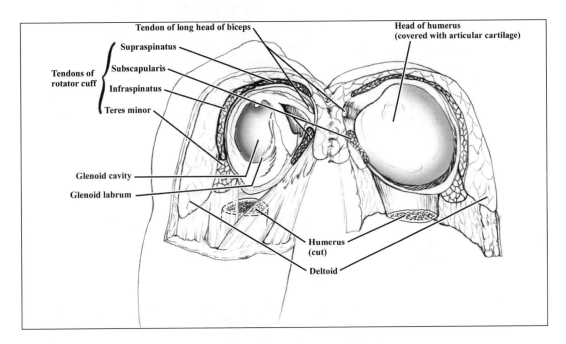

FIGURE 4–8. The Glenoid Labrum and Glenoid Fossa (lateral view).

Glenohumeral Capsule
- The capsule arises from the labrum and inserts on the neck of the humerus
- It covers the entire head of the humerus but is not quite adjacent to the glenoid fossa, leaving a small space that separates the two (capsule from the fossa)
- The capsule thickens anteriorly to form the glenohumeral ligaments

Glenohumeral Ligaments (Figure 4–9)
- These ligaments arise from folds of the anterior portion of the capsule and reinforce the joint
- They provide stability and prevent translation of the head of the humerus from the glenoid fossa
- They are composed of three segments, all located on the anterior aspect of the humeral head
  1. **Superior glenohumeral ligament**
     - Prevents translation in the inferior direction
     - This along with the middle glenohumeral ligament provides stability of the shoulder from 0–90° of abduction

2. **Middle glenohumeral ligament**
   – Prevents translation in the anterior direction
3. **Inferior glenohumeral ligament**
   – The primary anterior ligament stabilizer above 90°

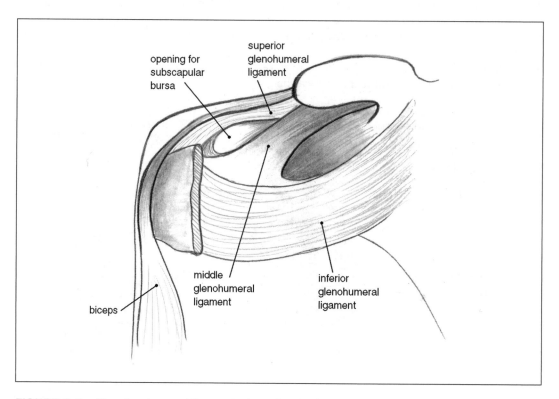

FIGURE 4–9. The glenohumeral ligaments (anterior view) depict a distinct Z pattern formed by the superior glenohumeral ligament, the middle glenohumeral ligament, and the inferior glenohumeral ligament. [Note: The opening for the subscapular bursa is variable.]

Shoulder Joint Stability

Dynamic Stabilizers (Muscles and Tendons)
• Surround the humeral head and help to approximate it into the glenoid fossa
   1. **Rotator cuff muscles (Figures 4–10, 4–11)**
      – "Minor S.I.T.S."
         ■ Supraspinatus
         ■ Infraspinatus
         ■ Teres minor
         ■ Subscapularis
   2. **Long head of the biceps tendon, deltoid, and teres major**

Static Stabilizers
• Include the articular anatomy, capsule, ligaments, as well as the glenoid labrum

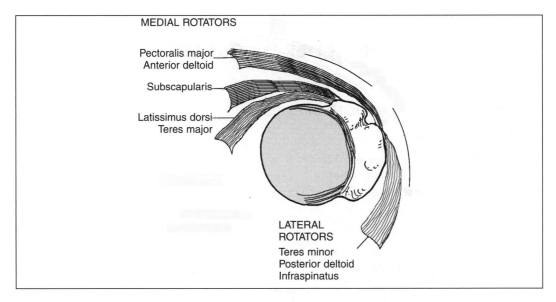

FIGURE 4–10. Right arm superior view: medial rotator; lateral rotators. This diagram depicts the relation of the rotators to the upper end of the humerus.

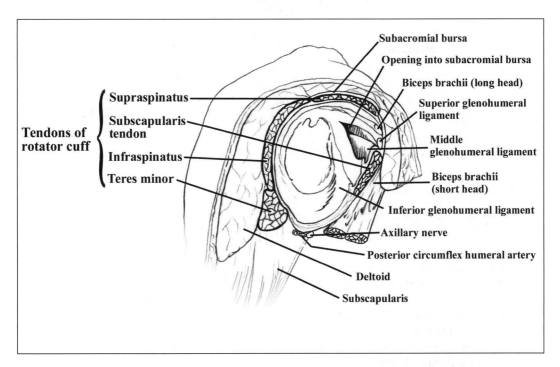

FIGURE 4–11. Right glenoid cavity of the scapula as viewed from the anteriolateral aspect. Note four short rotator cuff muscles (teres minor, infraspinatus, supraspinatus, and subscapularis).

■

SHOULDER DISORDERS

ACROMIOCLAVICULAR (AC) JOINT SPRAINS

General

Acromioclavicular Joint (Figure 4–12)
- Gliding joint that anchors the clavicle
- Disc between the two surfaces

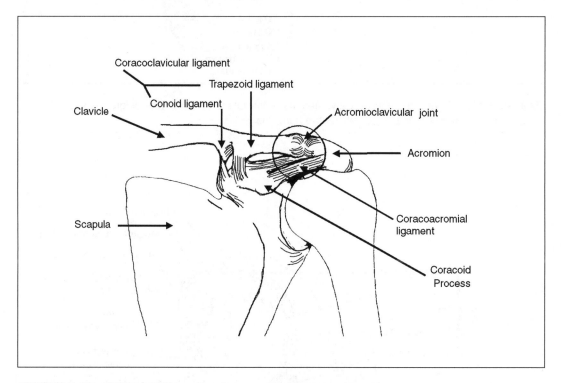

FIGURE 4–12. Anterioposterior view of the acromioclavicular joint. Note the contribution of the coraco-acromial ligaments to the inferior acromio-clavicular joint capsule.

Anatomy: Ligaments
1. **Acromioclavicular (AC) ligament**
   - Connects the distal end of the clavicle to the acromion, providing horizontal stability
2. **Coraco-clavicular (CC) ligament**
   - This ligament is made up of 2 bands: Conoid and trapezoid
   - Connects the coracoid process to the clavicle, providing vertical stability
3. **Coraco-acromial ligament**
   - Connects the coracoid process to the acromion

Mechanism of Injury
- A direct impact to the shoulder
- Falling on an outstretched arm

Classification of AC Joint Separations (See Figure 4–13)

TABLE 4–1

Ligament	Acromioclavicular	Coracoclavicular	Clavicular Displacement
Type I	Partial sprain	Intact	None
Type II	Complete tear	Partial sprain	None
Type III	Complete tear	Complete tear	Superior
Type IV	Complete tear	Complete tear	Posterior and superior into the trapezius, giving a buttonhole appearance
Type V	Complete tear	Complete tear More severe than type III with coracoclavicular space increased over 100%. This indicates disruption of the deltoid and trapezius fibers.	Superior and posterior
Type VI	Complete tear	Complete tear	Inferior

Clinical

- Patients generally complain of tenderness over the AC joint with palpation and range of motion
- AC joint displacement with gross deformity occurs in the later stages and is usually seen in a type III or greater

Provocative tests
- Cross-chest adduction
- Passive adduction of the arm across the midline causing joint tenderness

Imaging

- Weighted AP radiographs of the shoulders (10 lbs)
  - Type III injuries may show a 25% to 100% widening of the clavicular-coracoid area
  - Type V injuries may show a widening > 100%

Treatment

- Depends on the degree of separation
  Acute
  - **Types I and II**
    - Rest, ice, nonsteroidal anti-inflammatory (NSAIDs)
    - Sling for comfort
    - Avoid heavy lifting and contact sports
    - Shoulder-girdle complex strengthening
    - Return to play: When the patient is asymptomatic with full ROM
      - Type I: 2 weeks
      - Type II: 6 weeks
  - **Types III or greater: Controversial**
    - Conservative or surgical, depending on the patient's need (occupation or sport) for particular shoulder stability
    - Surgical: For those indicated (heavy laborers, athletes)
    - Generally, no functional advantage is seen between the two treatment regimens
  - **Types IV to VI**
    - Surgery is recommended: Open reduction internal fixation (ORIF) or distal clavicular resection with reconstruction of the CC ligament

Chronic AC joint pain
- Corticosteroid injection
- May require a clavicular resection and CC reconstruction

Complications
- Associated fractures and dislocations
- Distal clavicle osteolysis
  - Degeneration of the distal clavicle with associated osteopenia and cystic changes

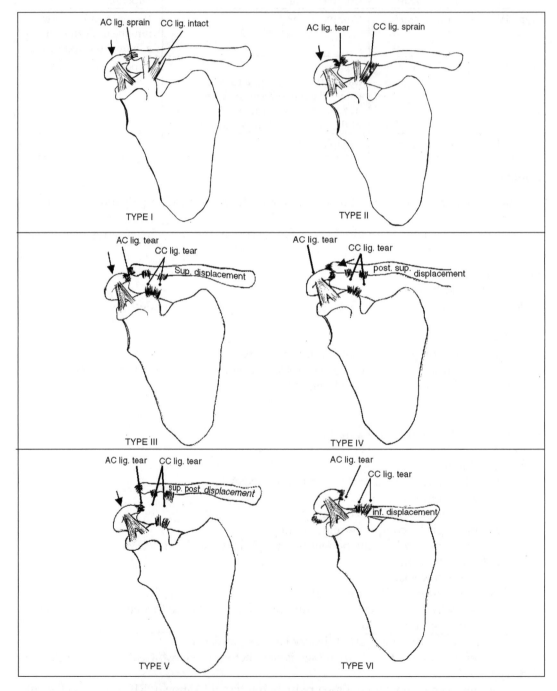

FIGURE 4–13. Classification of AC Joint Separations (Anterior Views) (see Table 4–1 for description).

- AC joint arthritis
  - May get relief from a lidocaine injection and conservative rehabilitative care should be sufficient

GLENOHUMERAL JOINT INJURIES (GHJ)

General

Glenohumeral joint type: Ball and socket
- **Scapulothoracic motion or glenohumeral rhythm**
  - Balance exists between the glenohumeral and scapulothoracic joint during arm abduction
  - There is a 2:1 glenohumeral: scapulothoracic motion accounting for the ability to abduct the arm (60° of scapulothoracic motion to 120° of glenohumeral motion)
  - The scapulothoracic motion allows the glenoid to rotate and permit glenohumeral abduction without acromial impingement

Classification of GHJ Instability

Definitions
- **Instability** is a translation of the humeral head on the glenoid fossa without complete separation. It may result in subluxation or dislocation
- **Subluxation** is a separation of the humeral head from the glenoid fossa with immediate reduction
- **Dislocation** is complete separation of the humeral head from the glenoid fossa without immediate reduction

📖 **Direction of Instability**
- **Anterior glenohumeral instability**
  - Most common direction of instability is anterior inferior
  - More common in the younger population and has a high recurrence rate
  - Mechanism: Arm abduction and external rotation
  - Complication may include axillary nerve injury
- **Posterior glenohumeral instability**
  - Less common than anterior instability
  - May occur as a result of a seizure
  - The patient may present with the arm in the adducted internal rotated position
  - Mechanism: Landing on a forward flexed adducted arm
- **Multidirectional Instability**
  - Rare with instability in multiple planes
  - The patient may display generalized laxity in other joints

Patterns of Instability
- **Traumatic: T.U.B.S.**

T.U.B.S.
T- Traumatic shoulder instability
U- Unidirectional
B- Bankart lesion
S- Surgical management
(Rockwood, Green, et al. 1996)

- **Atraumatic: A.M.B.R.I.**

> **A.M.B.R.I.**
> A- Atraumatic shoulder instability
> M- Multidirection instability
> B- Bilateral lesions
> R- Rehabilitation management
> I- Inferior capsular shift, if surgery
> (Rockwood, Green, et al. 1996)

Associated Fractures
- Anterior dislocations
  1. **Bankart lesion (Figure 4–14)**
     - Bankart lesion is a tear of the glenoid labrum off the front of the glenoid; this allows the humeral head to slip anteriorly
     - Most commonly associated with anterior instability
     - This type of lesion may be associated with an avulsion of a small fragment of bone from the glenoid rim
  2. **Hill-Sachs lesion (Figure 4–15)**
     - A compression fracture of the posterolateral aspect of the humeral head caused by abutment against the anterior rim of the glenoid fossa
     - Associated with anterior dislocations
     - A lesion that accounts for greater than 30% of the articular surface may cause instability
     - A notch occurs on the posterior lateral aspect of the humeral head due to the recurrent impingement
- Posterior dislocations
  - Reverse Hill-Sachs lesion
  - Reverse Bankart lesion

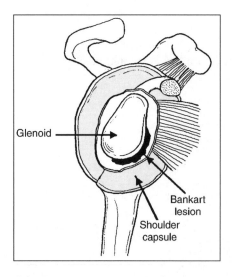

FIGURE 4–14. Bankart Lesion.

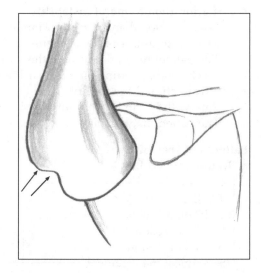

FIGURE 4–15. Hill-Sachs Lesion.

Clinical

The dead arm syndrome:
- These symptoms include early shoulder fatigue, pain, numbness, and paresthesias
- Shoulder slipping in and out of place, more commonly when the arm is placed in the throwing position (abducted and externally rotated)
- A syndrome of the shoulder and upper extremity usually seen in athletes (pitchers, volleyball servers) who require repetitive overhead arm motion
- **Laxity exam:** Some patients are double jointed, which is a lay term for capsular laxity. Ask the patient to touch the thumb against the volar (flexor) surface of the forearm. Patients with lax tissues are more likely than others to be able to voluntarily dislocate the shoulder

Provocative Tests

Anterior Glenohumeral Instability
- **Apprehension test (Figure 4–16)**
  - A feeling of glenohumeral instability on 90° of shoulder abduction and external rotation causing apprehension (fear of dislocation) in the patient
- **Relocation test**
  - Supine apprehension test with a posterior directed force applied to the anterior aspect of the shoulder not allowing anterior dislocation. This force relieves the feeling of apprehension
- **Anterior draw (load and shift)**
  - Passive anterior displacement of the humeral head on the glenoid

Posterior Glenohumeral Instability
- **Jerk test**
  - Place the arm in 90° of flexion and maximum internal rotation with the elbow flexed 90°. Adduct the arm across the body in the horizonal plane while pushing the humerus in a posterior direction. The patient will jerk away when the arm nears midline to prevent posterior subluxation or dislocation of the humeral head
- **Posterior draw (load and shift)**
  - Posterior displacement of the humerus

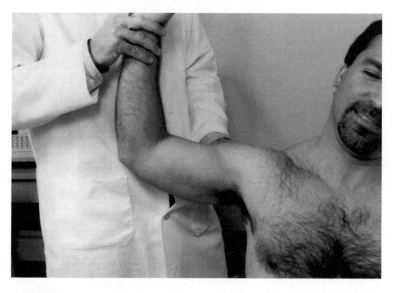

FIGURE 4–16. Apprehension Test. Photo courtesy of JFK Johnson Rehabilitation Institute, 2000.

Multidirectional Glenohumeral Instability
- **Sulcus sign (Figure 4–17)**
  - The examiner pulls down on the patient's arm with one hand as he stabilizes the scapula with the other. If an indentation develops between the acromion and the humeral head, the test is positive. This suggests increased laxity in the glenohumeral joint

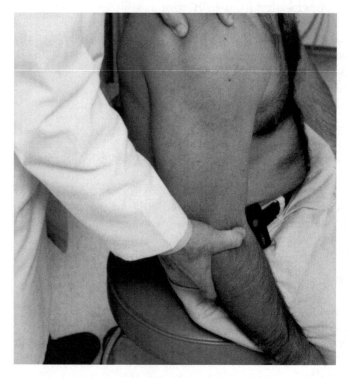

FIGURE 4–17. Sulcus Sign. Photo courtesy of JFK Johnson Rehabilitation Institute, 2000.

Imaging

- General films
  - Routine anteroposterior view (AP)
  - Scapular Y view
  - Axillary lateral view
    - Assess glenohumeral dislocations
  - Others views
    - West Point lateral axillary: Bankart lesions
    - Stryker notch view: Hill-Sachs lesions

Treatment

Anterior Glenohumeral Instability (T.U.B.S.)
- *Conservative*
  - Sling immobilization: Length of time is variable
  - Rehabilitation
    - Strengthening and range of motion of the shoulder-girdle complex should follow the brief stage of immobilization

- PROM (Pendulum-Codman's exercises): Isometric exercises early in the recovery course

Note: Muscle strengthening alone rarely prevents recurrent dislocations if there is sufficient capsular laxity; thus surgery should be considered if rehabilitation fails in active individuals

- *Surgical*

Note: After a third dislocation, the risk for another approaches 100%. Surgery may then be considered. In athletes or active individuals, surgery may be considered earlier

Posterior Glenohumeral Instability

- *Conservative*
  - Immobilize in a neutral position for roughly three weeks
  - Strengthening the posterior shoulder-scapula musculature is imperative
  - Infraspinatus, posterior deltoid, teres minor
    - This phase may last up to six months
- *Surgical*
  - Rehabilitation generally is adequate for the majority of these patients. In the event of a failed rehabilitation program, a posterior capsulorrhaphy is the surgical procedure of choice

Multidirectional Glenohumeral Instability (AMBRI)

- Greater than 80% of the patients obtain excellent results with rehabilitation
- Surgical treatment may be an option only when conservative measures fail. At that time, an inferior capsular shift may be indicated

Educating patients to avoid voluntarily dislocating the shoulder and to avoid positions of known instability should be a part of the treatment program

GLENOID LABRUM TEARS

General

- The labrum encircles the periphery of the glenoid fossa
- Tendons (rotator cuff and biceps) insert on the labrum and, as a result, any tear or instability of the labrum may be accompanied by rotator cuff or biceps tendon pathology
- Repetitive overhead sports (baseball, volleyball) or trauma are causative factors
- Tears may occur through the anterior, posterior, or superior aspect of the labrum
- SLAP lesion
  - **S**uperior glenoid **L**abral tear in the **A**nterior to **P**osterior direction
  - A tear encompasses the entire aspect of the glenoid labrum

Clinical

- Signs and symptoms are similar to that of shoulder instability (clicking, locking, pain)

Provocative Tests

- Load-and-shift test
  - The examiner grasps the humeral head pushes it into the glenoid while applying an anterior and posterior force. A positive test indicates labrum instability and is displayed by excess translation

Imaging and Treatment

- The same as glenohumeral joint instability

IMPINGEMENT SYNDROME AND ROTATOR CUFF TEAR

General

- Impingement syndrome (Figure 4–18)
  - Most likely the most common cause of shoulder pain
  - A narrowing of the subacromial space causing compression and inflammation of the subacromial bursa, biceps tendon, and rotator cuff (most often involving the supraspinatus tendon)
  - Impingement of the tendon, most commonly the supraspinatus, under the acromion and the greater tuberosity occurs with arm abduction and internal rotation
  - Impingement syndrome may progress to a rotator cuff tear (complete or partial)
  - Stages of subacromial impingement syndrome
    - Stage 1: Edema or hemorrhage—reversible (age < 25)
    - Stage 2: Fibrosis and tendonitis (ages 25–40)
    - Stage 3: Acromioclavicular spur and rotator cuff tear (Age > 40) (Miller, 2000)

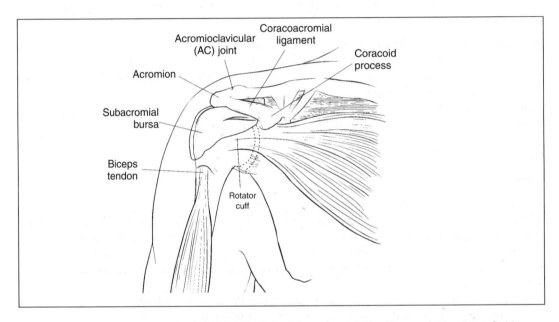

FIGURE 4–18. Anatomy of the Shoulder; Anterior View. Reprinted with permission from Snider RK. Essentials of Musculoskeletal Medicine. Rosemont IL, American Academy of Orthopaedic Surgeons, 1997.

- **Rotator cuff tear**
  Etiology
  - The rotator cuff is composed of four muscles (Figure 4–19):
    1. Supraspinatus
    2. Infraspinatus
    3. Teres minor
    4. Subscapularis
  - These muscles form a cover around the head of the humerus whose function is to rotate the arm and stabilize the humeral head against the glenoid

- Rotator cuff tears occur primarily in the supraspinatus tendon which is weakened as a result of many factors including injury, poor blood supply to the tendon, and subacromial impingement
- May be as a result of direct trauma or an end result from chronic impingement. This injury rarely affects people < 40 years of age

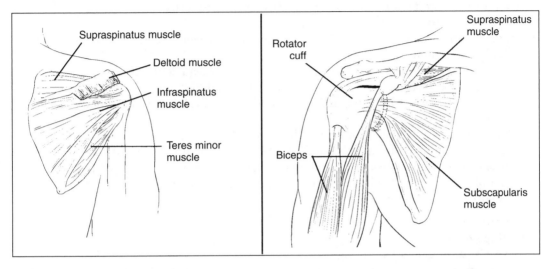

FIGURE 4–19. Rotator Cuff Muscles: Posterior View (Left); Anterior View (Right). Reprinted with permission from Snider RK. Essentials of Musculoskeletal Medicine. Rosemont IL, American Academy of Orthopaedic Surgeons, 1997.

Acromion Morphology and Its Association to Rotator Cuff Tears (Figure 4–20)
The anatomic shape of the patient's acromion has been linked with occurrence rates of rotator cuff tears—patients with curved or hooked acromions have a higher risk of rotator cuff tears
- Type I → flat
- Type II → curved
- Type III → hooked
(Brown and Neumann, 1999)

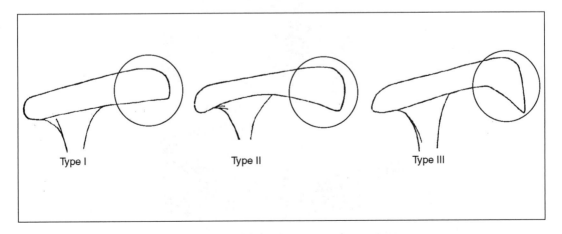

FIGURE 4–20. Three types of acromion morphology.

Clinical

- Pain during range of motion, specifically in repetitive overhead activities, such as:
  - Throwing a baseball
  - Swimming (occurs at the catch phase of the overhead swimming stroke)
    - Mechanism: flexion, abduction, internal rotation
    - More common strokes: freestyle, backstroke, and butterfly
    - Less common stroke: breast stroke
- Supraspinatus and biceps tendons are commonly affected secondary to their location under the acromion
  - Patients may feel crepitus, clicking, catching on overhead activities
  - Pain may be referred anywhere along the deltoid musculature
  - Weakness in forward flexion, abduction, and internal rotation indicating impingement (Hawkins sign)
  - Inability to initiate abduction may indicate a rotator cuff tear
  - Pain may be nocturnal. Patients often report having difficulty sleeping on the affected side
  - Tenderness over the greater tuberosity or inferior to the acromion on palpation
  - Atrophy of the involved muscle resulting in a gross deformity at the respective area, usually seen in chronic tears

Provocative Tests
- **Impingement test**
  - **Neer's impingement sign** (Figure 4–21)
    - Stabilize the scapula and passively flex the arm forward greater than 90° eliciting pain
    - Pain indicates the supraspinatus tendon is compressing between the acromion and greater tuberosity

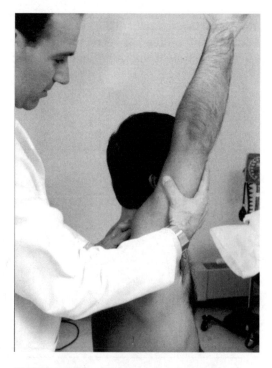

FIGURE 4–21. Neer's Impingement Sign.
Photo courtesy of JFK Johnson Rehabilitation Institute, 2000.

- **Hawkins Impingement Sign (Figure 4–22)**
  - Stabilize the scapula and passively forward flex (to 90°) the internally rotated arm eliciting pain
  - A positive test indicates the supraspinatus tendon is compressing against the coracoacromial ligament

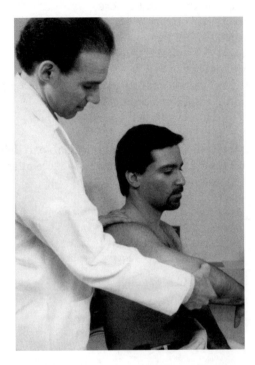

FIGURE 4–22. Hawkins Impingement Sign. Photo courtesy of JFK Johnson Rehabilitation Institute, 2000.

- **Painful arc sign**
  - Abducting the arm with pain occurring roughly between 60–120°
- **Rotator cuff tests**
  - **Supraspinatus test**
    - Pain and weakness with arm flexion abduction and internal rotation (thumb pointed down)
    - 📖 With abduction the humerus will naturally externally rotate. In assessing the integrity of the supraspinatus, the patient should internally rotate the humerus, forcing the greater tuberosity under the acromion. In this position, the maximum amount of abduction is to 120°
  - **Drop arm test**
    - The arm is passively abducted to 90° and internally rotated
    - The patient is unable to maintain the arm in abduction with or without a force applied
    - Initially the deltoid will assist in abduction but fails quickly
    - This indicates a complete tear of the cuff

Imaging

- Plain films (AP)
  - Impingement
    - Cystic changes in the greater tuberosity
  - Chronic rotator cuff tear
    - Superior migration of the proximal humerus
    - Flattening of the greater tuberosity
    - Subacromial sclerosis
- Supraspinatus outlet view (15° caudal tilt for a transcapular Y view) (Figure 4–23)
  - Assess acromion morphology
- MRI is the gold standard to evaluate the integrity of the rotator cuff
  - Full thickness tears and partial tears can be delineated
  - Gadolinium may be added to evaluate the labrum
- Arthrogram
  - ⬚ Beneficial in assessing full thickness tears but unable to delineate the size of the tear or partial tears; should not be used in patients who have allergies to dyes
- Ultrasound: Operator dependent

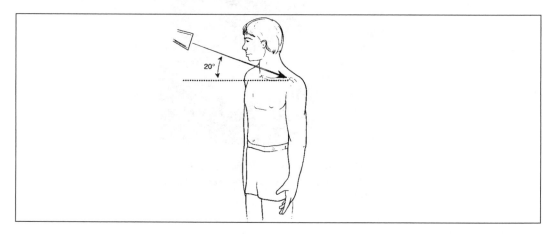

FIGURE 4–23. Radiograph of the Rotator Cuff: 15–20° Angled View. Reprinted with permission from Snider RK. Essentials of Musculoskeletal Medicine. Rosemont IL, American Academy of Orthopaedic Surgeons, 1997.

Treatment

Impingement, chronic-partial and full tears

- *Conservative: Rehabilitation*
  - Acute phase (up to 4 weeks)
    - Relative rest: Avoid any activity that aggravates the symptoms
    - Reduce pain and inflammation
    - Modalities: Ultrasound iontophoresis
    - Reestablish nonpainful and scapulohumeral range of motion
    - Retard muscle atrophy of the entire upper extremity
  - Recovery phase (months) (up to 6 months)
    - Improve upper extremity range of motion and proprioception
    - Full pain-free ROM

- Improve rotator cuff (supraspinatus) and scapular stabilizers
- Assess single planes of motion in activity related exercises
  – Functional phase
    - Continue strengthening increasing power and endurance (plyometrics)
    - Activity-specific training
    - Corticosteroid injection: Only up to three yearly
    - May weaken the collagen tissue leading to more microtrauma
- *Surgical*
  – Indications
    - Full thickness or partial tears that fail conservative treatment
    - Reduction or elimination of impingement pain is the primary indication for surgical repair in chronic rotator cuff tears. The patient should be made aware that restoration of abduction is less predictable than relief of pain
  – Partial tears (< 40% thickness)
    - Procedure: Partial anterior acromioplasty and coracoacromial ligament lysis (CAL)
  – Partial tears (> 40% thickness)
    - Excise and repair
  – Acute rotator cuff tears (i.e., athletes/trauma)
    - Statistics show that surgical repair of an acute tear within the first three weeks results in significantly better overall function than later reconstruction

DEGENERATIVE JOINT DISEASE OF THE SHOULDER (FIGURE 4–24)

General

- Destruction of the articular cartilage and narrowing of the joint space
- Arthritis may occur at the glenohumeral or acromioclavicular joint
- It is also seen in rheumatoid arthritis, posttraumatic lesions, chronic rotator cuff pathology, seronegative spondyloarthritis, Lyme disease and more

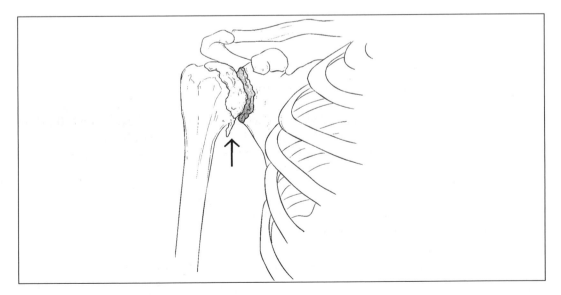

FIGURE 4–24. Degenerative Joint Disease of the Shoulder. Reprinted with permission from Snider RK. Essentials of Musculoskeletal Medicine. Rosemont IL, American Academy of Orthopaedic Surgeons, 1997.

Clinical

- Limitations and pain on active and passive range of motion affecting their ADLs
- Pain more commonly in internal rotation of the shoulder but may also be seen with abduction
- Manual muscle testing (MMT) may or may not be affected depending on the severity of the disease
- Pain may be nocturnal and relieved by rest
- Tenderness on palpation on the anterior and posterior aspects of the shoulder

Imaging

- AP view: Internal and external rotation and 40° of obliquity
- Axillary view
- Changes seen on X ray include
  - Irregular joint surfaces
  - Joint space narrowing (cartilage destruction)
  - Subacromial sclerosis
  - Osteophyte changes
  - Flattened glenoid
  - Cystic changes in the humeral head

Treatment

- *Conservative*
  - Decrease pain and inflammation
  - NSAID, Corticosteroid injection
- *Rehabilitation*
  - Range of motion and rotator cuff strengthening
- *Surgical*
  - **Total shoulder arthroplasty (TSA)**
    - Indications
      - Pain
      - Avascular necrosis
      - Neoplasm
    - Goals
      - Relieve pain, protect joint, and restore function
    - **Stage 1: (0–6 weeks)**
      - Precautions: status post TSA: avoid active abductions and extension > 0°, sling immobilization, no external rotation > 15°, no active ROM, NWB
      - Treatment: Pendulum exercises, isometrics (progressing), gentle passive and active ROM, such as wall-walking
    - **Stage 2: (6–12 weeks)**
      - Precautions: Discontinue sling, start light weights
      - Treatment: Isotonics, AAROM, AROM
    - **Stage 3: (Greater than 12 weeks)**
      - Treatment (previous ROM precautions cancelled)
        Start progressive resistive exercises, active ranging, stretching

- Shoulder arthrodesis
  - Definition
    - A surgical resection and fusion of the shoulder (glenohumeral) joint
    - Typical patient is a young heavy laborer with repetitive trauma to the shoulder
  - Indications
    - Severe pain in the shoulder secondary to osteoarthritis
    - Mechanical loosening of a shoulder arthroplasty
    - Joint infection
  - 📖 Fusion position
    - Abduction—50°
    - Forward flexion—30°
    - Internal rotation—50°

BICEPS TENDONITIS AND RUPTURE

General (Figure 4–25)

Tendonitis
- Inflammation of the long head of the biceps tendon at the insertion on the greater tuberosity
- The tendon may be impinged between the head of the humerus, acromion and coraco-clavicular ligaments with elevation and internal rotation of the arm

Rupture (Figure 4–26)
- The common site of rupture is at the long head of the biceps tendon at the proximal end
- Distal rupture is rare
- Seen in adults greater than 40 years old with a history of impingement syndrome
- Associated with rotator cuff tears in the elderly

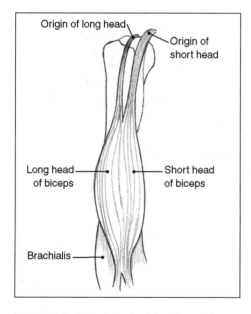

FIGURE 4–25. Anterior Muscles of the Right Arm.

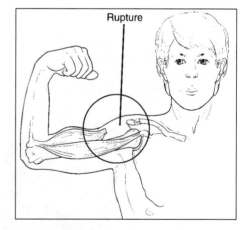

FIGURE 4–26. Rupture of the Biceps Tendon (Rupture is better appreciated on attempted contraction). Reprinted with permission from Snider RK. Essentials of Musculoskeletal Medicine. Rosemont IL, American Academy of Orthopaedic Surgeons, 1997.

Clinical

- Point tenderness in the bicipital groove (Figure 4–27)
- Positive impingement signs if associated with impingement syndrome
- Sharp pain, audible snap, ecchymosis and visible bulge in the lower arm (rupture)

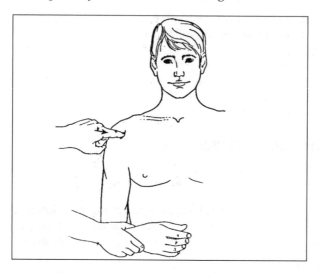

FIGURE 4–27. Point Tenderness of Biceps Tendon in Bicipital Groove. Reprinted with permission from Snider RK. Essentials of Musculoskeletal Medicine. Rosemont IL, American Academy of Orthopaedic Surgeons, 1997.

Provocative Tests

- Biceps tendonitis
  - Yergason's test (Figure 4–28)—This test determines the stability of the long head of the biceps tendon in the bicipital groove
    - Pain at the anterior shoulder with flexion of the elbow to 90° and supination of the wrist against resistance

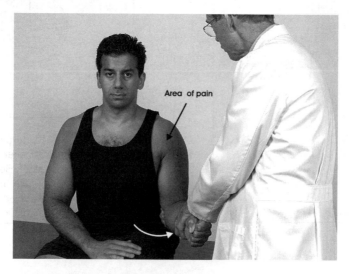

Area of pain

FIGURE 4–28. Yergason's Test.

- Speed's test
    - Pain at the anterior shoulder with flexion of the shoulder, elbow extended, and supinated against resistance
- **Biceps rupture**
    - Ludington's test (see Figure 4–26)
        - An obvious deformity seen with flexion of the biceps muscle

Imaging

- None specific

Treatment

- Tendonitis
    - Conservative treatment is appropriate for most patients
    - Range of motion and strengthening as tolerated
    - Modalities
    - Injection into the tendon sheath
- Rupture
    - It is not indicated for the tendon to be reattached in most patients
    - Biceps tenodesis: Younger individuals who require heavy lifting may need reattachment
    - Some patients may request reattachment of biceps tendon for cosmetic reasons

CALCIFIC TENDONITIS OF THE SUPRASPINATUS TENDON

General

- Calcium deposits most commonly involving the supraspinatus tendon
- Size of the deposit has no correlation to the symptoms

Clinical

- A sharp pain in the shoulder

Imaging

- AP X-ray of the shoulder will show calcium deposits usually at the site of tendon insertion

Treatment

- Symptoms will improve with subacromial injection and physical therapy
- Surgical treatment is rare and reserved for patients with severe pain and inability to perform ADLs

ADHESIVE CAPSULITIS (FROZEN SHOULDER) (Figure 4–29)

General

Definition
- Inflammation of the shoulder joint (glenohumeral)
- Painful shoulder with restricted glenohumeral motion

Etiology
- Unknown
- May be: Autoimmune, trauma, inflammatory

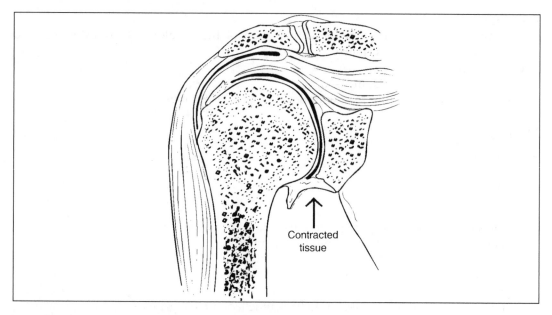

FIGURE 4–29. Genohumeral Joint in Frozen Shoulder. Note contracted soft tissue. Reprinted with permission from Snider RK. Essentials of Musculoskeletal Medicine. Rosemont IL, American Academy of Orthopaedic Surgeons, 1997.

Stages
- Painful stage: Progressive vague pain lasting roughly 8 months
- Stiffening stage: Decreasing range of motion lasting roughly 8 months
- Thawing stage: An increase of range of motion with decrease of shoulder pain

Pathology
- Synovial tissue of the capsule and bursa become adherent
- More common in women over the age of 40 years
- Associated with a variety of conditions:
    - Intracranial lesions: CVA, hemorrhage, and brain tumor
    - Clinical depression
    - Shoulder-hand syndrome
    - Parkinson's disease
    - Iatrogenic disorders
    - Cervical disc disease
    - Insulin dependent diabetes mellitus
    - Hypothyroidism

Clinical

- Pain, with significant reduction in range of motion both actively and passively

Imaging

- Plain films (AP)—indicated to rule out underlying tumor or calcium deposit
- Osteopenic, otherwise normal plain films are indicated in patients whose pain and motion do not improve after 3 months of treatment
- Arthrography will demonstrate a decreased volume in the joint, which can be realized by the small amount of contrast (less than 5 ml) that can be injected

Treatment

- Rehabilitation
    - Restoring passive and active range of motion
    - Decreasing pain
    - Corticosteroid injection: Subacromial and glenohumeral will decrease pain to maximize therapy
    - Home program: Stretches in all ranges of motion
    - Modalities: Ultrasound and electrical stimulation
- Surgical
    - Manipulation under anesthesia (MUA) may be indicated if there is no substantial progress after 12 weeks of conservative treatment
    - Arthroscopic lysis of adhesions—usually reserved for patients with IDDM who do not respond to manipulation

SCAPULA FRACTURES (Figure 4–30)

General

Mechanism
- Scapular fractures commonly occur in association with other serious injuries; therefore, the diagnosis is easily missed on initial exam
- Direct blow to the shoulder usually after a significant traumatic event (MVA, motorcycle accident)
- Associated with other significant injuries: Rib fractures, pulmonary pathology (contusions, pneumothorax)

Fracture sites: Glenoid, glenoid rim, coracoid, scapular neck and body, acromion

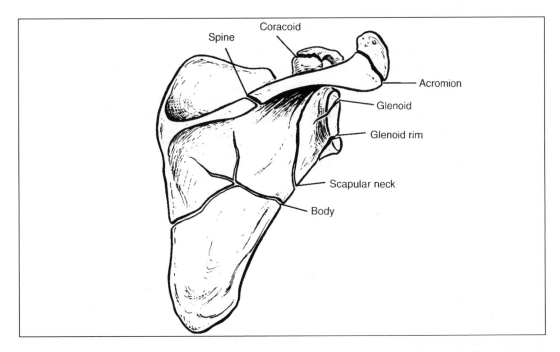

FIGURE 4–30.   Scapula Fracture Patterns. Reprinted with permission from Snider RK. Essentials of Musculoskeletal Medicine. Rosemont IL, American Academy of Orthopaedic Surgeons, 1997.

Clinical

- Tenderness over the scapular and acromial region

Imaging

- Plain films: AP, lateral (scapular Y), and axillary views
- CT scan

Treatment

- Closed treatment is adequate for nondisplaced fragments: sling, followed by early ROM exercises as tolerated, usually within 1 to 2 weeks after injury
- ORIF: Large displaced fragments
- **Note:** Patients with isolated scapular body fractures should be considered for hospital admission due to the risk of pulmonary contusion

CLAVICULAR FRACTURES

General

- Classification
  - Fracture location: Proximal, middle, and distal thirds

Clinical

- Pain in the shoulder region
- May or may not have an obvious deformity

Imaging

- Plain films: AP

Treatment

- Generally, most clavicular fractures can be treated conservatively
- > 1 cm displacement of lateral clavicle fractures at the AC joint are best treated surgically
- Closed reduction and figure eight sling immobilization
- Immobilization may range from 3 to 6 weeks depending on the age
- Progressive range of motion may be initiated after three weeks of immobilization
- Displacement of lateral clavicle fractures at the AC joint are best treated surgically

PROXIMAL HUMERUS FRACTURES (Figure 4–31)

General

Four-Part Classification: (Snider, 1997)
The four parts include:
  - Greater tuberosity
  - Lesser tuberosity
  - Head
  - Shaft
- A portion must be angulated by 45° or displaced at least one centimeter to be considered a fragment
- If the fracture is nondisplaced, it is considered a one part
  - One part: Nondisplaced, impacted fractures
  - Two part: One fragment is displaced in reference to the other three

- Three part: Two fragments are displaced
- Four part: All fragments are displaced
- Common locations for fractures include:
  - Greater tuberosity
  - Lesser tuberosity
  - 📖 Surgical neck (most common)
  - Anatomical neck

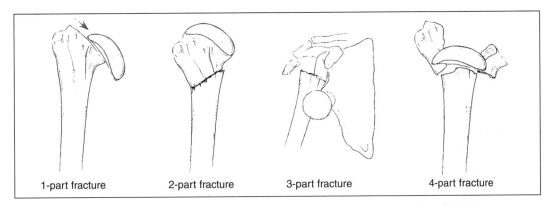

1-part fracture   2-part fracture   3-part fracture   4-part fracture

FIGURE 4–31. Displaced Proximal Humerus Fracture Patterns (Neer Classification). Reprinted with permission from Snider RK. Essentials of Musculoskeletal Medicine. Rosemont IL, American Academy of Orthopaedic Surgeons, 1997.

Clinical

- Typically occurs in elderly women with osteoporosis after a fall
- Pain, swelling and ecchymosis in the upper arm, which is exacerbated with the slightest motion
- 📖 In fracture at the surgical neck, the supraspinatus is the principle abductor, i.e., the supraspinatus causes abduction of the proximal fragment of the humerus
- Loss of sensation is seen if there is neurologic involvement
- Diminished radial pulse if the fracture compromises the vascular supply

Treatment

- One part: Nondisplaced, less than 1 cm apart
  - Early range of motion
  - Conservative: Sling immobilization and early rehabilitation (6 weeks)
  - AROM, pendulum exercises as early as tolerated
  - Greater than 1 part [displaced greater than 2 cm (2 part)]
- Surgical: ORIF (Open Reduction Internal Fixation)

Complications
- *Neurovascular*
  - 📖 **Brachial plexus injuries**
    - 📖 Axillary nerve is involved in surgical neck fractures
    - Radial and ulnar nerves may be affected as well
    - Median nerve is the least affected
    - Axillary artery compromise may be evident depending on the site of injury
  - **Avascular necrosis** of the humeral head may occur with anatomic neck fractures secondary to interruption of the humeral circumflex vasculature

■

UPPER EXTREMITIES—ELBOW REGION

FUNCTIONAL ANATOMY

Elbow Joint Articulations

- Humeroulnar joint
- Humeroradial joint
- Proximal radioulnar joint

Range of Motion

- Flexion: 135°
- Extension: 0–5°
- Supination: 90°
- Pronation: 90°

Elbow Motion

- **Flexion (Figure 4–32)**
  - Brachialis (musculocutaneus nerve, lateral cord, C5, C6, C7)
  - Biceps brachii (musculocutaneus nerve, lateral cord, C5, C6)
  - Brachioradialis (radial nerve, posterior cord, C5, C6, C7)
  - Pronator teres (median nerve, lateral cord, C6, C7)

- **Extension (Figure 4–33)**
  - Triceps (radial nerve, posterior cord, C6, C7, C8)
  - Anconeus (radial nerve, posterior cord, C7, C8, T1)
- **Supination (Figure 4–34)**
  - Supinator [posterior interosseus nerve (radial) posterior cord, C5, C6]
  - Biceps brachii (musculocutaneus nerve, lateral cord, C5, C6)
- **Pronation (Figure 4–35)**
  - Pronator quadratus [anterior interosseus nerve (median), C7, C8, T1]
  - Pronator teres (median nerve, lateral cord, C6, C7)
  - Flexor carpi radialis (median nerve, lateral cord, C6, C7)

Elbow Ligaments (Figure 4–36)

- **Medial (ulnar) collateral ligament (MCL)**
  - Key stabilizer of the elbow joint (anterior band)
- **Lateral (radial) collateral ligament (LCL)**
- **Annular ligament**
  - Holds the radial head in proper position

Common Muscle Origin of the Elbow Joint

- **Medial epicondyle of the humerus**
  - Flexor carpi radialis
  - Flexor carpi ulnaris

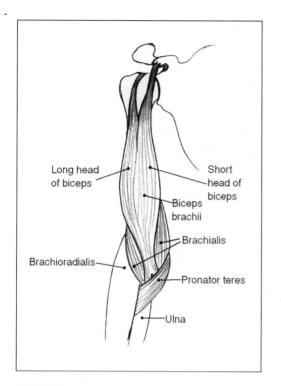

FIGURE 4–32. Elbow Flexors. (Anterior View)

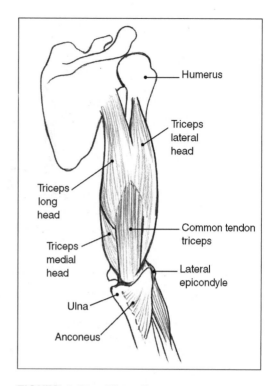

FIGURE 4–33. Elbow Extensors. (Posterior View)

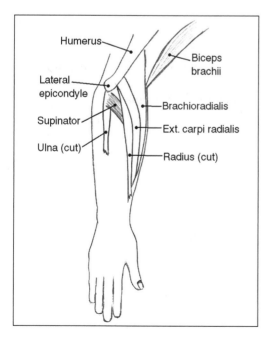

FIGURE 4–34. Forearm Supinators. (Dorsal View)

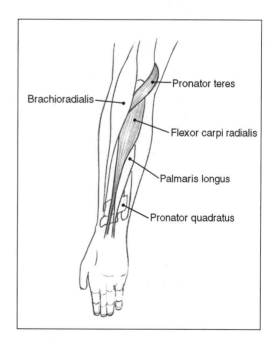

FIGURE 4–35. Forearm Pronators. (Volar View)

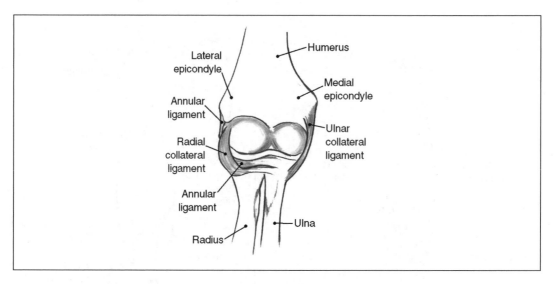

FIGURE 4–36. Elbow Ligaments (Anterior View of Right Elbow).

- – Flexor digitorum superficialis
- – Flexor digitorum profundus
- – Palmaris longus
- – Pronator teres
- **Lateral epicondyle of the humerus**
  - – Extensor carpi radialis longus
  - – Extensor carpi radialis brevis
  - – Extensor carpi ulnaris
  - – Extensor digitorum superficialis
  - – Supinator
  - – Anconeus

Mechanics of the Elbow: Carrying Angle

- The anatomic valgus angulation between the upper arm and forearm when the arm is fully extended
- It allows for the arm to clear the body when it is extended and supinated
- Normal carrying angle (from anatomical position)
  - – Males 5° of valgus
  - – Females 10–15° of valgus
  - – Angle > 20° is abnormal

Elbow Arthrodesis

- **Indications**
  - – Arthritis
  - – Failed surgical procedure
- **Fusion position**
  - – Unilateral: flexion—90°
  - – Bilateral: flexion—110° in one arm and 65° for the other

■

ELBOW DISORDERS

MEDIAL EPICONDYLITIS

General

Synonyms
- Golfer's elbow
- Little leaguer's elbow (children)

Mechanism
- A repetitive valgus stress more commonly seen in the throwing motion of a pitcher (especially in the late cocking and acceleration phase) (Figure 4–37)
- The back and downward motion of a golf swing just prior to the impact of the ball

Pathology
- **Medial epicondylitis**
  - Inflammation of the common flexor tendon, which may cause hypertrophy of the medial epicondyle
- **Little leaguer's elbow**
  - Hypertrophy of the medial epicondyle leading to microtearing and fragmentation of the medial epicondylar apophysis

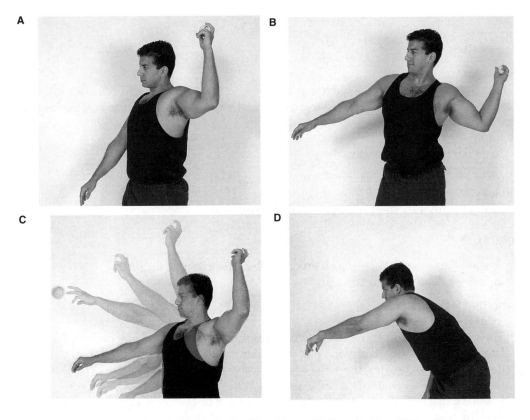

FIGURE 4–37. Throwing Mechanism. **A:** Cocking Phase. **B:** Acceleration Phase (Early). **C:** Acceleration Phase (Late). **D:** Follow-through.

Clinical

- Tenderness over the medial epicondyle
- Pain may be reproduced with wrist flexion and pronation

Imaging

- None needed

Treatment

- Conservative
  - Rest, ice, NSAIDs, immobilization
  - Activity and modification of poor throwing mechanics
- Surgical pinning
  - Reserved for an unstable elbow joint

Biomechanics of throwing a baseball—four phases:
- Cocking phase
- Acceleration early
- Acceleration late
- Follow-through

LATERAL EPICONDYLITIS

General

Synonyms
- Tennis elbow

Mechanism
- Sports that require repetitive movements
- Overuse and poor mechanics lead to an overload of the extensor and supinator tendons
- Poor technique with racquet sports
  - Improper backhand
  - Inappropriate string tension
  - Inappropriate grip size

Pathology
- Microtearing of the extensor carpi radialis brevis

CLINICAL

- Tenderness just distal to the lateral epicondyle at the extensor origin
- Pain and weakness in grip strength

Provocative test
- 📖 **Cozens test (Figure 4–38)**
  - The examiner stabilizes the elbow with a thumb over the lateral epicondyle. Pain in the lateral epicondyle is seen with patient making a fist, pronating the forearm, radially deviating and extending the wrist against resistance by the examiner. (The test may be more sensitive when done in full extension at the elbow) (Figure A).
  - Passive extension of the elbow with forced flexion of the wrist may precipitate pain at the lateral epicondyle (Figure B).

Imaging

- None needed
- Plain films of the elbow: Rule out arthritis and loose body fragments

Treatment

- Conservative
  - Relative rest, ice, NSAIDs for 10–14 days
  - Physical therapy (modalities)
  - Splinting, bands
  - Corticosteroid injection
  - Correct improper technique
- Operative
  - ECRB debridement

OLECRANON BURSITIS (Figure 4–39)

General

Synonyms
  - Draftsman's elbow
  - Student's elbow
  - Miner's elbow

Mechanism
  - Repetitive trauma, inflammatory disorder (gout, pseudogout, RA)

Pathology
  - Inflammation of the bursa located between the olecranon and skin

Clinical

- Swelling, pain, and a decreased range of motion in the posterior aspect of the elbow
- A hot, erythematous elbow may indicate infection

Imaging

- None needed

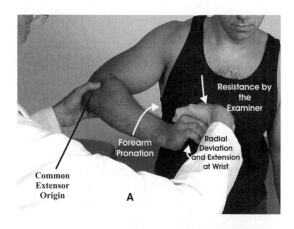

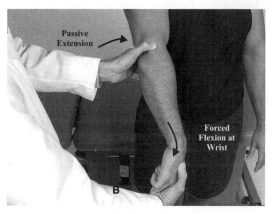

FIGURE 4–38. Cozens Test.

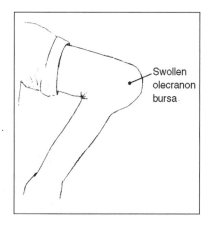

FIGURE 4–39. Olecranon Bursitis.

Treatment

- Aspiration of fluid and send it for culture if indicated
- Conservative: Rest, NSAIDs, elbow padding

DISLOCATION OF THE ELBOW

General

- The most common type of dislocation in children and the second most common type in adults, second only to shoulder dislocation
- Young adults between the ages of 25–30 years are most affected and sports activities account for almost 50% of these injuries
- Mechanism: Fall on the outstretched hand

Clinical

- Dislocation can be anterior or posterior with *posterior* being the most common, occurring 98% of the time (Figure 4–40)
- Associated injuries include fracture of the radial head, injury to the brachial artery and median nerve

Symptoms
- Inability to bend the elbow following a fall on the outstretched hand
- Pain in the shoulder and wrist
- On physical exam: The most important part of the exam is the neurovascular evaluation of the radial artery, and median, ulnar and radial nerves

Imaging

- Plain AP and lateral radiographs
- CT and MRI scans are seldom necessary

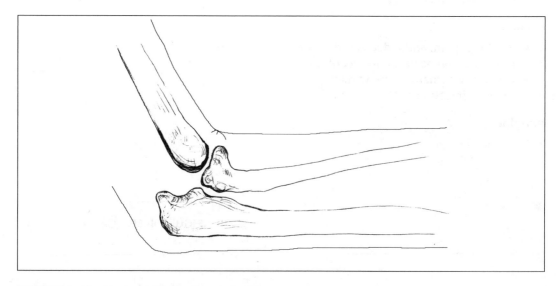

FIGURE 4–40. Posterior Dislocation of the Elbow.

Treatment

- Reduce dislocation as soon as possible after injury
- Splint for 10 days
- Initiate ROM exercises, NSAIDs

Adverse Outcomes

- Loss of ROM of elbow especially extension
- Ectopic bone formation
- Neurovascular injury
- Arthritis of the elbow

DISTAL BICEPS TENDONITIS

General

Mechanism
- Overloading of the biceps tendon commonly due to repetitive elbow flexion and supination or resisted elbow extension

Pathology
- Microtearing of the biceps tendon distally

Complication
- Biceps tendon avulsion

Clinical

- Insidious onset of pain in the antecubital fossa usually after an eccentric overload
- Audible snap with an obvious deformity, swelling, and ecchymosis if an avulsion is suspected

Imaging

- None needed

Treatment

- Conservative
- Relative rest, ice, NSAIDs
- Physical therapy: Modalities
- Correct improper technique
- Surgical: Reattachment

TRICEPS TENDONITIS/AVULSION

General

Mechanism
- Tendonitis: Overuse syndrome secondary to repetitive triceps extension
- Avulsion: A decelerating counterforce during active elbow extension

Clinical

- Posterior elbow pain with tenderness at the insertion of the triceps tendon
- Pain with resistive elbow extension
- Sudden loss of extension with a palpable defect in the triceps tendon (avulsion)

Imaging

- Plain films to rule out other causes, if indicated

Treatment

- Conservative
- Surgical: Reattachment

VALGUS EXTENSION OVERLOAD SYNDROME OF THE ELBOW

General

Synonyms
- Boxer's elbow

Mechanism
- An overuse disorder caused by repetitive and uncontrolled valgus forces demonstrated during the throwing motion, especially in late acceleration and deceleration
- Also may be seen in boxers

Pathology
- Osteophyte and loose body formation occurs secondary to a repetitive abutment of the olecranon against the fossa

Clinical

- Posterior elbow pain with lack of full extension
- Catching or locking during elbow extension

Imaging

- Plain films: AP/lateral may show a loose body or osteophyte formation at the olecranon

Treatment

- Conservative
- Surgical: Removal of the loose body

ULNAR COLLATERAL LIGAMENT (UCL) SPRAIN

General

Mechanism
- A repetitive valgus stress occurring across the elbow during the acceleration phase of throwing

Pathology
- Inflammation to the anterior band of the ulnar collateral ligament

Clinical

- Significant medial elbow pain occurring after the throwing motion
- A pop or click may be heard precipitating the pain
- Medial pain or instability on valgus stress with the elbow, flexed 20–30° if the UCL is torn

Provocative Test
- Valgus stress test
  - Tenderness over the medial aspect of the elbow which may be increased with a valgus stress

Imaging

- Plain films may reveal calcification and spurring along the UCL
- Valgus stress radiographs demonstrating a 2 mm joint space suggestive of UCL injury

Treatment

- Conservative
- Rest, ice, NSAIDs
- Rehabilitation program for strengthening and stretching
- Establishing return-to-play criteria
- Surgical reconstruction if needed

RADIAL COLLATERAL LIGAMENT (RCL) SPRAIN

General

Mechanism
- Elbow dislocation from a traumatic event

Clinical

- Recurrent locking or clicking of the elbow with extension and supination
- Lateral pain or instability on varus stress with the elbow flexed 20–30° if the RCL is torn

Provocative test
- **Varus stress test**
  - Tenderness over the lateral aspect of the elbow, which may be increased with a varus stress
- **Lateral pivot-shift test**
  - Assess the RCL for posterolateral instability

Imaging

- Varus stress radiographs demonstrating a 2 mm joint space suggestive of RCL injury

Treatment

- Conservative
  - Rest, ice, NSAIDs
  - Rehabilitation program for strengthening and stretching
  - Establishing return to play criteria
- Surgical reconstruction if needed

PRONATOR SYNDROME (Also see EMG/Nerve and Muscle Chapter)

General

📖 **Mechanism**
- Median nerve compression at the elbow by the following structures
  - Ligament of Struthers or supracondylar spur
  - Lacertus fibrosis
  - Pronator teres muscle
  - Between the two heads of the flexor digitorum superficialis (FDS)

Clinical

- Dull aching pain in the proximal forearm just distal to the elbow
- Numbness in the median nerve distribution of the hand
- Symptoms exacerbated by pronation

Imaging

- EMG/NCS
- Plain films: Rule out spur

Treatment

- Conservative
  - Modification of activities
  - Avoid aggravating factors
  - Stretching and strengthening program
- Surgical: Release of the median nerve at the location of the compression

ENTRAPMENT OF THE ULNAR NERVE (Also see EMG/Nerve and Muscle chapter)

General

Synonyms
- Cubital tunnel syndrome

Mechanism
- A hypermobility of the ulnar nerve, excessive valgus force or loose body/osteophyte formation, which aggravates the integrity of the ulnar nerve at the elbow

Pathology
- Hyperirritability of the ulnar nerve

Clinical

- An aching pain with paraesthesias, which may radiate distally to the fourth and fifth digits
- Positive Tinel's sign at the elbow
- Positive Froment's sign
- Weakness in the ulnar musculature of the hand, demonstrated by a weak grip strength and atrophy and poor hand coordination

Imaging

- EMG/NCS above and below the elbow

Treatment

- Conservative
- Relative rest, NSAIDs, elbow protection (splinting) and technique modification

OSTEOCHONDROSIS DISSECANS OF THE ELBOW

General

Synonyms
- Panner's disease (involving epiphysial aseptic necrosis of the capitellum)

Clinical

- Tenderness and swelling on the lateral aspect of the elbow
- Usually seen in young boys
- Limited extension seen on ranging

Imaging

- Plain films: Sclerosis, patchy areas of lucency with fragmentation

Treatment

- Conservative: Immobilization, then gradual range of motion

FRACTURE OF THE HUMERAL SHAFT

General

- Fairly common—constituting up to 5% of all fractures

Mechanism:
- MVA—direct trauma
- Fall on outstretched arm

Clinical

- Severe arm pain and swelling and deformity are characteristic of a displaced fracture of the humerus
- 📖 If the radial nerve has been injured, patients will exhibit a radial nerve palsy (Figure 4–41)

Imaging

- AP and lateral X rays—Confirm diagnosis

Treatment

- Humeral shaft fractures can be treated conservatively (i.e., splint for 2 weeks)
- 📖 Special problem associated with humeral shaft fracture is radial nerve injury

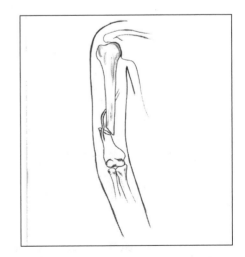

FIGURE 4–41. Radial Nerve Entrapment at the Humeral Shaft Fracture Site.

- **Note:** 95% of patients will regain their nerve function within 6 months. During this period of observation patient should wear a splint, work with a therapist, and EMGs are indicated if radial nerve function does not return

FRACTURE OF THE DISTAL HUMERUS
General

Classification—can be complex, the most useful way to consider them is displaced or nondisplaced. A displaced fracture involves one or both condyles, and the joint surface may or may not be involved (Figure 4–42).
- Complications
  - Neurovascular injury
  - Nonunion
  - Malunion
  - Elbow contracture
  - Poor range of motion

Clinical

- The patient will demonstrate swelling, ecchymosis, and pain at the elbow
- Inability to flex the elbow
- Inspect for an obvious deformity
- Examine the neurovascular status

Imaging

- Plain films: AP/lateral of the elbow

Treatment

- Orthopedic referral; displaced fractures—except severely comminuted fractures—required open reduction. Nondisplaced fractures can be treated by splinting and early motion

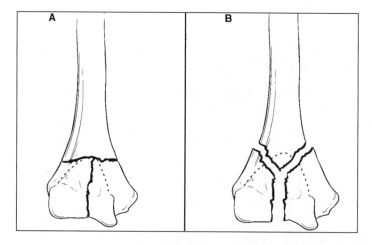

FIGURE 4–42.   A. Distal Humerus: Non-displaced Condylar Fracture.   **B.** Distal humerus: Displaced Intercondylar Fracture. Reprinted with permission from Snider RK. Essentials of Musculoskeletal Medicine. Rosemont IL, American Academy of Orthopaedic Surgeons, 1997.

RADIAL HEAD FRACTURE

General

Dislocations of the elbow are commonly associated with radial head fractures (Figure 4–43)
Classification: A commonly used classification separates these fractures into three types:
- Type I: Nondisplaced
- Type II: Marginal radial head fracture, minimal displacement
- Type III: Comminuted fracture

Clinical

- Fall on an outstretched arm causing pain, swelling, ecchymosis around the elbow
- Pain and decreased range of motion in elbow flexion and extension, pronation, and supination

Imaging

- Plain films of the elbow

Treatment—Orthopedic Referral

- Type I (nondisplaced): Conservative
  - Short period of immobilization approximately 3 to 5 days followed by early range of motion
- Type II (minimal displacement)
  - Surgical fixation: Greater than 2 mm displacement or 30% radial head involvement
- Type III: Surgical

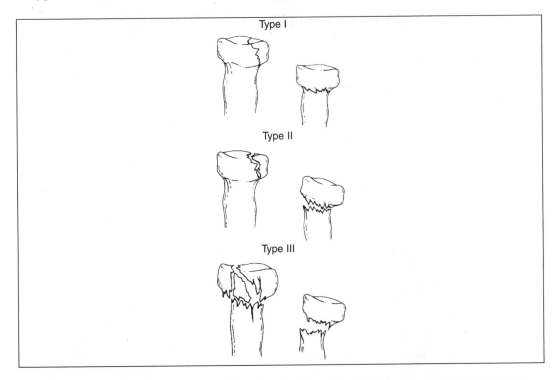

FIGURE 4–43. Radial Head Fracture Classification. Reprinted with permission from Snider RK. Essentials of Musculoskeletal Medicine. Rosemont IL, American Academy of Orthopaedic Surgeons, 1997.

FRACTURE OF THE OLECRANON

General

Mechanism
- Direct blow to the elbow
- Fall on the elbow with the elbow flexed
- Fall on an outstretched arm in association with a dislocation

Classification
- Nondisplaced
- Displaced

Clinical
- Swelling and ecchymosis with an obvious deformity
- Pain on gentle range of motion
- Numbness and paresthesias with radiation distally to the fourth and fifth digits with ulnar nerve involvement

Imaging
- Plain films: A/P lateral and oblique

Treatment
- Nondisplaced: Conservative (immobilization)
- Displaced: Surgical

■

UPPER EXTREMITIES—WRIST REGION

FUNCTIONAL ANATOMY

Range of Motion at the Wrist (Figure 4–44)

- Flexion: 80°
- Extension: 70°
- Ulnar deviation: 30°
- Radial deviation: 20°

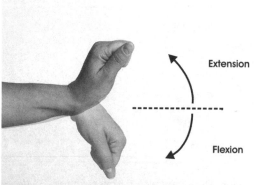

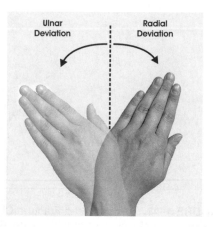

FIGURE 4–44. Wrist Range of Motion Terminology.

Carpal Bones (Figure 4–45)

- Proximal row: "Some Lovers Try Positions"
  - Scaphoid
  - Lunate
  - Triquetrum
  - Pisiform
- Distal row: "That They Can't Handle"
  - Trapezium
  - Trapezoid
  - Capitate
  - Hamate

Wrist Flexion (Fig. 4-46)

- Flexor carpi radialis (medial nerve, lateral cord, C6, C7)
- Flexor carpi ulnaris (ulnar nerve, medial cord, C8, T1)
- Palmaris longus (median nerve, C7, C8)
- Flexor digitorum superficialis (median nerve, C7, C8, T1)
- Flexor digitorum profundus (median nerve, C7, C8, T1 to second and third digit, ulnar nerve, C7, C8, T1 to fourth and fifth digit)
- Flexor pollicis longus (median, C8, T1)

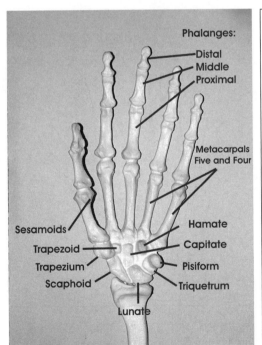

FIGURE 4–45. Palmar View—Bones of the Wrist and Hand.

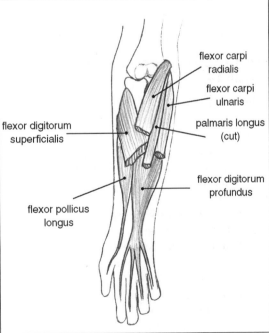

FIGURE 4–46. Wrist Flexors.

Wrist Extension (Figure 4–47)

- Extensor carpi radialis longus (radial nerve, posterior cord, C6, C7)
- Extensor carpi radialis brevis (radial nerve, posterior cord, C6, C7)
- Extensor carpi ulnaris (radial nerve, posterior cord, C7, C8)
- Extensor digitorum (radial nerve, C7, 8)
- Extensor digiti minimi (ulnar nerve, C8, T1)
- Extensor indicis (radial C6, C7, C8)
- Extensor pollicis longus (radial nerve, C6, C7, C8)

Ulnar deviation of the wrist (adduction)

- Flexor carpi ulnaris (ulnar nerve, medial cord, C8, T1)
- Extensor carpi ulnaris (radial nerve, posterior cord, C7, C8)

Radial deviation of the wrist (abduction)

- Flexor carpi radialis (medial nerve, lateral cord, C6, C7)
- Extensor carpi radialis longus (radial nerve, posterior cord, C6, C7)

Extensor Compartments of the Wrist (Figure 4–48)

- First Compartment
  - Abductor pollicis longus
  - Extensor pollicis brevis
- Second Compartment
  - Extensor carpi radialis longus
  - Extensor carpi radialis brevis
- Third Compartment
  - Extensor pollicis longus
- Fourth Compartment
  - Extensor digitorum communis
  - Extensor indices proprius
- Fifth Compartment
  - Extensor digiti minimi
- Sixth Compartment
  - Extensor carpi ulnaris

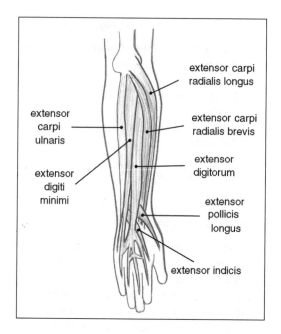

FIGURE 4–47. Wrist Extensors.

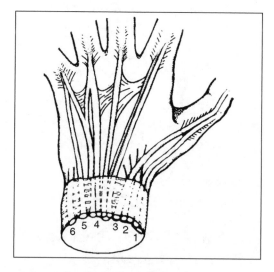

FIGURE 4–48. Extensor Tendons with the Six Tendon Sheath Compartments (Dorsum of the Wrist).

■
WRIST DISORDERS

ARTHRITIS

General

Types:
- Rheumatoid arthritis
  - Autoimmune attack on the synovial tissue destroying the articular cartilage leading to bone destruction
- Osteoarthritis
  - Noninflammatory disorder with deterioration of the articular cartilage and formation of new bone at the joint margins

Clinical

- Rheumatoid arthritis
  - Swelling of the joints of the hand and wrist (MCP and PIP joints)
  - Ulnar deviation of the wrist
  - Dorsal subluxation of the ulna
  - Erosion of the ulnar styloid at the end stage
  - Swan-neck deformity: Shortening and contracture of the intrinsic muscles of the hand causing:
    - Flexion of the MCP
    - Hyperextension of the PIP
    - Flexion of the DIP
  - Boutonnière deformity: Tearing of the extensor hood causing:
    - Hyperextension of the MCP
    - Flexion of the PIP
    - Hyperextension of the DIP
- Osteoarthritis
  - Heberden's and Bouchard's nodules involving the DIP and PIP, respectively
  - Tenderness along the area of involvement and crepitus with wrist ranging
    - Common in the first CMC joint of the thumb
  - Cyst formation in the joint space

Imaging

- Plain films of the wrist and digits

Treatment

- Conservative

DEQUERVAIN'S TENOSYNOVITIS

General

Mechanism
- Repetitive or direct trauma to the sheath of the extensor pollicis brevis and abductor pollicis longus tendons causing a tenosynovitis and inflammation
- **Involvement of the first compartment of the wrist**

Clinical

- Pain and tenderness on the radial side of the wrist associated with movement
- Edema and crepitus may also be present

Provocative Test

- **Finkelstein's test (Figure 4–49)**
  - Thumb is flexed into the palm of the hand with the fingers making a fist over the thumb
  - The examiner ulnar deviates the wrist, if this produces pain the test is positive and diagnostic for deQuervain's

Imaging

- None needed

Treatment

- Conservative
  - Immobilization of the thumb in a thumb spica splint
  - NSAIDs
  - Corticosteroid injection
- Surgical

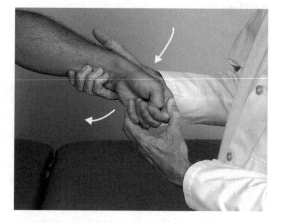

FIGURE 4–49. Finkelstein's Test.

GANGLION CYST (Figure 4–50)

General

Mechanism

- Cystic structure that arises from the synovial sheath of the joint space. Synovial fluid enters the cavity

Clinical

- Small smooth mass on the dorsal and volar aspect of the wrist
- Pain may occur with ranging the wrist or slight pressure

Imaging

- Plain films of the wrist

Treatment

- Immobilization
- Aspiration of the cyst (90% recurrence)
- Surgical removal if needed (10% recurrence)

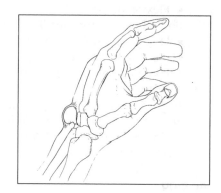

FIGURE 4–50. Wrist Ganglion. Reprinted with permission from Snider RK. Essentials of Musculoskeletal Medicine. Rosemont IL, American Academy of Orthopaedic Surgeons, 1997.

OSTEONECROSIS OF THE LUNATE (Figure 4–51)

General

Synonyms
- Kienböck's disease

Mechanism
- An idiopathic loss of blood supply to the lunate, which causes a necrosis of the bone and collapsing that results in degenerative changes in the wrist

Etiology
- The exact etiology is unidentified and is thought to be caused by trauma (repeated stress or fracture)
- Poor vascular supply to the area
- Short ulnar variance
  - Patients with a short ulna are thought to have an increased incidence of osteonecrosis of the lunate as compared to normal individuals. This is secondary to the increased shear forces that are placed on the lunate

Clinical

- Ulnar-sided pain, stiffness, and swelling over the dorsal aspect of the wrist directly over the lunate
- Reduced grip strength

Imaging

- Plain films: May see a compression fracture, flattening, or sclerosis of the lunate
- Bone scan: Increase, uptake
- MRI: Decreased signal intensity (T1)

Treatment

- Orthopedic referral

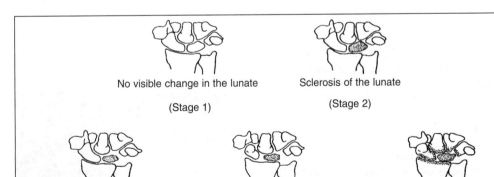

No visible change in the lunate
(Stage 1)

Sclerosis of the lunate
(Stage 2)

Sclerosis and fragmentation of the lunate (Stage 3A)

Stage 3A with proximal migration of the capitate or fixed rotation of the scaphoid (Stage 3B)

Stage 3A or 3B combined with degenerative changes at adjacent joints

FIGURE 4–51. Kienböck's Disease Classification. Reprinted with permission from Snider RK. Essentials of Musculoskeletal Medicine. Rosemont IL, American Academy of Orthopaedic Surgeons, 1997.

SCAPHOID FRACTURE

General

- One of the most common fractures of the wrist

Mechanism
- A fall or blow on a hyperextended (dorsiflexed) wrist
- Osteonecrosis of the bone may develop secondary to its poor blood supply
- The majority of the blood supply is to the distal one-third of the bone. Therefore, the middle and proximal portion of the bone have a large nonunion rate (one-third developing osteonecrosis)

Classification: Anatomical location (Figure 4–52)
- Tubercle (2%)
- Distal pole (10%)
- Waist (65%)
- Proximal pole (15%)

Complications
- Osteonecrosis, which may lead to carpal bones collapse (scapholunate) if not treated correctly

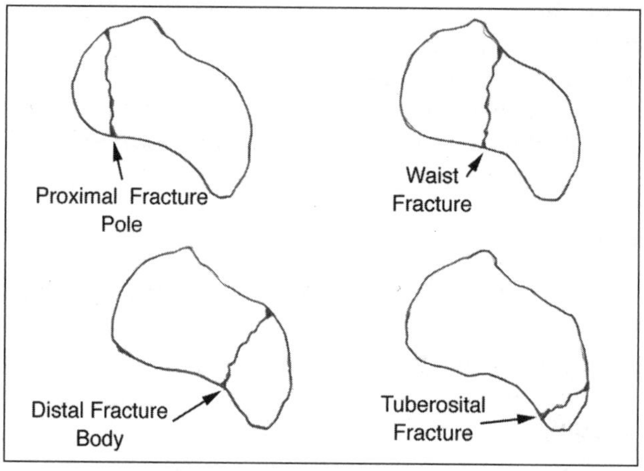

Clinical

- Swelling and tenderness in the areas of the thumb and wrist (anatomical snuff box)
- Anatomic snuff box: Borders (Figure 4–53)
  - Base: Scaphoid bone
  - Lateral: Abductor pollicis longus and extensor pollicis brevis
  - Medial: Extensor pollicis longus

FIGURE 4–52. Anatomic location of Scaphoid Fractures.

Proximal Fracture Pole

Waist Fracture

Distal Fracture Body

Tuberosital Fracture

Imaging

- Plain films: PA and oblique view of the wrist in ulnar deviation with comparisons of the opposite side if needed. Repeat in two weeks if no fracture is seen initially

Treatment

- A fracture may or may not be visualized initially on imaging, therefore, a patient with tenderness in the area of the anatomical snuff box has a fracture until proven otherwise and should be treated accordingly
- Depending on the location of the fracture, regarding which pole (proximal, middle or distal) is involved, will indicate how long immobilization with casting should occur

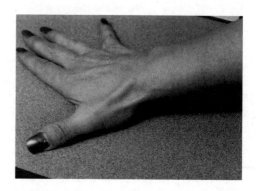

FIGURE 4–53. Anatomic Snuffbox.

- Nondisplaced fracture < 2mm
  - Immobilization of the wrist in a long thumb spica cast for 6 weeks with the wrist in a neutral position
  - At 6 weeks, change to a short thumb spica cast if the plain films show proper healing
  - If poor healing occurs at this time, surgical stabilization may be indicated
- Displaced fracture > 2mm
  - Surgical vs immobilization

FRACTURE OF THE DISTAL RADIUS

General

Types
- Colles' fracture (Figure 4–54A)
  - Most common type of fracture
  - Fracture of the distal radius with *dorsal* angulation
- Smith fracture (Figure 4–54B)
  - Fracture of the distal radius with *volar* angulation
  - Reverse Colles'

Clinical

- Acute pain, swelling at the wrist usually after a fall on an outstretched arm

Imaging

- Plain films of the wrist and hand: AP and lateral

Treatment

- Orthopedic referral for closed reduction depending on the location, degree of displacement, and reproducibility

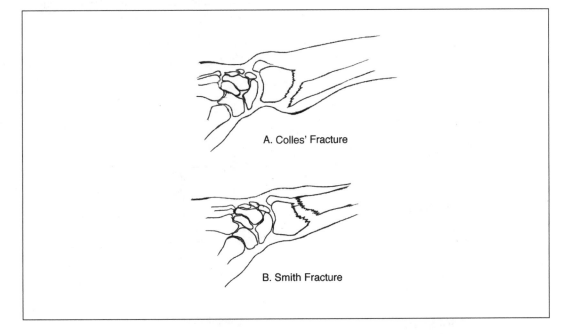

A. Colles' Fracture

B. Smith Fracture

FIGURE 4–54. **A:** Colles' Fracture (Note Radial Dorsal Angulation). **B:** Smith Fracture.

UPPER EXTREMITIES—HAND REGION

FUNCTIONAL ANATOMY

Bones of the Hand (Figure 4–55)

- Eight carpal bones
- Five metacarpals
- Fourteen phalanges
  - Five proximal
  - Four middle (not located in the thumb)
  - Five distal

Tendon Function "Pulley System"

- **Extensor system**
  - Extensor digitorum communis inserts in the terminal portion of digits 2 to 5
- **Flexor system**
  - Two-tendon pulley system made up of the flexor digitorum profundus and superficialis (Figure 4–56)

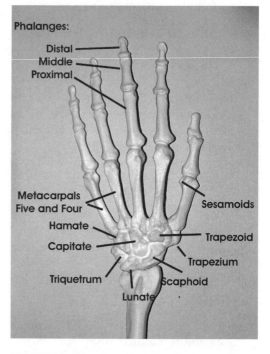

FIGURE 4–55. Dorsal View—Bones of the Wrist and Hand.

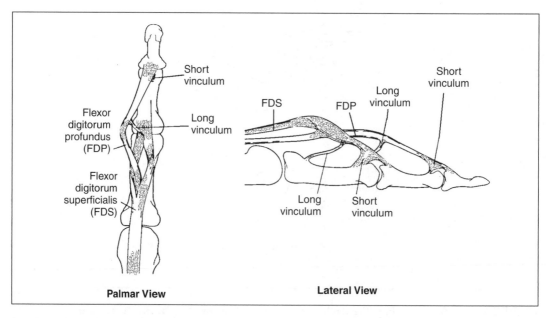

FIGURE 4–56. Flexor Tendon System.

Range of Motion of the Digits (Figure 4–57)

- **Flexion**
  - MCP: 90°
  - PIP: 90°
  - DIP: 90°
  - Thumb: MCP 50°, IP 90°
- **Extension**
  - MCP: 30°
  - PIP: 0°
  - DIP: 0–10°
  - Thumb: MCP 0°, IP 20°
- **Abduction**
  - Finger: 20°
  - Thumb: 70°
- **Adduction**
  - Finger: 0°, return of abduction
  - Thumb: 0°, return of abduction
- **Opposition**
  - Thumb: approximation of the palmar aspect of the thumb and fifth digit
- **Apposition**
  - Thumb: approximation between the thumb and other digit not using the palmar aspect

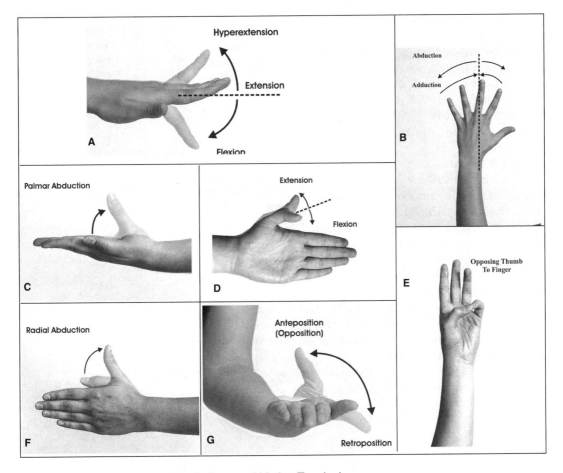

FIGURE 4–57. Finger and Thumb Range of Motion Terminology.

Digit Motion (Figure 4–58, 4–59, 4–60)

- **Finger flexors**
  - Flexor digitorum profundus [digits 2 and 3: anterior interosseus (median) nerve: digits 4 and 5: ulnar nerve, C8, T1]
  - Flexor digitorum superficialis (median nerve, C7, C8, T1)
  - Lumbricals (first and second: medial nerve; third and fourth: ulnar nerve, C8, T1)
  - Interossei (ulnar nerve, C8, T1)
  - Flexor digiti minimi (ulnar nerve, C8, T1)
- **Finger extensors**
  - Extensor digitorum communis [posterior interosseus (radial) nerve, C7, C8]
  - Extensor indicis proprius [posterior interosseus (radial) nerve, C7, C8]
  - Extensor digiti minimi [posterior interosseus (radial) nerve, C7, C8]
- **Finger abduction**
  - 4–Dorsal interossei (DAB) (ulnar nerve, C8, T1)
  - Abductor digiti minimi (ulnar nerve, C8, T1)
- **Finger adduction**
  - 3-Palmar interossei (PAD) (ulnar nerve, C8, T1)
- **Thumb flexors**
  - Flexor pollicis brevis (superficial head: median nerve; deep head: ulnar nerve, C8, T1)
  - Flexor pollicis longus [anterior interosseus (median) nerve, C8, T1]
  - Opponens pollicis (median nerve, C8, T1)
  - Adductor pollicis (ulnar nerve, C8, T1)
- **Thumb extensors**
  - Extensor pollicis longus [posterior interosseus (radial) nerve, C7, C8]
  - Extensor pollicis brevis [posterior interosseus (radial) nerve, C7, C8]
  - Abductor pollicis longus [posterior interosseus (radial) nerve, C7, C8]
- **Abduction of the thumb**
  - Abductor pollicis longus [posterior interosseus (radial) nerve, C7, C8]
  - Abductor pollicis brevis [median nerve, C8, T1]
- **Adduction of the thumb**
  - Adductor pollicis (ulnar nerve, C8, T1)

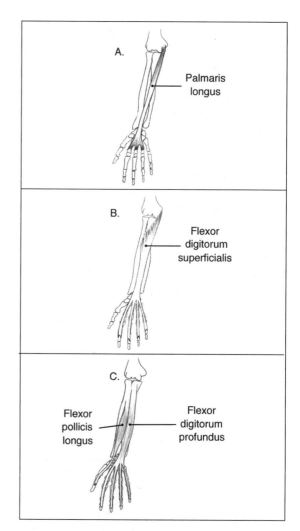

FIGURE 4–58. Hand Flexors: Muscles of the Forearm Anterior Compartment. A. 1st layer B. 2nd layer C. 3rd layer.

- **Opposition of the thumb to fifth digit**
  - Opponens pollicis (median nerve, C8, T1)
  - Flexor pollicis brevis (superficial head: median nerve, C8, T1)
  - Abductor pollicis brevis (median nerve, C8, T1)
  - Opponens digiti minimi (ulnar nerve, C8, T11)

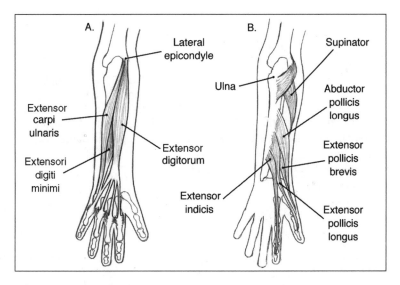

FIGURE 4–59. Muscle of the Forearm Posterior Compartment. **A.** Superficial layer and **B.** Deep layer.

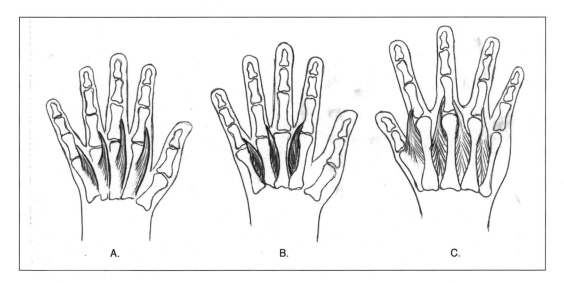

FIGURE 4–60. Palmar View: Intrinsic Muscles of the Hand A. Lumbricals B. Palmar interossei C. Dorsal interosse

■

HAND DISORDERS

DUPUYTREN'S CONTRACTURE (Figure 4–61)

General

Mechanism
- Thickening and contraction of the palmar fascia due to fibrous proliferation

Etiology
- Unknown
- Has dominant genetic component (Northern European descent), has also been called the Viking disease
- Commonly associated with: DM, ETOH, epileptics, pulmonary TB
- Seen in men > 40 years old

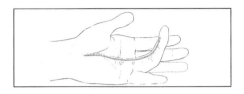

FIGURE 4–61. Dupuytren's Contracture. Reprinted with permission from Snider RK. Essentials of Musculoskeletal Medicine. Rosemont IL, American Academy of Orthopaedic Surgeons, 1997.

Clinical

- Painless nodules in the distal palmar crease. These nodules are initially nontender and may become tender as the disease progresses
- The involved finger may be drawn into flexion as the nodules thicken and contract
- Flexion is commonly seen at the MCP joint involving the ring finger

Imaging

- None needed

Treatment

- Conservative: Ultrasound, splinting, massage
- Surgical release: If severe and affects function

STENOSING TENOSYNOVITIS: TRIGGER FINGER (Figure 4–62)

General

Mechanism
- Repetitive trauma that causes an inflammatory process to the flexor tendon sheath of the digits
- This process forms a nodule in the tendon resulting in abnormal gliding through the pulley system. As the digit flexes, the nodule passes under the pulley system and gets caught on the narrow annular sheath resulting in the finger locked in a flexed position

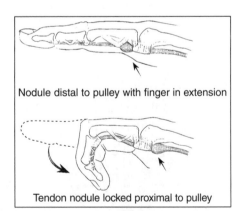

Nodule distal to pulley with finger in extension

Tendon nodule locked proximal to pulley

FIGURE 4–62. Trigger Finger. Nodule or thickening in flexor tendon, which strikes the proximal pulley, making finger extension difficult. Reprinted with permission from Snider RK. Essentials of Musculoskeletal Medicine. Rosemont IL, American Academy of Orthopaedic Surgeons, 1997.

Etiology
- Commonly associated with repetitive trauma, DM, RA
- Seen in persons > 40 years old

Clinical

- A catching or locking with finger flexion and/or extension
- The nodule may be tender on palpation

Imaging

- None needed

Treatment

- Conservative: Immobilization by splinting, NSAIDs, corticosteroid injection
- Surgical release: After failure of conservative treatment

LIGAMENTOUS INJURIES

General (Figure 4–63)

- Involves the ligaments of the digits (PIP and MCP) and the thumb (MCP)
  - Ligaments: Collaterals and volar plate
- Injury may result in a partial tear (sprain) or complete dislocation

Mechanism
- MCP and PIP ligamentous injury to the digits
  - Collateral ligament: Valgus or varus stress with the finger in an extended position
  - Volar plate: Hyperextension with dorsal dislocation, which is usually reducible

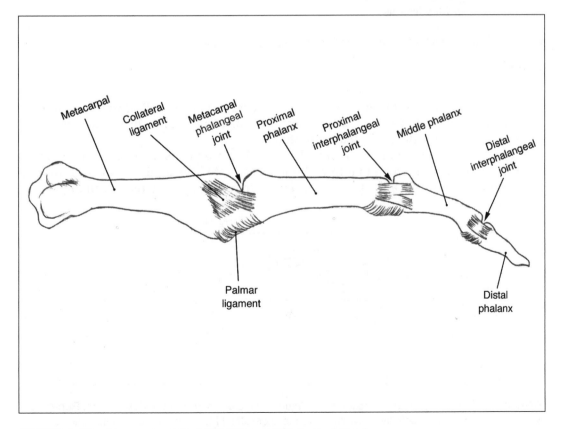

FIGURE 4–63. Ligaments of the MCP, PIP and DIP (Lateral View).

- MCP ligamentous injury to the thumb
  - Ulnar collateral ligament: Valgus stress of the thumb at the MCP joint
    - Synonyms
      - Gamekeeper's thumb
      - Skier's thumb
  - Radial collateral ligament: Uncommon

Clinical

- History of trauma to the finger with an immediate obvious deformity
- Local tenderness over the involved area with swelling of the joint
- Palpate both sides and assess the stability of the joint by applying a stress to the medial and lateral aspect

Imaging

- AP and lateral views to rule out fracture and ensure proper reduction and congruency of the joint

Treatment

- Conservative: Simple dislocations
  - Reduce the joint by stabilizing the proximal end and applying a distal traction
  - Buddy splinting of the finger should be done for approximately 2 weeks
  - Thumb spica 3 to 6 weeks for MCP injuries
- Surgical: Complex lesions

FLEXOR DIGITORUM INJURY: JERSEY FINGER (Fig. 4-64)

General

Mechanism

- Complete or incomplete injury to the flexor tendon (superficialis and/or profundus) which may be spontaneous as in the case of RA or more commonly due to a traumatic nature as seen in athletics (football, wrestling)
- The classic mechanism of injury in athletes is when a player's finger gets caught in the jersey of another in attempting to grab him. The profundus tendon is avulsed from its insertion and possibly accompanied by a bony fragment (usually the fourth digit)

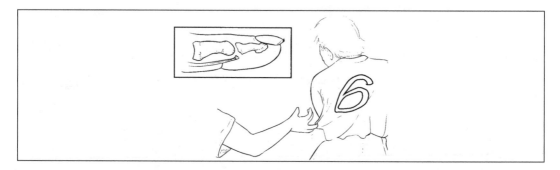

FIGURE 4–64. Jersey Finger: Mechanism of Injury Is Rupture of the Profundus Tendon. Reprinted with permission from Snider RK. Essentials of Musculoskeletal Medicine. Rosemont IL, American Academy of Orthopaedic Surgeons, 1997.

Clinical

- The patient is unable to actively flex the DIP joint
- Testing of the FDP (Fig. 4-65A)
  - In order to effectively test the function of the FDP, the patient must flex the DIP while the examiner holds the PIP joint in extension
- Testing flexion of the FDS (Fig. 4-65B)
  - The FDP can provide the same function of the FDS, which is MCP and PIP flexion, secondary to its attachment at the DIP
  - The examiner must isolate the FDS when testing its function secondary to the action of the FDP. This is done by eliminating the action of the FDP by holding the DIP of the non-involved digits in extension. The patient is then asked to flex the unrestrained digit, which can only be done with a normal FDS tendon

Imaging

- None needed
- Plain films may show an avulsed fragment near tendonous insertion

Treatment

- Orthopedic referral: Early surgical repair

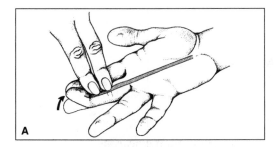 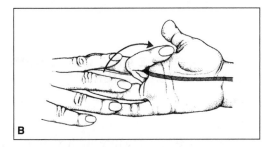

FIGURE 4–65. **A.** Test for FDP Function. **B.** Test for FDS Function. Reprinted with permission from Snider RK. Essentials of Musculoskeletal Medicine. Rosemont IL, American Academy of Orthopaedic Surgeons, 1997.

MALLET FINGER (Figure 4–66)

General

Mechanism
- Sudden passive flexion of the DIP joint when the finger is extended, causing a rupture of the tendon
- An avulsed fragment of the distal phalanx may also occur

Clinical

- A flexed DIP joint that cannot be actively extended
- DIP joint tenderness and edema at the distal dorsal area

Imaging

- None needed
- An avulsed fragment of the distal phalanx may be seen

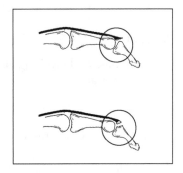

FIGURE 4–66. Mallet Finger. **Top:** Rupture of the extensor tendon at its insertion. **Bottom:** Avulsion of a piece of distal phalanx.

Treatment

- Conservative: Splinting of the DIP in extension for 6 to 8 weeks (Figure 4–67)
  - Maintaining the finger in extension is essential and should be done at all times
  - Weekly visits to assess full finger extension should be done
  - At the end of the six-week course, gentle active flexion with night splinting should be done for 2 to 4 weeks
- Surgical repair
  - Reserved for poor healing or if an avulsed fragment involves > one-third of the joint

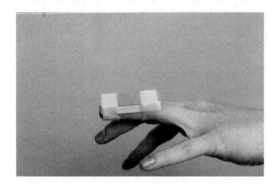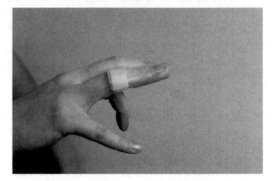

FIGURE 4–67. Splint for Treatment of Mallet Finger.

FRACTURE OF THE FIRST METACARPAL BASE: BENNET'S OR ROLANDO'S FRACTURE

General

Definitions

- *Bennet's:* Oblique fracture subluxation of the base of the thumb metacarpal
- *Rolando's:* Fracture at the base of the thumb metacarpal that may classified as a T, Y, or comminuted configuration

Complications

- An avulsed metacarpal fragment in a Bennet's fracture may subluxate secondary to the proximal pull of the abductor pollicis longus muscle

Clinical

- Tenderness and swelling at the base of the digit (thumb or fifth) following a direct blow to a flexed thumb or digit

Imaging

- Plain films: AP lateral and oblique

Treatment

- Orthopedic referral

METACARPAL FRACTURE TO THE NECK OR SHAFT: BOXER'S FRACTURE

General

Mechanism (Figure 4–68)

- Fracture of the metacarpal neck/shaft usually seen after a person strikes a wall or another with poor technique
- May occur at any digit but commonly seen at the fifth digit

Clinical

- Tenderness and swelling in the area of the hand seen after traumatic event

Imaging

- Plain films

Treatment

- Orthopedic referral

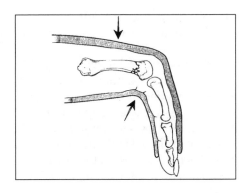

FIGURE 4–68. Boxer's Fracture. (Placed in an ulnar gutter splint). Reprinted with permission from Snider RK. Essentials of Musculoskeletal Medicine. Rosemont IL, American Academy of Orthopaedic Surgeons, 1997.

▪ LOWER EXTREMITIES—HIP

- The three hip joints of the pelvic girdle consist of the acetabular joint, the pubic symphysis, and the sacroiliac joint
- The hip is a very stable, multidirectional mobile ball and socket joint (enarthrosis)
- Due to high mobility, hip-joint pathology will be manifested during weight bearing, ambulation, or motion
- Pathology affecting the sacroiliac joint and pubic symphysis does not restrict motion to the extent that hip-joint pathology will
- The angle between the femoral neck and shaft of the femur is different in males (125°) than in females (115 to 120°). This difference is due to the female pelvis being wider to accommodate the birth canal and gravid uterus
  - Coxa vara occurs when the femoral neck and shaft angle is decreased. The affected leg is shortened and hip abduction is limited. The knee assumes a valgus deformity
  - Coxa valga occurs when the angle is increased. The affected limb is lengthened and the knees assumes a varus deformity

HIP AND PELVIC FUNCTIONAL ANATOMY (Figure 4–69)

Muscles

Flexor Group (Figure 4–70)
- Iliopsoas (nerve to iliopsoas or femoral nerve; L2, L3)
  - Prime hip flexor
- Sartorius (femoral nerve; L2, L3, L4)
- Rectus femoris (femoral nerve; L2, L3, L4)
- Pectineus (femoral nerve; L2, L3, L4)
- Tensor fasciae latae (superior gluteal nerve; L4, L5, S1)
- Adductor brevis (obturator nerve; L2, L3, L4)
- Adductor longus (obturator nerve; L2, L3, L4)
- Adductor magnus (obturator and sciatic nerves; L2, L3, L4, S1)
- Gracilis (obturator nerve; L2, L3, L4)

Adductor Group (Anteriorly Placed) (Figure 4–71)
- Gracilis (obturator nerve; L2, L3, L4)
- Pectineus (femoral nerve; L2, L3, L4)
- Adductor longus (obturator nerve; L2, L3, L4)
- Adductor brevis (obturator nerve; L2, L3, L4)
- Adductor magnus (obturator and sciatic nerves; L2, L3, L4, S1)

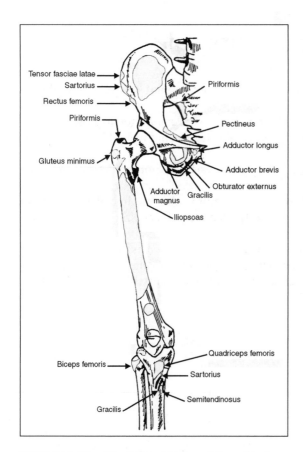

FIGURE 4–69. The Pelvis, Thigh and Knee Region.

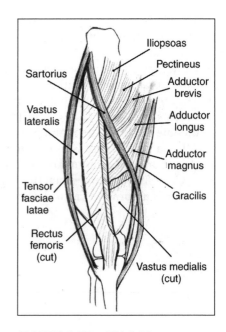

FIGURE 4–70. Thigh Flexors.

Adductor Group (Posteriorly Placed) (Figure 4–72)
- Gluteus maximus (inf. gluteal nerve, L5, S1, S2)
- Obturator externus (abturator n. L3, L4)
- Gracilis (obturator n. L2, L3, L4)
- Biceps long head (L5, S1, S2)
- Semitendinosus (L4, L5, S1, S2)
- Semimembranosus (L5, S1, S2)

Abductor Group (Figure 4–73)
- Gluteus medius (superior gluteal nerve; L4, L5, S1)
- Gluteus minimus (superior gluteal nerve; L4, L5, S1) abduction and medial rotation
- Tensor fascia latae (superior gluteal nerve; L4, L5, S1)
- Sartorius (femoral n. L2, L3, L4)
- Piriformis (nerve to piriformis; S1, S2)
- Gluteus maximus (upper fibers) (inferior gluteal n. L5, S1, S2)

Extensor Group (Fig. 4-73)
- Gluteus maximus (inferior gluteal nerve; L5, S1, S2)
  - Prime mover
- Gluteus medius (posterior part) (superior gluteal n. L4, L5, S1)
- Gluteus minimus (posterior part) (superior gluteal n. L4, L5, S1)
- Piriformis (nerve to piriformis, S1, S2)
- Adductor magnus (sciatic part) (obturator and sciatic n. L2, L3, L4)

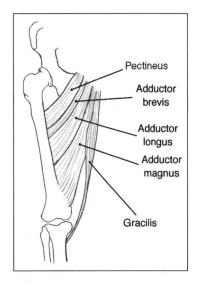

FIGURE 4–71. Adductors of the Thigh (Anteriorly Placed).

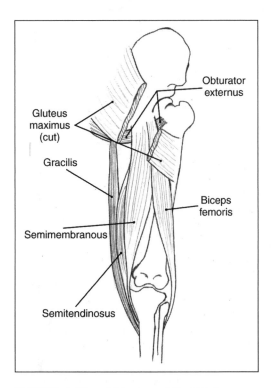

FIGURE 4–72. Adductors of the Thigh (Posteriorly Placed).

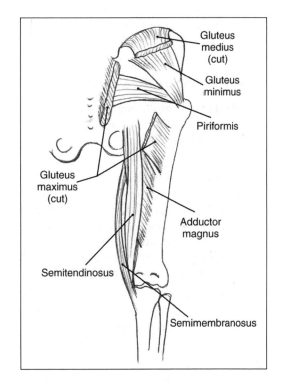

FIGURE 4–73. Extensors of the Thigh.

- Hamstring muscles:
- Biceps femoris long head (L5, S1, S2)
- Semimembranosus (L5, S1, S2)
- Semitendinosus (L4, L5, S1, S2)
- Sciatic nerve and tibial division for all

Lateral Rotation (Figure 4–74)

- Piriformis (nerve to the piriformis; S1, S2)
- Obturator internus (nerve to the obturator internus; L5, S1)
- Gemelli (nerve to the superior gemellus; L5, S1, S2, and inferior gemellus L4, L5, S1, S2)
- Obturator externus (obturator nerve; L3 and L4)
- Quadratus femoris (nerve to the quadratus femoris; L4, L5, S1)
- Gluteus maximus (inf. gluteal n. L5, S1, S2)
- Gluteus medius and minimus (superior gluteal n. L4, L5, S1)

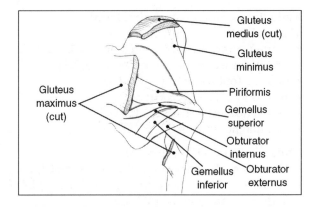

FIGURE 4–74. Lateral (External) Rotators of the Thigh (Quadratus femoris not shown) (Posterior view)

Medial Rotation (Figure 4–75)

- Pneumonic: TAGGG SS
- Tensor fasciae latae (superior gluteal n. L4, L5, S1)
- Adductor magnus, longus and brevis (add. magn; obturator n.; sciatic n. (L2, L3, L4, S1) (add. longus; add. brevis (L2, L3, L4)
- Gluteus medius (superior gluteal n. L4)
- Gluteus minimus (superior gluteal n. L4, L5, S1)
- Gracilis (obturator n. L2, L3, L4)
- Semitendinosus (L5, S1, S2)
- Semimembranosus (L5, S1, S2)

Ligaments (Figure 4–76A, B)

Acetabular Labrum (Glenoid Labrum)

- The acetabular labrum serves to deepen the acetabulum and its function is to hold the femoral head in place

Articular Fibrous Capsule

- The articular fibrous capsule extends from the acetabular rim to the intertrochanteric crest forming a cylindrical sleeve that encloses the hip joint and most of the femoral neck. Circular fibers around the femoral neck constrict the capsule and help to hold the femoral head in the acetabulum

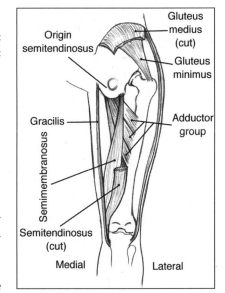

FIGURE 4–75. Medial (Internal) Rotators of the Thigh (Posterior View).

Iliofemoral

- Also known as the Y-ligament of Bigelow, it is the strongest ligament in the body
- The iliofemoral ligament extends from the anterior inferior iliac spine to intertrochanteric line
- Its function is to prevent overextension, abduction and lateral rotation

Ischiofemoral

- The ischiofemoral ligament extends from the ischium behind the acetabulum to blend with the capsule
- Its function is to check medial rotation

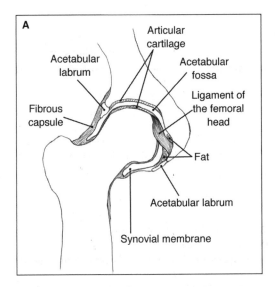

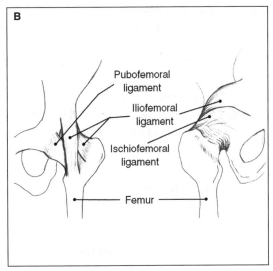

FIGURE 4–76. **A.** Frontal Section Through the Hip Joint. **B.** Anterior (a), and Posterior (b) View of the Left Hip Joint.

Pubofemoral
- The pubofemoral ligament extends from the superior pubic ramus and joins the iliofemoral ligament
- Its function is to check abduction

Ligamentum Capitis Femoris
- The capitis femoris ligament extends from the acetabular notch to the femur
- This ligament is fairly weak and does little to strengthen the hip
- In 80% of cases it carries a small artery to the femoral head

Normal Range of Hip Motion in the Adult

Flexion—120°
Extension—30°
Abduction—45–50°
Adduction—0–30°
External rotation—35°
Internal rotation—45°
- Osteoarthritis first limits internal rotation

Hip Tests

Fabere (Patrick) (Figure 4–77)
- This test is used to assess *F*lexion, *Ab*duction, *E*xternal *R*otation
- Perform this test with the patient supine, passively flex and externally rotate and abduct the hip
- The hip joint is now flexed, abducted, and externally rotated. In this position, inguinal pain is a general indication that there is pathology in the hip joint or the surrounding muscles

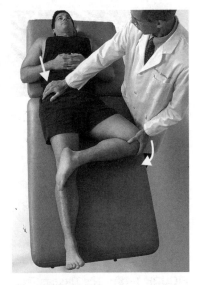

FIGURE 4–77. Fabere Test (or Patrick Test)

Thomas (Figure 4–78)

- This test is used to assess hip flexion contractures
- Perform this test with the patient supine, flex one hip fully reducing the lumbar spine lordosis, stabilizing the lumbar spine and pelvis, extend the opposite hip. If that hip does not fully extend, a flexion contracture is present

Ober (Figure 4–79)

- Tests for contraction of the fascia lata
- Perform the test as the patient is side lying with the involved leg uppermost. Abduct the leg as far as possible and flex the knee to 90°. If the thigh remains abducted, there may be a contracture of the tensor fascia lata or iliotibial band

Trendelenburg (Figure 4–80)

- Tests for gluteus medius weakness
- Performed with the patient standing erect, one foot is raised off the floor
- Strength of the gluteus medius of the supported side is assessed
- A positive test occurs when the pelvis on the unsupported side descends or remains level

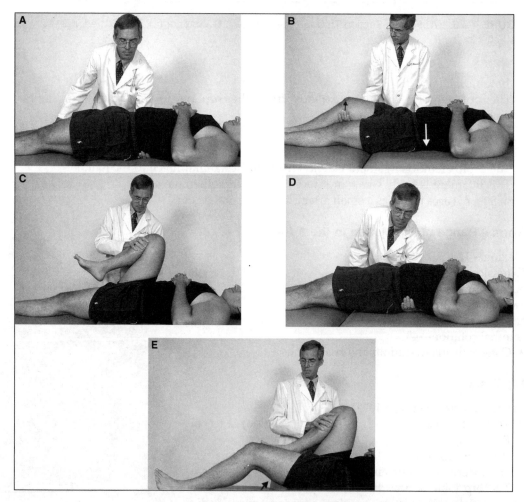

FIGURE 4–78. The Thomas Test. **A.** Patient is supine. **B.** Flex one hip, fully reducing the lumbar spine lordosis. **C.** The normal limit for hip flexion is approximately 135°. **D.** A fixed flexion contracture is characterized by the inability to extend the leg straight without arching the thoracic spine. **E.** The degree of the flexion contracture can be done by estimating the angle between the table and patient's leg.

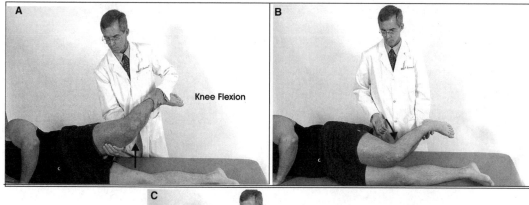

Knee Flexion

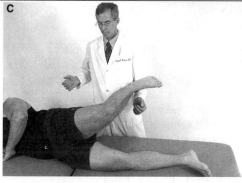

FIGURE 4–79. Ober Test. **A.** Test used to assess the contraction of the fascia lata. **B.** Negative Ober. **C.** Positive Ober.

- A negative test occurs when the pelvis on the unsupported side elevates slightly
- Conditions associated with gluteus medius weakness:
  - Radiculopathies
  - Poliomyelitis
  - Meningomyelocele
  - Fractures of the greater trochanter
  - Slipped capital femoral epiphysis
  - Congenital hip dislocation

Leg Length Discrepancy

True Leg Length Discrepancy (TLLD) (Figure 4–81)
- To assess TLL, measure from the ASIS to the medial malleoli. (Note there are two fixed bony landmarks.)
- To determine if the discrepancy is in the femur or the tibia:
  - With the patient supine, flex the knees to 90° and place feet flat on the table
  - If one knee is higher than the other, that tibia is longer (Fig. 4-81C(a))
  - If one knee projects further anteriorly, then that femur is longer (Fig. 4-81C(b))
  - True leg length shortening may be due to fractures crossing the epiphyseal plate in childhood or poliomyelitis

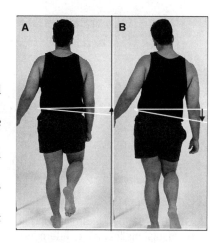

FIGURE 4–80. Trendelenburg Test. **A.** Negative. **B.** Positive

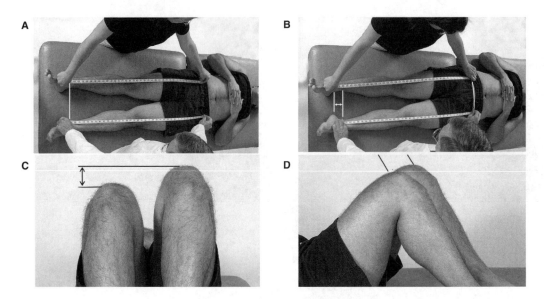

FIGURE 4–81. **A.** Examiner should measure from one fixed bony point (i.e., ASIS anterior superior iliac spine) to another (i.e., medial malleolus) to find true leg length. **B.** True leg length discrepancy. **C.** tibial length discrepancy; **D.** femoral length discrepancy.

Apparent Leg Length Discrepancy (Figure 4–82)

- First determine that no true leg length discrepancy exists
- With the patient supine, measure from the umbilicus to the medial malleoli, from a nonfixed to a fixed landmark
- Apparent discrepancy may be caused by pelvic obliquities or flexion or adduction deformity of the hip
- Pelvis obliquity may be assessed by observing the levelness of the anterior superior iliac spines or the posterior superior iliac spines

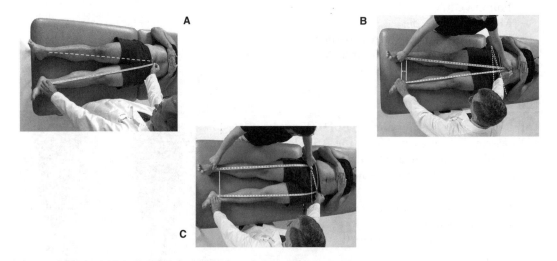

FIGURE 4–82. **A.** Examiner should measure from a nonfixed point (i.e., umbilicus) to a fixed point (i.e., medial malleolus) to determine an apparent leg length discrepancy. **B.** An apparent leg length discrepancy associated with pelvic obliquity. **C.** True leg length measurements are equal despite the apparent leg length discrepancy.

■
HIP DISORDERS

HAMSTRING STRAIN

General

- Predisposing factors associated with hamstring muscle strains include inadequate warm-up, poor flexibility, exercise fatigue, poor conditioning, and muscle imbalance
- A rehab program needs to modify these risk factors
- 📖 Note that the normal strength ratio of hamstrings to quadriceps is 3:5
- Injuries occur during the eccentric phase of muscle contraction
- Injuries range in severity from Grade I (strain) to Grade III (complete tear)
- Most commonly seen in track and gymnastics injuries

Clinical

- Presents as pain in the hamstring region after a forceful hamstring contraction or knee extension
- Pain may occur with loss of function
- There is tenderness over the muscle belly or origin
- Provocative test: Pain elicited in the ischial region with knee flexion

Imaging

- Generally not needed

Treatment

- Ice, compression, weight-bearing reduction if necessary, NSAIDs, gentle stretch
- Advance to strengthening when inflammation is reduced

PIRIFORMIS SYNDROME

General

- A painful muscle condition involving the piriformis muscle, an external hip rotator
- The piriformis can be stressed due to poor body mechanics in a chronic condition or injured acutely with forceful hip internal rotation
- In severe spasms the sciatic nerve may be involved to some degree because the nerve pierces the piriformis muscle fibers in some individuals
- Rehabilitation seeks to reduce pain and spasm and recover full hip internal rotation

Clinical

- Pain associated with piriformis injury may present in the lateral buttock, posterior hip and proximal posterior thigh, as well as the sacroiliac region
- The condition may be exacerbated by walking up stairs
- There is tenderness over the muscle belly that stretches from the sacrum to the greater trochanter
- Provocative test: Pain with internal hip rotation, adduction, and flexion

Imaging

- Radiographs of the low spine and hip may be necessary to rule out other sources of pathology

Treatment

- Stretching of the external rotator hip muscles, NSAIDs, and ultrasound are the initial therapies
- Local corticosteroids by injection can be used if more conservative measures fail

ILIOPSOAS BURSITIS AND TENDONITIS

Also known as iliopsoas snapping-tendon syndrome (Figure 4–83)

General

- Inflammation of the muscle tendon unit and bursa occur with overuse or trauma, causing muscle tightness and imbalance
- This condition may cause hip snapping
- The snapping is due to the iliotibial band snapping over the greater trochanter or the iliopsoas tendon subluxating over the pectineal eminence of the pelvis

Clinical

- Hip snapping may occur with flexion and may cause pain
- There is tenderness over the iliopsoas muscle
- Provocative test: Pain on hip flexion

Imaging

- Radiographs of the hip are useful to rule out underlying bony pathology

Treatment

- Ice, NSAIDs, stretching and strengthening
- Corticosteroid injection if conservative measures fail

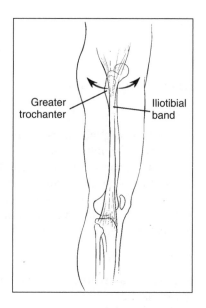

FIGURE 4–83. Iliopsoas Snapping Tendon Syndrome. Reprinted with permission from Snider RK. Essentials of Musculoskeletal Medicine. Rosemont IL, American Academy of Orthopaedic Surgeons, 1997.

HIP ADDUCTOR STRAIN—GROIN STRAIN

General

- A common injury in sports, groin strain occurs due to resisted forceful abduction of the hip
- The adductor groups are injured during eccentric contraction
- Predisposing factors include relative weakness and tightness of the adductor muscle groups
- It is important to distinguish muscle strain from adductor avulsion fracture

Clinical

- Presents as pain in the adductors distal to their origin at the ramus or adductor tubercle
- Provocative test: There is pain with resisted adduction and occasionally with hip flexion
- On palpation there is tenderness of the adductor muscle

Imaging

- Radiographs of the hip including the adductor tubercle to rule out avulsion

Treatment

- Rest, ice, NSAIDs, advance to stretching and strengthening

GREATER TROCHANTER BURSITIS (FIGURE 4–84)

General

- This condition is inflammation of the bursa located over the greater trochanter and deep to the gluteus medius and gluteus minimus and tensor fasciae latae
- It is associated with a number of conditions that cause altered gait mechanics, muscle imbalance and reduced flexibility including hip osteoarthritis, obesity, leg length discrepancy, direct trauma, overuse, herniated lumbar disc and hemiparesis
- This condition may also cause hip snapping

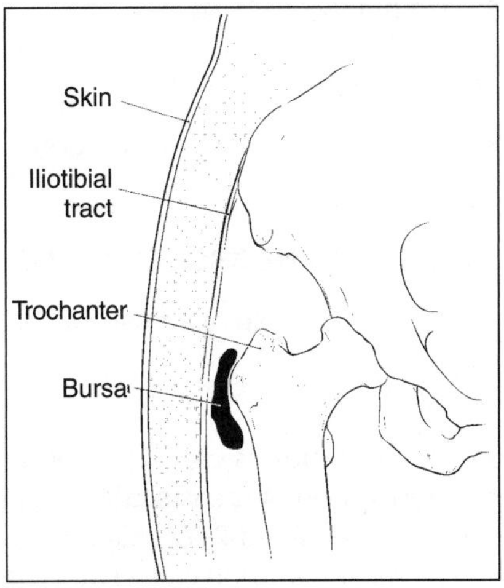

Clinical

- Patients report night pain and are unable to lie on the affected side
- Provocative test: Presents as pain over the greater trochanter during movement from full extension to flexion
- A snap may be palpable over the greater tubercle

Imaging

- Radiographs of the hip to rule out bony pathology

FIGURE 4–84. Trochanteric Bursa. Note relationship of the trochanteric bursa between the iliotibial band and the greater trochanter. Reprinted with permission from Snider RK. Essentials of Musculoskeletal Medicine. Rosemont IL, American Academy of Orthopaedic Surgeons, 1997.

Treatment

- Iliotibial band stretching, NSAIDs, and in severe cases, a cane may be needed for support and stability
- Strengthening of the hip adductor groups
- Local corticosteroid injection for resistant cases

POSTERIOR HIP DISLOCATION

General

- This is the most common type of hip dislocation and comprises 90% of the total
- It may occur during an automobile accident when the hip is flexed, adducted, and medially rotated. The knee strikes the dashboard with the femur in this position, driving it posteriorly. In this position, the head of the femur is covered posteriorly by the capsule and not by bone
- Due to the close proximity of the sciatic nerve to the hip posteriorly, the sciatic nerve may be stretched or compressed in posterior hip dislocations. **Note:** Anterior hip dislocations may result in femoral nerve compromise
- Avascular necrosis may occur in 10% to 20% of patients

Clinical

- The hip will be flexed, adducted, and internally rotated
- The affected leg appears shorter because the dislocated femoral head is higher than the normal side
- There will be an inability to abduct the affected hip

Imaging

- Hip radiographs

Treatment

- This is an orthopedic emergency due to potential vascular compromise and sciatic nerve injury

AVASCULAR NECROSIS OF THE FEMORAL HEAD (Figure 4–85)

Also known as osteonecrosis of the hip or aseptic necrosis of the hip

General

- This condition is characterized by death of the femoral head without sepsis
- Interruption of the vascular supply is the defining common pathway of the disease process
- In children aged 2–12 this is known as Legg-Calve-Perthes disease
- The most common causes in adults are steroid use and alcohol abuse

Clinical

- Pain may present in the groin, anterior thigh, or even the knee
- Symptoms are of insidious onset
- Short swing and stance phase on the affected side may be observed
- There is loss of external and internal rotation of the hip
- On hip flexion, the hip will externally rotate
- Pain is elicited on ROM

Imaging

- Irregular or mottled femoral head on plane films
  - MRI of both hips is indicated
  - There is low signal intensity on T1 imaging

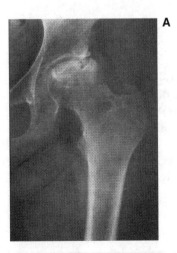

A

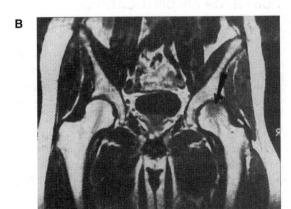

B

FIGURE 4–85. **A**. Sclerosis of the femoral head. **B.** MRI scan of hips consistent with osteonecrosis of left hip (arrow). Reprinted with permission from Snider RK. Essentials of Musculoskeletal Medicine. Rosemont IL, American Academy of Orthopaedic Surgeons, 1997.

Treatment

- The main objective is to maintain the femoral head within the acetabulum while healing and remodeling occurs
- Bracing and casting may help in the pediatric population to retain the femoral head within the acetabulum
- Osteotomy of the femoral head and pelvis may be used to treated symptomatically and monitored if the disease is not significantly advanced
- Adults may require total hip arthroplasty

HIP FRACTURES

General

- Osteoporosis of the hip carries increased incidence of fracture
- Osteoporosis of the hip is associated with both fixed and modifiable risk factors
  - Fixed risk factors include age, sex, and race
  - Approximately 60% of hip fractures occur in patients > 75 years of age
  - Females have higher incidence of hip fracture than males
  - Among females, there is a 2–3:1 higher rate of fracture in European Americans than in African Americans
  - Modifiable risk factors include: Alcohol and caffeine consumption, smoking, use of certain medications (antipsychotics, benzodiazepines), malnutrition, and body weight below 90% of ideal
- Surgery for hip fracture and degeneration carries considerable risks of morbidity and mortality
  - Venous thrombosis occurs in greater than 50% of unprotected patients. **Note:** The risk for pulmonary embolism is highest during the second and third week
  - The incidence of heterotopic ossification is high (> 50%) after total hip replacement and is the most common complication although less than 10% lose range of motion
  - The mortality rate for those who survive a hip fracture is 20% to 30% after one year and approximately 40% after two years
  - Approximately 50% of patients return to their premorbid level of functioning
- Classification is based on the anatomy of the proximal femur and consists of three main types: intracapsular, intertrochanteric and subtrochanteric (Figure 4–86)

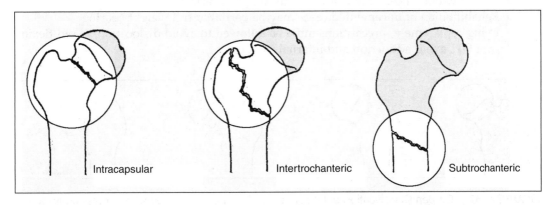

FIGURE 4–86. Classification of Hip Fractures Based on the Anatomy of the Proximal Femur.

INTRACAPSULAR OR FEMORAL-NECK FRACTURES

General

- Fractures of the femoral neck are classified by Garden Classification Stages I, II, III, IV (Figure 4–87)
  - Stage I—incomplete, nondisplaced with occasional valgus angulation
  - Stage II—complete, nondisplaced, occasionally unstable
  - Stage III—displaced with the hip joint capsule partially intact
  - Stage IV—displaced with the hip joint capsule completely disrupted
- Morbidity associated with the fracture involves disruption of the blood vessels to the femoral head causing necrosis
- Postoperatively, complications can include a nonunion or osteonecrosis

Clinical

- Common presentation of hip fracture are hip pain, limb external rotation greater than normal, and an apparent shortened limb on the affected side

Imaging

- Radiographs of the hip
- Bone scan may be necessary for occult fractures

Treatment

- Garden Stages I and II
  - Surgical
    - Pins across the fracture site or a cannulated hip screw is used for stabilization
  - Rehabilitation
    - Rehabilitation early with partial or full weight bearing
    - May be treated conservatively if the patient is unfit for surgery or in the case of an old impacted fracture
- Garden Stages III and IV:
  - Surgical
    - Replacement of the femoral head using cemented or noncemented hemiarthroplasty; total hip replacement or bipolar arthroplasty
  - Rehabilitation
    - Rehabilitation of cemented cases by full weight bearing
    - Rehabilitation of uncemented cases may be partial or full weight bearing
    - In hip replacement, precautions must be followed to avoid dislocation: Avoid flexion over 90°; avoid adduction and internal rotation

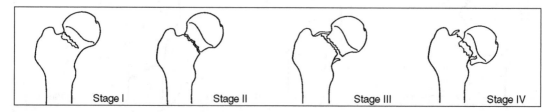

FIGURE 4–87. Garden Classification of Intracapsular Fractures. Reprinted with permission from Gerhart TN. Managing and preventing hip fractures in the elderly. J Musculo Med, 1987(4)60-8. Cliggott Publishers.

INTERTROCHANTERIC FRACTURES

General (Figure 4–88)

- This is the most common type of hip fracture
- Highly fragmented fractures may result in significant blood loss and hypovolemia
- Postoperatively, a leg length discrepancy may result due to comminution status post fixation
- Moderately high forces are generated in this area, and a strong fixation is required
- Fractures may be undisplaced, displaced two-part fractures, or unstable three-part fractures

Clinical

- The common presentation of hip fracture may be seen: Hip pain and an externally rotated and shortened limb

Imaging

- Radiographs and possible CT scan or MRI

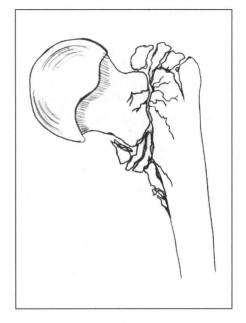

FIGURE 4–88. Intertrochanteric Hip Fracture. (Note fragmentation.)

Treatment

- Surgical
  - A compression screw or angle nail plate may be used
  - If the fixation is unstable, medial displacement osteotomy of the femur may be required
- Rehabilitation
  - Rehabilitation with progressive weight bearing from partial to full

SUBTROCHANTERIC FRACTURES

General (Figure 4–89)

- This region is subjected to very high mechanical stresses and is the most difficult to stabilize surgically
- Fractures may be simple, fragmented, or comminuted

Clinical

- The typical signs and symptoms of hip fracture are present: Hip pain, limb external rotation with possible shortening and malalignment

Imaging

- Radiographs of the hip and possible CT scan

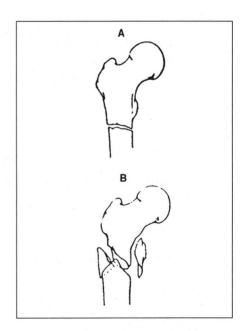

FIGURE 4–89. Subtrochanteric Femur Fractures. **A.** Simple. **B.** Comminuted.

Treatment

- Surgical
  - Open reduction and internal fixation will be necessary with several choices of fixation hardware
  - A blade plate and screws may be sufficient in some cases
  - An intramedullary rod may be required to make an extremely strong fixation through the proximal femur and trochanteric region
- Rehabilitation
  - In these fractures, rehabilitation may be delayed until fracture healing is evident
  - Weight bearing progresses from partial to full

FEMORAL-NECK STRESS FRACTURES

General

- There are two basic types of femoral-neck fractures: Compression and transverse
- Compression-type fractures are more common and generally occur along the inferior neck of the femur. They are more stable
- Transverse-type occurs with the fracture along superior aspect of the femur neck. These are more unstable and are also termed tension side fractures
- Endurance athletes, such as runners and military recruits, are susceptible to proximal femur stress fractures

Clinical

- Femoral-neck stress fractures present as groin pain made worse with activities of daily living
- There will often be pain at extreme ranges of internal and external rotation

Imaging

- Radiographs may be negative at first and in time may show periosteal thickening or a radiolucent line
- If plain films are negative, a bone scan should be done
- Bone scans may be positive 2–8 days after onset of symptoms

Treatment

- Compression type
  - Because they are more stable, they may be treated with bed rest
  - When there is no pain at rest, then weight bearing to limitation of pain is allowed
  - If compression-type fractures progress, they may require internal fixation
- Transverse or tension type
  - These fractures are generally treated with internal fixation due to the high risk of displacement

SLIPPED CAPITAL FEMORAL EPIPHYSIS (FIGURE 4–90)

General

- This is an injury to the epiphyseal growth plate at the head of the femur causing displacement of the plate
- The common ages of incidence are children 11–16
- The injury may be associated with a direct hip trauma

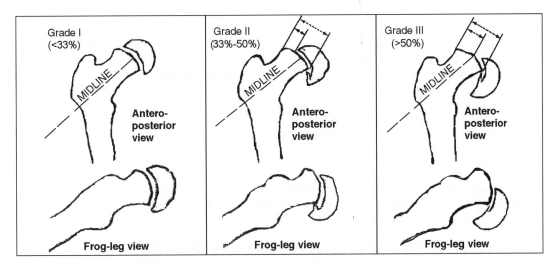

FIGURE 4–90. Slipped Capital Femoral Epiphysis Classification: Grade I, Grade II, Grade III. (% indicates degree of slippage for each grade)

Clinical

- Slipped capital femoral epiphysis presents as groin pain or hip pain but may also present as thigh or knee pain
- It is often associated with an antalgic gait
- Internal hip rotation is limited and the extremity externally rotates when the hip is flexed
- Muscle spasms and synovitis occur in the acute phase

Imaging

- Radiographs and/or CT will reveal medial and posterior displacement of the epiphysis

Treatment

- Immediate cessation of weight bearing
- Surgical stabilization is required
- Endocrine testing should be done to rule out:
  - Growth hormone deficiency
  - Hyperthyroidism
  - Hypothyroidism
  - Panhypopituitarism
  - Multiple endocrine neoplasia

AVULSION FRACTURES

ISCHIAL TUBEROSITY AVULSION FRACTURES

General

- Ischial tuberosity avulsion fractures generally occur with a forceful hamstring contracture with the knee in extension and the hip in flexion
- The origin of the hamstring is pulled away from the ischial tuberosity
- Ischial avulsion must be differentiated from ischial bursitis
- Ischial tuberosity bursitis (also known as weaver's bottom) is of insidious onset and is more progressive in presentation

Clinical

- Ischial tuberosity avulsion fractures present as pain and tenderness over the ischial tuberosity of sudden onset
- There will be reproduction or increased pain on straight leg raising

Imaging

- Radiographs should reveal the avulsion at the ischium

Treatment

- Generally, this avulsion is treated with rest, ice, and weight bearing as tolerated
- After achieving full range of motion, resistance exercises can be started
- Surgery may be required for a displaced apophysis

ANTERIOR SUPERIOR ILIAC SPINE (ASIS) AVULSION FRACTURES

General

- The ASIS is the point of attachment for the sartorius muscle
- This avulsion is caused by forceful contraction with the hip extended and the knee flexed
- If the lateral femoral cutaneous nerve is involved, paresthesias may involve the anterolateral thigh

Clinical

- These avulsions present as acute pain and tenderness over the ASIS
- There should be pain on hip flexion

Imaging

- Radiographs should demonstrate the avulsion fracture

Treatment

- ASIS avulsions are generally treated with rest, ice, and weight bearing as tolerated
- They may require the knee to be splinted in flexion to reduce tension on the avulsion segment
- Stretching and strengthening are instituted with reduction in pain
- Surgery may be required for a displaced apophysis

ANTERIOR INFERIOR ILIAC SPINE (AIIS) AVULSION FRACTURES

General

- The AIIS is the point of origin for the rectus femoris muscle
- Avulsions here may be caused by forceful kicking and contraction of the quadriceps

Clinical

- Avulsion here can present as pain over the AIIS or groin pain of acute onset
- Pain will be produced with quadriceps contraction, hip flexion, or hip extension

Imaging

- Radiographs should demonstrate the avulsion

Treatment

- These avulsions are generally treated with rest and ice with weight bearing as tolerated
- Strengthening may begin after full range of motion is achieved
- Surgery may be required for a displaced apophysis

OSTEITIS PUBIS

General

- This is an inflammatory condition of the joint of the pubic rami
- It is often caused by cumulative overuse of the adductors

Clinical

- Osteitis pubis presents as pubic symphysis or groin pain and may radiate into the thigh
- Normal ambulation may produce a popping in the pubic region
- Pain will be produced on resisted adduction
- Pain can be elicited in the groin or pubic area with one-legged hopping

Imaging

- Radiographs and/or CT may show periosteal thickening

Treatment

- Generally rest and NSAIDs are the first line of treatment
- Corticosteroid injection may be required in resistant cases
- Stretching and strengthening may proceed after reduction in pain
- Surgery for arthrodesis may be required in severe cases

MYOSITIS OSSIFICANS

General

- Myositis ossificans is the formation of heterotopic ossification within muscle
- This can be due to a direct blow to the hip
- Ultrasound, heat, massage, or repeated trauma at the onset of myositis ossificans can exacerbate the process

Clinical

- There will be pain and a palpable mass at the site of the lesion
- If the ossifying mass involves a nerve, related nerve impingement symptoms may occur

Imaging

- Initially radiographs will reveal a soft tissue mass
- Within 14 days calcific flocculations can develop
- Ossification can be seen between 2–3 weeks

Treatment

- Gentle range of motion
- Prevention of contractures is of prime importance
- Strengthening of the involved muscles should be done progressively

- Surgery may be necessary in cases resulting in nerve entrapment, decreased range of motion, or loss of function
- If possible, surgery should be delayed until the lesion matures at 10–12 months

■

LOWER EXTREMITIES—THE KNEE

KNEE FUNCTIONAL ANATOMY

- The knee joint is a modified hinge joint
- The knee is the largest joint in the body. It is susceptible to injury because it is at the end of the tibia and femur, two long lever arms

RANGE OF MOTION

Flexion—135°
Extension—0°
Internal Rotation—10°
External Rotation—10°

MUSCLES (Fig. 4–91)

Extensors

- Quadriceps (femoral nerve, L2, L3, L4):
  - Rectus femoris
  - Vastus lateralis
  - Vastus intermedius
  - Vastus medialis oblique
- All join with the patellar tendon
- The vastus medialis and lateralis draw the patellar in their direction

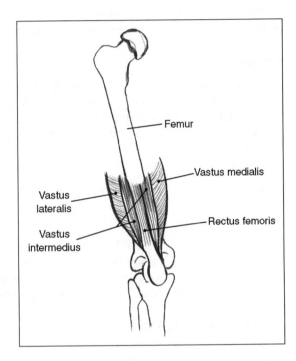

FIGURE 4–91. Anterior and Medial Aspects of the Thigh (Deeper Muscles).

Flexors (Fig. 4-92)

- Hamstrings:
  - Semimembranosus (sciatic, tibial portion, L4, L5, S1, S2)
  - Semitendinosus (sciatic, tibial portion, L4, L5, S1, S2)
  - Biceps femoris
    - Long head (sciatic, tibial portion, L5, S1, S2)
    - Short head (sciatic, common peroneal portion, L5, S1, S2)
- Sartorius (femoral nerve, L2, L3)
- Gracilis (obturator nerve, L2, L3, L4)
- Gastrocnemius (tibial, S1, S2)

Medial Rotators (Fig. 4-92)

- Semitendinosus
- Semimembranosus
- Sartorius
- Gracilis

Lateral Rotators (Fig. 4-92)

- Biceps femoris—long and short heads

Other

- Popliteus (tibial nerve, L4, L5, S1)—locks and unlocks the knee

BONY ANATOMY (Figure 4–93)

- The knee can be divided into the medial femoral tibial, lateral femoral tibial and patellofemoral regions
- The Q angle is formed by the long axes of the femur and the tibia and reflects the natural valgus attitude of the knee
  - Males ~13°
  - Females~18°
- Excessive valgum is termed genu valgum or knock knees
- Genu varum is bowed legs
- Hyperextension at the knees is termed genu recurvatum or back knee

Femoral/Tibial Joint
- The primary motion is flexion and extension
- The secondary motion is axial rotation when the knee is flexed
- The basic motion of the knee is rolling and gliding

Tibial Plateau
- Characterized by curved surfaces corresponding to the medial and lateral femoral condyles
- A raised prominence between the curved surfaces helps prevent rotation in extension
- The lateral tibial plateau is convex in shape. This allows the lateral femoral condyle to move further backward than the medial condyle. This causes internal tibial rotation with flexion

Patella
- The patella is a sesamoid bone embedded in the extensor muscle/tendon unit
- Efficiency of the extensor groups is increased by 150% due to the mechanical advantage provided by the patella
- The articular surface of the patella has two facets divided by a ridge, which helps with tracking over the condyles

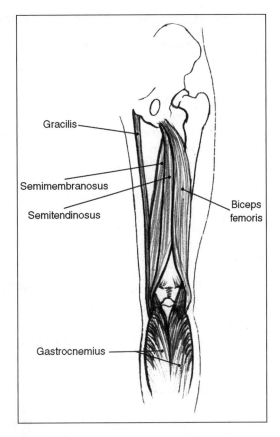

FIGURE 4–92. Posterior muscles of the thigh. (Sartorius not shown)

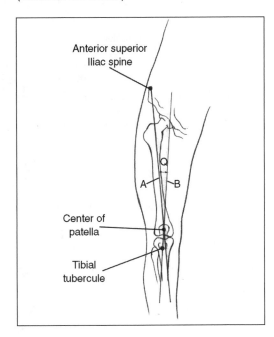

FIGURE 4–93. Q-angle. Illustration by Heather Platt, 2001.

LIGAMENTS (Figures 4–94, 4–95, and 4–96)

Anterior Cruciate Ligament (ACL)

Functional Anatomy

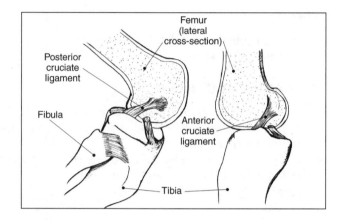

- The ACL attaches to the lateral intercondylar notch of the femur and to a point lateral to the medial tibial eminence
- The primary function is to restrain anterior tibial subluxation
- Prevents backward sliding of the femur and hyperextension of the knee
- Limits medial rotation of the femur when the foot is fixed
- The ACL tightens with full extension and loosens in flexion
- External rotation loosens the ACL and internal rotation tightens it

FIGURE 4–94. Cruciate Ligaments (Posterior Cruciate Ligament, Anterior Cruciate Ligament)

- 📖 In flexion, it draws the femoral condyles anteriorly
- ACL deficient knees create increased pressure on the posterior menisci

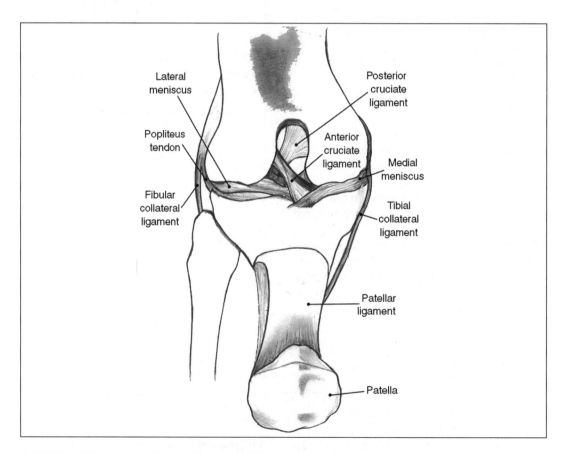

FIGURE 4–95. Anterior View—Ligaments of the Knee.

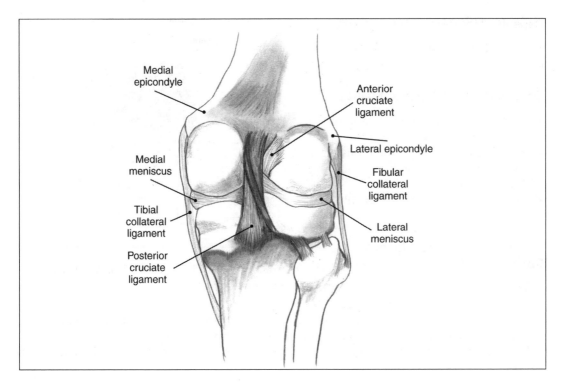

FIGURE 4–96. Posterior View—Ligaments of the Knee.

Posterior Cruciate Ligament (PCL)

Functional Anatomy
- The PCL attaches to the front of the medial intercondylar notch of the femur and to a point lateral to the posterior tibial plateau
- Its course is inferior, posterior, and lateral in direction
- The primary function is to restrain posterior tibial subluxation
- The ligament is looser in extension and tighter in flexion
- In extension, the PCL pulls the femur posteriorly
- PCL deficient knees place more force on the patellofemoral joint

Medial Collateral Ligament (MCL)

Functional Anatomy
- The MCL attaches to the medial femoral condyle and to the medial upper end of the tibia
- It has an attachment to the medial meniscus
- In full extension, the MCL tightens to full tension
- Tension is increased with abduction stress at increasing positions of flexion

Lateral Collateral Ligament (LCL)

Functional Anatomy
- The LCL attaches to the lateral femoral condyle posteriorly and superiorly and attaches to the upper end of the lateral fibula
- It does not have an attachment to the lateral meniscus
- It restrains varus stresses
- Peak stress is achieved with adduction when the knee is at 70° of flexion

Capsular Ligaments (Figure 4–97)

In general, the posterior capsule resists knee hyperextension

Oblique Popliteal Ligament (OPL)

- The OPL arises from the tendon of the semimembranosus
- It strengthens the fibrous posterior capsule of the knee joint
- It resists extension
- The OPL is attached to capsule and lateral meniscus

Arcuate Popliteal Ligament Complex (APLC)

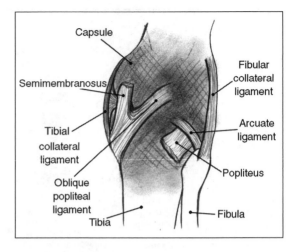

FIGURE 4–97. Knee Joint—Capsular Ligaments (Posterior View)

- The APLC provides attachment for the posterior horn of the lateral meniscus
- It reinforces the lateral aspect of the knee and gives posterior lateral rotary stability
- Also it provides restraint to posterior tibial subluxation
- Its attachment can be mistaken for a tear of the posterior horn of the lateral meniscus on MRI

Menisci of the Knee (Figure 4–98)

- The two menisci are fibrocartilage of crescent shape
- They deepen the articular surfaces of the tibia to provide more stability for the femoral condyles

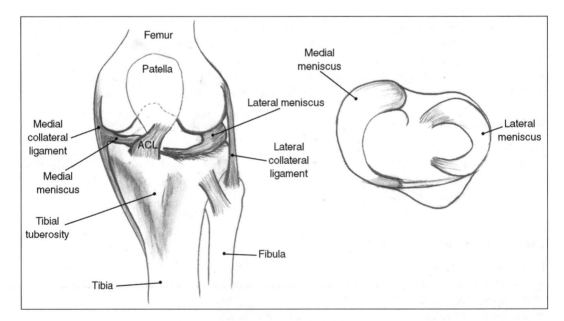

FIGURE 4–98. Major Structures of the Interior of the Knee Joint. **A.** Anterior View. **B.** View from above with the femur removed.

- The peripheral outer third of the menisci are well vascularized
- The inner two-thirds are not well vascularized and cannot usually be surgically repaired

Medial Meniscus
- The medial meniscus is longer than the lateral meniscus
- It is "C" shaped
- The peripheral border is adherent to the medial collateral ligament

Lateral Meniscus
- The lateral meniscus is nearly circular in shape
- It covers a larger area than the medial meniscus
- It is joined to the medial femoral condyle by the posterior meniscofemoral ligament

Bursae (Figure 4–99)

Anterior (4)
- Prepatellar bursa
  - The prepatellar bursa is located between the skin and the anterior patella
  - It is the most commonly damaged bursa
  - Inflammation of this bursa by prolonged kneeling is termed *housemaid's knee*
- Suprapatellar bursa
  - This bursa is located between the quadriceps femoris muscle and the femur and usually communicates with the joint capsule
- Deep infrapatellar bursa
  - This bursa is located between the patellar tendon and the tibia
- Superficial or subcutaneous infrapatellar bursa
  - This bursa is located between the skin and the tibial tuberosity
  - Associated with kneeling in upright position, termed *vicar's knee*

Lateral Bursae (3)
- There is a lateral bursa located between the biceps muscle and fibular collateral ligament
- A second lateral bursa is located between the popliteus muscle and the fibular collateral ligament
- A third lateral bursa is located between the lateral femur condyle and popliteus muscle

Medial Bursae (3)
- Pes anserinus bursa
  - Located between the tendons of the **s**artorius, **g**racilis, semi**t**endinosus muscles and medial collateral ligament. ("**S**ay **G**race before **T**ea")
  - May be misdiagnosed as a medial meniscus lesion when swollen and painful

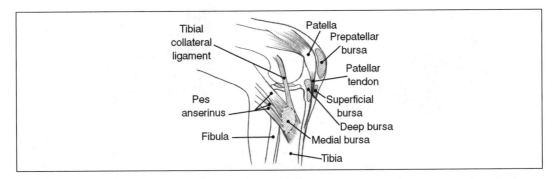

FIGURE 4–99. Bursae of the Knee that are Clinically Significant (medial view of knee).

- A second medial bursa is located between the MCL and the semitendinosus
- A third medial bursa is located between the semimembranosus and the tibia

Posterior Bursae (2)

- There is a posterior bursa located between the lateral head of the gastrocnemius and the capsule
- There is a second posterior bursa located between the medial head of the gastrocnemius and capsule and extending under the semimembranosus
  - It communicates with the joint cavity
  - It can be irritated by abnormal strain
  - When distended it is termed a *baker's cyst*
  - A baker's cyst is a distension of the bursa and outpocketing of the synovial membrane in this location. It can mimic a DVT due to the increased warmth and leg girth and associated pain

TESTS FOR THE KNEE

McMurray Test (Figure 4–100 A, B, C, D)

- This test is used to diagnose meniscal tears and is especially useful for diagnosing posterior meniscal tears
  - The patient lies supine with the knee flexed (Figure 4–100A)
  - The examiner palpates the medial joint line with his fingers and the lateral joint line with his thumb
  - With the knee flexed, rotate the tibia internally and externally on the femur (Figure 4–100B)

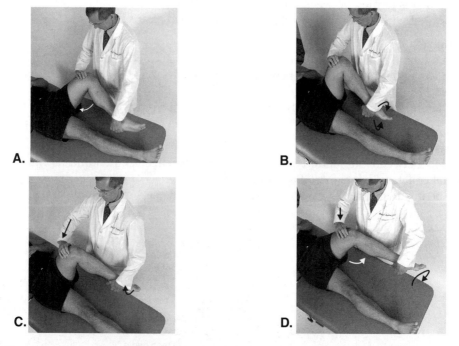

FIGURE 4–100. A. McMurray Test: Patient lies supine with the knee flexed. **B.** With flexed knee, internally and externally rotate the tibia on the femur. **C** Place a valgus stress on the knee with the leg externally rotated, and **D.** Slowly extend the leg with the leg externally rotated and in valgus position. If a click is heard or palpated, the test is positive for a torn medial meniscus, usually in the posterior position.

To Test for Medial Meniscal Damage:
- With the knee extended and the tibia externally rotated, push on the lateral side, while applying valgus stress to the medial side of the knee joint (Figure 4–100C)
- Externally rotating the tibia stresses the medial compartment for testing the medial meniscus
- With the leg externally rotated and in valgus, slowly extend the knee
- A positive test for a torn medial meniscus (usually in the posterior position) yields an audible or palpable click and pain (Figure 4–100D)

To Test for Lateral Meniscal Damage:
- Apply a varus stress and internally rotate the tibia while extending the knee. Pain and click should result if positive
- Internally rotating the tibia stresses the lateral compartment for testing the lateral meniscus
- A positive test for a torn lateral meniscus (usually in the posterior position) yields an audible or palpable click and pain

Apley's Grind Test (Figure 4–101)
This test is used to diagnose a torn meniscus
- The patient lies prone with the knee flexed to 90°
- The examiner places force downward on the heel compressing the menisci between the femur and tibia
- Pressure is maintained downward as the tibia is rotated
- A positive test should elicit pain; ask the patient to localize the pain to the medial or lateral compartment

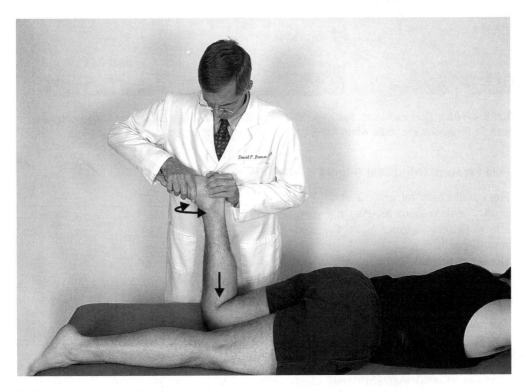

FIGURE 4–101. Apley's Grind Test.

Apley's Distraction Test (Figure 4–102)

- This is a test for ligamentous damage
- The patient lies prone with the knee flexed
- Traction force is applied while rotating the tibia internally and externally
- Pressure on the meniscus is reduced during this maneuver
- A positive test elicits pain indicating ligamentous rather than meniscal damage

Bounce Home Test (Figure 4–103)

- This is a test for decreased knee extension
- With the patient supine, the examiner flexes the knee while holding the heel (Figure 4–103A)
- The knee is allowed to extend passively and should have a definite endpoint. It should "bounce home" into extension (Figure 4–103B)

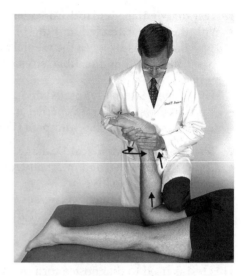

FIGURE 4–102. Apley's Distraction Test.

- A positive test occurs when full extension cannot be attained and a rubbery resistance is felt. Fluid in the knee joint prevents the joint from bouncing home (Figure 4–103C)
- Causes for a positive test may be a torn meniscus, loose body, intracapsular swelling, or fluid in the knee joint

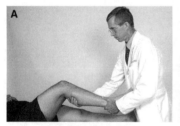 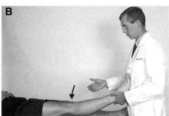 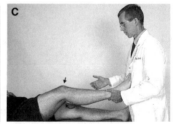

FIGURE 4–103. Bounce Home Test. **A.** Examiner flexes the knee. **B.** Let the knee passively extend. **C.** Positive test occurs when full extension cannot be attained.

Patella Femoral Grind Test (Figure 4–104)

- The patella femoral grind test evaluates the quality of the patella articulating surfaces
- The patient is supine with the legs in a neutral position
- The examiner pushes the patella distally and asks the patient to contract the quadriceps
- The patella should glide smoothly cephalad
- A positive test will yield pain and crepitation on patella movement

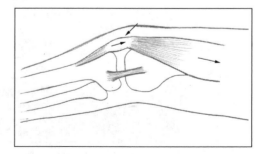

FIGURE 4–104. Patella Femoral Grind Test.

Anterior Draw Test (Figure 4–105)

- The anterior draw primarily tests the integrity of the anterior cruciate ligament

- With the patient supine, the knees flexed to 90°, and the foot stabilized by the examiner's body, the examiner grasps the patient's knee with the fingers in the area of the hamstring insertions and the thumbs on the medial and lateral joint lines. The tibia is drawn toward the examiner (Figure 4–105A)
- A positive test occurs when the tibia slides from under the femur. Some anterior motion is normal. A distinct endpoint should be encountered (Figure 4–105B)
- External rotation tightens the posteromedial portion of the joint capsule, reducing anterior movement. If the anterior movement with the leg in the neutral position is equal to the anterior movement with the leg externally rotated, the posteromedial joint capsule and the AC may be damaged

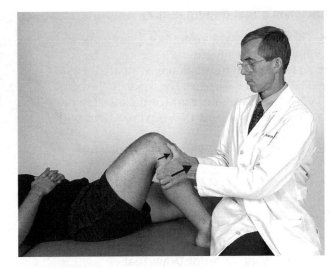

FIGURE 4–105. Anterior Draw Test. The tibia is drawn toward the examiner. Positive anterior draw sign: Torn anterior cruciate ligament.

- Internal rotation tightens the posterolateral joint capsule. If the anterior movement with the leg in the neutral position is equal to the anterior movement with the leg internally rotated, the posterior lateral joint capsule and the ACL may be damaged
- 📖 The test is not very sensitive because hemarthrosis, hamstring spasm, and other structures (i.e., the posterior capsule) can limit forward movement of the tibia

Posterior Draw Test (Figure 4–106)

- The posterior draw tests the posterior cruciate ligament
- The patient and examiner are in the same positions as for the anterior draw test
- The examiner pushes the tibia away from himself
- A positive test occurs when the tibia slides backward on the femur. Some posterior movement is normal; a distinct endpoint should be encountered

Sag Test

- This is a test for the patency of the posterior cruciate ligament
- The patient is supine with the knee flexed to 90° with the foot on the exam table
- The test is positive if the tibia is displaced posteriorly. Comparison should be done with the contralateral side
- The test can also be done with the patient supine with the hip and knee flexed to 90° and the heel held in the examiner's hand

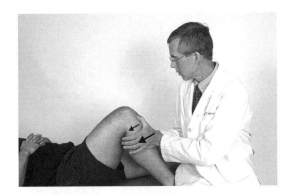

FIGURE 4–106. Positive Posterior Draw Sign: Torn Posterior Cruciate Ligament.

Lachman's Test (Figure 4–107)

- This test is used to assess ACL integrity and anterior knee integrity
- Anterior tibial translation is evaluated
- The patient is supine. The knee is flexed at 15–30°. The examiner grasps the distal femur with one hand and the proximal tibia with the other hand
- The femur is stabilized and anterior force is applied to the tibia
- 📖 A positive test yields significant anterior movement with no distinct endpoint
- A partial ACL tear may yield a test with a soft end point

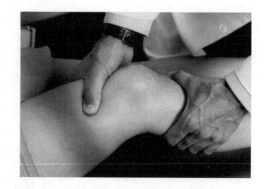

FIGURE 4–107. Lachman's Test. Photo courtesy of JFK Johnson Rehabilitation Institute, 2000.

Lachman's vs. Anterior Draw Test

- 📖 Lachman's test may be more difficult for clinicians to perform but tends to be more sensitive
- In the anterior draw test knee is positioned so that the hamstrings have a mechanical advantage. Increased hamstring activity can inhibit tibial translation, causing a false negative test
- A torn meniscus can act as a block to tibial motion, again causing a false negative while doing the anterior draw test

Collateral Ligament Testing (Figure 4–108)

- This tests the integrity at the medial and lateral collateral ligaments by imposing valgus and varus stress
- With the patient supine, the examiner tucks the patient's ankle under the examiner's arm. The thumbs of both hands palpate the medial and lateral joint lines
- If a valgus stress is applied and the medial joint line gaps, the medial collateral ligament may be damaged (Figure 4–108A)
- If a varus stress is applied and the lateral joint line gaps, the lateral collateral ligament may be damaged (Figure 4–108B)

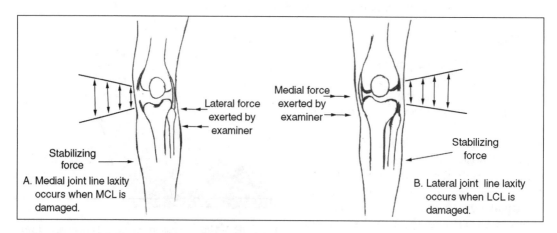

FIGURE 4–108. Collateral Ligament Testing. **A.** Test for integrity of the medial collateral ligament. (MCL) **B.** Test for integrity of the lateral collateral ligament (LCL).

- The knee may be tested in full extension and at ~25° of flexion to relax the fibers of the posterior joint capsules
- 5 mm of motion is considered a Grade I tear
- 5 to 10 mm is considered a Grade II tear
- > 10 mm is considered a complete interstitial tear
- Be aware that muscle guarding may cause a false negative test

▪

KNEE DISORDERS

MENISCAL INJURIES

General

- Medial meniscus injuries are associated with cutting injuries. They occur with tibial rotation while the knee is partially flexed during weight bearing (football, soccer)
- Lateral meniscus injuries occur during squatting. Full flexion with rotation is the usual mechanism (wrestling)

Clinical

- Acute tears
  - Acute tears are often associated with a pop after a specific inciting incident
  - They may cause true locking
  - Posterior horn tears of the medial meniscus are common and occur with valgus and external rotation
  - Effusions may occur within 24 hours
  - Patients frequently complain of knee stiffness
- Degenerative tears
  - These may involve minimal trauma
  - They usually occur in patients > 40 years old
  - Impingement episodes may be minimal
- PE
  - Range of motion is decreased
    - Effusion will limit flexion
    - Meniscal fragment impingement will limit extension
  - Tenderness
    - There will be tenderness of the medial joint line for medial meniscus damage
    - Lateral joint line tenderness indicates the lateral meniscus damage
  - Tests
    - Apley and McMurray

Imaging

- MRI is the gold standard in diagnosing meniscal tears
- Arthrograms are less expensive than MRI but more invasive because they require injections of dye into the joint to assess meniscal integrity

Treatment

- The inner two-thirds of the meniscus is not well vascularized. Therefore, injuries of that segment will often require surgical removal of the damaged tissue

- Injuries to the outer one-third of the meniscus are usually repaired due to better vascular supply
- If the meniscus is repaired, generally the patient is non-weight bearing for 4–6 weeks. Strengthening proceeds at that time
- If the meniscus is removed, generally the patient is weight bearing as tolerated in 1–2 days

ACL INJURIES (Figure 4–109)

General

- The ACL is the most commonly injured knee ligament in athletics (football, soccer, downhill skiing)
- The mechanism of injury is usually cutting, deceleration, and hyperextension of the knee
  - Noncontact injuries are most common
  - Contact injuries may often involve other structures
    - Greater than 50% of ACL tears occur with meniscal tears
    - The terrible triad or O'Donoghue's Triad involves simultaneous injury to the ACL, medial collateral ligament (MCL), and medial meniscus because of the attachment of the MCL to the medial meniscus
    - This injury occurs when a valgus force is applied to a flexed and rotated knee

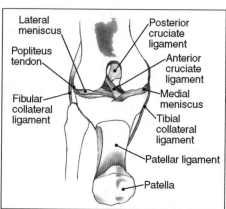

FIGURE 4–109. Anatomy of the Anterior Cruciate Ligament.

Clinical

- History
  - There is a sudden pop and anterior knee pain with posterior lateral joint line pain
  - Instability of the knee is common
  - Early swelling and, within 24 hours, a significant effusion will be present
- PE
  - An effusion is noted on clinical inspection
  - Tenderness is variable and associated with meniscal tears and avulsion fracture
  - The anterior drawer test may be positive or yield a false negative
  - 📖 Lachman's test may be positive or can yield a false negative ~10% of cases. It is examiner dependent and also influenced by muscle guarding

Imaging and Testing

- X rays may show an avulsion fracture of either the tibial insertion of the ACL or the lateral capsular margin of the tibia
- Arthrocentesis can be performed to relieve pressure and pain and will generally return blood or a sanguinous fluid in ACL tears
- MRI is considered to be 85% to 90% accurate
- Arthroscopy is close to 100% accurate

Treatment

- Initially partial weight bearing, ice, and compression are used while evaluation is ongoing
- If reconstruction is undertaken:
  - Partial weight bearing is maintained initially
  - Range of motion is instituted to regain flexion over the first 2 weeks

– Progress to closed chain kinetics is then undertaken
– Sports specific exercises may be started in 6–12 weeks
– Complete rehabilitation in one year is the goal with maximum range and strength and agility

PCL INJURIES

General

• The most frequent cause of PCL injury is impact to the front of the tibia with the knee flexed (dashboard injury)
• In athletics, hyperflexion is a common means of PCL injury
• PCL injuries are much less common than ACL injuries

Clinical

• History
  – The initial injury may or may not be associated with a pop
  – There may be minimal swelling initially, increasing over 24 hours
  – The ability to fully extend may be impaired
  – The patient may be able to bear weight without pain
• PE
  – An effusion may be present
  – Popliteal tenderness is a common finding in the acute phase
  – Posterior drawer test and sag tests may be positive (quadriceps spasms may cause a false negative)

Imaging

• X rays may show an avulsion
• MRI is less accurate than for ACL tears
• Arthroscopy has a higher accuracy than MRI

Treatment

• Surgical repair is indicated if the ligament is avulsed with a tibial fragment
• There is some controversy over surgical repair of an otherwise isolated PCL tear
• Attention to quadriceps strengthening is important

MCL TEARS

General

• MCL tears are common in football and skiing
• Impact force to the lateral knee is often the mechanism of injury
• However, MCL tears may occur without a direct blow. A sustained valgus force may also cause the injury

Clinical

• History
  – Often there is a lateral blow to the knee and a pop
  – Medial knee pain is often immediately present

  - Complete tears may allow walking and running after initial pain
  - The knee becomes stiff in several hours
- PE
  - Medial swelling and tenderness may be present and variable
  - Minimal effusion may be present
  - Medial instability on stress testing is present
  - The triad of MCL tear, ACL tear, and medial meniscal tear (O'Donaghue's Triad) is a possible complication and requires evaluation

Imaging

- Radiographs may reveal an epiphyseal fracture
- MRI is useful to delineate the MCL tear and also to investigate associated injuries (i.e., to the ACL and medial meniscus)

Treatment

- Isolated MCL tears may be treated conservatively
- The knee can be braced
- Rehabilitation focuses on strengthening and stability
- Epiphyseal fractures may be present with or without medial collateral tears

LATERAL COLLATERAL LIGAMENT TEARS

- Tears of the LCL usually are the result of knee dislocations
- Consideration should be made of associated vascular injuries and cruciate and peroneal nerve injuries
- Isolated LCL injuries are rare

ILIAL TIBIAL BAND SYNDROME (ITB SYNDROME)

General

- The ITB slides over the lateral femoral condyle with the knee in flexion and extension
- The ITB extends from the tensor fasciae latae distally in the lateral leg to insert on Gerdy's tubercle on the lateral tibia
- Inflexibility of the ITB and adductor/abductor muscle imbalances lead to the dysfunction

Clinical

- The patient presents with pain over the lateral femoral condyle, which is made worse by running and walking
- The patient adapts by externally rotating the hip, internally rotating the lower leg, and pronating the foot
- ITB tightness is evaluated by the Ober test. (For description of Ober test refer to the hip section.)
- Knee pain associated with ITB tightness is further assessed by the following: The patient extends the knee and at ~30° experiences pain over the lateral femoral condyle as the ITB crosses the bony prominence

Imaging

- Radiographs are useful to evaluate possible avulsion

Treatment

- Stretching the ITB, hip flexors, and gluteus maximus is central to rehabilitation
- Strengthening the hip adductors, gluteus maximus, and Tensor Fasciae Latae (TFL) is also important
- Orthotics may be helpful and foot overpronation must be corrected
- Injection at the lateral femoral condyle may be necessary in resistant cases

PATELLA RELATED INJURIES

The stability of the patella is dependent upon three main characteristics
1. Depth of the intercondylar groove
2. Proper contour of the patella
3. Adequate muscular control
- The normal patellar motion is vertical
- At full extension the applied force of the quadriceps approximating the patella to the condyles is reduced
- Patellofemoral weight bearing increases with knee flexion
  - Walking: 0.5 times body weight
  - Ascending or descending stairs: 3.3 times body weight
  - Squatting: 6.0 times body weight
- In hyperextension there is a tendency for the patella to separate from the femur. The lateral lip of the patellar surface of the femur acts to prevent subluxation

RECURRENT PATELLAR SUBLUXATION

General

- If a congenital malformation causes a less prominent lateral lip or a more prominent medial lip, the patella may dislocate laterally in full extension
- Increased genu valgum laterally displaces the patella
- Increased genu varum medially displaces the patella
- Excessive genu recurvatum elongates the patellofemoral structures causing loss of patella condylar contact
- Vastus medialis weakness allows lateral displacement
- Tibial external torsion can cause lateral displacement
- A shallow lateral femoral condyle can cause lateral displacement
- A laterally attached infrapatellar tendon on the tubercle can cause lateral displacement

Clinical

- The patella may be displaced medially or laterally in the acute phase
- The knee tends to buckle after a subluxation
- Pain and tenderness are present in the peripatellar region
- An effusion may be present
- Wasting of the vastus medialis may be present
- Full extension may be impaired
- The patella will often reset at 25–30° of flexion

Imaging

- Radiographs
  - The AP view visualizes the patellar position over the sulcus

 – The lateral view ascertains the patellar height and is done at 45° of knee flexion and in full extension
 – The sunrise or tunnel view ascertains the patellofemoral articulation and femoral condyle height

Treatment

See below for treatment of patellofemoral pain and overload syndrome

PATELLOFEMORAL PAIN AND OVERLOAD SYNDROME (RUNNER'S KNEE, BIKER'S KNEE)

General

- This may be the most common anterior knee pain syndrome
- It is an overuse injury caused by repeated microtrauma leading to peripatellar synovitis
- The predisposing conditions noted above in recurrent patellar subluxation apply for this syndrome. They are both patellar tracking problems

Clinical

- The syndrome presents as anterior knee pain of acute or insidious onset
- An effusion may be present
- Crepitus may be present on range of motion
- Ascending or descending stairs tends to aggravate the condition
- Patellar compression by the examiner produces the pain in the patellofemoral compartment
- Examination may reveal a high riding, laterally shifted patella (patella alta). This condition is due to vastus lateralis tightness and relative medial weakness causing tracking dysfunction
- A low patella (patella baja) is less common and may indicate quadriceps rupture
- Examination of the knee in the last 30° of extension is important
- A tight lateral retinaculum and/or VMO dysplasia can lead to lateral patellar shift or shear stress resulting in cartilage damage
- Rotation of the patella also indicates evidence of muscle imbalances:
  – Patellar internal rotation is given the term "squinting" patella
  – Patellar external rotation is given the term "frog's eye" patella
- Tight hip flexors can alter gait and cause symptoms
  – Check with the Thomas test (see the hip section)
- Measure Q angle. Normal: females should be ~18°, males should be ~13°
- Tight abductors can also alter gait
  – Check with the Ober test (see the hip section)
- Tight hamstrings can increase patellofemoral loading
- Check with the straight leg raise test

Imaging

Radiographs

- The AP view visualizes the patellar position over the sulcus
- The lateral view ascertains the patellar height and is done at 45° of knee flexion and in full extension
- The sunrise or tunnel view ascertains the patellofemoral articulation and femoral condyle height

MRI
- MRI is *not* often used to assess patellofemoral pain. Articular degeneration may be seen (see chondromalacia patella)

CT
- CT is useful if growth plate injury is suspected
- It can evaluate the stage of patellar subluxation present in the last 15° of flexion that plane films may not reveal
- CT can also reveal and delineate tumors

Bone Scan
- Bone scan is useful to evaluate symptoms present < 4 months of uncertain diagnosis
- It is a useful technique to detect intra-articular processes: Osteochondritis dissecans, osteomyelitis, or tumor

Treatment—Nonsurgical

- The vast majority is successfully treated by conservative means
- Controlling symptoms is of primary concern achieved by:
  - Decreasing pain
  - Increasing strength
  - Increasing range of motion
- Activity modification
  - For active individuals: Reduce the pace of activities that increase patellofemoral stress (climbing, jumping, squatting)
  - For inactive individuals: Institute baseline exercises and progress incrementally as tolerated
- Ice 10–15 minutes four to six times per day is used in the acute phase. This may be required before and after activity in the subacute phase
- Nonsteroidal anti-inflammatory medications should be used acutely and then tapered off as pain decreases
- Therapeutic exercise
  - Strengthening of the quadriceps, especially the VMO, is important
    - Short arc quadriceps activities (0–15°)
    - Isotonic quadriceps strengthening with eccentric loading in a nonpainful range of motion
    - Isometric quadriceps contractions (quad sets)
    - Straight leg raising
    - Stretching of the hamstrings, iliotibial band, adductors, and vastus lateralis is also important to balance forces
    - Proprioceptive exercises are used after initial strengthening and stretching
    - Increase activity when ROM is full and pain free and strength is 80% of normal
- Patellar taping
  - A very useful adjunct in therapy, the patella is taped in position to allow pain-reduced range of motion
    - It provides proprioceptive feedback to alter patellar tracking
    - Also it helps to balance contractile forces between the vastus lateralis and medialis
- Patellar bracing (knee sleeving with patellar cutout or strap)
    - Provides proprioceptive feedback
    - May prevent reinjury
    - Can allow the patient to resume activity

Treatment—Surgical

Consider surgical referral if:
- Conservative measures fail after 4–6 months
- An obvious surgical lesion exists
  - Surgery may involve:
    - Lateral release of the knee capsule and retinaculum
    - Patellar realignment
    - Patellar tendon transfer
    - Patellectomy

CHONDROMALACIA PATELLA

General

- Characterized by softening of the patellar articular cartilage
- It is the culmination of cartilage degeneration
- Chondromalacia patella is essentially an arthroscopic diagnosis. The cartilage appears roughened or fibrillated on arthroscopy
- Chronic patellofemoral overload and tracking dysfunctions may predispose to this condition. Therefore, the functional and anatomic conditions noted in recurrent patellar subluxation and patellofemoral overload syndrome apply
- Degradation of the articular cartilage of the patella may also result from infection, trauma, or autoimmune processes

Clinical

The presentation of chondromalacia patella is clinically the same as for patellofemoral pain and overload syndrome described previously

Imaging

- The imaging workup of chondromalacia patella is the same as for patellofemoral pain and overload syndrome as above. CT or MRI may detect defects in the articular cartilage of the patella which is the distinguishing characteristic of this disorder

Treatment

- Because abnormal patellar mechanics are often the cause of chondromalacia patella, treatment will follow the treatment already described for patellofemoral pain and overload syndrome

PLICA

General

- This is a condition marked by a redundant fold of the synovial lining of the knee
- The synovial lining extends from the infrapatellar fat pad medially around the femoral condyles and under the quadriceps tendon above the patella and lateral to the lateral retinaculum
- The redundant synovia is susceptible to tearing as it passes over the condyles
- Plica can occur in the mediopatellar, infrapatellar or suprapatellar regions

Clinical

- The patient may present with anterior knee pain of insidious onset

- There may be gradually increasing pain with prolonged knee flexion or sitting, made worse by standing and extension
- After direct trauma, such as ACL tears or meniscal tears, the plica can become inflamed and symptomatic
- The knee may give the sensation of buckling if the plica is trapped between the patella and medial condyle
- Careful palpation with knee flexion and extension may detect a plica
- Snapping with knee extension may occur if the plica is fibrosed

Imaging and Testing

- Because plica often accompanies patellofemoral dysfunction, the imaging workup correlates with that for patellofemoral pain and overload syndrome. MRI, arthrogram, and arthroscopy are all useful in evaluating for plica

Treatment

- The treatment would follow that of patellofemoral syndrome as previously outlined. Surgical excision can be done if conservative measures fail

JUMPER'S KNEE

General

- Jumper's knee is patellar tendinitis often associated with micro-tears of the tendon
- This is considered to be an overuse syndrome of the patellofemoral extensor unit. It is associated with high quadriceps loading: jumping, squatting, and kneeling
- The most common site of involvement is the inferior pole of the patella
- The superior pole of the patella or the insertion over the tibial tubercle may also be sites of involvement

Clinical

- The patient presents with pain on activity
- The pain may diminish during the course of the activity session and become more apparent afterward
- There will be tenderness on palpation over the inferior or superior pole of the patella

Imaging

- Generally the radiographic workup done for patellofemoral syndrome is done to evaluate bony anatomy

Treatment

- Treatment follows the guidelines for patellofemoral overload syndrome previously described

OSTEOCHONDRITIS DISSECANS

General

- This process is in a localized segmental area of avascular necrosis of the end of a long bone
- This results in the formation of dead subchondral bone covered with articular hyaline cartilage

- The overlying cartilage degenerates around the defect and an entire piece may detach from the rest of the bone, entering the joint space as a loose body
- The usual area of involvement in the knee joint is the medial femoral condyle
- The condition primarily tends to affect adolescents

Clinical

- The patient may experience joint pain and irritation, synovial effusion, and a buckling sensation
- The presence of a loose body may cause locking

Imaging

- The area of involvement may be visible on radiographs or CT

Treatment

- The healing of the defect may occur if the diagnosis is made before the fragment separates
  - The knee must be placed at rest and protected from weight bearing
- If healing does not occur or if the fragment becomes detached, the lesion will require surgical excision

■

LOWER EXTREMITIES—THE LOWER LEG

FUNCTIONAL ANATOMY

MUSCLE GROUPS

There are three groups of muscles in the leg, anterior, lateral, and posterior, defined by their relation to the tibia

Anterior Muscle Group (Figure 4–110)

- This group is composed of dorsiflexors of the ankle and extensors of the toes
- Dorsiflexors and invertors
  - Tibialis anterior (deep peroneal nerve, L4, L5)
  - Extensor hallucis longus (deep peroneal nerve, L4, L5) great toe extensor
- Dorsiflexors and everters
  - Extensor digitorum longus (deep peroneal nerve, L4, L5) toe extensor
  - Peroneus tertius (deep peroneal nerve, L4, L5)

Lateral Muscle Group (Figure 4–111)

- Peroneus brevis (superficial peroneal nerve, L5, S1) eversion, weak plantar flexor
- Peroneus longus (superficial peroneal nerve, L5, S1) eversion, weak plantar flexor

Posterior Muscle Group (Figure 4–112)

- Gastrocnemius (tibial nerve, L5, S1, S2) plantar flexor
- Plantaris (tibial nerve, L5, S1, S2) weak plantar flexor

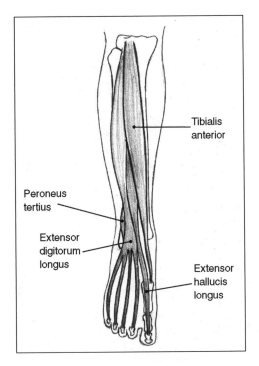

FIGURE 4–110. Anterior Muscle Group of the Leg.

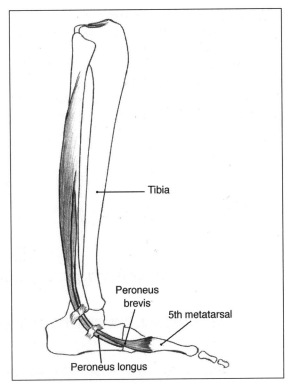

FIGURE 4–111. Lateral Muscle Group of the Leg.

- Soleus (tibial nerve, L5, S1, S2) plantar flexor
- Flexor digitorum longus (tibial nerve, L5, S1, S2) flexion lateral four toes, inversion, plantar flexor
- Tibialis posterior (tibial nerve, L5, S1, S2) inversion and plantar flexor
- Flexor hallucis longus (tibialis nerve, S2, S3)
- Popliteus (tibial nerve, L5, S1, S2) internal rotation of the leg on the femur

COMPARTMENTS (Figure 4–113)

There are four compartments of the lower leg:
- Anterior
- Lateral
- Deep posterior
- Superficial posterior

The anterior compartment comprises the tibialis anterior, extensor digitorum longus, extensor hallucis longus, and peroneus tertius muscles; the anterior tibial artery and vein; and the common peroneal nerve

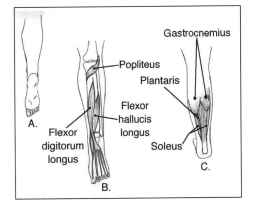

FIGURE 4–112. Posterior muscles of the leg. **A.** Posterior plantar flexion.
B. Posterior plantar flexion, Intermediate deep layer of posterior muscle group.
C. Posterior aspect, superficial layer of posterior muscle group.

The lateral compartment comprises the peroneus longus and brevis muscles; the superficial peroneal nerve; the common peroneal nerve dividing into the superficial and deep branches

The deep posterior compartment comprises the flexor digitorum longus, flexor hallucis longus, tibialis posterior, and popliteus muscles; the posterior tibial artery and vein; and the tibial nerve

The superficial posterior compartment comprises the gastrocnemius, plantaris, and soleus muscles

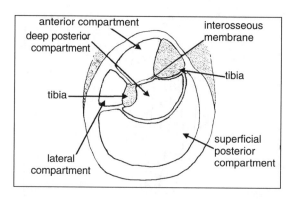

FIGURE 4–113. Lower Leg Cross Section. (Note: Compartments).

■ DISORDERS OF THE LOWER LEG

CHRONIC EXERTIONAL COMPARTMENT SYNDROME (CECS)

General

- This condition is marked by raised intracompartmental pressure
- Pressure increases have been measured during and after exercise
- Nerve impingement can result from high intracompartmental pressures during or after exercise
- Tissue ischemia may result due to restricted arterial inflow, obstruction of microcirculation, or arteriolar or venous collapse
- The pain associated with this syndrome could also be due to: Sensory receptor stimulation in fascia or periosteum caused by high pressure, or the release of biochemical factors caused by reduced blood flow
- Lower leg pain may also be caused by tibial stress fractures or periostitis. These syndromes may occur concurrently with CECS

Clinical

- Typically in CECS, pain will occur with exercise and progress as the activity increases in intensity
- Pain will usually diminish after the activity is stopped. Occasionally it may persist if the exercise session was particularly demanding
- Neurologic involvement can cause weakness and numbness
  - Anterior CECS can cause dorsiflexor weakness and numbness over the first web space of the dorsum of the foot (deep peroneal nerve)
  - Lateral CECS can cause dorsiflexor weakness and first web space numbness (deep peroneal nerve) or everter weakness and numbness of the dorsum of the foot and anterolateral distal shin
  - Deep posterior CECS can cause cramping of the foot intrinsics and numbness of the medial arch of the foot (tibial nerve)
  - On palpation, the compartment may be firm and, after exercise, deep palpation may be painful
  - Fascial hernias may be palpable
  - Rarely are distal pulses diminished

Imaging and Testing

- MRI has been found useful by some practitioners to diagnose CECS but a general consensus on its usefulness is pending
- Plain films, CT, bone scan, and MRI help to investigate other sources of leg pain
- EMG and nerve conduction studies may help diagnose unrelated sources of symptoms
- EMG/NCS pre- and post-exercise have been tried as a diagnostic tool with limited results
- Compartment pressure studies (using manometric technique) are the best means to evaluate CECS
  - Elevated pressures should coincide with reproduction of the exact pain syndrome
  - Pressures are measured pre- and post-exercise. A delay in return to pre-exercise pressure levels of 6–30 minutes is required for a positive test

Treatment

- At present, the most effective treatment for CECS is fasciotomy

ACUTE COMPARTMENT SYNDROME (ACS)

General

- Perfusion of muscle and nerve tissues decreases to a level inadequate to sustain the viability of these tissues
- In compartment syndrome, the intracompartmental tissue pressure becomes elevated and produces a secondary elevation in venous pressure that obstructs venous outflow. An escalating cycle of continued increase in intracompartmental tissue pressure occurs
- Necrosis of muscle and nerve tissue can develop in as little as 4–8 hours
- Thus, treatment of ACS constitutes a surgical emergency
- ACS most commonly follows trauma in association with fractures of the long bones of the leg or forearm
- The volar aspect of the forearm and the anterior compartment of the leg (shin area) are the most commonly affected
- If untreated, tissue necrosis can develop with secondary muscle paralysis, muscle contractures and sensory impairment. This process is called Volkmann's ischemic necrosis and results in claw hand or foot caused by contractures of the ischemic muscle

Clinical

- Intractable pain and sometimes sensory hypesthesia distal to the involved compartment [usually top of foot (and median distribution in the hand)] are the most important early symptoms
- The characteristics are pain, paresthisias, and paralysis (P characteristics)
- Exam:
  - Remove cast or dressing if present
  - Manometric measurement (with catheter insertion) of suspicious increases in compartment syndrome is mandatory
  - The most important physical sign is *extreme pain* on stretching the long muscles passing through a compartment (plantar flexion of toes or full extension of fingers will stretch muscles of the forearm or shin)
  - Note: Pulses are usually completely normal in ACS because the intracompartmental pressure rarely exceeds systolic or mean arterial pressure levels

Diagnostic Testing

- Manometric techniques are available to measure compartment pressure directly
- General guidelines indicate the presence of a compartment syndrome when the diastolic pressure minus the intracompartmental pressure is ≤ to 20 mmHg

Treatment

- In ACS muscle necrosis may develop in 4–8 hours
- When diagnosis is made, a surgical fasciotomy of the compartment is essential. The wound is left open with delayed closure or skin grafting performed after edema subsides
- Without immediate treatment, ACS may result in permanent loss of function. The muscles necrose, scar, and shorten. Fingers and toes often claw and have little motion

MEDIAL TIBIAL STRESS SYNDROME(MTSS)/"SHIN SPLINTS"

General

- This condition has been termed *shin splints* and is a common cause of exercise-induced leg pain
- It is a type of overuse injury that results from chronic traction on the periosteum at the periosteal-fascial junction
- The periosteum may become detached from the bone due to ballistic overload
- A fibrofatty filling may occur at the site of the defect
- The attachment of the soleus muscle along the medial tibia may be the most likely site of avulsion
- In some cases, the other deep flexors of the foot are involved
- The main predisposing factor to shin splints is hyperpronation

General

- The patient presents with the gradual onset of pain along the posteromedial border of the tibia
- Pain may decrease with exercise and then become more apparent after the completion of the activity and last until the next morning
- There will be tenderness on palpation along the medial tibial border, either of its entire length or for as little as 2–4 cm
- There may be a history of repetitive running on hard surfaces and inappropriate warm-up, or inappropriate footwear
- There may be a history of excessive use of the foot flexors, as in jumping
- Frequently linked with recent change of footwear

Imaging

- Plain films will be normal. Bone scan may reveal areas of uptake along the medial tibial border in the third phase. MRI will help rule out a stress fracture

Treatment

- Rest is the first point in management of MTSS
- Rest may involve decreasing the volume of the inciting activity (relative rest) or avoidance of the activity
- When pain is present at rest or with normal walking, crutch walking is indicated
- Icing and stretching is also done initially
- Return to activity should be gradual and occurs when the patient is pain free for several days
- Training should start at 50% of preinjury level for intensity and distance
- Soft level surfaces should be used initially
- Orthotics are useful to correct over-pronation or forefoot varus
- Fasciotomy of the posteromedial fascia may be required in resistant cases

STRESS FRACTURES

General

- Tibial stress fractures are the most commonly occurring stress fractures in running sports
- They are a common cause of lower leg pain in athletes with an incidence of 25% in those with lower extremity pain
- Stress fractures occur when repetitive loading causes irreversible bone deformation. Microfractures develop and with continued overuse they can coalesce and propagate through the bone to become a symptomatic stress fracture
- Conditions of low bone mineral density impose a higher risk for stress fractures. These include:
  - Females with late onset of menses
  - Individuals with low body weight (< 75% ideal body weight)
  - Poor nutrition correlates with lower calcium intake
  - Tobacco and alcohol use
- Biomechanical conditions can lead to a higher risk of stress fracture
  - Over-pronation places higher stress on the fibula and tibia (i.e., genu valgum and a wide gait pattern may cause over-pronation)
  - Leg length discrepancies, muscle imbalances, lack of flexibility, and malalignment factors can also place high forces on the lower leg
- Extrinsic factors can lead to stress fractures
  - The classic training errors of increasing intensity and length of activity abruptly or causing excessive fatigue increase the chances of stress fractures
  - Running on hard surfaces or using worn-out shoes may also be a cause

TABLE 4–2 Incidence of Lower Extremity Stress Fractures in Runners

Bone	Incidence (%)
Femoral neck	7
Femoral upper shaft	5
Distal femoral shaft	2
Fibula	24
Tibia metaphysis	7
Tibia upper shaft	12
Tibia midshaft	11
Tibia distal shaft	4
Metatarsals	20
Second	11
Third	7
Other	2
Sesamoid Os calcis, talus, navicular	2

(DeLisa 1993. Table 54-2 with permision)

Clinical

- There will be pain at the onset of activity that initially may be a deep ache
- As activity progresses, the pain becomes more severe
- The pain will be localized to the fracture site
- Night pain may occur

- On palpation, there is tenderness local to the fracture site
- There may be swelling and redness at the fracture site

Imaging

Plain Films
- This is the first line of investigation
- Stress fractures may not be seen for 2–3 weeks after symptoms develop
- Periosteal thickening appears first, followed by cortical lucency
- The linear stress fracture appears as a lucency within a thickened area of cortical hyperostosis during healing

Bone Scan
- Bone scans are used when radiographs are negative and stress fracture is highly suspected
- Bone scans are very sensitive (close to 100%) but low in specificity
- A positive scan will yield focal increased uptake in the third phase
- Tumors, osteomyelitis, bony infarct, and bony dysplasias can also cause localized increased uptake

CT Scan
- CT scan can reveal fracture lines not visualized with plain films
- CT can also differentiate other lesions that cause increased uptake on bone scan

MRI
- MRI is becoming the first-choice means of investigating stress fracture
- MRI has comparable sensitivity to bone scan
- MRI can also visualize the fracture and differentiate between fracture and other lesions

Treatment

- Treatment is dependent on the severity of the fracture, its site, and length of symptoms
- If there is pain on normal ambulation, the patient should be non-weight bearing for 7–10 days
- Those without pain on normal ambulation should avoid aggravating the injury
- NSAIDs and ice may be used initially to control pain
- Muscle strengthening and stretching can begin immediately
- Nonimpact activities such as cycling and swimming can be used to maintain cardiac fitness
- At least 1–2 weeks of pain-free normal ambulation should be achieved before returning to impact activity
- Impact activity is started cautiously at low intensity for short periods (10–15 minutes) in the first few days and increased incrementally as tolerated
- Orthotics are a useful adjunct to treatment and may decrease impact force and help correct excessive supination or pronation
- Softer running surfaces should be considered
- Calcium intake should be 1500 mg QD with 400–800 IU of vitamin D

LOWER EXTREMITY—ANKLE AND FOOT REGION

FUNCTIONAL ANATOMY

Ankle Mortise (Figure 4–114)

- **Distal tibia**
  - Forms the medial malleolus and the superior articular surface of the ankle mortise joint
- **Distal fibula**
  - Forms the lateral malleolus and its superior articular surface of the ankle mortise joint
    - The lateral malleolus extends more distally than the medial malleolus, making it very important in ankle stabilization
- **Talus**
  - The talus is made up of four parts
    - Body, neck, head, and dome
    - It has a fragile blood supply, which may lead to complications of healing

Bones of the Foot (Figure 4–115)

- **7 tarsals**
  - 1- Talus
  - 1- Calcaneus
  - 1- Navicular
  - 1- Cuboid
  - 3- Cuneiforms
    - Medial, intermediate, lateral
- **5 metatarsals (1–5)**
- **14 phalanges**
  - Proximal, middle, distal
  - The great toe has just proximal and distal phalanges
- **2 sesamoid**
  - located on the plantar surface of the head of the first metatarsal

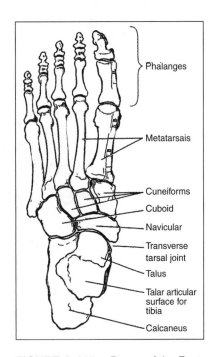

FIGURE 4–115. Bones of the Foot and Ankle: Dorsal View.

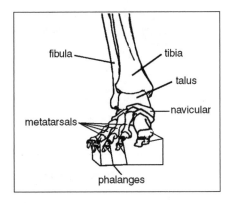

FIGURE 4–114. Ankle Mortise.

Ligaments of the Ankle (Figure 4–116)

- **Lateral aspect**
  - ▢ Anterior talofibular ligament (ATFL)
    - ▢ Primary lateral ankle ligament stabilizer
    - ▢ Most commonly injured ligament
  - Posterior talofibular ligament (PTFL)
  - Calcaneofibular ligament (CFL)
- **Medial aspect**
  - Deltoid ligament is one large ligament that consists of four parts broken down into deep and superficial areas
    - *Deep* (more important in maintaining stabilization)
      - Anterior tibiotalar
      - Posterior tibiotalar
    - *Superficial*
      - Tibionavicular
      - Tibiocalcaneal
    - The deltoid ligament maintains the close proximity of the medial malleolus and talus preserving the medial longitudinal arch of the foot
- **Anterior aspect**
  - **Syndesmotic ligaments**
    - Four ligaments that maintain the integrity of the distal tibia and fibula as well as resisting any forces that would separate the two bones
- **Ligaments**
  1. Anterior tibiofibular ligament
  2. Posterior tibiofibular ligament
  3. Transverse tibiofibular ligament
  4. Interosseous ligament

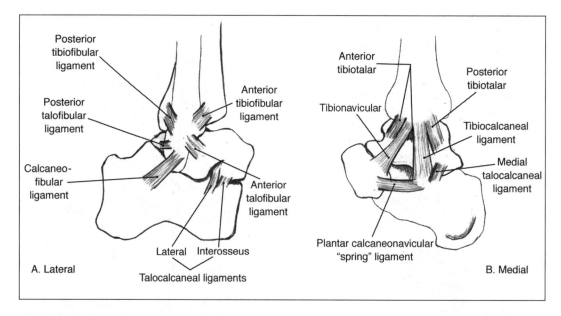

FIGURE 4–116. Ligaments of the Ankle and Subtalar Joint. **A.** Lateral View. **B.** Medial View.

Ligaments of the Foot

- **Lisfranc ligament**
  - Connects the second metatarsal head to the first cuneiform
- **Transverse metatarsal ligament**

Range of Motion of the Foot and Ankle
- **Ankle**
  - Dorsiflexion: 20°
  - Plantar flexion: 50°
- **Foot**
  - Subtalar joint
    - Inversion: 5°
    - Eversion: 5°
  - Forefoot
    - Abduction: 10°
    - Adduction: 20°
  - First MTP
    - Flexion: 45°
    - Extension: 80°

ANTERIOR		
	Inversion	**Eversion**
Dorsiflexion	• Tibialis anterior (Deep peroneal nerve, L4, L5) • Extensor hallucis longus (Deep peroneal nerve, L5, S1)	• Extensor digitorum longus (Deep peroneal nerve, L5, S1) • Peroneus tertius (Deep peroneal nerve, L5, S1)
Plantarflexion	• Tibialis posterior (Tibial nerve, L4, L5) • Flexor digitorum longus (Tibial nerve, S1, S2) • Flexor hallucis longus (Tibial nerve, S2, S3) • Plantaris (Tibial nerve, S1, S2) • Gastrocnemius (Tibial nerve, S1, S2) • Soleus (Tibial nerve, S1, S2)	• Peroneus longus (Superficial peroneal nerve, L5, S1, S2) • Peroneus brevis (Superficial peroneal nerve, L5, S1, S2)
	Posterior	**Lateral**

Foot Motion

- **Toe flexion**
  - Flexor digitorum longus (tibial nerve, S2, S3)
  - Flexor hallucis longus (tibial nerve, S2, S3)
  - Flexor digitorum brevis (medial plantar nerve [tibial], S2, S3)
  - Flexor hallucis brevis (medial plantar nerve [tibial], S2, S3)
  - Quadratus plantae (lateral plantar nerve [tibial], S2, S3)
  - Interossei (lateral plantar nerve [tibial], S2, S3)
  - Flexor digiti minimi brevis (lateral plantar nerve [tibial], S2, S3)
  - Lumbricals first lumbrical (medial plantar nerve [tibial]); second lumbrical; third lumbrical, fourth lumbrical (lateral plantar nerve [tibial] S2, S3)
- **Toe extension**
  - Extensor digitorum longus (deep peroneal, L5, S1)
  - Extensor hallucis longus (deep peroneal, L5, S1)
  - Extensor digitorum brevis (deep peroneal, S1, S2)
  - Lumbricals: first lumbrical (medial plantar nerve [tibial]); second lumbrical, third lumbrical, fourth lumbrical (lateral plantar nerve [tibial], S2, S3)

- **Toe abduction**
  - Abductor hallucis [medial plantar nerve (tibial), S2, S3]
  - Abductor digiti minimi [lateral plantar nerve (tibial), S2, S3]
  - Dorsal interossei [lateral plantar nerve (tibial), S2, S3]
- **Toes adduction**
  - Adductors hallucis [lateral plantar nerve (tibial), S2, S3]
  - Plantar interossei [lateral plantar nerve (tibial), S2, S3]

■

DISORDERS OF THE ANKLE

LATERAL ANKLE DISORDERS

LATERAL ANKLE SPRAINS (FIGURE 4–117)

General

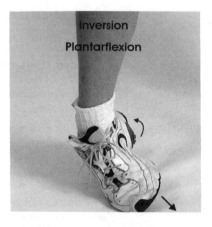

- Most common ankle sprain accounting for up to 85% of all ankle sprains result from plantar flexion inversion injuries causing lateral ankle sprains
- Anatomy: Ligaments
- Anterior talofibular ligament (ATFL)
  - Most common ligament injured
- Posterior talofibular ligament (PTFL)
  - Last to be injured
- Calcaneofibular ligament (CFL)
  - Second most common
    - Function: Stabilize the ankle during inversion

FIGURE 4–117. Lateral Ankle Sprain

- Mechanism of injury
  - 📖 Inversion on a plantarflexed foot is the most vulnerable position
  - History of "rolling over" the ankle
- Provocative Tests (Figure 4–118)
  - **Anterior draw**
    - Tests the integrity of the ATFL
  - **Talar tilt**
    - Tests the integrity of the CFL and ATFL

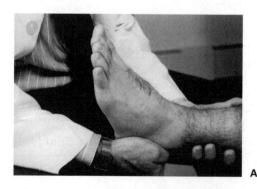
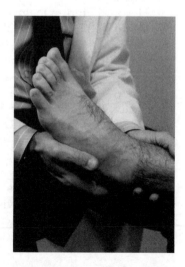

A   B

FIGURE 4–118. Stress Tests for Ligament Stability. **A.** Anterior Draw Sign. **B.** Inversion Test (Talar Tilt)

Clinical

- **Grade 1 (Mild)**
  - Partial tear of the ATFL
  - CFL and PTFL are intact
  - Mild swelling with point tenderness at the lateral aspect of the ankle
  - No instability
  - Stress tests
    - Anterior draw: Negative
    - Talar tilt: Negative
- **Grade 2 (Moderate)**
  - Complete tear of the ATFL
  - Partial tear of the CFL
  - Diffuse swelling and ecchymosis
  - Stress test
    - Anterior draw: Positive
      - ◆ Large anterior shift of the ankle or palpable clunk
    - Talar tilt: Negative
- **Grade 3 (Severe)**
  - Complete tear of the ATFL and CFL
  - Stress test
    - Anterior draw: Positive
    - Talar tilt: Positive
      - ◆ Inverting the talus on the tibia looking for a clinical asymmetry in comparison
- **Dislocation**
  - Complete tear of the ATFL, CFL, and PTFL

Imaging

- X ray; A/P, lateral, oblique
- Stress views: Anterior drawer and talar tilt
- Anterior drawer may show a > 5 mm displacement
- Talar tilt may show a 5–10° difference as compared to the contralateral extremity

Treatment

- **Grades 1 and 2**
  - Acute
    - Rest, ice, compression, elevation (RICE), NSAIDs, analgesics, immobilization
    - Early mobilization
  - Conservative: Rehabilitation
    - Range of motion, strengthening, proprioceptive exercises, taping, and bracing
    - Modalities
      - ◆ Moist heat, warm whirlpool, contrast baths, ultrasound, short wave diathermy
- **Grade 3**
  - Controversial: Conservative vs. surgical
    - Six month trial of rehabilitation and bracing
    - Ligament repair, tenodesis of the peroneus brevis
    - If patient is a high-performance athlete, and conservative Tx fails (i.e., patient has persistent critical instability), then surgical reconstruction of torn ligaments may be considered as early as 3 months post injury

Peroneal Tendon Injury

General

- Anatomy: Tendon insertion (Figure 4–119)
  - Peroneus longus inserts on the base of the first metatarsal
  - Peroneus brevis inserts on the base of the fifth metatarsal
- Function of the peroneus longus
  - Plantar flexes the ankle and everts the foot
- Mechanism
  - Tenosynovitis or rupture
    - Repetitive forceful eversion causing inflammation or degeneration of the tendon or synovium along its course, behind the lateral malleolus to its insertion point
  - Subluxation or dislocation
    - A sudden dorsiflexion of the ankle with the foot can cause a subluxation or dislocation of the peroneal tendon. This insult is commonly a skiing injury

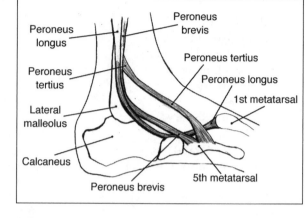

FIGURE 4–119. Anatomy of Peroneus Longus, Brevis, and Tertius.

Clinical

- Painful swelling in the retromalleolar area along the coarse of the peroneal tendons
- Sudden weakness with the inability to actively evert the foot if a subluxation or dislocation is suspected
- A popping sensation in the lateral aspect of the ankle
- *Provocative test*
  - Pain with resisted dorsiflexion and eversion

Imaging

- None needed. MRI if indicated

Treatment

- Tenosynovitis: Same treatment as for a lateral ankle sprain
- Rupture/subluxation/dislocation: Orthopedic evaluation
  - 4 to 6 weeks of immobilization in a plantarflexed position

MEDIAL ANKLE DISORDERS

Medial Ankle Sprain: Deltoid Ligament (Figure 4–120)

General

- Rare ankle injury associated with a 5% occurrence rate
- 📖 Medial collateral ligaments: Deltoid ligament is one ligament comprised of four parts
    - Anterior tibiotalar ligament
    - Posterior tibiotalar ligament
    - Tibionavicular ligament
    - Tibiocalcaneal ligament
  - Function is to stabilize the ankle during eversion

- Mechanism of injury
  - Pure eversion, which is rare
  - Foot caught in a pronated, everted position with internal rotation of the upper body. An example is when the foot strikes the ground instead of the ball in soccer or an extra-point in football.
  - Grade:
    - Grade 1: Stretch
    - Grade 2: Stretch partial tear
    - Grade 3: Full tear
- Complications
  - Syndesmosis ankle injuries and Maisonneuve fractures (see *Syndesmosis*)

Clinical

- Medial foot swelling and ecchymosis and pain on eversion
- Negative anterior drawer test

Imaging

- X ray; A/P, lateral, oblique
- MRI if indicated

Treatment

- Same as lateral ankle injuries

TIBIALIS POSTERIOR TENDON INJURY

General

- Anatomy—posterior tibialis (Figure 4–121)
  - Origin: Interosseus membrane and the posterior surface of the tibia and fibula
  - Insertion: Tuberosity of the navicular, cuboid, and base of the second to fourth metatarsals
- Function—Plantar flexes the ankle and inverts the foot
  - Maintains the medial longitudinal arch
- Mechanism of injury
  - Tenosynovitis or rupture
    - Repetitive forceful inversion causing inflammation or degeneration of the tendon or synovium along its course

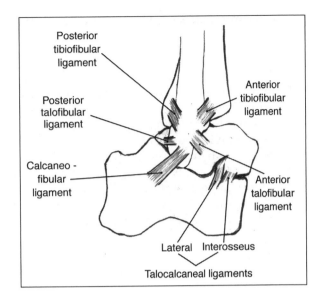

FIGURE 4–120. The Deltoid Ligament

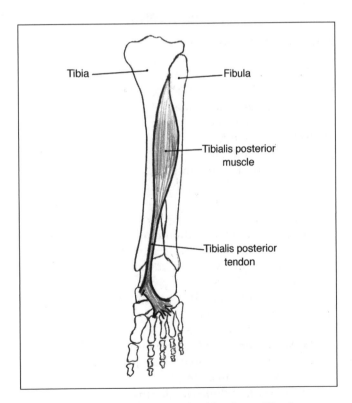

FIGURE 4–121. Tibialis Posterior Muscle and Tendon (posterior view).

- 5% to 10% associated with an accessory navicular

Clinical

- Insidious onset of posteromedial ankle pain increased by activity
- Medial hindfoot swelling
- Increase pain with push-off
- Weakness with inversion and plantar flexion
- The classic "too many toes" sign is seen with a tibialis posterior tendon rupture (Figure 4–122)
  - When viewing the patients' feet from behind, more toes are visible on affected side secondary to collapse of the medial longitudinal arch

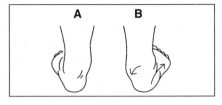

FIGURE 4–122. **A.** Normal. **B.** Positive "Too Many Toes" sign.

Imaging

- None needed

Treatment

- Acute: Same as lateral ankle sprains
- Conservative: Rehabilitation, orthotics
- Surgical: Tendon transfer, excising the accessory navicular

POSTERIOR ANKLE DISORDERS

ACHILLES TENDON DISORDERS

General

- Triceps surae function (Figure 4–123)
  - Plantar flexes the ankle
  - Supinate the foot
- Mechanism of injury
  - Achilles tendonitis
    - Repetitive eccentric overload causing inflammation and microtears of the tendon
  - Achilles tendon rupture
    - **Inflammatory:** Inflammation and degeneration causing a series of microruptures or breakdown in the collagen fibers
    - **Poor nutrition:** Inadequate vascularization 2–6 cm proximal to the insertion of the tendon
    - **Mechanical:** Sudden push-off with the foot in the extension position. (landing from a jump)
- Risk factors to Achilles tendonitis
  - Anatomic: Hyperpronation, tight hamstrings and heel cords, pes cavus and genu varum

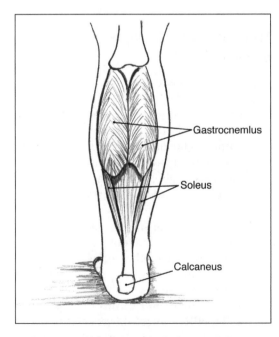

FIGURE 4–123. Anatomy of the Gastrocnemius and Soleus Muscles.

- Age: Leads to an inflexibility of the tendon and decreased tensile strength
- Training errors: Most common risk factor
  - Increase in mileage or intensity
  - Change in recent footwear

Clinical Presentation

- Tendonitis
  - Posterior ankle pain, swelling
  - Pain elicited on push-off
- Rupture
  - Sudden audible snap with immediate swelling, ecchymosis and weakness in plantar flexion
  - Positive Thompson's test is indicative of a ruptured Achilles tendon (Figure 4–124)
    - In an intact Achilles tendon squeezing the calf should elicit plantar flexion of the foot (i.e., negative Thompson's test)
    - In a rupture of the Achilles, the foot is unable to plantarflex secondary to the tendon separation (i.e,. positive Thompson's test)

Imaging

- None needed. MRI is helpful if the diagnosis is in question

Treatment

- ⌑ Achilles tendonitis
  - Relative rest, ice, anti-inflammatory medications
  - Rehabilitation: Short-term immobilization (splinting or bracing), stretching and strengthening, heel lifts
  - Corticosteroid injection. Do not inject into the tendon. This may cause rupture.
    - ⌑ Complication of rupture. The area of hypovascularity 2–5 cm proximal to the tendon insertion is where most ruptures occur. Corticosteroids decrease the metabolic rate of the chondrocytes and fibrocytes, weakening the structural integrity of the tendon and articular cartilage
- Rupture: Surgical vs. conservative
  - Conservative: Bracing in a plantar-flexed position for a period of 8–12 weeks. The dorsiflexion is increased gradually so

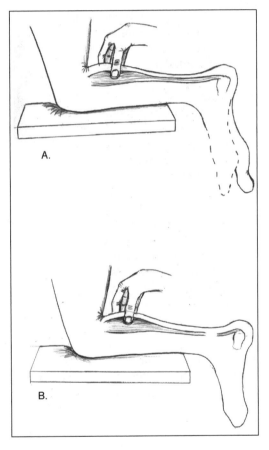

FIGURE 4–124. Thompson's Test.
A. Negative. **B.** Positive

that by the end of 12 weeks the patient is in a neutral position. Activity level is increased gradually (heel lifts may be used)

– Surgical: Tendon repair intraoperatively—patient is placed in a cast for 2 weeks, patient is then put in a plantar flexion dial lock brace for 4–6 weeks and slowly brought to neutral. Activity level is increased gradually (heel lifts may be used). Surgical repair is usually reserved for active individuals

FLEXUS HALLUCIS LONGUS INJURY

General

- Synonym: Dancer's tendonitis
- Flexor hallucis longus (Figure 4–125)
  - Origin: Distal fibula and interosseous membrane
  - Insertion: Base of the distal phalanx of the great toe
- Function
  - Flexes the great toe at all the joints
  - Plantar flexes the ankle
- Mechanism of injury
  - Repetitive push-off maneuvers causing inflammation of the synovium or tendon as it courses in the groove of the sustentaculum tali and behind the lateral malleolus to its insertion

Clinical

- Tenderness along the tendon at the posteromedial aspect of the great toe
- Decreased ability to flex the great toe
- Increased pain with active plantar flexion and passive dorsiflexion

Imaging

- None needed

Treatment

- Same as lateral ligament sprain

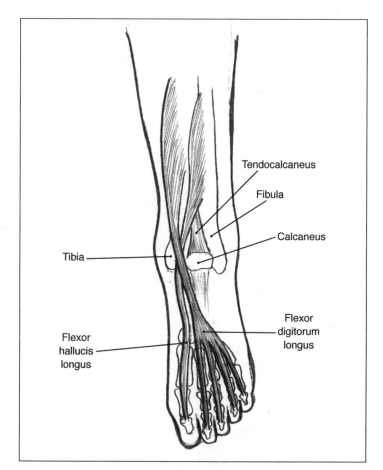

FIGURE 4–125. Anatomy of Flexor Hallucis Longus. (Posterior View—Plantar Flexed)

BURSITIS: RETROCALCANEAL, BONY EXOSTOSIS, CALCANEAL APOPHYSIS

General

- Common cause of heel pain, especially in women, secondary to high heel shoes
- Retrocalcaneal bursitis (Figure 4–126)
  - Inflammation of the bursae between the posterior superior portion of the calcaneus and the distal Achilles tendon or a bursa between the skin and the Achilles tendon causing pain

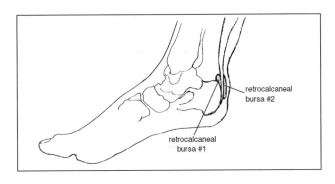

FIGURE 4–126. Retrocalcaneal Bursitis. Medial View.

- Mechanism of injury
  - Repetitive pressure and shearing forces from an object (i.e., shoes) causing thickening and inflammation of the bursae often resulting in a collection of fluid
- Associations
  - Haglund's deformity: Enlargement of the posterosuperior tuberosity
  - Sever's disease: Apophysitis, an independent area of ossification separated from the main bone at the cartilaginous plate. Occurring in the young population, especially female gymnasts from the stresses of the gastrocnemius pull

Clinical

- Tenderness and swelling in the posterior aspect of the tendon distally
- Small soft tissue swelling at the Achilles insertion can be palpated on exam, "pump bumps"
- Above symptoms may be exacerbated with the presence of a Haglund's deformity
- Similar type of pain can result from insertional Achilles tendonitis

Imaging

- None needed

Treatment

- Change or alter footwear
- Surgical excision of the bursae if conservative measures fail

ANTERIOR ANKLE DISORDERS

SYNDESMOSIS

Syndesmosis is a fibrous joint of the tibia and fibula united by ligaments

General

- Often related to a high ankle sprain
- Function

- Maintain the integrity of the ankle mortise. Resist the forces that attempt to separate the tibia and fibula
- Syndesmosis: Ligaments (Figure 4–127)
  - Anterior tibiofibular ligament
  - Posterior tibiofibular ligament
  - Interosseous ligament
  - Transverse tibiofibular ligament
- Mechanism of injury
  - Hyperdorsiflexion and forceful eversion of the ankle
  - Direct blow to the foot with the ankle held in external rotation

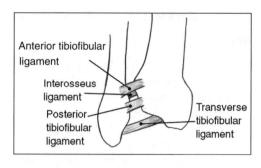

FIGURE 4–127. The Syndesmotic Ligaments of the Ankle.

Clinical

- Chronic in nature; pain and swelling on the anterior aspect just above the ankle
- Provocative tests
  - Squeeze test
    - Tenderness on compression of the distal tibia and fibula proximal to the injury
  - Stress test
    - With the knee held at 90° and ankle neutral, the patient experiences pain when the examiner attempts forcefully to externally rotate the foot

Imaging

- Plain films: A/P, lateral, oblique, mortise views; MRI, CT
- Rule out widening between the distal tibia and fibula
- Be sure to obtain plain films of the proximal fibula to rule out the possibility of a Maisonneuve fracture (Figure 4–128)
  - Definition: Rupture of the anterior tibiofibular ligament extending through the interosseus membrane which often results in a proximal fibula fracture

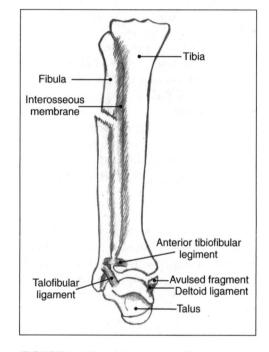

FIGURE 4–128. Maisonneuve Fracture.

Treatment

- Conservative
- Surgical: Screw fixation to stabilize the ankle mortise

SINUS TARSI SYNDROME

General

- Talocalcaneal ligament sprain
- Mechanism of injury
  - Excessive foot pronation causing adduction of the talus

– History of arthritis: Rheumatoid, gout, and seronegative spondyloarthropathy
– History of prior ankle injury: Inversion sprain or fracture of the tibia, calcaneal, or talar

Clinical

- Pain on the anterolateral aspect of the foot and ankle in the area of the sinus tarsi (Figure 4–129)
- Diagnosis: Resolution of symptoms with injection of local anesthetic into the sinus tarsi

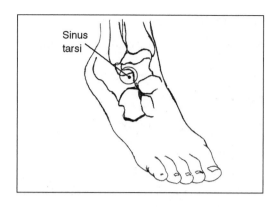

FIGURE 4–129. Sinus Tarsi Area.

Imaging

- None needed

Treatment

- Conservative: Same as lateral ankle sprain
- Surgical: Decompression of the tunnel contents

TIBIALIS ANTERIOR TENDON INJURY

General

- Tibialis anterior function: Dorsiflex and inversion of the foot
- Mechanism of injury
  - Tenosynovitis
    - Inflammation of the tendon or synovium as it courses under the superior retinaculum
  - Rupture
    - Degenerative process seen in the elderly
    - Eccentric overload

Clinical

- Tibialis anterior can be palpated distally upon its insertion onto the medial aspect of the base of the first metatarsal and the first cuneiform bones (Figure 4–130) and proximally along the tendon to the muscle belly on the lateral side of the tibial shaft
- Patient with a history of chronic ankle pain
- Painless foot slap that has gradually increased over time
- Increased tenderness and weakness with active dorsiflexion and passive plantar flexion
- Palpable defect may be noted over the anterior aspect of the ankle

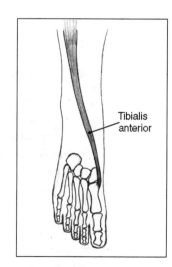

FIGURE 4–130. Palpation of the Tibialis Anterior Tendon.

Imaging

- None needed

Treatment

- Conservative vs. surgical, depending on the patient's age and functional needs

TIBIALIS ANTERIOR HYPERACTIVITY

General

- Typically hyperactivity of the tibialis anterior (TA) contributes to an equinovarus deformity

Clinical

- Commonly seen in patients with cerebral palsy (CP), cerebral vascular accidents (CVA), and traumatic brain injury (TBI). Any injury that may cause this hyperactivity/spasticity of the TA tendon
- Equinovarus deformity is present in physical exam
- Achilles tendon is frequently shortened, causing a toe-pointing equinus posture

Imaging

- Plain films AP lateral

Treatment

- 📖 Split Anterior Tibial Tendon Transfer (SPLATT)
  - Technique: Splitting the tibialis anterior tendon. Half is attached to its site of origin, while the distal end of the lateral half of the tendon is tunneled into the third cuneiform and cuboid bones. This provides an eversion force to counteract the dynamic varus deformity to provide a flat base for which weightbearing can occur
  - The SPLATT procedure is often done along with Achilles tendon lengthening to decrease plantarflexion

📖 OSTEOCHONDRAL FRACTURE OF THE TALAR DOME

General

- Etiology
  - Shear force on the anterior lateral surface of the talus resulting in a shallow lesion
  - Compressive force on the posterior medial surface of the talus resulting in a deep lesion
- Mechanism
  - Eversion and dorsiflexion
  - Inversion and plantar flexion
- Classification: (Hawkins)
  - Type 1: Nondisplaced vertical fracture of the talar neck
  - Type 2: Displaced fracture of the talar neck of the subtalar joint with the ankle joint remaining intact
  - Type 3: Displaced fracture of the talar neck with dislocation of the body of the talus from the subtalar and ankle joints
- 📖 Complication
  - Avascular necrosis, which most commonly occurs at the talar body. (The risk of AVN increases as the amount of displacement increases.)
  - Fracture of the talar dome may form a subchondral fragment that can detach and become displaced in the joint space

Clinical

- Chronic ankle injury
- Small effusion that may be painful
- Decreased range of motion

Imaging

- Plain films: Mortise view of the ankle; MRI

Treatment

- Conservative: Non-weight bearing
- Surgical: ORIF if indicated

■

FOOT DISORDERS

PLANTAR FASCITIS (FIGURE 4–131)

General

- Medial plantar heel pain, which may evolve from the bone (heel spur) or plantar fascia
- Females > males
- Mechanism
  - Tension on the plantar fascia leading to chronic inflammation most commonly at its origin
  - Disorders causing tension include: pes cavus (high arch), pes planus (flat foot), obesity, tight Achilles tendon
- Other associations: HLA-B27; seronegative spondyloarthropathy. Heel spurs may contribute to the etiology: 50% to 75% with heel spurs have plantar fascitis

Clinical

- Tenderness over the medial aspect of the heel and the entire plantar fascia
- Increased on awakening and decreases with activity
- Tight Achilles tendon frequently associated with plantar fascitis

Imaging

- Plain films to assess bony spur

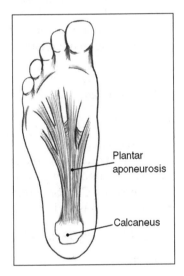

FIGURE 4–131. Plantar Aponeurosis.

Treatment

- Conservative: 90% to 95% effective and should be done for at least six months prior to considering surgery
  - Heel pads, cushion and lift
  - Achilles and plantar fascia stretching
  - Modalities, NSAIDs, night splints holding the foot in slight dorsiflexion
  - Injection: Do not inject anesthetic/corticosteroid into the subcutaneous tissue or fascial layer. Stay out of the superficial fat pad to avoid fat necrosis

- Surgical: Plantar fascia release, rarely indicated

📖 MORTON'S NEUROMA (Figure 4–132)

General

- Definition: Irritation and degeneration of the digital nerves in the toes producing a painful mass near the area of the metatarsal heads. The mass is secondary to the nerve fibrosing.
- More commonly between the second and third, and third and fourth digits
- Females > males

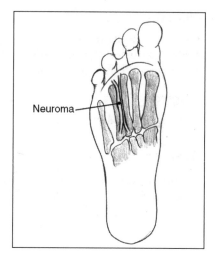

FIGURE 4–132. Morton's Neuroma, a perineural fibrosis of the interdigital nerves.

Clinical

- Sharp shooting forefoot pain radiating to the affected digits. Dysesthesias and numbness is common
- 📖 The exam is performed by applying direct pressure in the interdigit web space with one hand and then applying lateral and medial foot compression to squeeze the metatarsal heads together. Isolated pain on the plantar aspect of the web space is consistent with Morton's neuroma

Imaging

- None needed

Treatment

- Conservative
  - Shoes with a soft sole and wide toe box
  - Accommodative padding: Metatarsal pad
  - Injection: Corticosteroid and lidocaine may be diagnostic and therapeutic
- Surgical: Excision if indicated

HALLUX DISORDERS: VALGUS, RIGIDUS, AND SPRAINS

General

- Definitions
  - Metatarsal phalangeal (MTP) sprain
    - Acute injury to the ligaments and capsule of the MTP joint. "Turf toe" is commonly seen in athletes. Chronic sprains may lead to hallux rigidus
  - Hallux valgus
    - Lateral deviation of the first toe greater than the normal angle of 15 degrees between the tarsus and metatarsus. This may lead to a painful prominence of the medial aspect of the MTP joint (bunion)
  - Hallux rigidus
    - Degenerative condition of the first MTP joint leading to pain and stiffness (great toe arthritis of MTP joint)
- Female >> males

Clinical

- Valgus: Lateral deviation of the first toe with a large medial eminence of the MTP joint
- MTP sprain: Acute onset of pain, tenderness, and swelling of the MTP joint, particularly over the plantar aspect. Pain on passive dorsiflexion

- Rigidus: Pain and swelling with decreased range of motion of the MTP joint. Antalgic gait pattern
- Lesser toe deformities: The second toe usually will result in an overriding position

Imaging

- Plain films

Treatment

- Conservative: Rest, Ice, Compression, Elevation (RICE), taping, proper footwear (i.e., high toe box)
- Surgical debridement (rigidus)

■

TOE DISORDERS: HAMMER, CLAW, AND MALLET

HAMMER TOE (Figure 4–133)

📖 General

- Deformity of the lesser toes in which there is flexion of the proximal interphalangeal (PIP) joint
- A passive extension of MTP joint occurs when the toe is flat on the ground. The DIP joint is usually not affected
- Caused by chronic tight shoe wear that crowds the toes, but may be seen after trauma

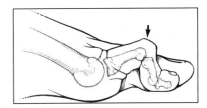

FIGURE 4–133. Hammer Toe. Reprinted with permission from Snider RK. Essentials of Musculoskeletal Medicine. Rosemont IL, American Academy of Orthopaedic Surgeons, 1997.

Clinical

- Obvious deformity as described previously
- Pain is present in the toe and patient has difficulty with footwear

Imaging

- Standing AP and lateral help exclude other diagnosis

Treatment

- Shoes with roomy toe boxes. Shoes should be 1/2 inch longer than the longest toe
- Home exercise program of passive manual strengthening

CLAW TOE (Figure 4–134)

📖 General

- Characterized by extension of MTP and flexion of the PIP and flexion of the DIP
- Deformity is usually the result of the incompetence of the foot intrinsic muscles, secondary to the neurologic disorders affecting the strength of these muscles (i.e., diabetes, alcoholism, peripheral neuropathies, Charcot-Marie-Tooth disease and spinal cord tumors)

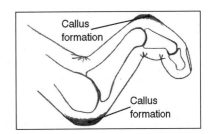

FIGURE 4–134. Claw Toe

Clinical Symptoms

- Pain is the principle symptom
- If progression is rapid, this suggests a related neurologic condition

Imaging

- Radiographs of foot confirm the diagnosis

Treatment

- Shoes with soft, roomy, high toe boxes
- Splints available
- Surgical correction may be necessary if conservative treatment fails

MALLET TOE (Figure 4–135)

General

- Flexion deformity at the DIP joint with normal alignment at the proximal interphalangeal (PIP) and MTP joint
- Usually the result of jamming type injury—or wearing tight shoes

Clinical Symptoms

- Obvious deformity, pain, callus at tip of toe

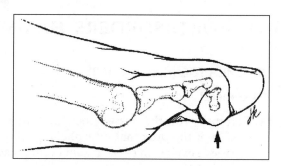

FIGURE 4–135. Mallet Toe. Reprinted with permission Snider RK. Essentials of Musculoskeletal Medicine. Rosemont IL, American Academy of Orthopaedic Surgeons, 1997.

Imaging

- AP and lateral radiographs may be indicated to rule out fracture

Treatment

- The callus should be trimmed
- Shoes with high toe boxes

LISFRANC JOINT INJURY

General

- Traumatic disruption of the tarsometatarsal joints involving fracture, dislocation, or both (Figure 4–136)
- Mechanism of injury
  - Direct: Less common; trauma—direct impact
  - Indirect: Positional, commonly seen in athletes
    - Force applied to the heel in line with the axis of the foot and toes in a flexed position

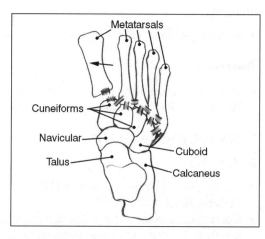

FIGURE 4–136. Isolated Lisfranc Dislocation.

Clinical

- Vague ankle pain. Pain and swelling localized to the dorsum of the foot
- This injury is easily missed and often misdiagnosed as a lateral ankle sprain
- Pain may be exacerbated by stabilizing the hind foot and rotating the forefoot

Imaging

- X rays: A/P, lateral, oblique of the ankle and the entire foot. Look for a shift commonly between the first and seconds metatarsals
- MRI, CT if needed

Treatment

- Conservative
  - Nondisplaced joint: Non-weight-bearing, immobilization for 6–8 weeks with continued support thereafter
- Surgical
  - Stabilization is integral to maintaining the bony architecture of the entire foot

FOOT FRACTURES

General

- Definitions
  - Jones fracture: Transverse fracture through the base of the fifth metatarsal
  - Nutcracker fracture: Cuboid fracture
  - March fracture: A fatigue fracture of one of the metatarsals

Clinical

- Pain to palpation, swelling and ecchymosis over the involved area
- Usually a result of trauma

Diagnosis

- Plain films of foot and ankle, MRI or CT

Treatment

- Jones: Non-weight-bearing cast for six weeks. ORIF if nonunion occurs
- Nutcracker: ORIF
- March: Cast if needed

■

SPINE REHABILITATION

INTRODUCTION

Neck and back pain are leading musculoskeletal complaints that contribute to impairment and disability. Injury to the lumbar region in particular has a 5% to 10% annual incidence and 60% to 90% lifetime prevalence, reaching more than 100 million people in the United States alone. Fortunately, the natural course is favorable, as symptoms are usually self-limited. Though resolution remains likely, recurrence of symptoms is possible because of structural and functional pathological adaptations. These can be addressed and limited with adequate comprehensive treatment programs.

📖 Clinical Course

Outcome	Time
~ 50 % resolve	~ 1–2 weeks
~ 90 % resolve	~ 6–12 weeks
~ 85 % recur	~ 1–2 years

Approximately 10% of patients with low back pain continue with residual complaints. Due to its morbidity, this subgroup constitutes the second most common reason for primary care physician office visits. Proper treatment of these patients depends on an accurate diagnosis, which may be elusive due to the complexity of the structures involved. Diagnostic testing may be indicated to further define pathology and focus care. Regardless, proper screening begins with a complete history and physical examination. Assessment for the presence of red flags, representing conditions requiring more immediate attention, is imperative.

📖 Red Flags

Clinical Presentation	Condition
Gait ataxia/Upper motor neuron changes	Myelopathy
Bowel/Bladder/Sexual dysfunction	Cauda equina syndrome
Night pain/Weight loss	Tumor
Fevers/Chills	Infection

In the work force, low back pain is second to upper respiratory infections as the most frequent cause of absenteeism. Due to the cost of medical care, time lost from work, disability payments, production loss, staff retraining, and litigation expenses, its economic impact reaches into the billions annually. It will cause approximately 25 million Americans to lose one or more days from work a year. Over five million people are disabled from low back pain and the yearly prevalence continues to grow at a rate greater than that of the size of the general U.S. population.

📖 Absenteeism

Time Missed from Work	Return to Work Expectations (%)
~ 6 months	50
~ 1 year	25
~ 2 year	0

This section focuses on board-related topics with regard to musculoskeletal spinal disorders and is to be used as a study guide. It is not intended to be an all-inclusive composite. However, for more elaborate coverage of the subject matter, the reader is directed to the suggested references at the end of this chapter.

FUNCTIONAL ANATOMY

CERVICAL VERTEBRAE

Typical: C3 to C7 (Figure 4–137)

Unique Characteristics
- **Anterior region**
  - Vertebral body
    - Uncinate processes: The lateral aspect of the vertebral body has a superior projection (the uncinate process). As the disks become degenerative these projections approximate with the body of the next higher vertebrae. The end result is the degenerative joint change called the Joint of Luschka (uncovertebral joint).📖 The Joints of Luschka function to limit lateral translation (Figure 4-138).

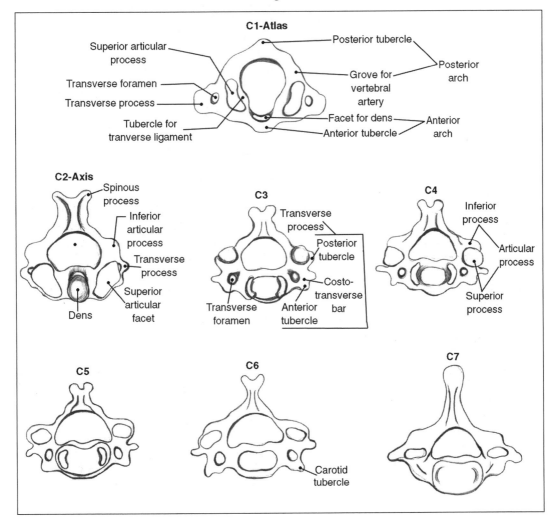

FIGURE 4–137. The Typical Cervical Vertebrae —(Superior View)

- **Posterior region**
  - Pedicles, superior and inferior articular pro-cesses, laminae, transverse processes, foramen transversarium and spinous process
    - C3, C4, C5, C6: Bifid spinous process
    - C7: Nonbifid spinous process

Atypical: C1 and C2

Unique Characteristics
- C1 (atlas) (Figure 4–139)
  - Ring shaped bone containing two lateral masses
  - No vertebral body or spinous process

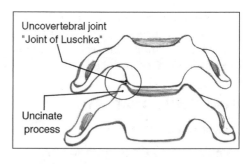

FIGURE 4–138. Joints of Luschka.

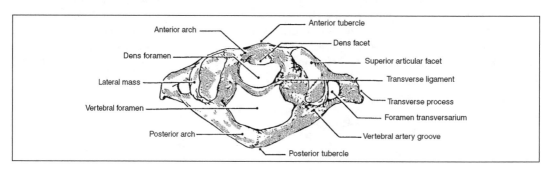

FIGURE 4–139. The Atlas—Superior View.

- C2 (axis) (Figure 4–140)
  - Its vertebral body has an odontoid process
  - Bifid spinous process

THORACIC VERTEBRAE

Typical: T1 to T12 (Figure 4–141)

Unique Characteristics
- **Anterior region**
  - Vertebral body with articulations for the rib heads
- **Posterior region**
  - Pedicles, superior and inferior articular pro-cesses, laminae, trans-verse processes with articulations for rib tubercles and spinous process

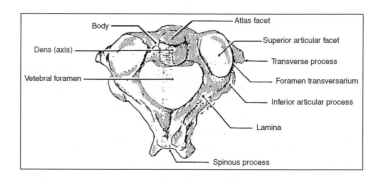

FIGURE 4–140. The Axis—Superior View.

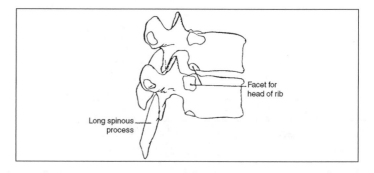

FIGURE 4–141. The Thoracic Vertebrae—Lateral View.

Lumbar Vertebrae

Typical: L1 to L5 (Figure 4–142)

Unique Characteristics
- **Anterior region**
  - Vertebral body
- **Posterior region**
  - Pedicles, superior and inferior articular processes, transverse processes, mamillary process, laminae and spinous process

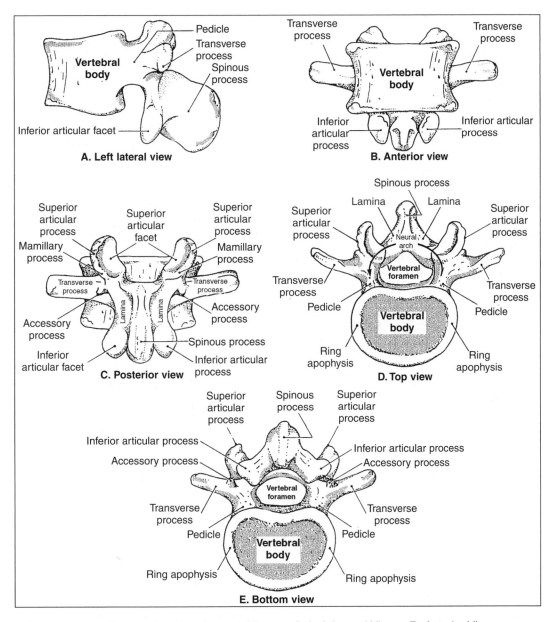

FIGURE 4–142. The Lumbar Vertebrae—5 Views. **A.** Left Lateral View. **B.** Anterior View. **C.** Posterior View. **D.** Top View. **E.** Bottom View

Atypical: Sacralization

- An anomalous fusion of the fifth lumbar vertebrae with the sacrum. Incidence: 1% complete, 6% incomplete

The Motion Segment Figure (Figure 4–143)

- A three-joint complex is formed between two lumbar vertebrae

Joint 1	Disc between two vertebral bodies
Joint 2	Zygapophyseal joint (facet joint)
Joint 3	Zygapophyseal joint (facet joint)

SACRAL VERTEBRAE

Typical (Figure 4–144)

Unique Characteristics
- A triangular-shaped bone consisting of five fused vertebrae.
- Four pairs of foramina (anterior and posterior), sacral promontory, ala, hiatus, cornua, medial, intermediate, and lateral crests which are analogous to the spinous process

Atypical: Lumbarization
- An anomalous partial or complete nonunion of the first and second segment of the sacrum. This forms an additional lumbar segment (L6), and leaves four remaining fused sacral segments. Incidence ~ 4%

Ligaments (Figure 4–145)

COCCYGEAL VERTEBRAE

Typical

Unique Characteristics
- Three to four fused segments, with transverse processes, hiatus and cornua

ZYGAPOPHYSEAL JOINT (Z-JOINT/FACET JOINT)

Characteristics (Figure 4–146)

- Superior articular process (SAP)
- Inferior articular process (IAP)
- Joint capsule (C)
- Articular Carticular (AC)
- Meniscus (M)

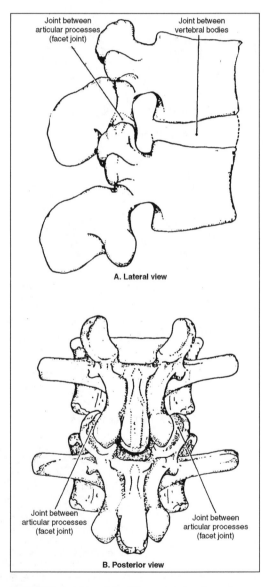

A. Lateral view

B. Posterior view

FIGURE 4–143. The Three—Joint Complex.

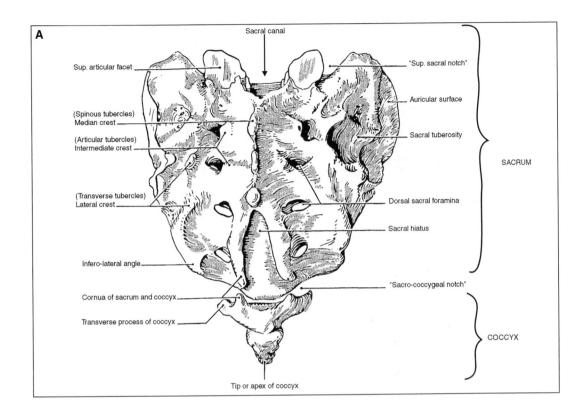

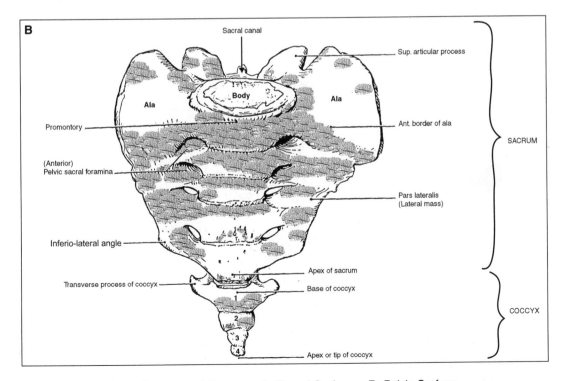

FIGURE 4–144.   The Sacrum and Coccyx.   **A.** Dorsal Surface.   **B.** Pelvic Surface.

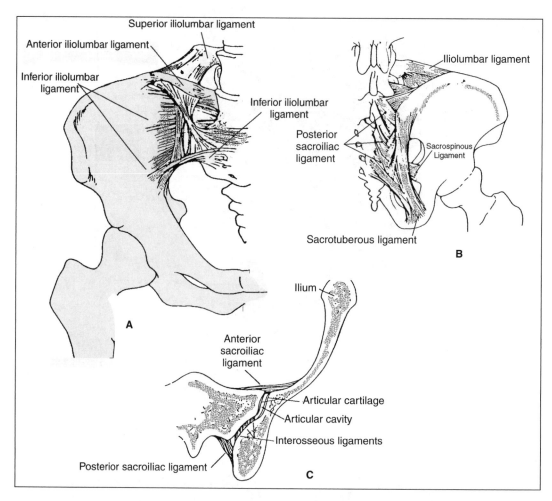

FIGURE 4–145. The Sacral Ligaments. **A.** Anterior View. **B.** Posterior View. **C.** Axial View.

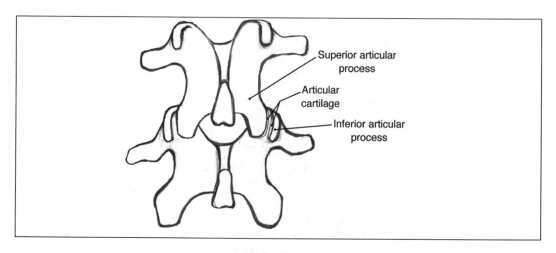

FIGURE 4–146. The L3-L4 Zygapophyseal Joint —Posterior View. The posterior capsule has been resected to reveal the joint cavity.

Orientation

- Cervical: AA and OA have no true Z-joints due to their atypical anatomy. C3 to C7 are positioned in the frontal (coronal) plane
- Thoracic: Positioned in the frontal plane.
- 📖 Lumbar: Begins in the sagittal plane and progresses to the frontal plane at L5 to S1

Function

- Direct vertebral motion
- Resist shearing and rotational forces
- Weight bearing: Increased with extension

📖 INTERVERTEBRAL DISC

Characteristics (Figure 4–147)

- **Nucleus pulposus**
  A viscous muco-protein gel mixture of water and proteoglycans in a network of type II collagen that braces the annulus to prevent buckling
- **Annulus fibrosus**
  Type I collagen fibers arranged in obliquely running lamellae that encase the nucleus pulposus and are attached to the vertebral endplate plates. This orientation withstands distraction and bending but is relatively weaker for torsional stresses
- **Vertebral endplate**
  Cartilaginous covering of the vertebral body apophysis, forming the top and bottom of the disc

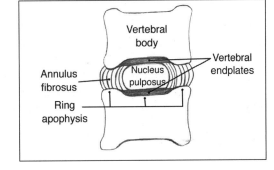

FIGURE 4–147. The Intervertebral Disc.

Vascular Supply

- Essentially avascular by adulthood

Function

- Allows for vertebral body motion
- Weight bearing (Figure 4–148)

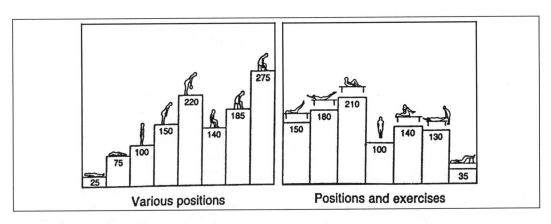

FIGURE 4–148. Disc Pressure Changes. Relative change in pressure (or load) in the 3rd lumbar disc in various positions in living subjects. Note: Neutral erect posture is considered 100% in the figures; other postures and activities are calculated in relationship to this. From Nachemson AL. The lumbar spine: an orthopaedic challenge. Spine 1976; 1:59.

Aging Effects

Decreases	Increases
• Nuclear water content	• Fibrous tissue
• Ratio of chondroitin-keratin	• Cartilage cells
• Proteoglycan molecular weight	• Amorphous tissue

INNERVATIONS (FIGURE 4–149)

Nerve	Contributions
Ventral Primary Rami	Trunk musculature, plexus contributions
Dorsal Primary Rami	Lateral: Iliocostalis, skin Intermediate: Longissimus Medial: Multifidus, rotators, interspinalis, intertransversei, posterior spinal ligaments, zygapophyseal joints
Sinuvertebral Nerve	Posterior longitudinal ligament, posterior disc, anterior dura vertebral body and anterior-lateral disc (with the grey rami communicantes)

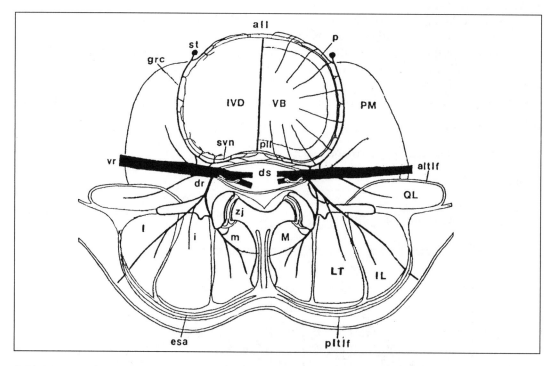

FIGURE 4–149. The Lumbar Spine Innervations. Cross-sectional view, which incorporates the level of the vertebral body (VB), and the periosteum (P) on the right and the intervertebral disc (IVD) on the left. The following abbreviations are used in the above diagram:

(PM) psoas muscle, (QL) quadratus lumborum, (IL) iliocostal lumborum, (LT) longissimus thoracic, (M) multifidus, (altlf) anterior layer of thoracolumbar fascia, (pltlf) posterior layer of thoracolumbar fascia, (esa) erector spinal aponeurosis, (ds) dural sac, (zj) zygapophyseal joint, (pll) posterior longitudinal ligament, (all) anterior longitudinal ligaments, (vr) ventral ramus, (dr) dorsal ramus, (m) medial branch, (i) intermediate branch, (l) lateral branch, (svn) sinuvertebral nerve, (grc) grey ramus communicans, (st) sympathetic trunk.

LIGAMENTS (Figure 4–150)

- **Anterior longitudinal ligament (ALL)**
  - Course: Runs the entire length of the spine, covering the anterior aspect of each vertebral body and disc
  - Function: Limits hyperextension and forward movement
- **Posterior longitudinal ligament (PLL)**
  - Course: Attaches to the posterior rim of the vertebral bodies and disc from C2 to sacrum. It continues superiorly with the tectorial membrane to the occiput
  - Function: Prevents hyperflexion of the vertebral column
- **Ligamentum nuchae (LN)**
  - Course: Continuation of the supraspinous ligament extending from the occipital protuberance to C7
  - Function: Boundary of the deep muscle in the cervical region
- **Ligamentum flavum (LF)**
  - Course: Connects adjacent vertebral arches longitudinally, attaching laminae to laminae
  - Function: Maintains constant disc tension and assists in straightening the column after flexion
- **Interspinous ligament and supraspinous ligament (ISL, SSL)**
  - 📖 Course: Runs from spinous process to spinous process
  - Function: Weakly resists both spinal separation and flexion. The supraspinous ligament runs from C7 to L3
- **Intertransverse ligament (IL)**
  - Course: Connects transverse process to transverse process
  - Function: Resists lateral bending of the trunk

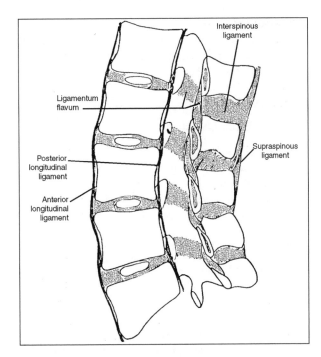

FIGURE 4–150. The Lumbar Spine Ligaments. A median sagittal section of the lumbar spine.

LANDMARKS

Cervical Region

- Anterior
  - C2: Transverse process palpated at the angle of the mandible
  - C3: Hyoid bone
  - C4, C5: Thyroid cartilage
  - C6: First cricoid ring, carotid tubercle
- Posterior
  - C2 First palpable midline spinous process, two finger breadths below the occiput
  - C7: Vertebral prominens (largest spinous process, nonbifid)
  - Articular pillars: lateral off the spinous process bilaterally

Thoracic Region
- T3: Spine of the scapula
- T8: Inferior angle of the scapula
- T12: Lowest rib

Lumbar Region
- L4: Iliac crests
- S2: Posterior superior iliac spine (PSIS)

BACK MUSCULATURE (Figure 4–151)

Extrinsic Back Muscles

- Superficial layer
  - Trapezius
  - Latissimus dorsi
- Intermediate layer
  - Serratus posterior: Superior, inferior

Intrinsic Back Muscles

- Superficial layer
  - Splenius: Capitis, cervices
- Intermediate layer
  - Erector spinae
    - Iliocostalis: Lumborum, thoracis, cervices
    - Longissimus: Thoracis, cervicis, capitis
    - Spinalis: Thoracis, cervicis, capitis
- Deep layer
  - Transversospinal muscles
    - Semispinalis: Thoracis, cervicis, capitis
    - Multifidus
    - Rotators
  - Interspinalis, intertransversarii

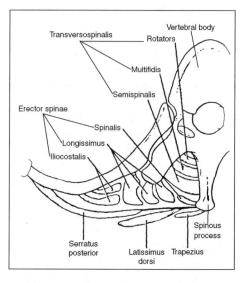

FIGURE 4–151. The Back Muscles: transverse section, thoracic region.

PERTINENT BIOMECHANICS

	Spine Flexion
Erect posture	Mild activity in the erector spinae muscles
Initial flexion phase	Increased activity in the erector spinae muscles
Mid flexion phase	Increased activity in the gluteus maximus
Late flexion phase	Increased activity in the hamstrings
Terminal flexion phase	Electrical silence

	Cervical Joint Range of Motion
Occipitoatlantal joint	📖 50% of flexion and extension of the entire cervical spine
Atlantoaxial joint	📖 50% rotation of the entire cervical spine
C3–C7 joints	The remaining motion is distributed over the typical cervical segments

PATHOPHYSIOLOGY

THE DEGENERATIVE CASCADE (FIGURE 4–152)

General

- Kirkaldy-Willis presented a functional degenerative classification of the three-joint complex. It is initiated by a rotational strain or compressive force to the spine during lumbar flexion. This cascade consists of three phases: 1) dysfunction, 2) instability, and 3) stabilization, but initial symptoms may present at any phase. Pathology of one component (disc or Z-joint) influences deterioration of the other components (Z-joint or disc) and adjacent vertebral body. This overall degeneration of the spine may be referred to as *Spondylosis*.

Phase

Dysfunction	This initial stage is a typically a result of repetitive trauma. However, the pathologic changes that occur can be reversible. The Z-joints undergo minor capsular tears, cartilage degeneration and synovitis, causing abnormal motion. The disc may have annular tears and/or endplate separation. The segmental spinal muscles become hypertonic, splinting the spine, resulting in hypomobility.
Instability	Due to scar formation, each successive injury causes incomplete healing of the Z-joint capsules and annular fibers. With increased dysfunction, the joints have further degeneration of cartilage, attenuation, stretching, and laxity of the capsule. The disc has a coalescence of its tears, loss of nuclear substance, and bulging of the annulus. Overall, this results in hypermobility of the segments.
Stabilization	Progression leads to Z-joint articular cartilage destruction, internal fibrosis, hypertrophy, erosion, locking, and periarticular fibrosis. The disc has further loss of nuclear material, vertebral body approximation, endplate destruction, fibrosis, and osteophyte formation. Ankylosis can occur at the motion segment as well entrapping spinal nerves. The patient may have an overall feeling of spinal stiffness.

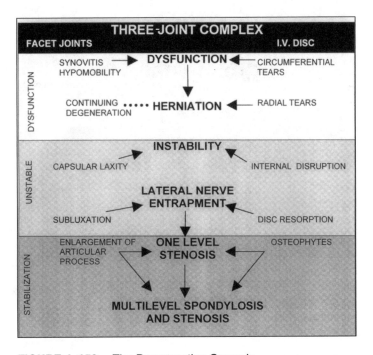

FIGURE 4–152. The Degenerative Cascade.

■

DISC DISORDERS

HERNIATED NUCLEUS PULPOSUS (HNP)

General

- A disc injury in which the nuclear pulposus migrates through the annular fibers. It may also initiate the release of enzyme phospholipase A2, which activates inflammatory mediators, such as leukotrienes, prostaglandins, platelet activating factors, bradykinins, and cytokines. ▢ This most commonly happens at 30 to 40 years of age. A higher prevalence occurs for the lumbar region at the L4–L5 or L5–S1 followed by the C5–C6 disc. Fortunately, approximately three-fourths of these injuries will resolve with conservative care in six months to one year.

Classification (Figure 4–153)

A. Bulging disc	No annulus defect. Disc convexity is beyond vertebral margins
B. Prolapsed disc	Nuclear material protrudes into an annulus defect
C. Extruded disc	Nuclear material extends to the posterior longitudinal ligament
D. Sequestered disc	Nuclear fragment free in the canal

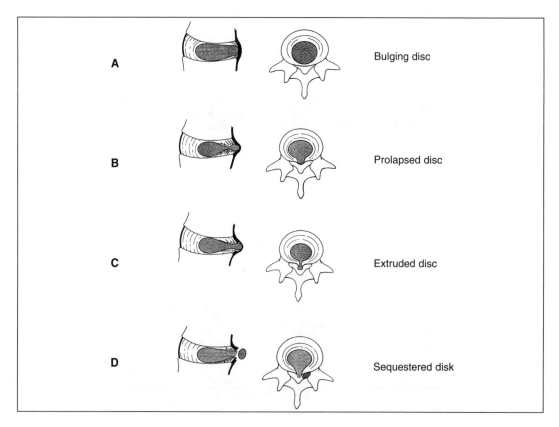

FIGURE 4–153. Disc Classifications. **A.** Bulging Disc. **B.** Prolapsed Disc. **C.** Extruded Disc. **D.** Sequestered disc.

Location (Figure 4–154)

Central	May or may not have radicular symptoms. Possible multiroot involvement if affecting the cauda equina, or myelopathy if involving the spinal cord.
📖 Posterolateral	More common in the lumbar spine due to tapering presentation of the posterior longitudinal ligament, e.g., the L4, L5 HNP injures the L5 nerve root.
Far-lateral/foraminal	May or may not have low back pain. Possibly affects the exiting root of that level, e.g., an L4, L5 HNP injures the L4 nerve root.

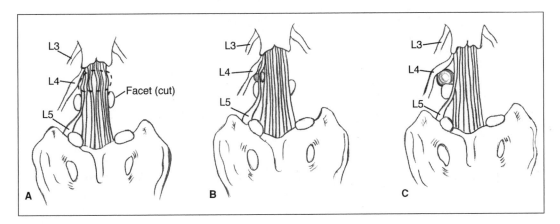

FIGURE 4–154. Herniation Location. **A.** Central. **B.** Posterolateral. **C.** Far Lateral.

Etiology

- Spontaneous
- Lifting activities
- Coughing/sneezing
- Bending/twisting activities

Clinical Presentation

- Acute neck or back discomfort radiating down the upper or lower limbs
- Weakness, numbness, paresthesias or pain secondary to chemical or mechanical stimuli to the disc or nerve root. A lateral lumbar list or shift may be noted
- Exacerbation occurs with lumbar motion (forward flexion: central and posterior-lateral HNP; extension: lateral HNP), sitting, sneezing, coughing, or Valsalva maneuvers, as well as neural tension tests
- Symptoms are dependent on herniation location

Distribution (Figure 4–155)

Root	Muscle Weakness	Reflex Abnormalities	Sensory Deficits
C5	Biceps brachii	Biceps brachii	Lateral arm
C6	Extensor carpi radialis	Brachioradialis	Lateral forearm
C7	Triceps brachii	Triceps brachii	Middle finger
C8	Flexor digitorum profundus	None	Medial forearm
T1	Interossei	None	Medial arm

Root	Muscle Weakness	Reflex Abnormalities	Sensory Deficits
T2, T4	None	None	• Bandlike presentation based on segmental innervation
T5–T10	Upper rectus abdominus		• Abdominal or chest pain. T2—apex of axilla T4—nipple line T6—xiphisternum
T10–L1	Lower rectus abdominus		T10—umbilicus T12—inguinal ligament

Root	Muscle Weakness	Reflex Abnormalities	Sensory Deficits
L2	Iliopsoas	Cremaster	Anterior thigh
L3	Quadriceps	Patellar	Anterior and lateral thigh
L4	Tibialis anterior	Patellar	Medial malleolus
L5	Extensor hallucis longus	? Medial hamstring	Dorsum of the foot
S1	Gastrocnemius-soleus	Achillis	Lateral foot and little toe

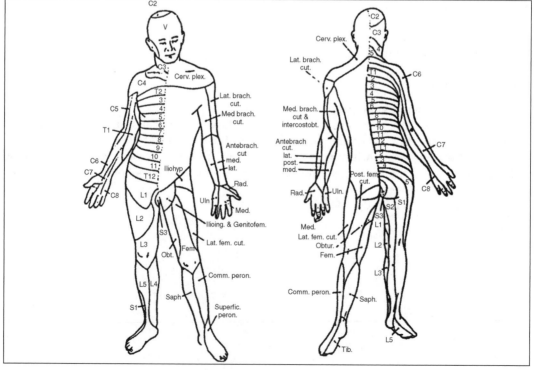

FIGURE 4–155. Dermatome and Peripheral Nerve Distribution. Reprinted with permission from Gilroy J, Holliday PT. Basic Neurology. New York: Macmillan, 1982.

Provocative tests

CERIVICAL SPINE

📖 *Spurling's Test (Figure 4–156)*
Reproduction of radicular symptoms with cervical spine extension, rotation, and lateral flexion of the seated patient

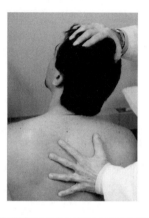

FIGURE 4–156.
Spurling's Test.
Photo courtesy of JFK Johnson Rehabilitation Institute. George Higgins, 2000.

📖 *Compression test (Figure 4–157)*
Reproduction of radicular symptoms with a downward compression on top of the head

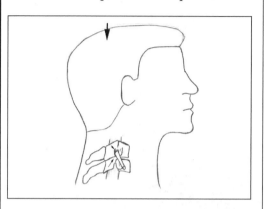

FIGURE 4–157. Cervical Compression Test.

LUMBAR SPINE

Straight Leg Raising Test, Lasegue's Test (Figure 4–158)
Reproduction of radicular symptoms with passive hip flexion of the supine patient, which creates sciatic nerve tension at 30–60° (A). This may be increased with dorsiflexion of the ankle, Lasegue's Sign (B). (A crossed Straight Leg Raise Test reproduces pain on the involved side with flexion of the opposite hip.)

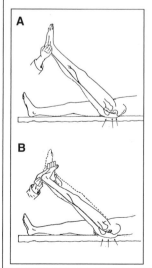

FIGURE 4–158.
Straight Leg Raising Test.
A. Sciatic Nerve Tension at 30-60° of Hip Flexion.
B. Dorsiflexion of Ankle May Produce Lasegue's Sign.

Bowstring Test (Figure 4–159)
After a positive SLR is elicited, decrease the angle of hip elevation to decrease the radicular pain. Then add pressure to the popliteal fossa over the nerve to reproduce symptoms.

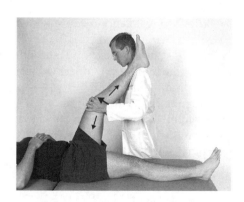

FIGURE 4–159. Bowstring Test.

LUMBAR SPINE (continued)	
Femoral Stretch Test/Reverse SLR Test (Figure 4–160) Reproduction of anterior thigh pain in the prone patient with knee flexion and hip extension. This will stretch the femoral nerve and L2–L4 roots. 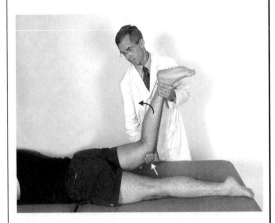 **FIGURE 4–160.** Femoral Stretch Test.	**Sitting Root Test (Figure 4–161)** Reproduction of radicular symptoms with a seated patient in a slumped posture, with cervical spine flexion and knee extension. 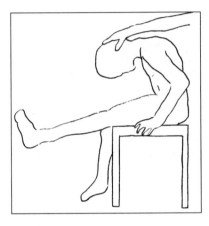 **FIGURE 4–161.** Slump Test. Illustration by Heather Platt, 2000.

Diagnostic Studies

- Imaging: X rays, CT/myelogram, MRI
- Decreased disc height, vertebral osteophytosis, and sclerosis are seen on radiographs
- Disc desiccations, annular tears, and HNPs are best demonstrated on MRI

Treatment

- **Conservative care**
  - Relative rest
    - Strict bed rest is not recommended.
  - Medications
    - NSAIDs, analgesics, oral steroids, adjuvants (tricyclic antidepressants, serotonin reuptake inhibitors), muscle relaxants, etc.
  - Rehabilitation program
    - Patient education
    - Stretching program with a focus on hamstring flexibility
    - Strengthening program with a focus on abdominal exercises
    - Spinal stabilization
      - Mackenzie program to centralize extremity pain. Extension-biased programs may be used for posterior-lateral HNP. Neutral or flexion-biased program may be used for far lateral HNP.
    - Modalities
      - Thermal therapies (heat, cold), electric stimulation, etc.
      - Traction

    ▲ Vertebral distraction may relieve nerve compression
- ▶ 📖 Cervical region: 20–30° of flexion with 25 pounds of resistance. Less flexion is required for treatment of muscle spasm
- ▶ 📖 Lumbar region: May require increased force or a split table to overcome friction

    ▲ Indications
- ▶ Radicular pain (most widely accepted)
- ▶ Paraspinal muscle spasm

    ▲ Contraindications
- ▶ Ligamentous instability
- ▶ Radiculopathy of uncertain etiology
- ▶ Acute injury
- ▶ Rheumatoid arthritis
- ▶ Vertebrobasilar arteriosclerotic disease
- ▶ Spinal infections (Pott's disease)

- **Bracing**
  - ▪ Lumbar corsets. (Note: Address abdominal/trunk musculature weakness from disuse atrophy.)
- **Home exercise program**
- **Other**
  - ▪ Epidural steroid injections. Recommendation: Fluoroscopically guided, contrast-enhanced procedures
    - ◆ Mechanism: To decrease inflammation causing nerve-root irritation
    - ◆ Complications/side effects: Needle placement—bleeding, infection, tissue damage. Anesthetic—confusion, anaphylaxis, convulsions, seizures, or death with intravascular placement. Corticosteroid—immunosuppression, fluid and electrolyte imbalance, adrenal suppression, symptom flare. Exacerbation of underlying medical conditions: Diabetes, congestive heart failure or hypertension
  - ▪ 📖 Chymopapain injections
    - ◆ Mechanism: Dissolve subligamentous herniations contained by the posterior longitudinal ligament
    - ◆ Complication/side effects: Anaphylactic reaction, chronic pain, poor efficacy
  - ▪ Psychologic interventions, muscle relaxation techniques, acupuncture
- • **Surgical care**
  - May demonstrate quicker initial resolution of radicular pain but has not been shown to have any greater statistical advantage over conservative measures with time
  - Considered for progressive weakness, unremitting pain, cauda equina syndrome or myelopathy

CAUDA EQUINA SYNDROME (Figure 4–162) (See Spinal Cord Injury Chapter)

General

- • Injury to the nerve roots forming the cauda equina. Usually a result of a large central disc herniation. Other causes may include epidural tumors, hematomas, abscesses, and trauma

Clinical Presentation

- • Lumbar, buttock, perianal discomfort, and lower limb weakness
- • Bowel and bladder abnormalities (retention, frequency, incontinence); sexual dysfunction
- • Saddle anesthesia including the back of the legs, buttocks, and soles of the feet

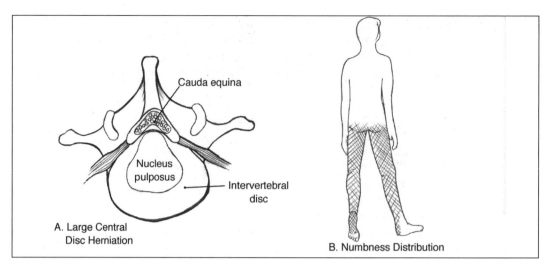

FIGURE 4–162. Cauda Equina Syndrome.

MYELOPATHY

General

- 📖 Injury to the spinal cord. Patients can have a history of radiculopathy, disc herniation, or spondylosis. Tumors, arterio-venous malformations, multiple sclerosis, syphilis, syringomyelia, amyotrophic lateral sclerosis, or rheumatoid arthritis may also be considered.

Clinical Presentation

- Spastic or ataxic gait abnormalities, weakness, sensory changes, bowel or bladder dysfunction, bilateral radiculopathy
- Upper motor neuron signs including: Hyperreflexia, clonus, spasticity, Lhermitte's phenomenon, up-going plantar response, Hoffmann's sign

UPPER MOTOR NEURON SIGNS	
Plantar Responses (Figure 4–163)	**Hoffmann's Sign (Figure 4–164)**
Rub the sole of the foot from a lateral to medial direction up the arch and monitor for an up-going great toe	Flick the patient's middle finger and monitor for twitching of the thumb

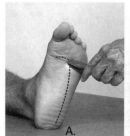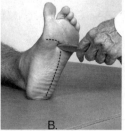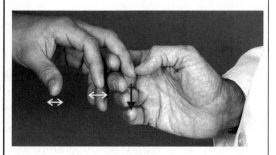

FIGURE 4–163. Babinski Test—Plantar Responses. A. Negative B. Positive

FIGURE 4–164. Hoffmann's Sign.

INTERNAL DISC DISRUPTION

General

- This is the degradation of the internal architecture of the disc without a gross herniation. It is associated with annular fissures and nuclear tissue disorganization. The degradation of nuclear material can lead to radial fissures and erosion of the annulus, causing chemical and mechanical stimulation of nociceptive fibers

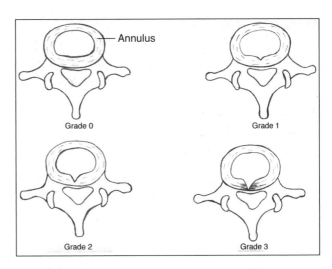

FIGURE 4–165. Internal Disc Disruption. Grades of radial fissures in internal disc disruption. (See text for description of grades.)

	Grading (Figure 4–165)
0	No annular disruption
1	Inner 1/3 annular disruption
2	Inner 2/3 annular disruption
3	Outer 1/3 annular disruption ± circumferential spreading

Etiology (Figure 4–166)

- Endplate fractures from excessive loads

Clinical Presentation

- Constant deep aching axial discomfort, increased with mechanical stresses, i.e., sitting
- May have absent neurologic involvement

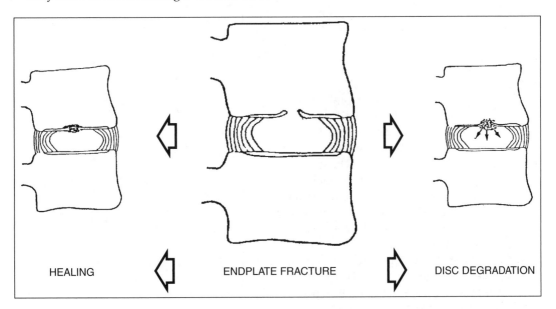

HEALING ENDPLATE FRACTURE DISC DEGRADATION

FIGURE 4–166. Possible Outcome of Endplate Fractures: Compression of the intervertebral disc results in fracture of a vertebral end-plate. The fracture may heal or trigger intervertebral disc degradation.

Diagnostic Studies

- Imaging: CT/discogram, MRI
- Radial fissures are best demonstrated on postdiscogram CT
- A high-intensity zone (HIZ) in the annulus may be seen on T2 weighted MRI images.

Treatment

- Conservative care
  - Relative rest, medications; rehabilitation program; epidural steroid injections. Intradiscal corticosteroids have demonstrated limited success in discs with HIZs. Intradiscal electrothermography annuloplasty or radio-frequency treatments may also prove beneficial
- Surgical care
  - Spinal procedures including stabilization may be considered for patients with unremitting pain

■

BONE DISORDERS OF THE SPINE

SPINAL STENOSIS

General

- Degenerative changes occur to the spine resulting in disc space narrowing, vertebral body osteophytosis, and joint arthropathy. This narrows the central canal, lateral recess, or neuroforamina, which produces stenosis. Neural compression or ischemia is possible, causing associated limb pain syndromes that usually present at ~50 years of age. Involvement of the lumbar region is most common, affecting the L3 and L4 levels

Classification

- **Central stenosis** (Figure 4–167)
  - Decreased size of the vertebral canal secondary to hypertrophic facets, hypertrophic ligamentum flavum, disc encroachment, or degenerative spondylolistheses
  - Cervical spine AP diameters: The spinal cord is approximately 10 mm; the spinal canal—17 mm. Neurologic sequelae may begin with a central canal less than 12 mm (relative stenosis) to 10 mm (absolute stenosis)
- **Lateral stenosis** (Figure 4–168)
  - Lumbar spine: Lateral stenosis has been further subdivided into three areas of entrapment, across the motion segment
    - A) Lateral Recess
    - B) Mid Zone
    - C) Intervertebral Foramen

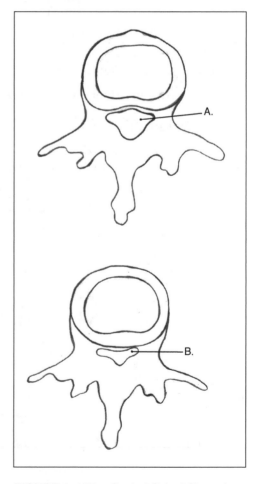

FIGURE 4–167. Central Spinal Stenosis **A.** Normal. **B.** Canal Stenosis

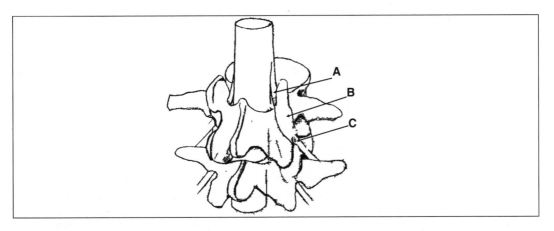

FIGURE 4–168. Lateral Stenosis. **A.** Lateral Recess. **B.** Mid Zone. **C.** Intervertebral Foramen.

Zones	Entrance Zone (Lateral recess)	Midzone (Pars region)	Exit Zone (Intervertebral foramen)
Borders	Posterior: Superior articular process Anterior: Posterior vertebral body and disc Medial and lateral walls: Open	Posterior: Pars interarticularis Anterior: Posterior vertebral body Medial wall: Open	Posterior: Z-joint (inferior level) Anterior: Posterior disc (inferior level)
Contents	Lumbar nerve root	Dorsal root ganglia Ventral motor root	Spinal nerve
Etiology	Hypertrophic facet joints (SAP)	Osteophytes under the pars	Hypertrophic facet joints (SAP)
Root Level	Same as the vertebrae (L3 SAP involve L3 roots)	Same as the vertebrae (L3 pars involve L3 roots)	One level up from the vertebrae (L4 SAP or L3–L4 disc involve L3 roots)

SAP = Superior Articulate Process

Etiology

- Congenital
  - Hereditary
  - Achondroplastic
- Acquired
  - Degenerative (most common)
  - Spondylotic/spondylolisthetic
  - Iatrogenic (postlaminectomy/fusion)
  - Posttraumatic
  - Metabolic (Paget's disease)

Clinical Presentation

- Gradual neck or back discomfort with upper or lower limb involvement
- Neurogenic claudication (pseudoclaudication): Pain in the buttock, thigh, or leg with standing or walking relieved with sitting or leaning forward. This may be due to neural ischemia or venous congestion
- Myelopathic changes may be noted with higher spinal involvement

Claudication		
Types	**Neurogenic (pseudoclaudication)**	**Vascular**
Discomfort	Numbness, aches, pain	Cramping, tightness
Location	Thigh and calf	Calf
Exacerbation	Standing, walking, lying flat	Walking, cycling
Bicycle test	Painless	Painful
Downhill walking	Painful	Painless
Uphill walking	Painless	Painful
Remission	Flexed position, bending, sitting	Standing, resting, lying flat
Associated factors	Back pain, decreased spine motion, atrophy, weakness, normal pulses	Rare back pain, normal spine motion, Rare atrophy or weakness; abnormal pulses; loss of hair; shiny skin

Diagnostic Studies

- Imaging: X-rays, CT, myelogram, MRI
  - Findings include multilevel vertebral body osteophytosis, ligamentum flavum hypertrophy, and Z-joint arthropathy compromising the vertebral canal or foramen

Treatment

- Conservative care
  - Relative rest; medications. Rehabilitation program: Focus on a flexion based or neutral positioned program and spinal stabilization; epidural steroid injections; aquatic therapy
- Surgical care
  - Spinal procedures including decompression and/or stabilization.

SPONDYLOLYSIS (Figure 4–169)

General

- A vertebral defect most commonly seen in children and adolescents at the L5 vertebral level. It occurs at the pars interarticularis, which is formed at the junction of the pedicle, transverse process, lamina and the two articular processes. This can lead to a spondylolisthesis

Etiology

- Hyperextension forces (Sports: gymnastics, football)

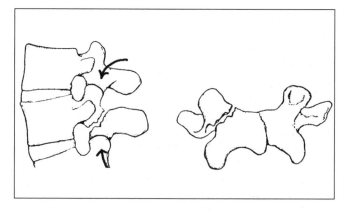

FIGURE 4–169. Lumbar Spondylolysis.

Clinical Presentation

- Localized back pain exacerbated by motion (hyperextension), standing, lying prone, and relieved with flexion
- Neurologic exam should be normal

Diagnostic Studies

- Imaging: 📖 X rays, bone scan with single Photon Emission Computed tomography (SPECT), CT, MRI
  - Oblique X rays demonstrate a pars defect represented by a collar on the "Scotty dog" (Figure 4–170)
  - Bone scans may be hot (positive) at 5 to 7 days and last up to 18 months, aiding in distinguishing between acute and chronic fractures
- SPECT increase bone scanning sensitivity

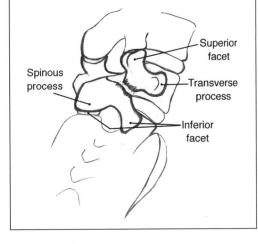

FIGURE 4–170. Spondylolysis ("Scotty Dog with Collar" Defect in the Pars Interarticularis)

Treatment

- See the treatment for spondylolisthesis

SPONDYLOLISTHESIS (Figure 4–171)

General

- A forward (anterolisthesis) or backward (retrolisthesis) slippage of one vertebral body on another. It can present at any vertebral level but is most commonly seen in the lumbar region. Occurrence is 2 to 4 times greater in males.

CLASSIFICATION

- Lumbar slippage: Measured according to the percentage of displacement of the adjacent vertebrae (Figure 4–172)

MEYERDING GRADING OF SLIPPAGE

Grade 0	0% slippage
Grade 1	1–25% slippage
Grade 2	26–50% slippage
Grade 3	51–75% slippage
Grade 4	76–100% slippage
Spondyloptosis	> 100% slippage

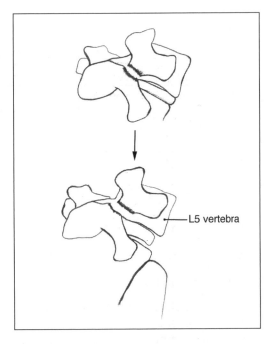

FIGURE 4–171. Spondylolisthesis ("Scotty Dog Decapitated"). In this instance the apparent collar on the scotty dog widens because the vertebra has slipped.

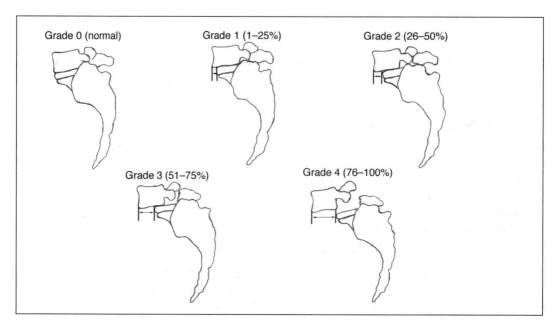

FIGURE 4–172. Meyerding Grading of Slippage—See text for grading description (previous page).

Etiology

Class	Type	Age	Criteria
I	Dysplastic (congenital)	Child	Congenital abnormality of the lumbosacral Z-joint
📖 II	Isthmic (most common)	5–50	Pars interarticularis fracture (subtype A), which is most common at L5–S1 or an elongation (subtype B)
III	Degenerative	Elderly	Facet arthrosis causing subluxation. Common location: L4–5
IV	Traumatic	Young	Acute fracture in surrounding location other than the pars
V	Pathological	Any	Generalized disease: Cancer, infection, metabolic disorder
VI	Postsurgical	Adult	Excessive resection of neural arches or facets causing an unstable structure

Clinical Presentation

- Low back pain exacerbated with motion; hamstring tightness; palpable step-off noted at the slippage site
- Radicular symptoms may occur with marked slippage

Diagnostic Studies

- Imaging: X rays, bone scan with SPECT, CT, MRI
- Flexion and extension views may demonstrate signs of segmental instability

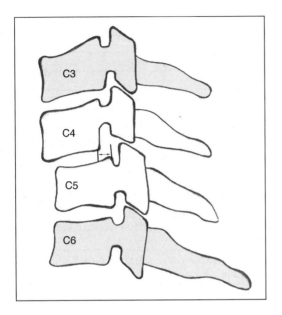

FIGURE 4–173. Increased Cervical Translation—Sagittal Plane.

Cervical instability is translation >3.5 mm

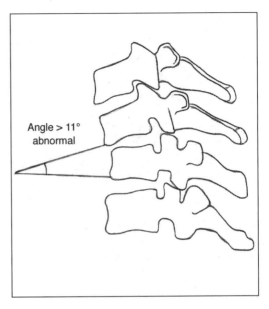

FIGURE 4–174. Increased Cervical Rotation—Sagittal Plane.

Instability is translation >3.5mm

- Instability: Translation > 3.5 mm (cervical) or > 5 mm (thoracic or lumbar). Rotational motion of two adjacent vertebrae > 11° (cervical) and 15° (lumbar) (Fig. 4–173 and 4–174)

Treatment
- **Conservative care**
  - Grade 1, Grade 2, and asymptomatic Grade 3
    - Relative rest, eliminate aggravating activities. Rehabilitation program: Focus on spinal stabilization exercises in a flexion biased position and hamstring flexibility. Asymptomatic Grade 1 slips may return to any activity but asymptomatic Grade 2 and 3 slips are restricted from contact sports. Slip progression is uncommon and treatment will depend on risk factors and degree of angulation
    - TLSO bracing is used if increased pain occurs despite decreased activity or an increase slippage is suspected
- **Surgical care**
  - Symptomatic Grade 3 and Grades 4 and 5
  - Spinal procedures including a bilateral posterolateral fusion with or without decompression

SCOLIOSIS (See also Pediatric Chapter)

General

- A general spinal deformity characterized by lateral curvatures and vertebral rotation. It may be associated with a fixed structural curve or reducible functional curve. Correlation with discomfort is unclear but low back pain is usually the initial symptom. It is related to curve severity and usually begins at the convexity

Etiology

Structural Scoliosis			
Idiopathic	Most common		
	Subtypes		
	Infantile	Birth to 3 years: Associated with congenital defects	
	Juvenile	4 years to 10 years: High risk of curve progression	
	Adolescent	Most common; 10 years to maturity; high risk of progression	
Congenital	May be due to an early embryologic developmental defect		
	Subtypes		
	Open	Caused by myelomeningocele	
	Closed	May be associated with neurologic deficits Associated with a wedged vertebra, hemivertebra, congenital bar, or block vertebrae	
Neuromuscular	Certain neuromuscular disorders may have a rapid curve progression with associated pulmonary and spinal cord complications		

Clinical Presentation

Patterns	Characteristics
📖 **Right thoracic curve**	Most common; the apex can typically be seen at T7 or T8
Double major curve	Right thoracic with a left lumbar curve; little cosmetic deformity
Lumbar curve	Left lumbar curves are greater than right lumbar curves.
Thoracolumbar curve	Less cosmetic deformity than thoracic curve, may have rib and flank distortion
Left thoracic curve	Rare; may be associated with spinal cord abnormalities

Diagnostic Studies

- Imaging: X rays help establish diagnosis and prognosis
  - Follow-up X rays will depend on skeletal maturity, patient age, and degree of curvature
  - Younger patients with rapidly progressing curves will warrant earlier X ray follow-up
- Rotation (Figure 4–175)
  - Pedicle portion estimates the amount of vertebral rotation on the PA view
  - Grading: 0 (no rotation) to 4 (complete pedicle rotation out of view)
- Curve: Cobb Angle (Figure 4–176)
  - An angle formed by the perpendicular lines drawn from the endplates of the most tilted proximal and distal vertebrae to measure the scoliotic curve

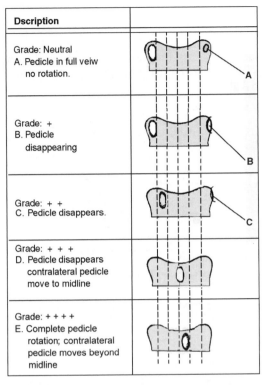

Dscription	
Grade: Neutral A. Pedicle in full veiw no rotation.	A
Grade: + B. Pedicle disappearing	B
Grade: + + C. Pedicle disappears.	C
Grade: + + + D. Pedicle disappears contralateral pedicle move to midline	
Grade: + + + + E. Complete pedicle rotation; contralateral pedicle moves beyond midline	

FIGURE 4–176. Cobb Angle.

FIGURE 4–175. Measurement of vertebral rotation using pedicle method. Vertebral body is divided into 6 segments and grades from 0 to 4+ are assigned, depending on location of the pedicle within the segments.

Treatment
- **Conservative care**
  - Rehabilitation program
  - Bracing

Treatment	Degree of Angulation
Observation	< 20°
Bracing	20–40°
Surgery	> 40° (< 35° neuromuscular disease)

- **Criteria**: Worn 23 hours a day until spinal growth is completed. Weaning off can begin when radiographs display signs of maturity and curves are stable. Patients should be evaluated at 2 to 3 year intervals for life after the brace is discontinued
- **Types:**

Milwaukee brace	High thoracic curves (apex at T8)
Low profile TLSO	Lower thoracic, thoracolumbar, and lumbar curves (apex below T8)

- **Surgical care**
  - Spinal procedures are indicated for curves with: Relentless progression, > 40° in the skeletally immature, < 35° in neuromuscular disease, > 50° in the skeletally mature or progressive loss of pulmonary function

SCHEUERMANN'S DISEASE (EPIPHYSITIS)

General

- 📖 An adolescent disorder of the vertebral endplates and apophysis resulting in an increased thoracic kyphosis. The kyphosis is generally > 45° and usually involves three sequential vertebrae

Etiology

- Failure of endochondral ossification causing:
  - Intervertebral disc herniation
  - Anterior wedging of the vertebral bodies
  - Fixed thoracolumbar kyphosis

Clinical Presentation

- More common in adolescent males
- Can present with a progressive nonpainful thoracic kyphosis
- The thoracic kyphosis remains fixed and does not correct with hyperextension
- Back pain may occur in young athletes due to localized stress injury to the vertebral growth plates

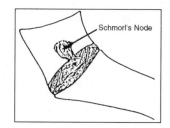

FIGURE 4–177. Schmorl's Node.

Diagnostic Studies

- Imaging: X rays, CT, MRI
  - Irregular endplates, spondylosis, scoliosis, 📖 Schmorl's nodes (herniation of disc material through the vertebral endplate into the spongiosa of the vertebral body), and vertebral wedging (~ 5°) (Figure 4–177)

Treatment
- Conservative Care
  - Rehabilitation program: Focus on thoracic extension and abdominal strengthening exercises.
  - Bracing may be used for kyphosis ≤ 74° for a length of time dependent on skeletal maturity
- Surgical Care
  - Correction may be indicated if kyphosis is > 75° or > 65° in the skeletally mature

COMPRESSION FRACTURE (FIGURE 4–179)

General

- Typically associated with osteoporosis, these fractures are more commonly seen in the thoracolumbar junction. This is due to the transition between the fixed rigid thoracic and the highly mobile lumbar vertebra. Denis described a three-column model for evaluating thoracolumbar fractures and determining their stability (Figure 4–178). (See Spinal Cord Injury chapter.)

Column	Components	Stability
Anterior	• Anterior longitudinal ligament • Anterior two-thirds of the vertebral body and annulus fibrosis	Stable
Middle	• Posterior longitudinal ligament • Posterior one-third of the vertebral body and annulus fibrosis	Unstable
Posterior	• Ligamentum flavum, supraspinous and infraspinous ligament • Posterior elements: pedicles, facets, spinous process	Stable

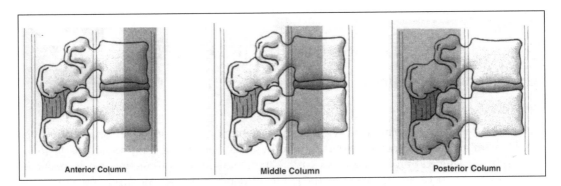

FIGURE 4–178. The Three-Column Model of Spine Stability. Reprinted with permission from Nesathurai S, ed. The Rehabilitation of People With Spinal Cord Injury: A House Officer's Guide. Boston: Arbuckle Academic Publishers, 1999.

Etiology

- Trauma
- Osteoporosis
- Osteomalacia
- Medication related: corticosteroids
- Neoplasm (see Cancer chapter)

Clinical Presentation

- Sudden onset of constant thoracolumbar pain
- Exacerbated with Valsalva maneuvers, turning in bed, coughing, or incidental trauma such as stepping off a curb

Diagnostic Studies

- Imaging: X rays, bone scan with SPECT, CT, MRI
- Vertebral body wedging on imaging studies. Bone scan with SPECT may have increased sensitivity

Treatment

- **Conservative care**
  - Indicated for fractures causing < 25% decrease of vertebral height. Short-term bed rest followed by activity restriction. Medications for pain control. Rehabilitation program: Focus on hyperextension exercises
  - Bracing

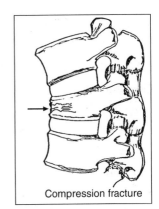

Compression fracture

FIGURE 4–179. Thoracic Compression Fracture.

Elastic binder	• Acts as a reminder to limit motion • Increases intraabdominal pressure
Custom molded TLSO/ Jewett brace	• Greater immobilization • Places patient in slight hyperflexion • Jewett should be used with caution in the osteoporotic patient

- **Surgical care**
  - Spinal procedures are indicated for fracture causing > 50% decrease of vertebral height, instability, and late kyphotic deformity leading to neurologic compromise

JOINT DISORDERS OF THE SPINE

FACET SYNDROME (FIGURE 4–180)

General Facet Joints

- The facet joints (Z-joints) are true synovial joints containing a capsule, meniscus, and a synovial membrane. These joints also sustain progressively increasing compressive loads down the spine, reaching approximately 12% to 25% in the lumbar region. As the disc decreases in height, greater loads are imparted on the joints influencing the degenerative cascade.

Etiology

- Somatic dysfunction/facilitated segment
- Positional overload
- Capsular tears/injury
- Meniscoidal/synovial impingement
- Spondylosis

Clinical Presentation

- Neck or back pain exacerbated with rotation and extension
- Referred pain pattern can be seen in a nondermatomal presentation
- No neurologic abnormalities

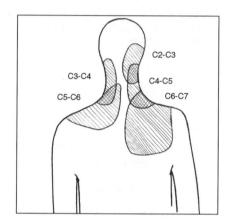

FIGURE 4–180. Cervical Z-Joint Referral Pain Patterns. (Posterior View)

Diagnostic Studies

- Imaging: Xray, CT, MRI
  - Degenerative changes may be noted but are not diagnostic
  - MRI may show hypertrophy of the capsule and facets
  - Fluoroscopic Z-joint injections or medial branch blocks may have a higher diagnostic value

Treatment

- **Conservative care**
  - Relative rest. Medications. Rehabilitation program: Focus on lumbar spine stabilization with flexion and neutral postures, proper body mechanics. Manual medicine. Interventional procedures may include facet joint injections or dorsal rami medial branch radiofrequency ablation.

SACROILIAC JOINT DYSFUNCTION/SACROILIITIS

General

- 📖 The L-shaped articulation between the sacrum and the ilium has a synovial joint anterior and syndesmosis posterior. It is innervated by the L5 dorsal ramus and lateral S1 to S3 (S4) dorsal rami

Etiology

- Hyper/hypomobile joint patterns
- Repetitive overloads
- Trauma
- Capsular tears/injury

Clinical Presentation

- Acute or gradual back, buttock, leg, or groin pain with tenderness over the joint
- Abnormal sacroiliac joint motion patterns, increased discomfort with positional changes
- Discomfort within associated muscles, which may include the quadratus lumborum, erector spinae, and piriformis
- No neurologic abnormalities

PROVOCATIVE TESTS	
Patrick's (Faber) Test (Figure 4–181) Pain reproduction with flexion, abduction and external rotation of the hip joint. Ipsilateral pain occurs in a degenerative hip, contralateral pain occurs in the dysfunctional SI joint	***Gaenslen Test (Figure 4–182)*** SI joint pain is reproduced with dropping the involved leg off the table while the contralateral hip is held in flexion

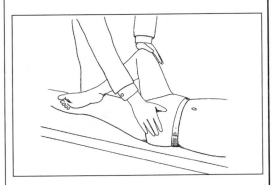

FIGURE 4–181. Patrick's (Faber) Test.

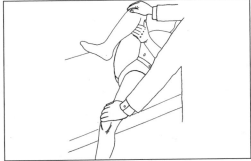

FIGURE 4–182. Gaenslen Test.

Iliac Compression Test (Figure 4–183)

SI joint pain with downward force placed on the iliac crest

Yeoman's Test (Figure 4–184)

SI joint pain with hip extension and ilium rotation

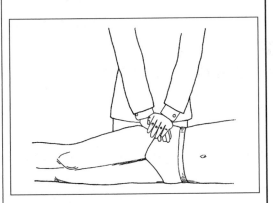

FIGURE 4–183. Iliac Compression Test.

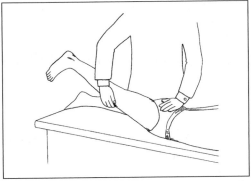

FIGURE 4–184. Yeoman's Test.

PROVOCATIVE TESTS *(Continued)*	
Gillet Test (Figure 4–185)	*Seated Flexion Test (Figure 4–186)*
Monitor posterior superior iliac spine (PSIS) motion when the patient raises the leg to 90°. The PSIS on raised leg should rotate down. Restriction of this motion is considered abnormal	Monitor the PSIS of the seated patient as they bend forward. Asymmetric cephalad motion of the PSIS indicates a sacroiliac dysfunction. Use the Standing Flexion Test to distinguish the side of the dysfunction
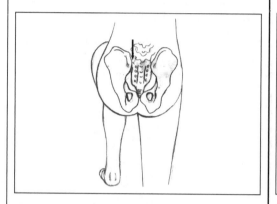	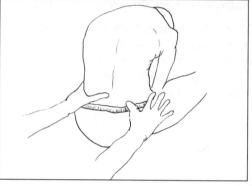
FIGURE 4–185. Gillet Test.	**FIGURE 4–186.** Seated Flexion Test. Illustration by Heather Platt, 2000.

Diagnostic Studies

- Imaging: X ray, bone scan, CT, MRI
- These studies can be considered to rule out alternative pathologies in resistant cases
- Fluoroscopic sacroiliac joint injections can have higher diagnostic value
- Serology workup can be indicated for underlying arthropathies

Treatment

- **Conservative care**
  - Relative rest. Medications. Rehabilitation program: Manual medicine, SI joint injections, SI joint belt

■

SOFT TISSUE DISORDERS OF THE SPINE

SPRAIN/STRAIN

General

- This may be an overutilized term pertaining to muscular or ligamentous disruption due to overload injuries

Etiology

- Overuse syndromes
- Excessive eccentric contraction
- Acceleration-deceleration injuries
- Acute trauma

Clinical Presentation

- Muscle aches with associated spasm and guarding in the region of injury
- Delayed onset muscle soreness can occur within 24–48 hours after an eccentric overload injury
- Facilitated segmental or somatic dysfunction may be more commonly involved then actual tissue disruption
- Normal neurologic exam

Diagnostic Studies

- None available. Strengthening of lordotic curves may be seen on lateral X rays due to muscle spasm

Treatment

- Conservative care
  - Relative rest. Medication. Rehabilitation program: Manual medicine, focus on flexibility, range of motion, strengthening, and spinal stabilization exercises

MYOFACIAL PAIN SYNDROMES

General

- Regional pain with local muscle tenderness and associated trigger points (Figure 4–187)

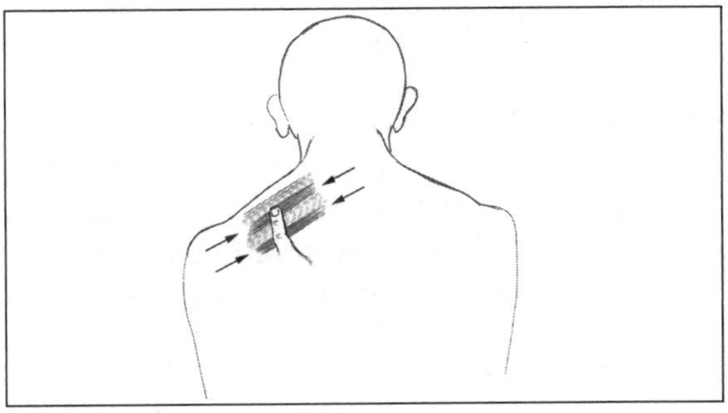

Etiology

- Postural mechanics
- Overuse injuries
- Trauma
- Stress

FIGURE 4–187. Myofascial Trigger Point: Pulling the taut band under the finger tip at the trigger point (dark stippled area) produces a "local twitch response" with shortening of the band of muscle.

Clinical Presentation

- Muscle tenderness. Trigger points: Palpable taut band with twitch response and referred pain patterns
- Other nonmuscular symptoms including paresthesias, poor sleep patterns, and fatigue may occur
- Normal neurologic exam

Diagnostic Studies

None available. Further work-up may be considered to rule out other potential alternative pathologies

Treatment

- **Conservative care**
  - Correct underlying causes. Medications (analgesics, tricyclics) for discomfort or sleep. Rehabilitation program: Focus on flexibility, strengthening and aerobic exercises. Spray and stretch or trigger point injections may be beneficial. Psychologic counseling

FIBROMYALGIA (SEE RHEUMATOLOGY CHAPTER)

■

OTHER INFECTIOUS DISORDERS OF THE SPINE

VERTEBRAL BODY OSTEOMYELITIS AND DISCITIS (Figure 4–188)

General

- 📖 An embolic infection of the vertebral body metaphysis causing ischemia, infarct, and bony destruction with disc involvement. Risk factors include advanced age, diabetes, immunodeficiency, penetrating trauma, GU procedures and invasive spinal procedures. It is most commonly seen in the lumbar spine, but increases in the cervical region with intravenous drug abuse and in the thoracolumbar junction with tuberculosis

Etiology

- Staphylococcus aureus—most common
- Pseudomonas—intravenous drug abuse
- 📖 Mycobacterium tuberculi—Pott's disease

Clinical Presentation

- Fever and back pain exacerbated with extension
- Spinal deformity evolves with collapse of vertebral body
- Neurologic involvement including radicular pain, myelopathy, or paralysis can occur due to direct dural invasion with compression from an epidural abscess

Diagnostic Studies

- Imaging: X rays, bone scan and SPECT, CT, MRI, or labs
  - By 2 weeks, radiographs demonstrate disc space narrowing and blurred endplates. CT shows hypodensity with trabecular, cortical, and endplate destruction. MRI is the most sensitive and specific with T1 hypointensity, T2 hyperintensity and gadolinium enhancement
  - Serology: Blood: Leukocytosis, increased ESR and C-reactive protein, positive Gram stain and cultures
  - Positive bone biopsy

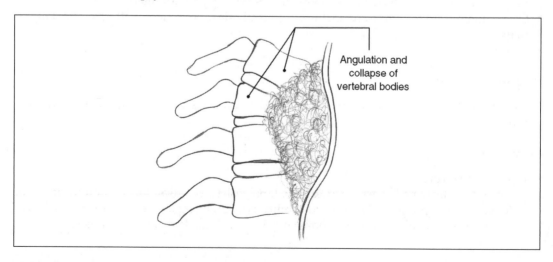

Angulation and collapse of vertebral bodies

FIGURE 4–188. Pott's Disease: Spinal Tuberculosis.

Treatment

- **Conservative care**
  - Spinal immobilization with casting or bracing. Intravenous and oral medication. Early ambulation.
  - Medications:
    - Staphylococcus aureus—Penicillin, first or second generation cephalosporins
    - Pseudomonas—Extended spectrum penicillins
    - Tuberculosis—12 months mycobacterial agents (rifampin, INH, ethambutol, pyrazinamide)
- **Surgical care**
  - Spinal procedure including decompression and/or fusion

NONORGANIC SOURCES

MALINGERING

General

- Patients may misrepresent their condition due to secondary gain issues. More than pure symptom magnification or a deceptive distortion of events, malingering is a DSM-IV disorder. It is defined as an intentional production of falsely or grossly exaggerated physical and psychological symptoms

Etiology

- Motivated by external incentives
- Avoiding work
- Avoiding military duty
- Obtaining financial compensation
- Obtaining drugs
- Evading criminal prosecution

Clinical Presentation

- Exaggerated complaints with nonanatomical basis and without an organic pathology
- Multiple screening tests exist. In particular for patients with low back pain are the Waddell signs. Demonstration of more than three of five presentations may be cause for suspicion. These can be remembered with the acronym **DO ReST**

Waddell Signs

Signs	Comments
Distraction	Presentation of severe radicular pain with the supine straight leg raising test but no pain in the seated straight leg raising test. Both should be positive
Overreaction	Inappropriate, disproportionate reactions to a request. This may manifest with exaggerated verbalizations, facial expressions, tremors, or collapsing
Regionalization	Motor or sensory abnormalities without anatomic basis such as in a stocking-glove distribution, give-way weakness or cog-wheel type of rigidity
Simulation	Leg or lumbar pain with a light axial load on the skull. Or a presentation of lumbar pain with simultaneous pelvis and shoulder rotation in unison
Tenderness	Exaggerated sensitivity or dramatic reproduction of pain with light touch of the soft tissue or with skin-rolling

Diagnostic Studies

- There are no specific studies to determine if a patient is malingering or demonstrating associated disorders. Certain psychological tests may offer insight on a patient's condition but diagnosis rests mainly on clinical suspicion

Treatment

- This rests on addressing the underlying issues involved with each patient's individual situation. It may require a multidisciplined approach incorporating diverse aspects of the medical field, as well as confronting certain social matters

MEDICAL SOURCES

Visceral disorders	GU (prostatitis, renal stones), bladder, gynecological (endometriosis, PID, ectopic pregnancy), GI (pancreatitis, cholecystitis, PUD)
Psychological disorders	Depression, anxiety, hysteria, somatization disorders
Neoplastic disorders	Primary tumors, metastatic tumors. See Cancer chapter
Vascular disorders	Aortic aneurysm (back pain associated with pulsatile abdominal mass)
Rheumatologic disorders	See Rheumatology chapter
Hematologic disorders	Sickle cell anemia, thalassemia

RECOMMENDED READING

Aprill C, Bogduk N. The prevalence of cervical zygapophyseal joint pain: A first approximation. *Spine* 1992; 17:744–747.

Bergquist-Ullman M, Larsson U. Acute low back pain in industry. A controlled prospective study with special reference to therapy and confounding factors. *Acta Orthop Scand* 1977; (170):1–117.

Bigos SJ, Spengler DM, Martin NA, Zeh J, Fisher L, Nachemson A. Back injuries in industry: A retrospective study. III. Employee-related factors. *Spine* 1986 Apr; 11(3):252–6

Boden SD, Davis DO, Dina TS, Patronas NJ, Wiesel SW. Abnormal magnetic-resonance scans of the lumbar spine in asymptomatic subjects. A prospective investigation. *J Bone Joint Surg Am* 1990 Mar; 72(3):403–8

Boden SD, McCowin PR, Davis DO, Dina TS, Mark AS, Wiesel S Abnormal magnetic-resonance scans of the cervical spine in asymptomatic subjects. A prospective investigation. *J Bone Joint Surg Am* 1990; 72(8):1178–84

Bogduk N, Twomey LT. *Clinical Anatomy of the Lumbar Spine and Sacrum*, 3rd ed. New York: Churchill Livingstone; 1997.

Bohlman HH, Emery SE. The pathophysiology of cervical spondylosis and myelopathy. *Spine* 1988; 13:843–846.

Botwin KP, Gruber RD, Bouchlas CG, Torres-Ramos FM, Freeman TL, Slaten WK. Complications of fluoroscopically guided transforaminal lumbar epidural injections. *Arch Phys Med Rehabil*. 2000 Aug; 81(8):1045–50.

Braddom RL. *Physical Medicine and Rehabilitation*. W.B. Saunders; 1992: 3–42, 728–754, 813–850.

Brinker, MR. Miller M. *Fundamentals of Orthopaedics*. Philadelphia: W.B. Saunders; 1999.

Brown, DE. Neumann, RD. *Orthopedic Secrets*, 2nd ed. Philadelphia: Hanley and Belfus; 1999.

Calliet, R. *Shoulder Pain*. 3rd ed. Phildaelphia: F.A. Davis; 1991.

Cole AJ, Herring SA, eds. *The Low Back Pain Handbook: A Practical Guide for the Primary Care Clinician*. Philadelphia: Hanley & Belfus; St. Louis: Mosby; 1997.

DeLisa JA, Gans BA. *Rehabilitation Medicine: Principles and Practice*, 2nd ed. Philadelphia: JB Lippincott; 1993.

DeLisa JA, Gans BA. *Rehabilitation Medicine: Principles and Practice*, 3rd ed. Philadelphia: Lippincott-Raven; 1999:1423–1451, 1599–1625.

Denis F. The three column spine and its significance in the classification of acute thoracolumbar spinal injuries. *Spine* 1983; 8(8):817–31.

Frymoyer JW. *The Adult Spine: Principles and Practice.* Philadelphia: Lippincott-Raven, 1997.

Gonzalez EG, Materson RS. *The Nonsurgical Management of Acute Low Back Pain.* New York: Demos Vermande; 1997.

Gordon SL, Weinstein JN. A review of basic science issues in low back pain. *Phys Med Rehabil Clin N Am* 1998; 9(2):323–42.

Greenman PE. *Principles of Manual Medicine,* 2nd ed. Philadelphia: Williams & Wilkins; 1996.

Herkowitz HN. Rothman-Simeone, *The Spine,* 4th ed. Philadelphia: W.B. Saunders; 1999.

Hoppenfeld, S. Physical *Examination of the Spine and Extremities.* New York: Appleton-Century Crofts; 1976.

Jenkins, DB. *Hollinshead's Functional Anatomy of the Limbs and Back,* 7th ed. Philadelphia: W.B. Saunders; 1998.

Kannus P, Restrom P. Treatment for acute tears of the lateral ligaments of the ankle. Operation, cast, or early controlled mobilization. *J Bone Joint Surg Am* 1991; 73(2):305–12.

Kibler WB, Herring SA, Press JA. *Functional Rehabilitation of Sports and Musculoskeletal Injuries.* Gaithersburg, Maryland: Aspen Publishers; 1998.

Kirkaldy-Willis WH, Burton CV, eds. *Managing Low Back Pain,* 3rd ed. New York: Churchill Livingstone; 1992.

Magee D. *Orthopedic Physical Assessment.* Philadelphia: W.B. Saunders; 1987.

Miller MD. *Review of Orthopaedics,* 3rd ed. Philadelphia: W.B. Saunders; 2000.

Modic MT, Masaryk TJ, Ross JS. *Magnetic Resonance Imaging of the Spine.* Chicago: Year Book Medical Publishers; 1989.

Moore KL, Dalley AF. *Clinically Oriented Anatomy,* 4th ed. Philadelphia: Williams & Wilkins; 1999.

Nachemson AL. Disc pressure measurements. *Spine* 1981; 6:93–97.

Nesathurai S, ed. *The Rehabilitation of People With Spinal Cord Injury: A House Officer's Guide.* Boston: Arbuckle Academic Publishers; 1999.

Netter, FH. *Musculoskeletal System,* Vol 8, Part 1: *Anatomy, Physiology and Metabolic Disorders.* Summit, New Jersey: Ciba-Geigy Corp; 1991.

O'Young B, Young MA, Stiens SA. *PM&R Secrets.* Philadelphia: Hanley & Belfus; 1997.

Reid, DC. *Sports Injury Assessment and Rehabilitation.* Philadelphia: Churchill Livingstone; 1992.

Rockwood CA, Green DP, Bucholz RW, Heckman JD. *Rockwood and Green's Fractures in Adults,* 4th ed. Philadelphia: Lippincott-Raven; 1996.

Saal JA, Dillingham MF. Non-operative treatment and rehabilitation of disk, facet and soft-tissue injuries. In Nicholas JA, Hershman EB. *The Lower Extremity and Spine in Sports Medicine,* 2nd ed. St. Louis: Mosby; 1995.

Saal JS, Saal JA, Yurth EF. Nonoperative management of herniated cervical intervertebral disc with radiculopathy. *Spine* 1996; 21(16):1877–83.

Saal JS, Saal JS, Herzog RJ. The natural history of lumbar intervertebral disc extrusions treated nonoperatively. *Spine* 1990; 15(7):683–6.

Sinaki, Mehrsheed, Mokri, Bahram. Low back pain and disorders of the lumbar spine. In Braddom RL. *Physical Medicine and Rehabilitation.* Philadelphia, W.B. Saunders, 1996.

Snider, RK. *Essentials of Musculoskeletal Care.* Rosemont, Il: American Academy of Orthopaedic Surgeons; 1997.

Travell JG, Simon DG. *Myofascial Pain and Dysfunction: The Trigger Point Manual.* Baltimore: Williams & Wilkins; 1992.

Waddell G, McCulloch JA, Kummel E, Venner RM. Non-organic physical signs in low back pain. *Spine* 1980; 5(2):117–25.

White AA, Punjabi MM. *Clinical Biomechanics of the Spine,* 2nd ed. Philadelphia: J.B. Lippincott; 1990.

5

ELECTRODIAGNOSTIC MEDICINE AND CLINICAL NEUROMUSCULAR PHYSIOLOGY

Ted L. Freeman, D.O., Ernest Johnson, M.D., Eric D. Freeman, D.O., and David P. Brown, D.O.

■

INTRODUCTION

Electrodiagnostic medicine incorporates a patient's history and physical examination with an electrophysiologic evaluation. Combining data found on electromyography (EMG) and nerve conduction studies (NCS), the pathophysiology of a disease process can be defined to further illustrate location, duration, severity, and prognosis. It can function as a valuable aid in patient management, serving as an extension of the clinical exam, but not a substitute.

This chapter focuses on board-related topics about neuromuscular disorders and associated electrophysiologic changes. It is to be used as a study guide. It is not intended to be an all-inclusive composite. However, for more elaborate coverage of the subject matter, the reader is directed to the recommended reading at the end of this chapter.

■

BASIC ANATOMY/PHYSIOLOGY

MOTOR UNIT (MU)

Definition

This anatomic structure is the basic functional element of the neuromuscular system (Figure 5–1).

Components

- **Alpha Motor Neuron (AMN)**
  Description: This is the cell body, or soma, of the motor nerve. It is located in the anterior horn region of the spinal cord and regulates the characteristics of the entire motor unit.

- **Axon (Spinal Nerve)**
  Description: This is the neural branch of the cell body that propagates current flow and transports cell nutrition (axonal transport). It can be unmyelinated or myelinated by the Schwann cells.

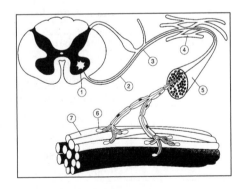

FIGURE 5–1. The Motor Unit. 1–Anterior Horn Cell. 2–Nerve Root. 3–Spinal Nerve. 4–Plexus. 5–Peripheral Nerve. 6–Neuromuscular Junction. 7–Muscle Fiber. (Reprinted with permission from Dumitru D. Electrodiagnostic Medicine. Philadelphia, Hanley & Belfus, 1995)

- **Terminal Nerve Branches (Peripheral Nerve)**
  Description: These are multiple neural extensions from the distal portion of the axon. They innervate individual muscle fibers. The amount of muscle fibers belonging to an axon is the innervation ratio (IR). This ratio varies, depending on the function of the motor unit. Muscles of gross movement have a larger amount of their fibers innervated by one axon (high ratio). Muscles of fine movement have a smaller amount of their fibers innervated by one axon (low ratio). 📖 The axons innervating leg muscles can have a ratio of 600 muscle fibers to 1 axon (600:1) while the IR of the eye muscles can be 1 muscle fiber to 1 axon (1:1). The higher the IR the greater the force generated by that motor unit.

- **Neuromuscular Junctions**
  Description: This is the site where the electric impulse propagated along the axon is converted into a chemical reaction to initiate a muscle action potential.

- **Muscle Fibers**
  Description: These extrafusal fibers are the final components of the motor unit. Their characteristics, including twitch response, depend on the alpha motor neuron by which it is innervated.

Alpha Motor Neuron (AMN)

The three motor neurons listed in Table 5–1 innervate specific fibers, extrafusal or intrafusal. Needle electromyography monitors factors related to the motor unit and thus is limited to evaluating the alpha motor neurons. The alpha motor neurons and associated motor unit parameters have been described based on size and physiology (Figure 5–2). The order of recruitment is related to their size, starting with the smaller motor units. This sequential activation allows for a smooth increase of contractile force and is described by the Henneman Size Principle.

TABLE 5–1   Three Types of Motor Neurons

Motor Neuron	Innervations
Alpha	Extrafusal Fibers—Skeletal muscle
Gamma	Intrafusal Fibers—Muscle spindle
Beta	Intrafusal and Extrafusal Fibers

Descriptions	Characteristics
Type I	Smaller cell body
	Thinner diameter axon
	Lower innervation ratio
	Slower twitch muscle fibers
Type II	Larger cell body
	Thicker diameter axon
	Higher innervation ratio
	Faster twitch muscle fibers

Henneman Size Principle 📖

A smaller alpha motor neuron has a lower threshold of excitation, causing it to be recruited first during voluntary contraction.

A larger alpha motor neuron has a higher threshold of excitation and is recruited when more motor units are needed to generate greater contractile force.

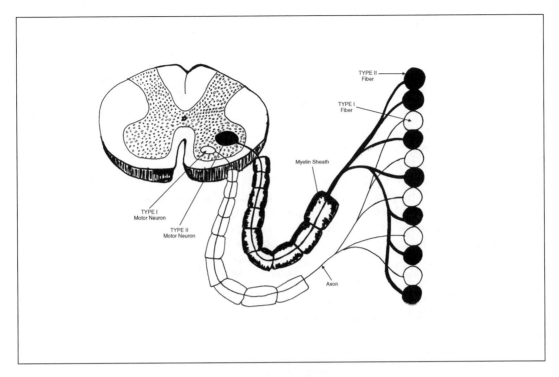

FIGURE 5–2. Description of Type I and Type II Alpha Motor Neurons

Axons

These are long cellular processes that make up the nerve. Their diameter and function vary, along with impulse propagation velocity. Two classic classifications describing the different nerve fibers are listed below, but the electrodiagnostic evaluation only tests the 📖 Ia fibers.

Nerve Fiber Classification (Table 5-2)

TABLE 5–2

Lloyd and Hunt (Sensory)	Erlanger and Gasser (Sensory and Motor)	Diameter (μm)	Velocity (m/s)	Function
Ia fibers	A-alpha fibers	10–20 largest	50–120 fastest	Motor: alpha motor neurons Sensory: muscle spindle
Ib fibers	A-alpha fibers	10–20	50–120	Sensory: Golgi tendon organ, touch, pressure
II fibers	A-beta fibers	4–12	25–70	Motor: intrafusal and extrafusal muscle fibers Sensory: muscle spindle, touch, pressure
III fibers	A-gamma fibers	2–8	10–50	Motor: gamma motor neurons, muscle spindle
	A-delta fibers	1–5	3–30	Sensory: touch, pain, temperature
IV fibers	B-fibers	1–3	3–15	Motor: preganglionic autonomic fibers
	C-fibers	<1	<2	Motor: postganglionic autonomic fibers Sensory: pain, temperature

Connective Tissue (Figure 5–3)

Endoneurium
Description: This is the connective tissue surrounding each individual axon and its myelin sheath.

Perineurium
Description: This is the strong, protective, connective tissue surrounding bundles or fascicles of myelinated and unmyelinated nerve fibers. It helps strengthen the nerve and acts as a diffusion barrier. Individual axons may cross from one bundle to another along the course of the nerve.

Epineurium
Description: This is the loose connective tissue surrounding the entire nerve that holds the fascicles together and protects it from compression.

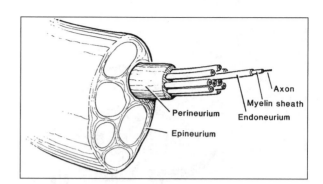

FIGURE 5–3. Neuronal Connective Tissue: The Internal Anatomy of the Nerve. (From Buschbacher RM: Basic tissue organization and function. In Buschbacher RM (ed): Musculoskeletal Disorders: A Practical Guide for Diagnosis and Rehabilitation. Stoneham, Mass,, Butterworth-Heinemann. 1994, p.17.)

Function
- **Resting Membrane Potential (RMP)**
  Description: This is the voltage of the axon's cell membrane at rest.

Leak Channels
These are openings that allow sodium (Na^+) and potassium (K^+) to move passively in and out of the cell membrane.

Na^+–K^+ ATP-Dependent Pumps
The RMP of the nerve would dissipate from diffusion through the leak channels; however, a negative potential is maintained inside the cell by actively exporting three ions of Na^+ and importing two ions of K^+ through a *semipermeable membrane*. This keeps each ion against a concentration gradient with a deficit of positive ions inside the cell (Figure 5–4).

Normal RMP: –70 to –90 mV

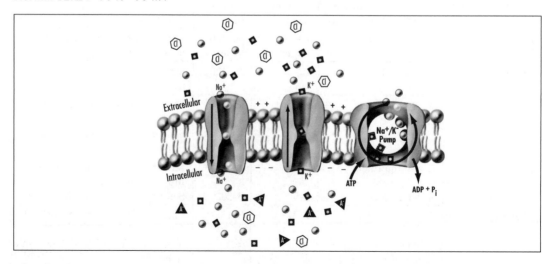

FIGURE 5–4. Na^+–K^+ ATP–dependent pump: (2) K^+ ions are imported. (3) Na^+ ions are exported, therefore a negative potential is maintained inside the cell.

- **Depolarization**

  Description: When an outside current is applied to a nerve by a stimulator consisting of a negative pole (cathode) and a positive pole (anode), positive charges on the axon become attracted under the cathode and lower the membrane potential. The membrane becomes increasingly permeable to Na⁺, which rushes into the cell through the opened voltage-gated channels toward an equilibrium. This process of 📖 **sodium conductance** (Figure 5–5) is the most important event in generating an action potential.

  - **Action Potential (AP)**

    This is a voltage change occurring from an excited cell. The electric impulse propagates along an axon or muscle membrane. It can also be evoked by a stimulator. The all-or-none response travels in both directions along the axon.

  - **All-or-None Response**

    A stimulus must be strong enough to reach a certain threshold of activation. Once reached, the AP generated remains at a constant size and configuration. If it is below this

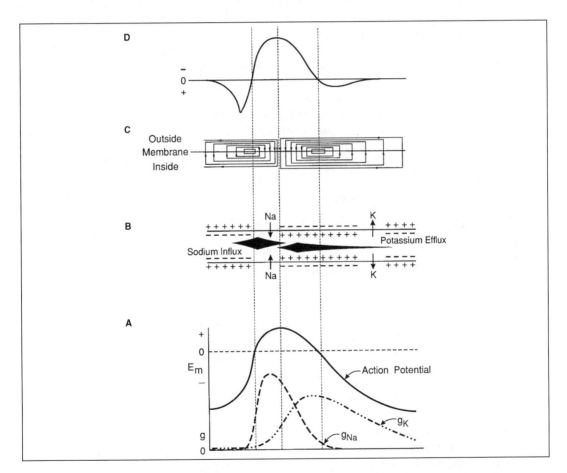

FIGURE 5–5. **A:** Sodium (gNa) and Potassium (gK) ion conductances are depicted over time, resulting in an alteration of the transmembrane potential and creating an action potential. **B:** The spatial relationship of the sodium and potassium ion influx during an action potential is schematicallly depicted. Note the alteration of the transmembrane ionic potential differences corresponding to the depolarization and repolarization. **C:** Local circuit currents describe the pathways of extracellular sodium ions entering the cell and then migrating longitudinally within the cell. **D:** Triphasic extracellular waveform associated with the intracellular monophasic action potential. (Reprinted with permission from Dumitru D. Electrodiagnostic Medicine. Philadelphia, Hanley & Belfus, 1995.)

threshold, no potential will occur. Furthermore, any stimulus intensity greater than the threshold will not generate a larger potential.

- **Na⁺ Voltage Gated Channels**
These are protein channels used for ion exchange. They have activation and inactivation gates, that undergo conformational changes from a depolarization. This allows increased Na⁺ influx into the cell (Figure 5–6).

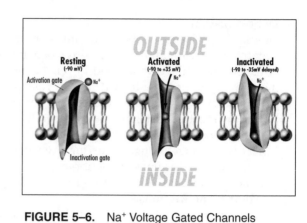

FIGURE 5–6. Na⁺ Voltage Gated Channels

- **Absolute Refractory Period**
This pertains to the time after closure of the inactivation gates. They will not immediately reopen. No action potential can be formed at this time, no matter how strong a repeated stimulus is used.

- **Relative Refractory Period**
This pertains to the period of time after the absolute refractory period. At this time an action potential can be elicited with more intense stimulation.

- **Temperature Effects**
The Na⁺ channels will remain open for approximately 25 microseconds (μs). A decrease in temperature affects the protein configuration and causes a delay in opening and closing of the gates. This typically changes the waveform appearance, as described below. However the amplitude can drop due to an increase in temporal dispersion or phase cancellation. Also, note the difference in focal cooling compared to generalized limb cooling (Figure 5–7).

Parameters	Change
Latency 📖	Prolonged
Amplitude 📖	Increased
Duration	Increased
Conduction Velocity 📖	Decreased

- **Propagation**
Description: As Na⁺ goes into the cell from a depolarization, it moves away from the membrane and spreads the current down a path of least resistance along the length of the axon. 📖 The affinity to flow back out through the membrane is low due to the myelin sheath covering. Thus, the potential "jumps" to the next group of Na⁺ channels, located between the myelin, to areas called the *Nodes of Ranvier*. This process of propagating a current from one node to another is known as *saltatory conduction*.

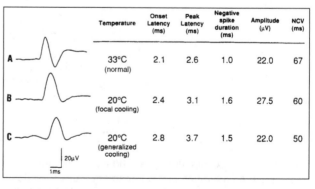

	Temperature	Onset Latency (ms)	Peak Latency (ms)	Negative spike duration (ms)	Amplitude (μV)	NCV (ms)
A	33°C (normal)	2.1	2.6	1.0	22.0	67
B	20°C (focal cooling)	2.4	3.1	1.6	27.5	60
C	20°C (generalized cooling)	2.8	3.7	1.5	22.0	50

FIGURE 5–7. Decreased Temperature Effects. **A:** Normal. **B:** Focal Cooling. **C:** Generalized Cooling. (Reprinted with permission from Dumitru D. Electrodiagnostic Medicine. Philadelphia, Hanley & Belfus, 1995.)

Direction

Orthodromic

The action potential is monitored traveling in the direction of its typical physiologic conduction. The conduction along motor fibers is monitored away from the spinal cord, and sensory fibers are monitored toward the spinal cord.

Antidromic

The action potential is monitored traveling in the opposite direction of its typical physiologic conduction. The conduction along motor fibers is monitored toward the spinal cord, and sensory fibers are monitored away from the spinal cord.

- **Repolarization**
  Description: This is the process of bringing the depolarized membrane back to its resting state. It is dependent on Na^+ inactivation and K^+ activation.
  - **K^+ Voltage-Gated Channels**
    These are protein channels, which, after a slight delay, open from a depolarization. This allows K^+ to move out of the cell to establish a charge equilibrium. A delay exists in channel closure, which results in a membrane with a hyperpolarized state called an *overshoot phenomenon*. This process of *potassium conductance* eventually returns the waveform to its baseline due to the K^+ leak channels restoring the RMP (Figure 5–8).

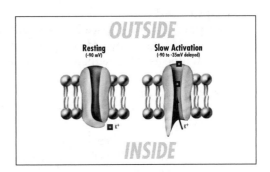

FIGURE 5–8. K^+ Voltage Gated Channels

Neuromuscular Junction

The distal portion of a motor axon has small twig-like projections that innervate individual muscle fibers. This portion of the nerve and single muscle fiber forms the motor endplate. The axon terminal, containing various neural structures, including mitochondria and synaptic vesicles with acetylcholine (ACh), does not contact its muscle fiber. Rather, it remains separate from it by primary and secondary synaptic clefts (Figure 5–9).

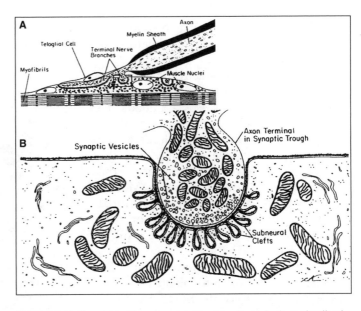

FIGURE 5–9. The Neuromuscular Junction. **A:** Longitudinal Section of the Junction. **B:** Enlarged View. (From Fawcett DW: Bloom and Fawcett: A Textbook of Histology. Philadelphia, W.B. Saunders, 1986, Edward Arnold Publishing, © Don W. Fawcett.)

Components
- ### Presynaptic Region
  Description: This is the bulbous area at the axon's terminal zone. It is comprised of three storage compartments containing acetylcholine. They are contained in packets called quanta consisting of approximately 5,000–10,000 molecules. The acetylcholine migrates from the main and mobilization storage compartments to replenish the immediate storage compartment, which is depleted in the process of generating each action potential. This migration of acetylcholine takes approximately 4–5 seconds.

Storage Compartments	Content
Main store	300,000 quanta
Mobilized store	10,000 quanta
Immediate store	1,000 quanta

- ### Synaptic Cleft
  Description: This is a space 200–500 angstroms wide where acetylcholine crosses from the presynaptic region toward receptors on the postsynaptic region. It contains an enzyme, acetylcholine esterase, which degrades acetylcholine into acetate and choline as it crosses the cleft.

- ### Postsynaptic Region
  Description: This is a membrane lined with acetylcholine receptors. It has convolutions to increase its surface area by approximately 10 times the surface of the presynaptic membrane. At the crests of each fold, receptors are located across from the presynaptic active zones, which are the sites of acetylcholine release. Each postsynaptic acetylcholine receptor requires two molecules of acetylcholine to become activated.

Function

ACh Release
- ### Resting State
  During the periods of inactivation, a spontaneous release of a quanta occurs every 5 seconds. This results in one miniature endplate potential (MEPP).
- ### Excited State
  During the periods of activation, a nerve depolarization opens voltage-gated calcium (Ca^{++}) channels. Ca^{++} floods the nerve terminals and remains there approximately 200 ms. This leads to the release of multiple quanta into the synaptic cleft, which increases the amount of MEPPs. These MEPPs summate and form an endplate potential (EPP), which generates a motor unit action potential (MUAP) (Figure 5–10).
- ### Safety Factor (SF)
  Description: The amplitude of an EPP must be high enough to initiate an action potential. Normally, the EPP's amplitude is four times the amount needed to initiate an action potential. However, the EPP's amplitude drops each time the EPP is created, due to a drop in immediate available acetylcholine. This initial excess

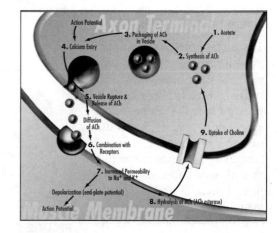

FIGURE 5–10. Acetylcholine Release and Recycling

amplitude of the EPP is called the **safety factor** and allows time for acetylcholine to move from the main and mobilizing storage compartments to replenish the immediate storage compartment. This avoids a drop of the EPP's amplitude below the threshold needed to cause an action potential. The safety factor depends on two parameters:

- **Quantal Content**
  This is the number of ACh quanta released with each nerve depolarization.
- **Quantal Response**
  This is the ability of the ACh receptors to respond to the ACh molecules that are released.

Muscle Fiber

This is a cylindrical multinucleated cell containing contractile elements composed of actin and myosin. The muscle cell (sarcomere) runs from Z line to Z line (Figure 5–11). Its size changes during contraction. (Figure 5–12)

Muscle Fiber Classification

Description: The characteristics of these fibers depend on the MU by which it is innervated. If a muscle fiber becomes denervated it will take on the characteristics of the alpha motor neuron that reinnervates it. (Table 5-3)

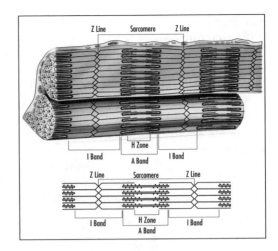

FIGURE 5–11. The Sarcomere

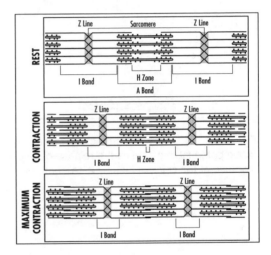

FIGURE 5–12. Sarcomere Positional Changes

TABLE 5–3 Muscle Fiber Classification

Characteristics	Type I (SO) Slow Twitch Oxidative	Type II-A (FOG) Fast Twitch Oxidative/Glycolytic	Type II-B (FG) Fast Twitch Glycolytic
Alpha motor neuron	Small	Large	Large
Color	Dark	Dark	Pale
Recruitment	Early	Late	Late
Fatigue	Highly resistant	Resistant	Sensitive
Effort	Mild (4–8 Hz)	Intermediate (20–30 Hz)	High (20–30 Hz)
Firing frequency	Slow, prolonged	Fast, unsustained	Fast, unsustained
Movements	Fine, precise	Gross	Gross
Innervation ratio	Small	Large	Large
Amplitude/duration	Small	Large	Large
O_2 capacity	Aerobic	Anaerobic	Anaerobic

Function

- **Contraction** 📖

  An action initiated by muscle fiber depolarization. The stimulus spread in both directions on the fiber at 3–5 meters/second. It penetrates deeper into the muscle through the *T-tubule system*. This causes Ca^{++} to be released from the *sarcoplasm reticulum (SR)*. It binds to the troponin–tropomyosin complex and exposes actin's active sites. Myosin heads, powered by ATP, bind with the active sites. The actin and myosin filaments slide over each other to shorten the muscle (Figure 5–13).

- **Relaxation**

  Powered by ATP, Ca^{++} is actively pumped back into the SR. This allows the tropomyosin to block actin's active sites. Absence of ATP results in rigor mortis due to the actin and myosin filaments remaining permanently joined.

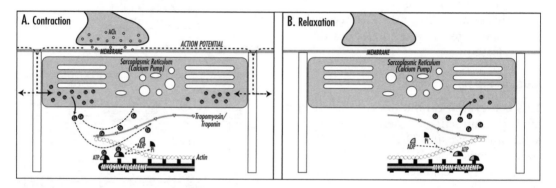

FIGURE 5–13. Muscle Contraction: Excitation–Contraction Coupling in the Muscle. This shows an action potential that causes the release of calcium ions from the sarcoplasmic reticulum and then reuptake of the calcium ions by a calcium pump.

CLINICAL INSTRUMENTATION

Electrodiagnostic Instruments (Figure 5–14)

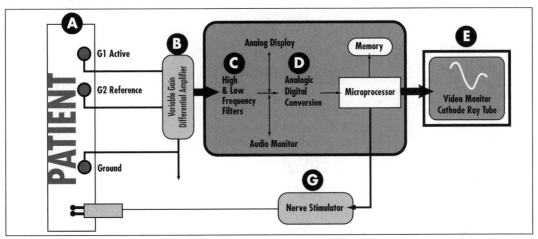

FIGURE 5–14. Electrodiagnostic Instrumentation. **A:** A patient with recording electrodes has a peripheral nerve excited with a stimulator (G). **B:** The differential amplifier receives the action potential. **C:** The signal is filtered. **D:** The analog signal is converted to a digital representation while being fed to a loud speaker. **E:** The signal is displayed on a cathode ray tube. **G:** Stimulator is used to excite the peripheral nervous system.

Electronic Circuitry (Ohm's Law)

Definition
An electric current passes through a wire at an intensity of the current **(I)** measured in amperes, equal to the electro-motor source **(E)** measured in volts, divided by the resistance **(R)** measured in ohms.

$$\text{📖} \quad I = E/R \text{ or } E = I\,R$$

Electrodes

Definition
These devices are used to record or stimulate the skin surface, muscle, or nerve.
- **Recording Electrode**
  Description: This is a device placed on or through the skin to pick up muscle or nerve electrical activity.
  - **Active Site**
    This pickup is placed over the endplate region of the muscle for a Compound Muscle Action Potential (CMAP), or over the nerve for a Sensory Nerve Action Potential (SNAP).
  - **Reference Site**
    This pickup is placed over the tendon for a CMAP or nerve for a SNAP. To obtain a proper reading, the impedance (resistance) between electrode and skin must be kept low by removing skin lotions, oils, gels, etc.
  - **Surface Electrode (Figure 5-15)**
    This is an electrode placed on the skin to record nerve or muscle action potentials.

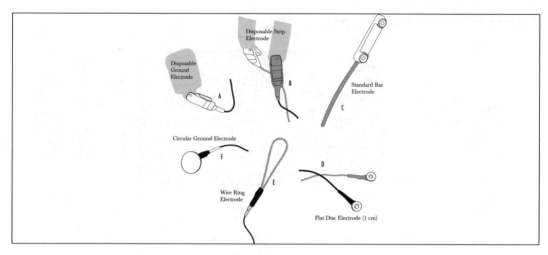

FIGURE 5–15. Various Types of Surface Electrodes. **A:** Square ground electrode. **B:** Lead strips mounted in a plastic bar. **C:** Circular ground electrode. **D:** Non-lead plastic bar electrode. **E:** Flat disc electrodes (1 cm). **F:** Flat disc electrodes mounted in a plastic bar. **G:** Wire ring electrodes. **H:** Pipe cleaner electrodes. **I:** 1 mm tip plug.

Components (Figure 5–15)

• Needle Electrode

This is an electrode inserted through the skin to record muscle or nerve action potentials. If used for NCS, the waveform's amplitude and conduction velocity cannot be assessed because the needle samples only a few fibers.

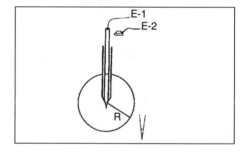

FIGURE 5–16. Monopolar Needle Electrode. (Reprinted with permission from Dumitru D. Electrodiagnostic Medicine. Philadelphia, Hanley & Belfus, 1995.)

– **Monopolar Needle Electrode (Figure 5–16)**
This is a 22–30 gauge Teflon® coated needle with an exposed tip of 0.15–0.2 mm².
Advantage:
■ Inexpensive
■ Conical tip: omnidirectional recording
■ Less painful (Teflon® decreases friction)
■ Larger recording area (2 × concentric)
■ Records more positive sharp waves (PSW)
Disadvantage:
■ Requires a separate surface reference
■ Unstandardized tip area
■ Teflon® fraying
■ More interference

– **Standard Concentric (Coaxial) Needle Electrode (Figure 5–17)**
This is a 24–26 gauge needle (reference) with a bare inner wire (active).
Advantage:
■ Standardized exposed area
■ Fixed location from reference

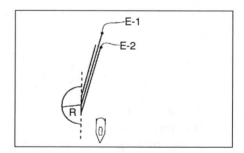

FIGURE 5–17. Concentric Needle Electrode. (Reprinted with permission from Dumitru D. Electrodiagnostic Medicine. Philadelphia, Hanley & Belfus, 1995.)

- Less interference
- No separate reference
- Used for quantitative EMG

Disadvantage:
- Beveled tip: unidirectional recording
- Smaller recording area
- *Motor unit action potentials (MUAP) have smaller amplitudes*
- More painful

- **Bipolar Concentric Needle Electrode (Figure 5–18)**
  This is a needle with the active and reference wires within its lumen.
  Advantage:
  - Best for isolating MUAP
  - Less artifact

  Disadvantage:
  - Expensive
  - More painful

- **Single Fiber Needle Electrode (Figure 5–19)**
  This is a needle (reference) consisting of an exposed 25 μm diameter wire (active).
  Advantage:
  - Looks at individual muscle fibers
  - Used to assess fiber type density
  - Used to assess jitter
  - Used to assess fiber blocking
  - Helpful in neuromuscular junction disorders
  - Helpful in motor neuron disorders

  Disadvantage
  - Not used for traditional EMG

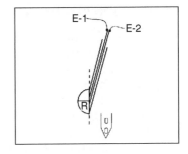

FIGURE 5–18. Bipolar Needle Electrode. (Reprinted with permission from Dumitru D. Electrodiagnostic Medicine. Philadelphia, Hanley & Belfus, 1995.)

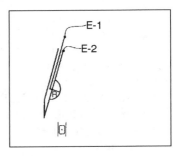

FIGURE 5–19. Single Fiber Electrode. (Reprinted with permission from Dumitru D. Electrodiagnostic Medicine. Philadelphia, Hanley & Belfus, 1995)

- **Ground Electrode**

Description: This is a zero-voltage, neutral, surface reference point placed between the recording electrode and the stimulating electrode.

- **Stimulating Electrode**

Description: This is a bipolar device used to apply an electrical impulse to a nerve initiating an AP (Figure 5–20).

- **Poles**
  - **Cathode**
    This terminal generates a negative impulse, which attracts positive charges from the axon.
  - **Anode**
    This terminal generates a positive impulse, which attracts negative charges from the axon.

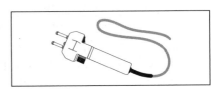

FIGURE 5–20. Bipolar Stimulator

Anodal Block 📖

A theoretical local block that occurs when reversing the stimulator's cathode and anode. This hyperpolarizes the nerve, thus inhibiting the production of an action potential.

STIMULATION INTENSITY

- **Threshold Stimulus**
  This is an electrical stimulus occurring at an intensity level just sufficient enough to produce a detectable evoked potential from the nerve.
- **Maximal Stimulus**
  This is an electrical stimulus at an intensity level in which no further increase in an evoked potential will occur from the nerve with added stimulus intensity.
- **Submaximal Stimulus**
  This is an electrical stimulus at an intensity below the maximal stimulus level but above the threshold level. This can lead to a falsely lower recorded amplitude and prolonged latency reading since all the axons of the nerve are not being discharged. During a distal stimulation, these false readings can mimic axonal loss due to the decreased appearance of the action potential. During a proximal stimulation they can mimic conduction block by the appearance of a drop in action potential amplitude.
- **Supramaximal Stimulus**
  This is an electrical stimulus at an intensity 20% above the maximal stimulus and is typically used for nerve conduction studies. 📖 Waveform changes can occur if the intensity is too high. This can cause a decreased latency due to increasing the surface area stimulated, thus decreasing the distance the stimulus must travel. However, the amplitude would remain unchanged. Also, volume conduction can occur from unwanted stimulation of surrounding nerves and muscles, altering the waveform.
- **Stimulation Duration**
  This should be at 0.1–0.3 milliseconds. If it is higher, it can falsely prolong the distal latency due to stimulating the nerve for a longer period of time.
- **Stimulation Number**
  - **Averaging**
    This is a process that extracts the desired neurophysiologic signal from larger noise and interference signals. These unwanted signals can occur from biological or environmental sources, such as EMG audio feedback, needle artifact, 60 Hz line interference, preamplifier proximity to the machine, fluorescent lights, or the patient.
  - **Signal-to-Noise Ratio (S:N)**
    The process of *averaging* improves the S:N by a factor that is the square root of the number of averages performed. The number of averages must be increased by a factor of 4 to double the S:N.

    $$\text{📖 S:N} = \frac{\text{Signal Amplitude} \times \sqrt{\text{\# of Averages Performed}}}{\text{Noise Amplitude}}$$

  - **Stimulus Artifact**
    This is a defect seen at the time the stimulus is applied to the skin and represents current spread to the electrode. It can be reduced by:
    - Placing the ground electrode between the recording electrode and stimulator
    - Appropriate anode and cathode placement
    - Cleansing the skin from dirt, perspiration, and lotions

DIFFERENTIAL AMPLIFIER

Definition

This is a device within a preamplifier that responds to alternating currents (AC) of electricity. It cancels waveforms recorded at both the active and reference pickups and amplifies the remaining potentials (Figure 5–21). It should have a high impedence and common mode rejection but low noise from within the system.

Common Mode Rejection Ratio (CMRR)
This refers to selectively amplifying different signals and rejecting common ones. It is usually expressed as decibels (dB) and should be 90 dB or greater. The larger the CMRR, the more efficient the amplifier.

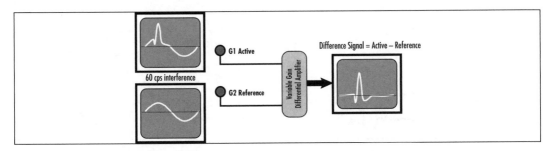

FIGURE 5–21. Schematic Representation of Differential Amplifier Function. A difference amplifier only amplifies the difference in the signal present at the active and reference inputs. When 60 cps interference is the same at both inputs, it is eliminated, leaving only the difference signal, this is the action potential, being measured.

FILTERS

• **Definition**

This is a device composed of resistors and capacitors that function to exclude un- wanted waveforms from being recorded (Figure 5–22).

• 📖 **Types**

– **High Frequency (Low Pass) Filter**
Description: This affects the faster portion of the summated waveform. It removes the signals with frequencies above its cut-off setting but allows lower frequencies to be recorded.

– **Low Frequency (High Pass) Filter**
Description: This affects the slower portion of the summated waveform. It removes the signals with frequencies below its cut-off setting but allows higher frequencies to be recorded.

• **Settings**

Sensory NCS:	20 Hz– 2 kHz
Motor NCS:	2 Hz–10 kHz
EMG:	20 Hz–10 kHz

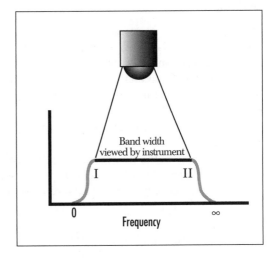

FIGURE 5–22. The Frequency Bandwidth. This is a schematic representation of the fre- quencies the filters have "allowed" the instru- ment to "view." **I:** Low Frequency Filter. **II:** High Frequency Filter.

Elevating the Low Frequency Filter (Figure 5–23 I–IV)	**Reducing the High Frequency Filter** (Figure 5–24 I–IV)
• Shortens the peak latency • Reduces the amplitude • Changes potentials from bi- to triphasic • Does not change the onset latency	• Prolongs the peak latency • Reduces amplitudes • Creates a longer negative spike • Prolongs the onset latency

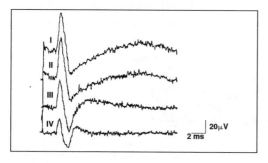

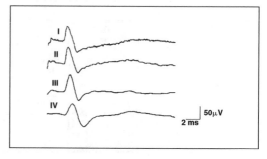

FIGURE 5–23. Elevating the Low Frequency Filter: Sequential elevation of the low frequency filters (I–IV).

FIGURE 5–24. Reducing the High Frequency Filter: Sequential reduction of high frequency filters (I–IV).

SCREEN

Definition

Once a signal has been recorded, amplified, filtered, and passed through, the analogue to digital converter is displayed on a cathode ray tube (CRT). A grid is projected on the monitor with divisions consisting of a horizontal axis (x axis) allocated as *sweep speed* and a vertical axis (y-axis) allocated as *sensitivity*. Each of these parameters can be adjusted to manipulate the recorded waveform for an accurate measurement.

- **Sweep Speed**

  This pertains to the time allocated for each x-axis division and is measured in milliseconds.
- **Sensitivity**

  This pertains to the height allocated for each y-axis division and is measured in millivolts (mV) or microvolts (μV). The term *gain* is sometimes used interchangeably with sensitivity. The gain is actually a ratio measurement of output to input and does not have a unit value such as mV or μV.
- **Settings**

  The following equations represent a simple way to remember possible screen settings.

$$
\begin{array}{llll}
\textbf{Sweep Speed:} & 5 \text{ ms} & \times \quad 2 \text{ ms} & = \quad 10 \text{ ms} \\
& \text{Sensory} & \text{EMG} & \text{Motor} \\
\textbf{Sensitivity:} & 10 \text{ μV} & \times \quad 100 \text{ μV} & = \quad 1000 \text{ μV (1 mV)} \\
& \text{Sensory} & \text{EMG} & \text{Motor}
\end{array}
$$

▪ PATHOPHYSIOLOGY

DEMYELINATION

Definition

This is a nerve injury that can cause motor and sensory abnormalities in which the myelin is impaired but the axon remains intact. The membrane capacitance increases due to the loss of myelin insulation, thus hindering saltatory conduction. The trophic factors of the nerve are maintained and myelin regeneration is possible due to Schwann cell proliferation (Figure 5–25).

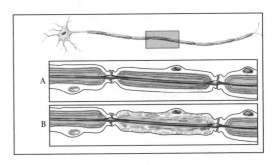

FIGURE 5–25. Demyelination. **A:** Normal Nerve. **B:** Injured Segment with Myelin Breakdown.

Conduction Block

This is the failure of an action potential to propagate past an area of demyelination along the structurally intact axons comprising the nerve. It can present as a greater than 50% drop in CMAP amplitude between proximal and distal stimulation sites across the area of injury.

- **Etiology**

  📖 (a) Compression causing a transient ischemic episode, edema, or 📖 myelin invaginations with paranodal intussusception (Figure 5–26), or (b) peripheral neuropathies

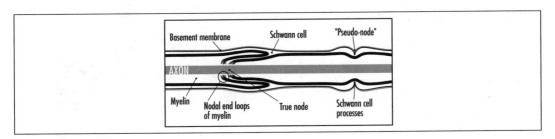

FIGURE 5–26. Paranodal Intussusception. Diagram of an invaginating paranode into an adjacent one.

- **Electrodiagnostic Findings (EDX)**

NCS	EMG
Latency: Prolonged	Insertional activity: Normal
Amplitude: Decreased across the site of injury	Resting activity: Normal, ± myokymia
Temporal dispersion: Increased	Recruitment: ± Decreased
Conduction velocity: Decreased	MUAP: Normal

- **Recovery**

  - **Self Limited**
    Description: The pathology can reverse with cessation of the insulting event. Transient ischemia can be immediately reversed but edema can take several weeks.

– **Remyelination**

Description: This is a process of repair in which the demyelinated region develops new myelin by the Schwann cells. 📖 This new myelin is thinner with shorter internodal distances, it can cause an improved but slower than normal conduction velocity (Figure 5–27).

AXONAL INJURY

Definition

An injury to the axon may present in one of two typical forms: axonal degeneration or Wallerian degeneration. Both of these can affect the cell body and cause a central chromatolysis (Figure 5–28).

• **Axonal Degeneration**

Description: A nerve injury that begins presenting in a "dying back" fashion, affecting the nerve in a length-dependent manner. It begins distally and ascends proximally. (Figure 5–29)

• **Wallerian Degeneration (WD)**

Description: A nerve injury that begins presenting 4–5 days postfocal or multifocal nerve damage. It completes in 7 days for motor nerves or 11 days for sensory nerves. The axon degenerates distally from the site of injury, leaving the proximal portion intact (Figure 5–29).

• **Etiology**

Pathology can occur from: (a) focal crush, (b) stretch, (c) transection, or (d) peripheral neuropathies.

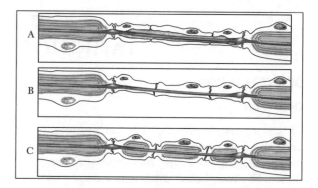

FIGURE 5–27. Remyelination. **A:** Myelin digestion and Schwann cell proliferation. **B:** Myelin is removed. **C:** Remyelination is complete.

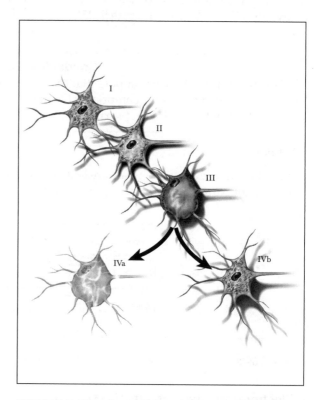

FIGURE 5–28. Axonal Injury. I: Normal nerve cell. II: Post-injury: Nissl substance degenerates. III: Swollen cell body with eccentric nucleus. IV **A:** Cell death. IV **B:** Cell recovery.

• **EDX Findings**

NCS	EMG
Latency: Normal	Insertional activity: Abnormal
Amplitude: Decreased throughout the entire nerve	Resting activity: Abnormal
Temporal dispersion: Normal	Recruitment: Decreased
Conduction velocity: Decreased	MUAP: Abnormal

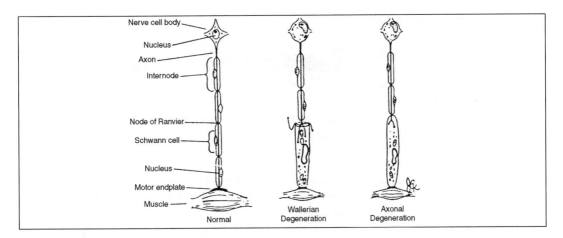

FIGURE 5–29. Schematic representation of axonal injuries. (From Asbury AK, Johnson PC: Pathology of Peripheral Nerve, v.9. In Bennington, JL (ed): Major Problems in Pathology. W.B. Saunders, Philadelphia, 1978.)

- **Recovery**

  - **Collateral Sprouting (Figure 5–30)**
    Description: This is a process of repair in which a neurite sprouts off the axon of an intact motor unit and innervates denervated muscle fibers of an injured motor unit. The sprouts connect with smaller terminal branches, thinner myelin, and weaker neuromuscular junctions. Increased fiber type grouping occurs as muscle fibers become part of the new motor unit and take on its characteristics, increasing the size of its territory. This remodeling results in motor units with poor firing synchronicity, secondary to the immature terminal sprouts. This results in polyphasic waveforms with increased amplitudes.

  - **Axonal Regrowth** 📖
    Description: This is a process of repair in which the axon will regrow down its original pathway toward its muscle fibers. It will travel approximately *1 mm/day* or *1 inch/month* if

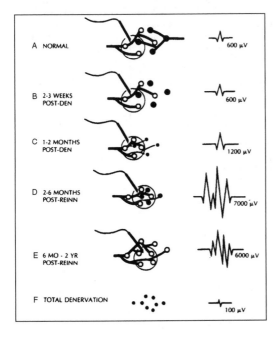

FIGURE 5–30. Motor Unit Remodeling. **A:** Type I: light circles; Type II: dark circles. Depolarization of one of the motor unit results in a 600 µV MUAP. **B:** Following degeneration of the Type II MU at 2–3 weeks, the Type I MUAP still yields a 600 µV potential. **C:** Within 1–2 months the Type II muscle fibers have atrophied and collateral sprouting from Type I is beginning to reinnervate them. The Type I motor unit territory has subsequently "collapsed" due to Type II fiber atrophy, causing a larger MUAP (1200 µV). **D:** As the connections mature, the MUAP demonstrates a further increase in amplitude (7000 µV) and number of phases. By 6 months, all muscle fibers belonging to the Type I motor units are of the same fiber type; i.e., Type II fibers have been converted to Type I fibers. **E:** As maturity continues the MUAP may decrease its amplitude and phases due to the collaterals conducting potentials more rapidly. **F:** An example of complete dennervation. (Copyright ©1995 American Association of Electrodiagnostic Medicine)

the supporting connective tissue remains intact. These axons will have a decreased diameter, thinner myelin, and shorter internodal distance (Figure 5–31). With reinnervation, low amplitude, long duration, and polyphasic potentials

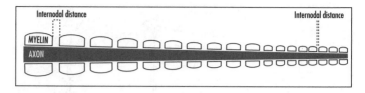

FIGURE 5–31. Axonal Regrowth. The axons: Diameter is decreased. Myelin is thinner. Internodal distance is shorter.

known as *nascent potentials* are formed. If the connective tissue is not intact to guide proper nerve re-growth, a neuroma can form with failure to reach the final end organ.

- **Collateral Sprouting vs. Axonal Regrowth**
  If an axon regrows to innervate its original muscle fibers and collateral sprouting to these fibers has occurred, the recovery process possessing the largest axon, thickest myelin, and strongest neuromuscular junction will prevail and keep the muscle fibers.

NERVE INJURY CLASSIFICATION

Definition

Two classification systems categorizing nerve injuries are listed below.
- **Seddon Classification** 📖 **(Table 5–14)**

TABLE 5–4

	Characteristics	Neuropraxia		Axonotmesis		Neurotmesis	
	Etiology	Nerve compression injury		Nerve crush injury		Nerve transection injury	

	Description	Axon is intact
		Local myelin injury
		
		Conduction block
				Axonal interruption
				Connective tissue/
				  Schwann cell intact
				Conduction failure
						Axonal interruption
						Connective tissue
						  disruption
						Conduction failure	

	Nerve Conduction Studies	The signal is normal
		  distal to the lesion and
		  abnormal across it
				Conduction resembles
				  neuropraxia for 4 to 5
				  days, until Wallerian
				  degeneration occurs
						Conduction intially
						  resembles axonotmesis,
						  but does not
						  demonstrate recovery	

		Wave Form Distal to Lesion	**Wave Form Proximal to Lesion**	**Wave Form Distal to Lesion**	**Wave Form Proximal to Lesion**	**Wave Form Distal to Lesion**	**Wave Form Proximal to Lesion**
		Immediate		Immediate		Immediate	
		2 weeks		2 weeks		2 weeks	
		> 2 weeks		weeks-months		2 years	
	EMG	Normal/decreased recruitment		Abnormal activity		Abnormal activity	

- **Sunderland Classification**   (Figure 5–32) (Table 5-5)

TABLE 5–5

Type 1	Conduction block (neuropraxia)
Type 2	Axonal injury (axonotmesis)
Type 3	Type 2 + Endoneurium injury
Type 4	Type 3 + Perineurium injury
Type 5	Type 4 + Epineurium injury (neurotmesis)

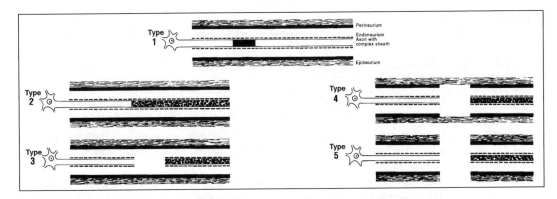

FIGURE 5–32. Sunderland Classification. (From Sunderland S. Nerve Injuries and Their Repair: A Critical Appraisal. Edinburgh, Churchill Livingstone, 1991, with permission.)

■

NERVE CONDUCTION STUDIES (NCS)

Definition

These studies assess the ability of peripheral nerve to conduct electrical impulses. A representative waveform is generated by nerve stimulation and its parameters are evaluated to monitor neuronal function.

- **Waveforms**

Description: The recorded potential represents a compilation of multiple sinusoidal waves. The different phases and amplitudes of each waveform summate or cancel to create a final potential. The final potential displayed represents an average of all the subcomponent's frequencies (Figure 5–33). Frequency is defined as the number of times the same event or cycle occurs in one second (cycles/second). They are measured in Hertz (Hz).

PARAMETERS (Figure 5–34)

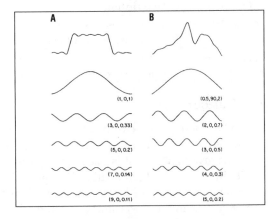

FIGURE 5–33. Waveform Subcomponents (Summation). **A:** A square wave and five subcomponent sine waves, which, when added together, result in the square wave. **B:** A more "biologic" appearing potential and its subcomponent sine waves. The frequency, phase shift, and relative amplitude are described below each subcomponent waveform. (Reprinted with permission from Dumitru D. Electrodiagnostic Medicine. Philadelphia, Hanley & Belfus, 1995.)

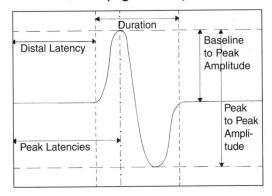

FIGURE 5–34. Waveform Parameters

• **Latency**

This is the time required for an electrical stimulus to initiate an evoked potential. (Table 5-6)

TABLE 5–6 Nerve Responses of Motor and Sensory Nerve Fibers

Nerve Fiber	Nerve Response
Motor	**Latency of activation:** This is the time between the initiation of the electrical stimulus and the beginning of saltatory conduction. It is typically 0.1 ms or less.
	Conduction: This is the saltatory conduction of an action potential along the myelinated axons to its terminal branches, unmyelinated twigs, and neuromuscular junction.
	Synaptic transmission: This is the chemical transmission of the signal across the neuromuscular junction to initiate a single fiber action potential. It takes 0.2–1.0 ms.
Sensory	**Latency of activation:** Same process as above.
	Conduction: Same process as above.
	Synaptic transmission: This does not apply due to absence of a neuromuscular junction.

Measurements	Description
Onset latency	• This represents conduction along the fastest axons • It is recorded at the initial deflection from baseline
Peak latency	• This represents conduction along the majority of the axons • It is recorded at the peak of the waveform response

• **Calculation**

  – **Conduction Velocity (CV)**

  This is the speed an impulse travels along a nerve and is primarily dependent on the integrity of the myelin sheath. It is calculated by dividing the change in distance (proximal stimulation site in mm – distal stimulation site in mm) by the change in time (proximal latency in ms – distal latency in ms). Normal values are 50 meters per second in the upper limbs and 40 meters per second in the lower limbs. It can be decreased with nerve injury; however, it can remain normal even if only a few axons are intact due to impulses traveling in surviving faster fibers.

  – **CV Variations** 📖

  Age
  CV is 50% of an adult for newborns, 80% of adult by 1 year and equal to an adult by 3–5 years. Above 60 years the CV decreases 1.5% per decade.

  Temperature
  Normal is approximately 32°C for the upper limbs and 30°C for the lower limbs. It decreases 2.4 m/s per 1°C dropped. Also a 5% decrease in CV has been described for each 1°C drop below 29°C.

  – **Amplitude**

  This is the maximum voltage difference between two points. It reflects the number of nerve fibers activated and their synchronicity of firing. Recordings are measured as peak-to-peak or baseline-to-peak.

– **Duration**

This is measured from the initial deflection from baseline to the final return. It depends on the summation and rate of firing of numerous axons.

– **Area**

This is a function of both the amplitude and duration of the waveform.

– **Temporal Dispersion (TD)**

(Figure 5–35)

This reflects the conduction velocities of the fastest and slowest nerve fibers. It is seen as a spreading out of the waveform with proximal compared to distal stimulation. This is due to slower fiber conduction reaching the recording electrode later than faster fibers. This is not usually seen with more distal stimulation when slow and fast fibers reach the recording electrode at relatively the same time. The area under the waveform remains essentially constant.

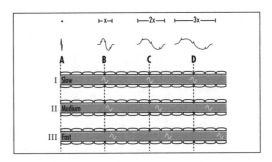

FIGURE 5–35. Temporal Dispersion. Three axons of various conduction speed. I: Fast conduction axon. II: Medium conduction axon. III: Slow conducting axon. The signal is measured at different points along the nerve at site **A, B, C** then. Conduction begins at the left and proceeds to the right. At point **A**, the signal of each axon arrives almost simultaneously, producing a very compact recorded response. At point **B**, the signals are less well synchronized, producing a smaller amplitude and longer duration response, and this spreading is increased by the time the signals arrive at point **C** and point **D**.

– **Phase Cancellation**

When comparing a proximal to distal stimulation, a drop in amplitude and increase in duration occurs. This is most notable with a Sensory Nerve Action Potential (SNAP) because of its short duration. When the nerve is stimulated, the action potentials of one axon may be out of phase with neighboring ones. The negative deflections of one axon can then cancel the positive deflection of another, reducing the amplitude. The summation of these axons creates an action potential that appears as one long prolonged wave. 📖 For this reason a drop of 50% is considered normal when recording a proximal SNAP. The Compound Motor Action Potential (CMAP) does not have as much a drop in amplitude because it has a longer duration waveform. Thus, a smaller decrease in amplitude of approximately 15% is expected (Figures 5–36 and 5–37).

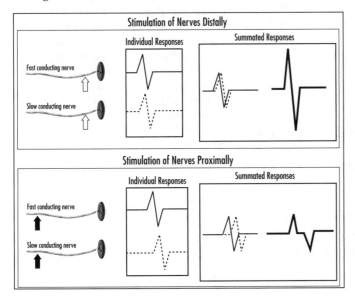

FIGURE 5–36. Sensory—SNAP Phase Cancellation. Open arrows indicate stimulation of the nerve distally; the phases from the individual SNAPs summate. Closed arrows indicate stimulation of the nerve proximally; with the increased distance the phases separate enough by the time they reach the recording electrodes to summate less or even cancel.

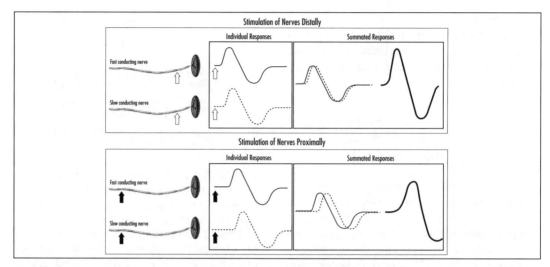

FIGURE 5–37. Motor—CMAP Phase Cancellation. Open arrows indicate stimulation of the nerve distally resulting in the discharge of two MUAPs that produce a potential with twice the size. Closed arrows indicate stimulation of the nerve proximally resulting in two MUAPs that still summate in phase because of the long duration of the MUAPs' negative phases.

SENSORY NERVE ACTION POTENTIAL (SNAP)

Definition

This NCS represents the conduction of an impulse along the sensory nerve fibers. It can also be useful in localizing a lesion in relation to the dorsal root ganglion (DRG). 📖 The DRG is located in the neural foramen and contains the sensory cell body. Lesions proximal to it (root, spinal cord) preserve the SNAP despite clinical sensory abnormalities (Figure 5–38). This is because axonal transport from the cell body to the axon continues to remain intact. SNAPs are typically considered more sensitive than CMAPs in the detection of an incomplete peripheral nerve injury.

- **Technical Considerations**
  - **Antidromic Studies**
    - Are easier to record a response than orthodromic studies
    - Are less uncomfortable when orthodromic studies secondary to less stimulation required
    - Have larger amplitudes due to the nerve being more superficial at the distal recording sites
  - **Recording Electrodes**

The active and reference pickup should be at least 4 cm apart. Less than this distance will alter the waveform in the following manner (Figure 5–39).

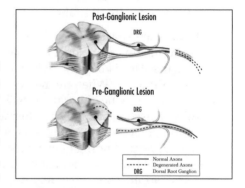

FIGURE 5–38. Post-ganglionic injury: results in Wallerian Degeneration of both motor and sensory axons. There is physical separation of the axon from the cell bodies in the DRG and the ventral portion of the spinal cord. CMAP and SNAP responses are diminished or absent. Pre-ganglionic injury: produces the same injury to the motor fibers but allows the peripheral sensory fibers to remain in contact with their cell body. SNAPs are normal in this injury.

Parameters	Change
📖 Peak Latency	Decreased
Amplitude	Decreased
Duration	Decreased
Rise Time	Decreased

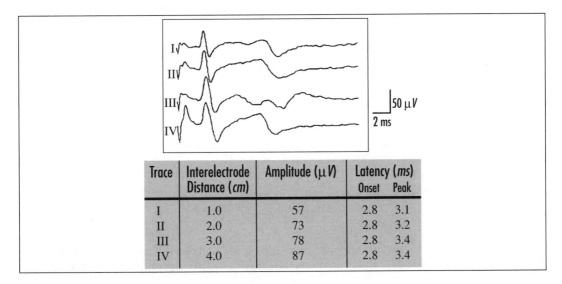

Trace	Interelectrode Distance (*cm*)	Amplitude (μ*V*)	Latency (*ms*) Onset	Peak
I	1.0	57	2.8	3.1
II	2.0	73	2.8	3.2
III	3.0	78	2.8	3.4
IV	4.0	87	2.8	3.4

FIGURE 5–39. Active and Reference Interelectrode Distance. Median nerve SNAP and the effect of varying the interelectrode separation. (I–IV show a sequential increase in the electrode separation.)

COMPOUND MOTOR ACTION POTENTIAL (CMAP)

Definition

This NCS represents the conduction of an impulse along motor nerve fibers. It is recorded as a compound evoked potential from a motor point within the muscle. It corresponds to the integrity of the motor unit but cannot distinguish between pre- and postganglionic lesions because the cell body is located in the spinal cord. It can be abnormal with normal SNAPs if the lesion is proximal to the DRG or affecting a purely motor nerve (Figure 5–40).

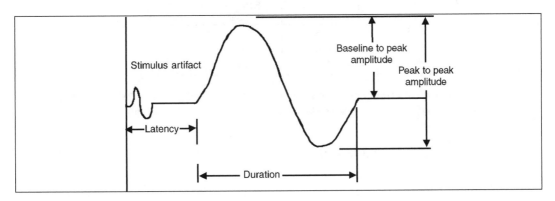

FIGURE 5–40. Compound Motor Action Potential

- **Technical Considerations**
    - ▪ Phases
        - ◆ The potential should be biphasic with an initial negative deflection. If an initial positive deflection exists, it may be due to:
            - ▲ Inappropiate placement of the active electrode from the motor point (Figure 5–41).
            - ▲ Volume conduction from other muscles or nerves.
            - ▲ Anomalous innervations.

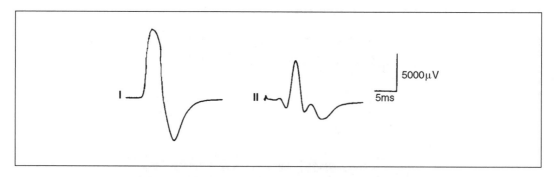

FIGURE 5–41. CMAP Electrode Placement. **I:** Over the endplate region. **II:** Off the endplate region

Recording Electrode

The active and reference pickup should not be too close together. If this occurs, similar waveforms are recorded at both sites and rejected, dropping the amplitude of the waveform (Figure 5–42).

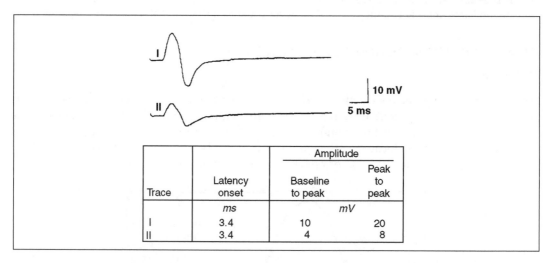

Trace	Latency onset	Amplitude	
		Baseline to peak	Peak to peak
	ms	*mV*	
I	3.4	10	20
II	3.4	4	8

FIGURE 5–42. Active and Reference Interelectrode Distance. Median nerve CMAP and the effect on the amplitude of varying the interelectrode separation. **A:** Normal. **B:** Pickups are too close.

Measurement Differences (Table 5–7)

TABLE 5–7

NCS	SNAP	CMAP
Anatomy examined:	Sensory nerve fibers	Motor nerve fibers, NMJ, muscle fibers
Pertinent latencies:	Peak or onset latency	Onset latency
Amplitude measurements:	Peak to peak, Microvolts (uV)	Baseline to peak, millivolts (mV)

Conduction Values

Description: The following normal values are proposed for the basic motor and sensory nerve conduction studies. Each electrodiagnostic lab may have different normal values and a space has been provided for those used in your lab. (Table 5-8)

TABLE 5–8 Normal Values Proposed for Basic Motor and Sensory NCS

Nerve	Values	Nerves	Values
Median Motor		**Sup. Radial Sensory**	
Distal latency	3.7 ± 0.3	Distal latency	2.3 ± 0.4
Amplitude	13.2 ± 5.0	Amplitude	31.0 ± 20.0
Conduction velocity	56.7 ± 0.2	Conduction velocity	58 ± 6.0
Median Sensory		**Peroneal Motor**	
Distal latency	3.2 ± 0.5	Distal latency	4.5 ± 0.8
Amplitude	41.2 ± 25.0	Amplitude	4.4 ± 1.4
Conduction velocity	56.9 ± 4.0	CV below fibula head	51.6 ± 4.1
		CV Above fibula head	53.9 ± 4.3
Ulnar Motor			
Distal latency	3.2 ± 0.5	**Tibial Motor**	
Amplitude	6.0 ± 1.9	Distal latency	3.4 ± 0.5
CV below elbow	61.8 ± 5.0	Amplitude	11.8 ± 4.5
CV above elbow	62.7 ± 5.5	Conduction velocity	53.9 ± 4.3
Ulnar Sensory		**Sural Sensory**	
Distal latency	3.2 ± 2.5	Distal latency	3.5 ± 0.2
Amplitude	34.0 ± 12.1	Amplitude	16.6 ± 7.5
Conduction velocity	57.0 ± 5.0	Conduction velocity	39.6 ± 2.3
Radial Motor		**Sup. Per. Sensory**	
Distal latency	2.4 ± 0.5	Distal latency	2.9 ± 0.3
Amplitude	14.0 ± 8.8	Amplitude	20.5 ± 6.1
Conduction velocity	61.9 ± 5.9	Conduction velocity	65.7 ± 3.7

H-REFLEX

Definition

This NCS creates a late response that is an electrically evoked analogue to a *monosynaptic reflex*. It is initiated with a 📖 *submaximal stimulus* at a long duration (0.5–1.0 milliseconds). This preferentially activates the *IA afferent* nerve fibers, causing an *orthodromic sensory* response to the spinal cord, and then an *orthodromic motor* response back to the recording electrode. The waveform can be potentiated with agonist muscle contraction and abolished with antagonist contraction or increased stimulation causing collision blocking. 📖 The morphology and latency remains constant with each stimulation at the appropriate intensity (Figure 5–43).

- **Function**
  It reflects a proximally traveling evoked potential. It is typically used to monitor for an S1 radiculopathy

- **Formula**
  H-reflex = 9.14 + 0.46 (Leg length in cm from the medial malleolus to the popliteal fossa) + 0.1 (age)

- **Latency**
  Normal: 28–30 mseconds
  Side to side difference: Greater than 1.0–2.0 milliseconds is significant
  Above 60 years: Adds 1.8 milliseconds.

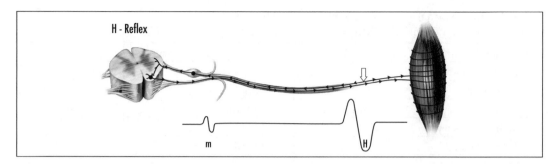

FIGURE 5–43. H-Reflex. The H response is obtained by stimulation of the afferent sensory fiber (top) resulting in orthodromic conduction to the spinal cord. In the spinal cord, there is synaptic stimulation of the alpha motor neuron, this results in the evoked H response in the muscle. A rudimentary M response is produced when a few motor axons are directly stimulated.

- **Location**
  Gastrocnemius/Soleus Complex: Tibial nerve; S1 pathway
  📖 Flexor Carpi Radialis: Median nerve; C6–C7 pathway
  📖 Possibly obtained in all nerves in adults with UMN (corticospinal tract) lesion and infants.

- **Limitations**
  This evaluates a long neural pathway, which can dilute focal lesions and hinder specificity of injury location. It can be normal with incomplete lesions. It does not distinguish between acute and chronic lesions. Once it is abnormal, it is always abnormal.

📖 F-WAVE

Definition

This NCS evokes a small late response from a short duration *supramaximal* stimulation. It initiates an *antidromic motor* response to the spinal cord followed by an *orthodromic motor* response to the recording electrode 📖 (Figure 5–44). It is approximately 5% of the CMAP height. The configuration and latency change with each stimulation. This is due to a *polysynaptic* response in the spinal cord, where Renshaw cells inhibit impulses from traveling the same path each time (Figure 5–45).

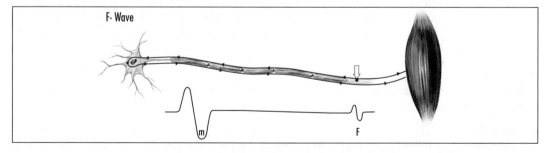

FIGURE 5–44. F-Wave. F response: Stimulation (dot) is followed by the source of depolarization (arrows). Initially depolarization travels in both directions: first directly to the muscle fiber producing the M response, and retrograde up to the axon and to the neuron, where it is repropogated in a small percentage of neurons back down the axons to produce the delayed F response.

- **Function**
  Helpful in polyneuropathies and plexopathies, but not overly useful in radiculopathies

- **Latency**
  Normal: Upper limb: 28 msec, Lower limb: 56 msec.
  Side to side difference: 2.0 msec difference in the upper limbs is significant.
  4.0 msec difference in lower limbs is significant.

- **Location**
  It can be obtained from any muscle.

- **Limitations**
  This evaluates a long neural pathway, which can dilute focal lesions and hinder specificity of injury location. It only accesses the motor fibers.

A-(AXON) WAVE

Definition

When performing a CMAP study, a response can be evoked by a submaximal stimulation and abolished with a supramaximal level. The stimulus can travel antidromically along the motor nerve and becomes diverted along a neural branch formed by collateral sprouting, due to a previous denervation and reinnervation process. 📖 It typically occurs between the CMAP and F-wave at a constant latency (Figure 5–46).

- **Function**
  This is not a NCS but does represent nerve damage with subsequent collateral sprouting.

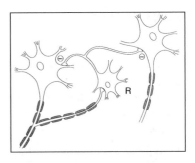

FIGURE 5–45. Renshaw Cell Activation. Inhibitory neurons, Renshaw cells (R), are activated by a stimulus and in turn, suppresses (-) firing of the alpha motor neuron. (Reprinted with permission from Dumitru D. Electrodiagnostic Medicine. Philadelphia, Hanley & Belfus, 1995.)

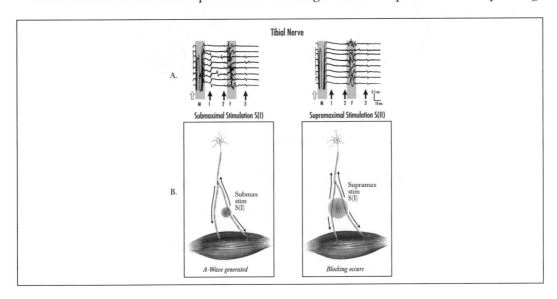

FIGURE 5–46. A-Wave. **A:** Arrows 1, 2, and 3 represent the A-waves. M is the CMAP and F is the F-wave. S(I)—weak stimulus, S(II) strong stimulus. (Note A-waves seen in S(I) are abolished.) **B:** S(I) A-wave generated, S(II) blocking occurs.

BLINK REFLEX

Definition

This NCS is an electrically evoked analogue to the corneal reflex. It is initiated by stimulating the *supraorbital branch* of the trigeminal nerve. The response propagates into the pons and branches to the lateral medulla. It then branches to innervate the ipsilateral and contralateral orbicularis oculi via the facial nerve. Two responses are evaluated, an ipsilateral R1 and bilateral R2. The blink is associated with the R2 response (Figures 5–47, 5–48, and Table 5–9).

TABLE 5–9   Blink Reflex Pathways

Pathway	Nerve Fibers
Afferent	Sensory branches of CN V (trigeminal nerve)
Efferent	Motor branches of CN VII (facial nerve)

Response	Course
R1 (Early)	Through the pons
R2 (Late)	Through the pons and lateral medulla

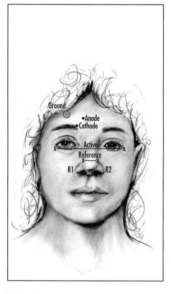

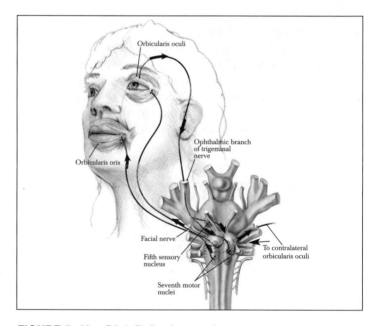

FIGURE 5–47.   Blink Reflex Study

FIGURE 5–48.   Blink Reflex Innervation

R1 is affected by lesions of the:	R2 is affected by:	
Trigeminal nerve	Consciousness level	Valium
Pons	Parkinson's disease	Habituation
Facial nerve	Lateral medullary syndrome	
	Contralateral hemisphere	

- **Function**

- **Latency (Figure 5–49)**
  Normal: R1 < 13 milliseconds
  R2 Ipsilateral (direct) < 40 milliseconds
  R2 Contralateral (consensual) < 41milliseconds

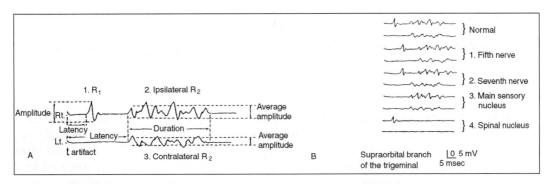

FIGURE 5–49. Blink Reflex Responses. **A:** The pons (1) is the pathway for R1. The pons and lateral medulla (2 and 3) is the pathway for R2. **B:** Different lesion sites along the reflex pathway.

DIRECT FACIAL NERVE STUDY

Definition

The NCS of CN VII (facial nerve) is performed by stimulating it distal to the stylomastoid foramen at the angle of the mandible. The response is recorded over the nasalis muscle. The patient can present with equal weakness in the upper and lower facial muscles with a peripheral nerve injury. If the lesion is rostral to the facial nerve nucleus (central), the lower facial muscles are more severely affected than the upper (Figure 5–50).

> **Synkinesis**
> An aberrant regeneration of axons can occur with facial nerve injuries leading to reinnervation of inappropriate muscles. This may present as lip twitching when closing an eye or crocodile tears when chewing.

- **Function**
  This monitors for injury to the facial nerve such as seen in Bell's palsy, neoplasms, fractures, middle ear infection, diabetes mellitus, mumps, Lyme disease, etc.

- **Findings**
  This can be monitored periodically over

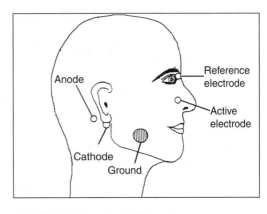

FIGURE 5–50. Facial Nerve Study

two weeks to access prognosis; better outcomes are anticipated for demyelinating vs. axonal injuries. Also, absence of an evoked potential in seven days indicates poor prognosis.

NCS	Amplitude Height
CMAP	Less then 10% of the unaffected side indicates a poor outcome. Recovery > 1 year to incomplete.
CMAP	Between 10–30% of the unaffected side indicates a fair prognosis. Recovery within 2–8 months.
CMAP	Greater than 30% of the unaffected side indicates a good prognosis. Recovery within 2 months.

Treatment
📖 Interventions may include: Prednisone, massage, or electrical stimulation

■

SOMATOSENSORY EVOKED POTENTIALS (SSEP)

DEFINITION

This study evaluates time-locked responses of the nervous system to an external stimulus. They represent the function of the ascending sensory pathways using an afferent potential, which travels from the peripheral nerve to the plexus, root, spinal cord (posterior column), contralateral medial lemniscus, thalamus, to the somatosensory cortex. It is initiated by a repetitive submaximal stimulation of a sensory nerve, mixed nerve or dermatome and is recorded from the spine or scalp (Figure 5–51).

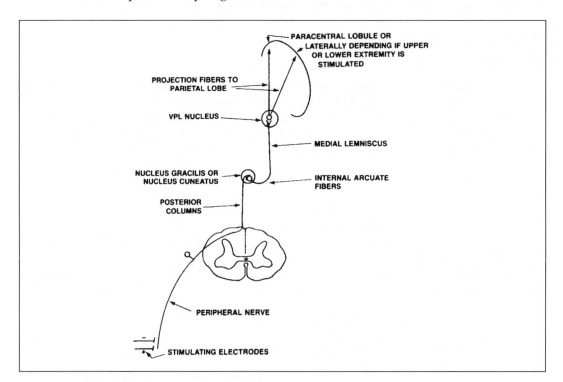

FIGURE 5–51. Somatosensory Evoked Potential Pathways from the Peripheral Nerve to the Parietal Cortex. The fasciculus gracilis is monitored when a lower extremity nerve is stimulated and the fasciculus cuneatus is monitored when an upper extremity nerve is stimulated. (Reprinted with permission from Dumitru D. Electrodiagnostic Medicine. Philadelphia, Hanley & Belfus, 1995.)

• Function

SSEP monitors for problems such as: (a) peripheral nerve injuries, (b) CNS lesions such as 📖 multiple sclerosis (increased interpeak latency), or (c) intra-operative monitoring of spinal surgery. 📖 During spinal surgery the loss of the tibial nerve potentials with preservation of the median nerve indicates an injury. Anesthesia will affect both the upper and lower limbs.

Recording Sites:

Median Nerve (Figure 5–52)
- N9—Erb's point
- N11—Roots
- N13—Cervical medullary junction (nucleus cuneatus)
- N20—Cortical

Tibial Nerve (Figure 5–53)
- PF—Popliteal Fossa
- L3—Third Lumbar
- N22—T12 and lumbosacral spine
- N45—Cortical

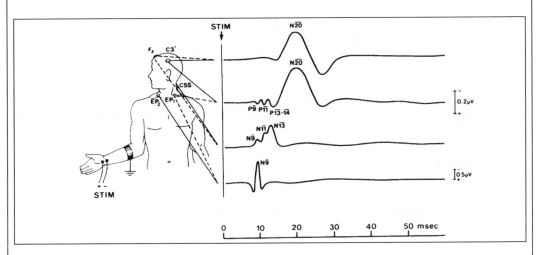

FIGURE 5–52. Median Nerve SSEP. (From Spehlmann R. Evoked Potential Primer. Boston, Butterworth Publishers, 1985, with permission.)

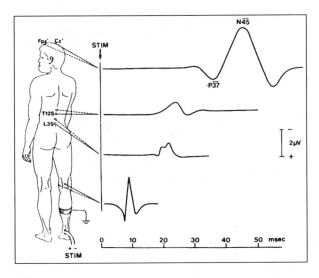

FIGURE 5–53. Tibial Nerve SSEP. (From Spehlmann R. Evoked Potential Primer. Boston, Butterworth Publishers, 1985, with permission.)

- **Advantages**

SSEP theoretically evaluates the sensory components of the peripheral and central nervous systems. Abnormal results occur immediately.

- **Limitations**
  - It only evaluates the nerve fibers, sensing vibration and proprioception.
  - It evaluates a long neural pathway, which may dilute focal lesions and hinder specificity of injury location.
  - It can be adversely affected by sleep and high dose general anesthetics (halothane, enflurane, isoflurane). This may be avoided with nitrous oxide or low dose isoflurane.

■

BASIC NEEDLE EMG

DEFINITION

This study accesses nerve and muscle function. A needle electrode is placed into a muscle and parameters including insertional activity, resting activity, and voluntary electric activity are monitored.

INSERTIONAL ACTIVITY

Definition

This is an electrical injury potential. It represents discharges mechanically provoked by disrupting the cell muscle membrane with a needle electrode (Figure 5–54 and Table 5-10).

TABLE 5–10 Insertional Activity

Characteristic	Normal	Increased	Decreased
Duration	300ms	> 300–500ms	< 300ms
Etiology	• Muscle depolarization	• Denervation • Irritable cell membrane	• Fat • Fibrosis • Edema • Electrolyte abnormalities

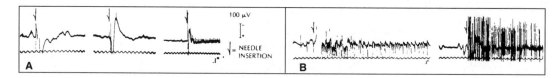

FIGURE 5–54. Insertional Activity. **A:** Normal. **B:** Increased.

RESTING ACTIVITY

- **Normal Spontaneous Activity**

Definition

After a needle is inserted into a normal muscle, there should be electrical silence at rest. However, if it is placed into the neuromuscular junction, two waveforms can occur: miniature endplate potentials (MEPP) and end plate potentials (EPP). Needle placement in this area is painful but these waveforms also indicate that the muscle has maintained its innervation (Figure 5–55 and Table 5–11).

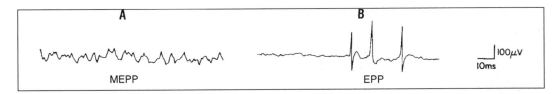

FIGURE 5–55. Endplate Activity: **A:** MEPP—Monophasic negative potentials primarily present as baseline irregularities because of their small amplitude. **B:** EPP—Biphasic, usually negative single fiber action potential.

- **Miniature Endplate Potentials (MEPP)**
  Description: This "endplate noise" is due to spontaneous quanta release, which occurs every five seconds. It results in a 10-50µV non-propagated potential seen on the screen as an irregular baseline when they are recorded with a standard extracellular needle electrode.

- **Endplate Potentials (EPP)**
  Description: This endplate spike is due to increased acetylcholine release, provoked by needle irritation of the muscle fiber, or synchronization of several MEPPs. It results in a propagated single muscle fiber action potential. Its hallmark sign is its irregularity and it can present with a positive deflection if the needle electrode is placed in the endplate.

TABLE 5–11   Normal Spontaneous Activity

Characteristics	MEPP	EPP
Initial Deflection	Negative (monophasic)	Negative (biphasic)
Duration	0.5–1.0 ms	2.0–4.0 ms
Amplitude	10–50 µV	<1000 µV (1 mV)
Rate	150 Hz	50–100 Hz
Rhythm	Irregular	Irregular
Origin	Endplate	Endplate/provoked
Sound	Sea shell murmur	Sputtering fat in a frying pan

- **Abnormal Spontaneous Activity**

Definition
These pathologic waveforms can be generated from a muscle or neural source. If originating from a muscle source, the activity can represent lack of muscle fiber innervation. The RMP becomes less negative and unstable, causing it to approach the threshold to activate an action potential. It either fires independent of external stimulation or is induced by needle movement. If neural in origin, it can have the appearance of (MUAPs).

1. Muscle Generated

- **Fibrillation Potentials (FIB) (Figure 5–56) (Table 5–12, 5–13)**
  Description: These are spontaneously firing action potentials originating from denervated single muscle fibers, secondary to uncontrolled ACh release. Its hallmark sign is its regularity of firing.

2. Neural Generated

- **Positive Sharp Waves (PSW) (Figure 5–57) (Table 5–12, 5–13)**
  Description: These are spontaneous firing action potentials stimulated by needle movement of an injured muscle fiber. There is propagation to, but not past, the needle tip. This inhibits the display of the negative deflection of the waveform.

TABLE 5–12   Characteristics of Fibrillations and Positive Sharp Waves

Characteristics	FIB	PSW
Initial Deflection	Positive (biphasic)	Positive (Biphasic)
Duration	1–5 ms	10–30 ms
Amplitude	Early: > 300 μV, Late: < 25 μV	< 1 mV
Rate	1–10 Hz	1–20 Hz
Rhythm	Regular	Regular
Origin	Postjunctional	Postjunctional
Sound	Rain on a tin roof	Dull thud or chug

TABLE 5–13   Grading of Fibrillation Potentials and Positive Sharp Waves

Grade	Characteristics
0	None
1+	Persistent single runs > 1 second in two areas
2+	Moderate runs > 1 second in three or more areas
3+	Many discharges in most muscle regions
4+	Continuous discharges in all areas of the muscle

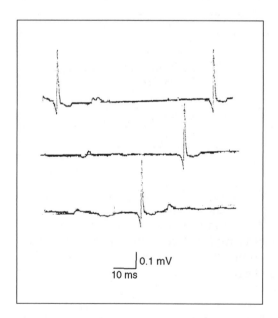

0.1 mV
10 ms

FIGURE 5–56.   Fibrillation Potential.

+ PSW   ++ PSW

+++ PSW   ++++ PSW

0.1 mV
10 ms

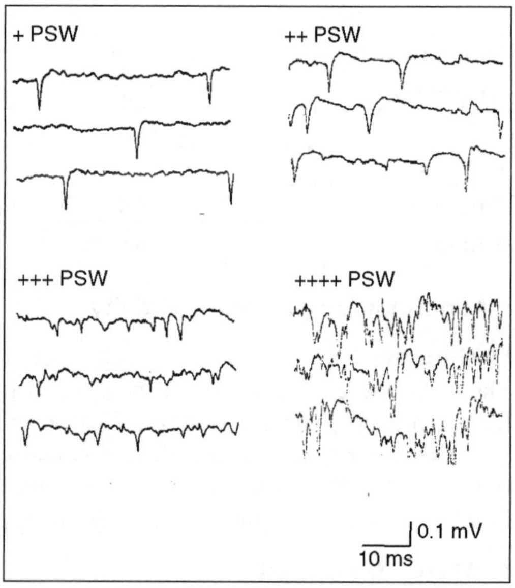

FIGURE 5–57.   Positive Sharp Waves.

Etiology
Examples: *Nerve disorders:* Anterior horn cell disease, radiculopathy, plexopathy, peripheral neuropathy, mononeuropathy. *Neuromuscular junction disorders:* Myasthenia gravis, botulism. *Muscle disorders:* Muscular dystrophy, polymyositis, dermatomyositis, hyperkalemic periodic paralysis, acid maltase deficiency.

- **Complex Repetitive Discharges (CRD) (Figure 5–58) (Table 5–14)**
Description: These bizarre high frequency discharges are action potentials originating from a principle pacemaker, initiating a group of single muscle fibers to fire in near synchrony.

The current spreads to the other muscle fibers by ephaptic transmission. This results from a process in which denervated muscle fibers are reinnervated by collateral sprouting from axons of a neighboring motor unit. When these fibers, in turn, become denervated, a population of muscle fibers now belonging to one motor unit lacks neural control. These muscle fibers lie in close proximity to each other and serve as a circuit for the pacemaker fiber. *Its hallmark sign is its regular interval between each discharge and within each discharge* (Figure 5–59).

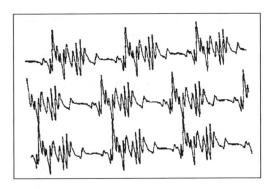

FIGURE 5–58. Complex Repetitive Discharges.

TABLE 5–14 Complex Repetitive Discharges

Characteristics	CRD
Initial deflection	Resembles: FIB, PSW, MUAP
Amplitude	50–1000μV
Rate	10–100Hz
Rhythm	Regular/abrupt start and stop
Origin	Postjunctional/ephaptic transmission
Sound	Motor boat

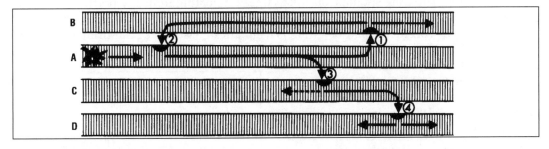

FIGURE 5–59. Ephaptic Transmission. Fiber A acts as the pacemaker. It transmits an impulse to B, C, and D, which perpetuates the cycle. (From Trontelji J, Stalberg EV. Bizarre repetitive discharges recorded with single fiber EMG. J Neurol Neurosurg Psychiatry 1983;46:310-16, with permission from BMJ Publishing Group.)

Etiology
Examples: *Nerve disorders:* Anterior horn cell disease, chronic radiculopathy, peripheral neuropathy. *Muscle disorders:* Polymyositis, dermatomyositis, muscular dystrophy, limb-girdle dystrophy, myxedema. *Normal variant.*

- **Myotonic Discharges (Figure 5–60) (Table 5–15)**

  Description: These are single muscle fiber action potentials triggered by needle movement, percussion, or voluntary contraction. They are caused by an alteration of the ion channels in the muscle membrane and can be seen with or without clinical myotonia. Its hallmark sign is the smooth change in rate and amplitude.

TABLE 5–15   Myotonic Discharges

Characteristics	Myotonic Discharges
Initial Deflection	Resembles: EPP, FIB, PSW
Duration	>5–20ms
Amplitude	20–300µV
Rate	20–100Hz
Rhythm	Wax and wane
Origin	Postjunctional
Sound	Dive bomber

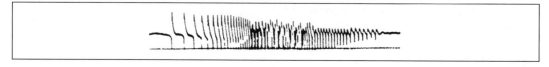

FIGURE 5–60.   Myotonic Discharges.

Etiology

Examples: *Nerve disorders:* Chronic radiculopathy, peripheral neuropathy. *Muscle disorders:* Myotonic dystrophy, myotonia congenita, paramyotonia, polymyositis, dermatomyositis, maltase deficiency, hyperkalemic periodic paralysis. *Medications:* Propranolol.

2. Neural Generated

- **Fasciculations (Figure 5–61) (Tables 5–16)**

  Description: These are spontaneous discharges originating from any portion of a single motor unit and result in intermittent muscle fiber contraction. If associated with FIB or PSW they are considered pathological. Its hallmark sign is an irregular firing motor unit. Normal voluntary motor unit firing does not occur at the slow rates seen with pathological fasciculations.

TABLE 5–16   Fasiculations

Characteristics	Fasciculations
Initial Deflection	Resembles: MUAP
Duration	5–15 ms
Amplitude	<300 µV
Rate	0.1–10 Hz
Rhythm	Irregular
Origin	Prejunctional
Sound	Variable

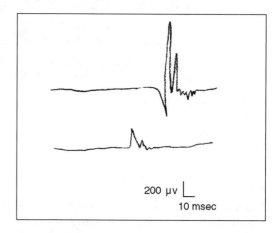

200 µv

10 msec

FIGURE 5–61.   Fasciculations.

TABLE 5–17   Grading of Fasciculations

Grade	Characteristic
0	None
+/-	Equivocal
1+	In two areas, 2–10/minute
2+	In many areas, 10–15/minute
3+	All areas, < 60/minute
4+	All areas, > 60/minute

Etiology
Examples: Nerve disorders: Anterior horn cell disease, tetany, Creutzfeldt-Jakob syndrome, radiculopathy, mononeuropathy. *Metabolic disorders:* Thyrotoxicosis, tetany. *Normal variant.*

- **Myokymic Discharges (Figure 5–62) (Table 5–18)**
  Description: These are groups of MUAPs firing repetitively. They can be associated with a clinical myokymia, which presents as slow continuous muscle fiber contractions. This gives a rippling appearance to the overlying skin. Its hallmark sign is the semiregularity between each discharge and within each discharge.

TABLE 5–18   Myokymic Discharges

Characteristics	Myokymic Discharges
Initial Deflection	Groups of MUAPs
Amplitude	100 µV–2 mV
Rate	Discharge: 40–60 Hz, Interdischarge: 0.1–10 Hz
Rhythm	Semi-regular
Origin	Prejunctional
Sound	Marching soldiers

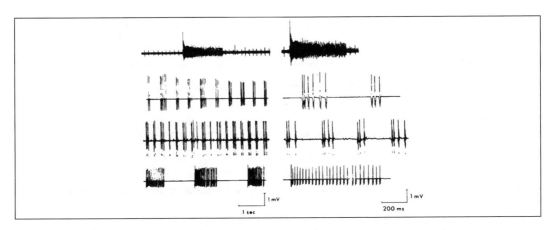

FIGURE 5–62.   Myokymic Discharges. (From Albers JW, Allen AA, Bastron JD, et al.: Limb myokymia. Muscle Nerve 1981: 4;494-504, John Wiley & Sons, Inc., with permission.)

Etiology
Examples: Nerve disorders: Facial Myokymia—Multiple sclerosis, brainstem neoplasm, polyradiculopathy, Bell's palsy. *Extremity Myokymia*—Radiation plexopathy, compression neuropathy, rattlesnake venom.

- **Neuromyotonic Discharges (Figure 5–63) (Table 5–19)**
  Description: These are discharges originating from motor axons. They are classically seen in neuromyotonia (Isaac's syndrome). This is a disorder associated with continuous muscle fiber activity resulting in the appearance of muscle rippling and stiffness, secondary to irritable nerves. The progressive decrement of its waveform is due to single muscle fiber fatigue and drop off.

TABLE 5–19 Neuromyotonic Discharges

Characteristics	Neuromyotonic Discharges
Duration	Discharges continuously or in bursts
Amplitude	Progressive decrement
Rate	100–300 Hz
Sound	Ping or Kawasaki motorcycle sound
Appearance	Tornadolike

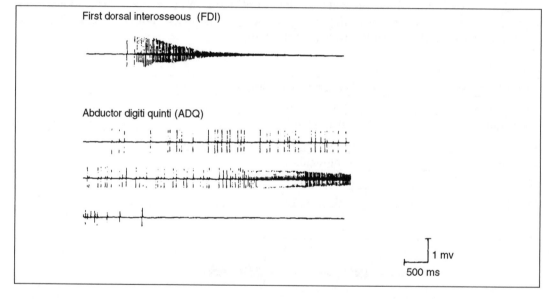

FIGURE 5–63. Neuromyotonic Discharges in Spinal Muscular Atrophy.

Etiology
Examples: *Nerve disorder:* Anterior horn cell disease, tetany. *Toxins:* Anticholinesterase.

- **Cramp Discharges (Figure 5–64) (Table 5–20)**
  Description: These are discharges associated with involuntary repetitive firing of MUAPs in a large area of muscle. They are usually associated with a painful muscle contraction.

TABLE 5–20 Cramp Discharges

Characteristics	Cramp Discharges
Duration	Gradual start and stop
Amplitude	Up to 1 mV
Rate	40–150 Hz
Rhythm	Irregular

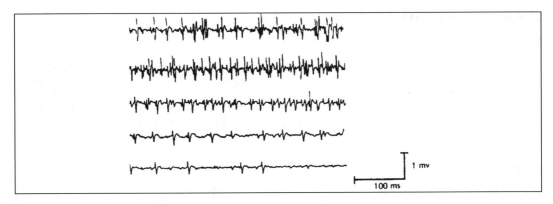

FIGURE 5–64. Muscle Cramp Discharges.

Etiology
Examples: Salt depletion, uremia, pregnancy, myxedema, prolonged muscle contraction, myotonia congenita, myotonic dystrophy, Stiff-man's syndrome.

- **Artifact Potentials**
  Description: These are waveforms that obscure the neurophysiologic signals. Interference potentials are unwanted signals occurring from outside the system being studied. Noise is described as unwanted signals occurring from within the system. They arise from the EMG instrument, printer, unshielded power cords, electrical outlets or fluorescent lights (Figures 5–65 and 5–66).

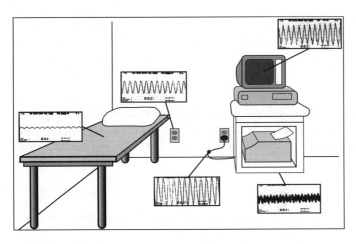

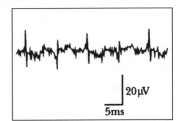

FIGURE 5–66. Fluorescent Light Interference. (Reprinted with permission from Dumitru D. Electrodiagnostic Medicine. Philadelphia, Hanley & Belfus, 1995.)

FIGURE 5–65. Source of Noise and Interference. Noise is greatest near electrical outlets, power cords, and equipment including the EMG instrument itself.

EXERTIONAL ACTIVITY

Definition

Voluntary muscle activity can be electrically recorded as a motor unit action potential.

- **Motor Unit Action Potential (MUAP)**
  Description: This is a compound action potential from muscle fibers belonging to a single motor unit, within the recording range of the needle electrode. Its territory is typically 5–15 mm (Figure 5–67) (Table 5–21).

Parameters

- **Amplitude**
This represents the muscle fibers recorded near the needle electrode. It is measured from the most positive to the most negative peak. It can be increased from a reinnervation process, decreased from loss of muscle fibers, or variable due to blocking associated with neuromuscular junction disorders.
Normal: 1 mV.

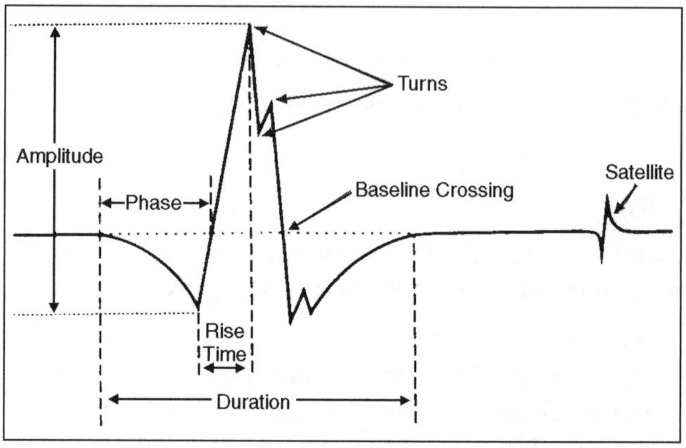

FIGURE 5–67. Motor Unit Action Potential

- **Rise Time**
This represents the time it takes the MUAP to go from its baseline to the peak of the negative wave. It represents proximity of the needle to the motor unit.
Normal: Less than 500 μs

- **Duration**
This represents the number of muscle fibers within the motor unit. It is measured from the waveform's initial departure from baseline to its final return. It increases (< 15 msec) as the motor unit territory increases from collateral sprouting or decreases (> 5 msec) with the loss of muscle fibers.
Normal: 5–15 ms

- **Turns**
These are changes in the direction of the waveform that do not cross the baseline. They are also called serrations.

- **Phases**
This represents the synchronicity of muscle fiber action potentials firing. They are calculated as the number of baseline crossings plus 1. Five or more baseline crossings represent *polyphasicity*. This can result from pathology causing muscle fiber dropout, alterations in fiber conduction velocity, or reinnervation from collateral sprouting. However, this can occur normally 15% (concentric needle) or 30% (monopolar needle) of the time in adults or higher in the elderly.
Normal: 2–4

TABLE 5–21 Motor Unit Action Potentials (MUAPs)

Characteristics	MUAP
Initial deflection	Positive/negative
Duration	5–15 ms
Amplitude	1 μV – 2 mV
Rise Time	< 500 ms
Phases	2–4
Rate	Exertion dependent
Rhythm	Exertion dependent
Origin	Prejunctional

Abnormalities

- **Long Duration, Large Amplitude Polyphasic Potentials (LDLA)**
  Description: These typically occur from collateral sprouting. This reinnervation process causes an increased number of muscle fibers per motor unit. It is most commonly seen in neuropathic diseases but can also occur in chronic myopathic disease from fiber splitting, as seen in an inflammatory or dystrophic myopathy. The recruitment patterns help distinguish between a myopathic or neuropathic process.

- **Short Duration, Small Amplitude Polyphasic Potentials (SDSA)**
  Description: These typically occur from a dropout or dysfunction of muscle fibers. It is most commonly seen in myopathic diseases and neuromuscular junction disorders. It can also occur from a severe neuropathic injury leading to nascent motor unit potentials resulting from axon regrowth. Again, the two processes are differentiated by their recruitment patterns.

- **Neuropathic Potentials**
  Description: This refers to long duration, large amplitude MUAPs that occur from a denervation and reinnervation process typically seen in neuropathies. This terminology lacks the appropriate quantitative description of the motor unit parameters. It is not considered accurate because certain disease processes mimic MUAP features, regardless of whether the pathology originated in nerve or muscle.

- **Myopathic Potentials**
  Description: This refers to short duration small amplitude MUAPs that occur from muscle disorders. This terminology lacks the appropriate quantitative description of the motor unit parameters. It is not considered accurate because certain disease processes mimic MUAP features, regardless if the pathology is muscle or nerve in origin.

- **Unstable Potentials**
  Description: This refers to the occurrence of variations in the MUAP's amplitude and duration. Most commonly it is seen in neuromuscular junction disorders, which cause blocking of discharges. It also can occur in motor neuron disorders, neuropathic disorders, or muscle trauma.

- **Satellite Potentials**
  Description: This is a small potential originating from a few muscle fibers. They are time-locked to occur approximately 10–15 milliseconds after a MUAP. It can be due to incomplete myelin formation and immature terminal sprouts from chronic reinnervation or a myopathy.

- **Doublet/Multiplet Potentials**
  Description: This refers to two or more MUAPs firing recurrently and together in a semirhythmic fashion. It is seen in ischemia, hyperventilation, tetany, motor neuron disorder or metabolic diseases.

- **Giant Potentials**
  Description: This refers to the extremely large MUAPs (> 5 mV) that occur in disease process, such as poliomyelitis. These are also described as large amplitude potentials.

MINIMAL CONTRACTION

RECRUITMENT

Definition

This is the successive activation of additional motor units to increase the force of a contraction.

- **Types (Figure 5–68) (Table 5–22)**
  - **Normal**
  The Rule of Fives—The onset frequency of the first MUAP begins at approximately 5 Hz. To generate more force, the firing rate and recruitment of more motor units must be increased. When the firing rate reaches approximately 10 Hz, a second MUAP begins at approximately 5 Hz. When the first MUAP reaches a rate of 15 Hz, the second should be at 10 Hz and a third will begin at 5 Hz. As more force is needed, the firing rate of the first may reach 20 Hz, the second 15 Hz, the third 10 Hz, and a fourth will begin at approximately 5 Hz.

TABLE 5–22   Normal Recruitment

First (A)	Second (B)	Third (C)	Fourth (D)
A—5 Hz			
A—10 Hz	B—5 Hz		
A—15 Hz	B—10 Hz	C—5 Hz	
A—20 Hz	B—15 Hz	C—10 Hz	D—5 Hz

- **Reduced**
  The firing of only a few MUAPs with even a maximal contraction is most commonly seen in neuropathic conditions. However, this can also be due to any disorder that destroys or blocks axonal conduction or muscle fibers.

- **Early**
  The firing of many MUAPs with a mild contraction is most commonly seen in myopathic conditions that result in a loss of muscle fibers. This loss causes less force to be generated per motor unit, thus more motor units must now be called upon.

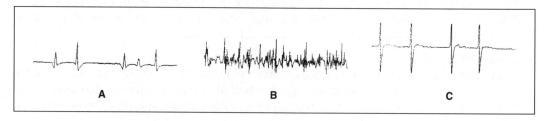

FIGURE 5–68.   Motor Unit Recruitment. **A:** Normal. **B:** Early ("Myopathic"). **C:** Decreased ("Neuropathic").

FIRING PATTERNS

- **Firing Rate (FR)**
  This is the number of times an MUAP fires per second. It is expressed in Hertz (Hz) and is calculated by dividing 1000 by the Interspike Interval (II), measured in milliseconds. The FR = 1000/Interspike Interval (Figure 5–69).

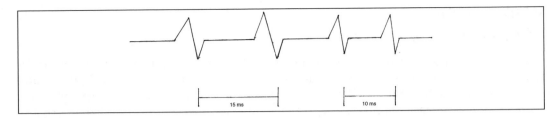

FIGURE 5–69. Firing Rate (FR): 100/13 = ~75.

- ### Recruitment Frequency (RF)

  This is the FR of the first MUAP when a second MUAP begins to fire. It is initiated by an increase in the force of a contraction. Normal is considered 20 Hz or below. Values above this correlate with a neuropathic process.

- ### Recruitment Interval (RI)

  This is the interspike interval (in milliseconds) between two discharges of the same MUAP when a second MUAP begins to fire. It is initiated by an increase in the force of a contraction. Normal is considered approximately 100 ms.

- ### RI vs. RF

The following parameters help distinguish between a neuropathic and myopathic process.

Firing Pattern	Neuropathy	Myopathy
Recruitment Interval	↓	↑
Recruitment Frequency	↑	↓

- **Decreased RI (Increased RF)**
  A loss of motor units restricts additional motor unit activation to increase contractile force. This causes the first motor unit to fire more rapidly until a second motor unit finally joins in. This shortens the interval between successive MUAPs from one motor unit.

- **Increased RI (Decreased RF)**
  A loss of muscle fibers causes a second motor unit to join in early to help increase contractile force. This occurs before the first motor unit has the opportunity to increase its firing frequency. This lengthens the interval between successive MUAPs from one motor unit.

- **Recruitment Ratio (RR)**
  Description: This has been used to represent recruitment capabilities, especially when a patient demonstrates difficulty in controlling a contractile force. It is calculated by dividing the FR of the first MUAP by the number of different MUAPs on the screen. A motor unit firing at 10 Hz when two different MUAPs are viewed on the screen demonstrates a RR of 5. 10 Hz/2 different MUAP = 5. The normal RR is considered less than 10 (Figure 5–70).

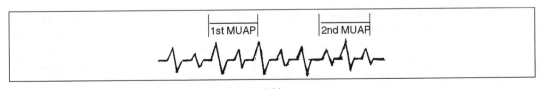

FIGURE 5–70. Recruitment Ratio: $\dfrac{10\ Hz}{2\ different\ MUAP} = 5$

MAXIMAL EFFORT

• Interference Pattern

Description: This is a qualitative or quantitative description of the sequential appearance of MUAPs. It is the electrical activity recorded from a muscle during a maximum voluntary contraction. It is comprised of *recruitment* plus *activation*. Activation is the ability of a motor unit to fire faster to produce a greater contractile force and is controlled by a central process. It can be decreased in CNS diseases, pain, and hysteria. Furthermore, if a patient is asked to generate a force and only a few MUAPs are seen while the Hz continue to remain low, it can indicate decreased activation from poor patient cooperation and is not the result of abnormal recruitment.

Patterns (Figure 5–71)	Presentation
Complete	No individual MUAPs can be seen. A full screen represents 4–5 MUAPs
Reduced	Some MUAPs are identified on the screen during a full contraction
Discrete	Each MUAP can be identified on the screen during a full contraction
Single Unit	One MUAP is identified on the screen during a full contraction

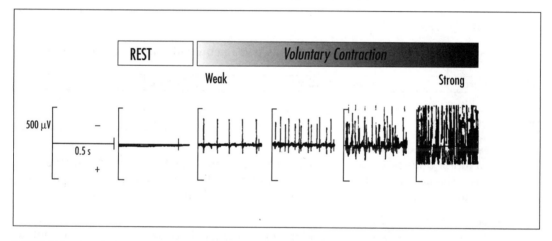

FIGURE 5–71.   Interference Patterns: Representation of Normal Recruitment Patterns.

■

RADICULOPATHY

DEFINITION

This is a pathologic process affecting the nerves at the root level. In descending order, it most commonly presents as pure sensory complaints, sensorimotor complaints, or pure motor complaints. This is due to the larger size of the sensory fibers rendering them more prone to injury. A pure sensory injury would demonstrate a negative EMG. Sensory NCS would be normal due to sparing of the DRG (Figure 5–72).

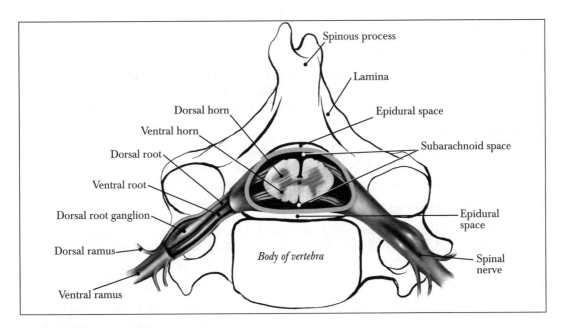

FIGURE 5–72. Cervical Spine Cross Section.

ETIOLOGY

• Common

Herniated nucleus pulposus: Most common. Typically seen in adults below 50 years of age.
Spondylosis: Typically seen more commonly in adults above 50 years of age.

• Uncommon: "Hi Madam"

H—Herpes Zoster
I—Inflammatory: TB, Lyme disease, HIV, syphilis, cryptococcus, and sarcoidosis

M—Metastasis
A—Arachnoiditis: Myelogram, surgery, steroids, and anesthesia
D—Diabetes mellitus
A—Abscess
M—Mass: Meningioma, neurofibroma, leukemia, lipoma, cysts, and hematoma

CLINICAL PRESENTATION (Table 5–23)

TABLE 5–23 Clinical Presentation of Radiculopathy

Nerve Root	Reduced Reflex	Weakness	Numbness/Paresthesias
C5	Biceps brachii	Elbow flexion	Lateral arm
C6	Brachioradialis	Wrist extension	Lateral forearm
C7	Triceps brachii	Elbow extension	Middle finger
C8	None	Finger flexion	Medial forearm
T1	None	Finger adduction	Medial elbow
L4	Patella tendon	Knee extension	Medial ankle
L5	?—Hamstring	Hallux extension	Dorsal foot
S1	Achilles tendon	Plantar flexion	Lateral ankle

EDX FINDINGS

• Nerve Conduction Studies

SNAP: Normal. The lesion is located proximal to the dorsal root ganglion.
CMAP: Reduced amplitude. The lesion is distal to the motor neuron. It can be normal if the injury is purely demyelinating, incomplete, or reinnervation has occurred.

• Late Responses

H-reflex: Possibly abnormal in an S–1 radiculopathy.
F-waves: This is not overly sensitive or specific for a radiculopathy. Muscles have more than one root innervation, which can result in a normal response.

• Somatosensory Evoked Potentials

Advantage: It monitors sensory pathways and proximal demyelinating injuries.
Disadvantage: The long pathway monitored can mask focal lesions between the recording sites.

• EMG

📖 Classically FIBs or PSWs should be found in two different muscles innervated by two different peripheral nerves originating from the same root. They may not be found if the lesion is demyelinating, purely sensory, post reinnervation, or missed by random sampling.

• Cervical Myotomes (Table 5–24)

TABLE 5–24

Root	C3/C4	C5	C6	C7	C8/T1
Etiology	C2/C3 disc lesion	C4 disc lesion	C5 disc lesion	C6 disc lesion	C7 disc lesion
Muscles Involved	Clinical diagnosis No discrete myotomal patterns Innervates the posterior and lateral scalp Patient may complain of headaches C2 and C3 nerve becomes the greater and lesser occipital nerve	Rhomboids Deltoid Biceps brachii Supraspinatus Infraspinatus Brachialis BR Supinator Paraspinals	Deltoid Biceps brachii BR Supraspinatus Infraspinatus Supinator PT FCR EDC Paraspinals	PT FCR EDC Triceps brachii Paraspinals	Triceps Brachii (8) FCU FDP ADM FDI PQ APB Paraspinals

• Lumbosacral Myotomes (Table 5–25)

TABLE 5–25

Roots	L2/3/4	L5	S1	S2/3/4
Etiology	L1/L2/L3 disc lesion	L4 disc lesion	L5 disc lesion	Iatrogenic
Muscles Involved	Iliopsoas Iliacus Gracilis Adductor longus Vastus medialis TA Paraspinals Difficult to distinguish between radiculopathy and alternate lesions due to only two peripheral nerves	Gluteus maximus Gluteus medius TFL TA MG Medial hamstring TP PL Paraspinals	Gluteus maximus Gluteus medius TFL MG Medial hamstring PL TP Paraspinals	Abductor hallucis ADQ Needle exam of the external anal sphincter Other clinical presentations to monitor: Bulbocavernosus reflex, anal wink, external sphincter tone, and bowel and bladder function

- 📖 **Dual Innervated Muscles (Table 5–26)**

TABLE 5–26

Muscle	Nerves	
Pectoralis major	Medial pectoral	Lateral pectoral nerve
Brachialis	Musculocutaneus nerve	Radial nerve
Flexor digitorum profundus	Median nerve (AIN)	Ulnar nerve
Lumbricals	Median nerve	Ulnar nerve
Flexor pollices brevis	Median nerve	Ulnar nerve
Pectineus	Femoral nerve	Obturator nerve
Adductor magnus	Sciatic nerve (tibial portion)	Obturator nerve
Biceps femoris	Sciatic nerve (tibial portion)	Sciatic nerve (peroneal portion)

- **Chronology of Findings (Table 5–27)**

TABLE 5–27

Time	Abnormality
0	Decreased recruitment Decreased recruitment interval Prolonged F-wave. Abnormal H-reflex (S1 radiculopathy)
4 days	Decreased CMAP amplitude (~50% compared to opposite side)
1 week	Abnormal spontaneous activity occurs first in the paraspinals. They can be normal if: • They become reinnervated • The posterior primary rami are spared They can be the only abnormal finding 10–30% of the time
2 weeks	Abnormal spontaneous activity beginning in the limbs
3 weeks	Abnormal activity present in the paraspinals and limbs
5–6 weeks	Reinnervation
6 months–1 year	Increased amplitude from reinnervated motor unit

■

PLEXOPATHY

DEFINITION

This is a pathologic process typically occurring distal to the DRG and proximal to the peripheral nerves. Abnormalities can appear diffuse and will not follow any particular dermatomal or myotomal distribution.

ETIOLOGY

Pathology can occur from: (a) Trauma (stretch, traction, transection, obstetrical injuries, compression, and hemorrhage); (b) Cancer (tumor and radiation therapy); (c) Idiopathic (neuralgic amyotrophy)

EDX FINDINGS

- **NCS**
  SNAP: Abnormalities depend on the site of plexus injury
  CMAP: Abnormalities depend on the site of plexus injury

- **Late Response**

  F-wave: Possibly useful
  H-reflex: Possibly useful

- **EMG**

  Normal paraspinal activity. Abnormal activity in the peripheral muscles

BRACHIAL PLEXUS

Anatomy

- **Origin**

These nerve fibers originate from the anterior rami of the C5–T1 nerve roots, which further divide to form the trunks, division, cords, and branches.

- **Course**

The anterior rami emerge between the anterior and middle scalene muscles. In the posterior triangle of the neck C5 and C6 form the upper trunk, C7 forms the middle trunk, and C8 and T1 form the lower trunk. The trunks pass the clavicle and form anterior and posterior divisions to become cords. The cords are named in their relation to the axillary artery. The three posterior divisions of the upper, middle, and lower trunk form the posterior cord. The lateral cord is formed from the anterior divisions of the upper and middle trunk and the medial cord is formed by the anterior divisions of the lower trunk. The lateral cord splits to form the musculocutaneous branch and also fuses with the medial cord to form the median branch. The posterior cord splits into the radial and axillary branches and the medial cord splits to contribute to the median branch and the ulnar branch (Figure 5–73).

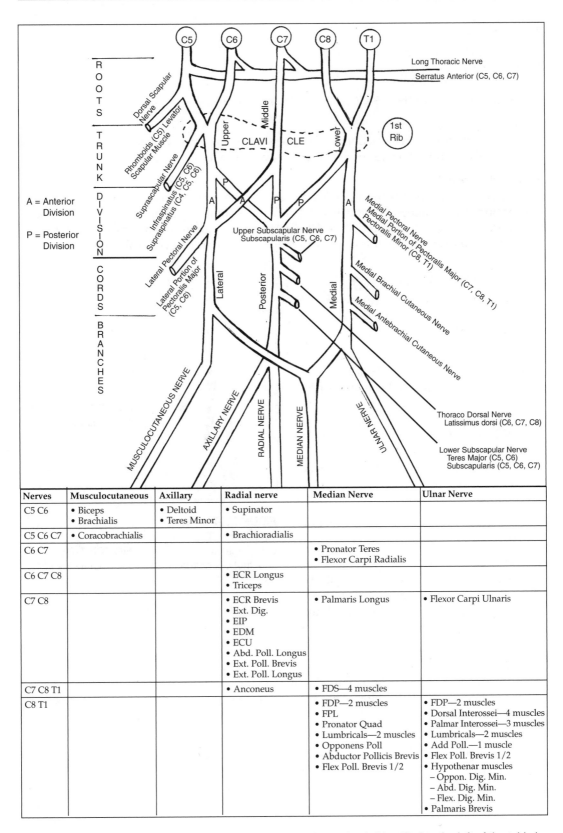

Nerves	Musculocutaneous	Axillary	Radial nerve	Median Nerve	Ulnar Nerve
C5 C6	• Biceps • Brachialis	• Deltoid • Teres Minor	• Supinator		
C5 C6 C7	• Coracobrachialis		• Brachioradialis		
C6 C7				• Pronator Teres • Flexor Carpi Radialis	
C6 C7 C8			• ECR Longus • Triceps		
C7 C8			• ECR Brevis • Ext. Dig. • EIP • EDM • ECU • Abd. Poll. Longus • Ext. Poll. Brevis • Ext. Poll. Longus	• Palmaris Longus	• Flexor Carpi Ulnaris
C7 C8 T1			• Anconeus	• FDS—4 muscles	

C8 T1				• FDP—2 muscles
				• FPL
				• Pronator Quad
				• Lumbricals—2 muscles
				• Opponens Poll
				• Abductor Pollicis Brevis
				• Flex Poll. Brevis 1/2
					• FDP—2 muscles
					• Dorsal Interossei—4 muscles
					• Palmar Interossei—3 muscles
					• Lumbricals—2 muscles
					• Add Poll.—1 muscle
					• Flex Poll. Brevis 1/2
					• Hypothenar muscles
					  – Oppon. Dig. Min.
					  – Abd. Dig. Min.
					  – Flex. Dig. Min.
					• Palmaris Brevis

FIGURE 5–73. Brachial Plexus. (Root level of individual muscles is identified to the left of the table.)

Injury

Erb's Palsy

- *General*
  This injury involves the C5–C6 nerve roots or upper trunk.

- *Etiology*
  It can occur from nerve traction or compression or from an obstectrical injury. It can be sports-related (Stinger) and involve the cervical nerve roots.

- *Clinical Presentation*
  A classic manifestation is the *Waiter's tip* position. The arm becomes adducted (deltoid and supraspinatus weakness), internally rotated (teres minor and infraspinatus weakness), extended (bicep and brachioradialis weakness), pronated (supinator and brachioradialis weakness), with the wrist flexed (extensor carpi radialis longus and brevis weakness) (Figure 5–74).

- *EDX Pearl*
  📖 Stimulate at the tip of the C6 transverse process over the trunks of the bracial plexus to assess Erb's point (Figure 5–75).

- *Treatment*
  Interventions may include: Rehabilitation, intermittent splinting and activity restriction.

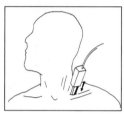

FIGURE 5–75. Erb's Point Stimulation.

Klumpke's Palsy

- *General*
  This injury involves the C8–T1 nerve roots or lower trunk.

- *Etiology*
  It can occur from an obstetrical traction injury.

- *Clinical Presentation*
  The patient may have wasting of the small hand muscles and a claw hand deformity (lumbrical weakness) (Figure 5–76). The shoulder girdle muscle function is preserved.

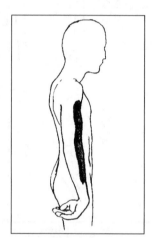

FIGURE 5–74. Waiter's Tip Position: The area of skin that is usually anesthetic is shaded.

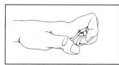

FIGURE 5–76. Ulnar Claw Hand.

- *EDX Pearl*
  The preservation of a SNAP potential may indicate a nerve root avulsion. Avulsions may be associated with this location of injury due to the lack of protective support at the C8 and T1 roots.

- *Treatment*
  Interventions may include: Rehabilitation with incomplete lesions or a surgical exploration with an avulsion.

Thoracic Outlet Syndrome (TOS)

- *Vascular TOS*
  - **General**
    This injury involves the subclavian artery, subclavian vein, or axillary vein.
  - **Etiology**
    It can occur from a pathology resulting in arterial or venous compromise.
  - **Clinical Presentation**
    Arterial involvment may manifest as limb ischemia, necrosis, vague pain, fatigue, with decreased color and temperature. Venous involvement can manifest as a bluish, swollen, achy limb.

- *Neurogenic TOS*
  - **General**
    This injury is rare and may actually be seen in only 1 in 1,000,000 patients.
  - **Etiology**
    It can occur from compression of the lower trunk of the brachial plexus between a cervical rib, fibrous band, or muscular entrapment by the scalenes or pectoralis minor (Figure 5–77).
  - **Clinical Presentation**
    The patient may have pain and numbness along the medial aspect of the forearm and hand, which increases with overhead activity. Intrinsic hand muscle wasting may also be noted (median < ulnar). A maneuver to assess the neurovascular bundle is Adson's test (Figure 5–78). This is performed by abduction, extending and externally rotating the patient's arm. While monitoring the radial pulse, have the patient rotate the head toward the arm (the side of the lesion). A decrease or loss of pulse may be related to a compression of the subclavian artery, indicating compromise to the complex.

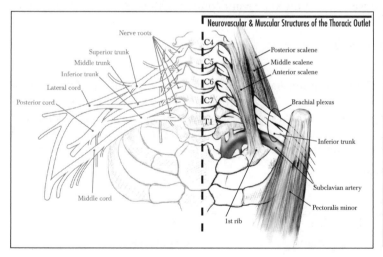

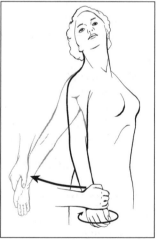

FIGURE 5–77. The Thoracic Outlet.

FIGURE 5–78. Adson's Test.

- **EDX Pearl**
  📖 Abnormal findings can be noted on median CMAP and ulnar CMAP/SNAP NCS. Abnormal spontaneous activity can also occur in the median and ulnar hand muscles on EMG.
- **Treatment**
  Interventions may include: Rehabilitation with a focus on range of motion exercises and strengthening of the trapeizus and rhomboids and postural mechanics.

Neuralgic Amyotrophy

- *General*
  This injury can include various nerves of the brachial plexus. Other names include: Brachial neuropathy, brachial neuritis, idiopathic brachial plexopathy, Parsonage–Turner syndrome, shoulder-girdle neuritis, and paralytic brachial neuritis.

- *Etiology*
  Unknown

- *Clinical Presentation*
  The patient may complain of an acute onset of intense pain and weakness at or about the shoulder girdle region. It can be exacerbated by abduction and rotation. Two-thirds may present bilaterally with recovery taking up to two to three years.

- *EDX Pearl*
  Abnormal spontaneous activity can occur in a variety of combinations: Mononeuropathy (suprascapular nerve, long thoracic nerve, axillary nerve, anterior interossei nerve, spinal accessory nerve) or plexopathy.

- *Treatment*
  Interventions may include: Rehabilitation to prevent contractures or it can resolve spontaneously.

Neoplastic vs. Radiation Plexopathy

- *General*
  These nerve injuries are related to tumors and their treatments. A primary plexus tumor can arise from schwannomas, neuromas, and neurofibromas. Secondary plexus involvement can arise from a Pancoast tumor from the lung or breast. Radiation therapy can cause neural fibrosis and constriction of the vasa nervorum, leading to destruction of the axon and Schwann cells. This can occur months or years post radiation treatment. (Table 5–28)

- *Clinical Presentation/EDX Pearl*

TABLE 5–28   Neoplastic vs. Radiation Plexopathy

Characteristics	Radiation	Tumor
Site of injury	Upper trunk	Lower trunk
Clinical presentations	Myokymia	Horner's syndrome
Sensation	Painless	Painful

Root Avulsion

- *General*

  A severe plexus injury can lead to disruption of the nerve roots. This can occur from a traction injury that disrupts the protective connective tissue support. The C8 and T1 roots have less protection and are the most common site of being torn from their spinal cord attachments (Figure 5–79).

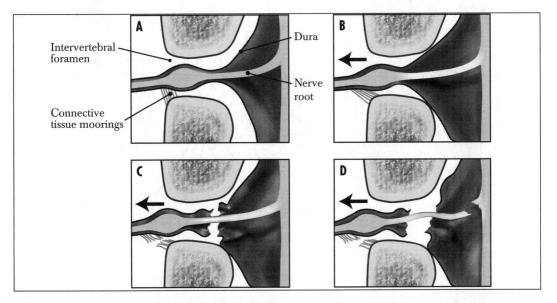

FIGURE 5–79. Nerve Root Avulsion. **A:** Normal nerve root exiting the intervertebral foramen. **B:** Slight traction with dura plugging the foramen and support by tissue moorings. **C:** Ruptured dura and moorings. **D:** Ruptured roots. Note: arrows depict direction of traction forces.

- *Clinical Presentation*

  The patient complains of absent sensation or muscle contraction from the muscles innervated by the roots involved. This may manifest as a flail shoulder.

- *EDX Pearl*

  ☐ The SNAPs remain normal but the CMAPs are absent. Needle exam reveals absent recruitment and abnormal spontaneous activity in myotomic distribution, including the paraspinals.

LUMBOSACRAL PLEXUS

Anatomy

- **Origin**

  The nerve fibers originating from the anterior rami of L1, L2, L3, and L4, roots form the lumbar plexus. The nerve fibers originating from the anterior rami of L4, L5, S1, S2, S3, and S4 roots form the sacral plexus (Figure 5–80).

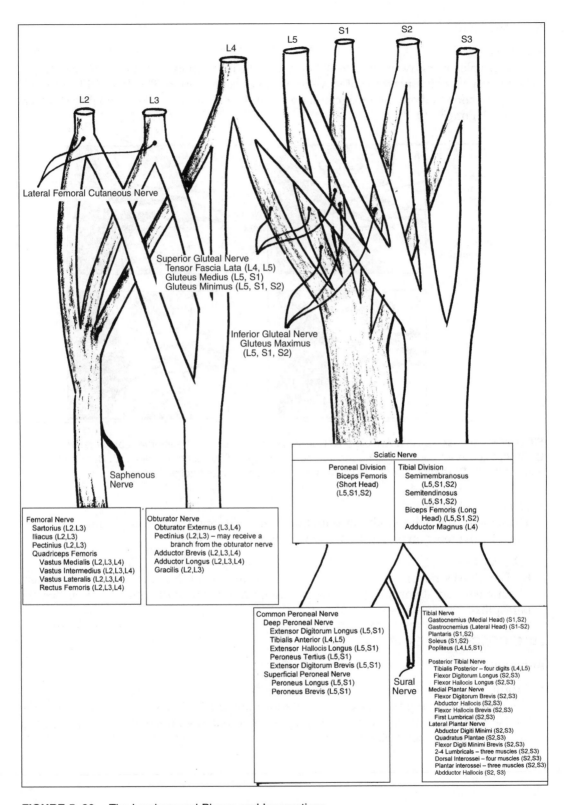

FIGURE 5–80. The Lumbosacral Plexus and Innervations.

- **Course**

  The anterior rami divide to form posterior and anterior divisions. The femoral nerve and lateral femoral cutaneous nerve originate from the posterior division of the lumbar plexus. The obturator nerve originates from the anterior division. The common peroneal nerve originates from the posterior division of the sacral plexus, while the tibial portion originates from the anterior division. The lumbosacral trunk forms from the L4 and L5 nerve fibers connecting the lumbar to the sacral plexus and travels over the pelvic brim.

Injury

- Neuralgic amyotrophy: Similar to brachial plexus pathology
- Neoplastic vs. radiation plexopathy: Similar to brachial plexus pathology
- Retroperitoneal bleed: Can involve a hematoma formation in the psoas muscle
- Hip dislocation
- Obstetric injuries/cephalopelvic disproportion: Presents as a postpartum foot drop

▪

UPPER LIMB MONONEUROPATHY

MEDIAN NERVE

Anatomy

- **Origin**

  These nerve fibers originate from the C5, C6, C7, C8, and T1 roots. They continue on to contribute to the upper, middle, and lower trunks, medial and lateral cords, and finally form the median branch (Figure 5–81).

- **Course**

Arm

The nerve runs medial to the axillary artery. It continues down the humerus to the Ligament of Struthers at the medial epicondyle of the elbow.

Forearm

Innervations and cutaneous branches:

- Pronator Teres (PT)
- Flexor Carpi Radialis (FCR)
- Palmaris Longus
- Flexor Digitorum Superficialis (FDS)
- Palmar Cutaneous Branch

  The anterior interosseus nerve branches from the median nerve to innervate the:

  – Flexor Pollicis Longus (FPL)
  – Flexor Digitorum Profundus (FDP)
  – Pronator Quadratus (PQ)

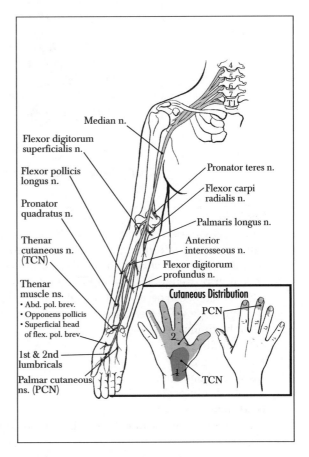

FIGURE 5–81. The Median Nerve (Cutaneous branches in hand supply: 1. Thenar eminence. 2. Palmar surface as indicated).

Hand

Through the carpal tunnel the median nerve innervates the "LOAF" muscles 📖:

- *Lumbricals (1,2)*
- *Opponens Pollicis*
- *Abductor Pollicis Brevis*
- *Flexor Pollicis Brevis (Superficial)*
- Digital Cutaneous Branches

Injury

Arm

- *Ligament of Struthers (LOS)*
  - **General**
    There is a 2 cm bone spur 3 to 6 cm proximal to the medial epicondyle. It is connected to the epicondyle by a ligament in 1% of the population (Figure 5–82).

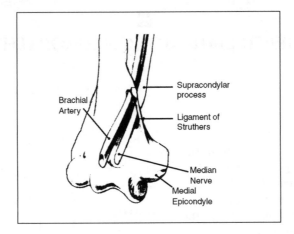

FIGURE 5–82. The Ligament of Struthers

  - **Etiology**
    The nerve can become entrapped with the brachial artery under the ligament.
  - **Clinical Presentation and Muscles Involved**
    The patient may have involvement of all median nerve innervated muscles. It can manifest as weakness in grip strength (FDP and FDS weakness) and wrist flexion (FCR weakness). A dull, achy sensation can occur in the distal forearm. There may be difficulty in flexing the second and third digit (FDP weakness) resulting in an active benediction sign. The brachial pulse is possibly diminished.
  - **EDX Findings**
    NCS
    SNAP: Abnormal
    CMAP: Abnormal
  - **Treatment**
    Interventions may include: Rehabilitation or surgical release.

- *Bicipital Aponeurosis (Lacertus Fibrosis)*
  - **General**
  This is a thickening of the antebrachial fascia attaching the biceps to the ulna. It overlies the median nerve in the proximal forearm. (Figure 5–83)
  - **Etiology**
  The nerve can be injured by entrapment or hematoma compression resulting from an arterial blood gas or venipuncture.
  - **Clinical Presentation and Muscles Involved**
  This is similar to the previous pathology.
  - **EDX Findings**
  This is similar to the previous pathology.
  - **Treatment**
  Interventions may include: Rehabilitation or surgical release

Forearm

- *Pronator Teres Syndrome (PTS)*
  - **General**
  The median nerve passes between the two heads of the pronator teres muscle and continues down under the FDS muscle. An entrapment is commonly named for the muscle compressing the nerve. The muscle is usually spared because it receives its innervation before it is pierced by the nerve. However, the nerve can also contribute to the innervations as it courses through the muscle.
  - **Etiology**
  The nerve can be injured by compression between the heads of the pronator teres muscle or the bridging fascial band of the flexor digitorum superficialis muscle. (Figure 5–84)

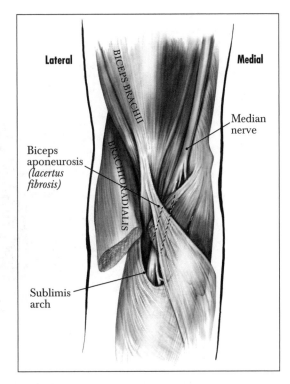

FIGURE 5–83. The Lacertus Fibrosis.

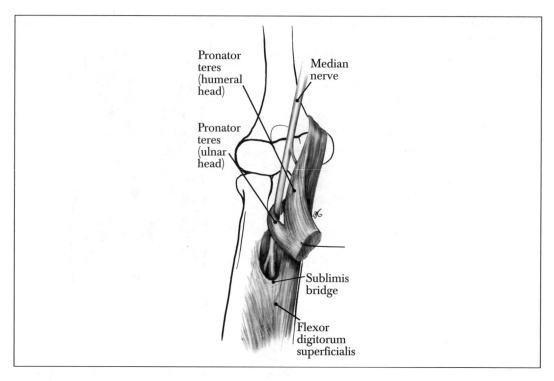

FIGURE 5–84. Median Nerve Entrapment at the Pronator Teres or Flexor Digitorum Superficialis (Flexor Sublimis).

- **Clinical Presentation and Muscles Involved**
  The muscles involved include all median innervated muscles except the pronator teres. The patient may complain of a dull ache of the proximal forearm exacerbated by forceful pronation (PT) or finger flexion (FDS). The forearm and hand muscles may become easily fatigued.
- **EDX Findings**
  NCS
  SNAP: Abnormal
  CMAP: Abnormal
  EMG
  Abnormal activity in all median nerve innervated muscles distal to the pronator teres
- **Treatment**
  Interventions may include: Rehabilitation or surgical release.

- *Anterior Interosseus Syndrome (AIS)*
  - **General**
    This is an injury to a motor branch of the median nerve. It lacks cutaneous innervations but has sensory branches to the wrist joint. It supplies the 🕮 FPL, **PQ**, and FD**P 2, 3** (the 4 P muscles). The FPL is usually the first muscle affected. It is a motor syndrome.
  - **Etiology**
    The nerve can be injured by an idiopathic process (neuralgic amyotrophy), fracture of the forearm or humerus, lacerations, or compression.
  - **Clinical Presentation and Muscles Involved**
    The muscles involved include FPL, PQ, second FDP, and third FDP (the 4 P muscles).

The patient may demonstrate a positive "OK" sign (Figure 5–85) or have difficulty forming a fist (Figure 5–86) because of an inability to approximate the thumb and index finger (FPL, FDP weakness). Sensation is spared.

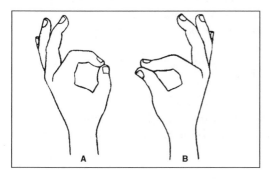

FIGURE 5–85. **A:** Normal. **B:** Positive OK sign (or pinch sign).

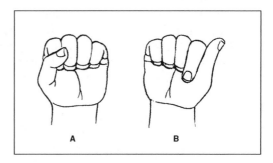

FIGURE 5–86. **A:** Normal. **B:** Inability to make a fist due to problems incorporating the thumb and index finger.

- **EDX Findings**
  NCS
  SNAP: Normal
  CMAP: Possible abnormal activity to the pronator quadratus
  EMG
  Abnormal activity in the muscles innervated by the anterior interosseus nerve
- **Treatment**
  Interventions may include: Rehabilitation or surgical exploration

• *Carpal Tunnel Syndrome (CTS)*
  - **General**
  This is a median neuropathy with associated abnormal clinical symptoms

📖 **Contents** (Figure 5–87)
Flexor digitorum superficialis tendons (4)
Flexor digitorum profundus tendons (4)
Flexor pollicis longus tendon (1)
Median nerve (1)

Borders
Carpal bones
Transverse carpal ligament

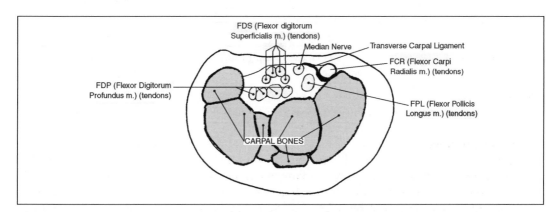

FIGURE 5–87. Cross Section of the Carpal Tunnel (at level of the first row of the carpal bones).

- Etiology

  The nerve can be injured by: (a) an idiopathic process; (b) increased canal volume from: thyroid disease, CHF, renal failure, mass (tumor, hematoma) and 📖 pregnancy (it usually occurs at 6 months and resolves post delivery); (c) decreased canal volume from: a fracture, arthritis, and rheumatoid tenosynovitis; or (d) double crush syndrome from: diabetes mellitus, cervical radiculopathy, and thoracic outlet syndrome.

- Clinical Presentation and Muscle Involvement

  The muscles involved include the muscles that pass through the carpal tunnel FDS (4), FDP (4), FPL (1), and the median nerve. (Table 5–29)

Mild

The patient may complain of numbness, paresthesias, or dysesthesias radiating to the first, second, third, and lateral fourth digits. Symptoms may be exacerbated during sleep and relieved with wrist shaking.

Moderate

The patient may complain of continuous sensory deficits in the median nerve distribution, involving the entire palm and radiating proximally. The ability to handle fine objects is impaired.

Severe

The patient may complain of severe sensory loss and muscular atrophy of the thenar eminence.

TABLE 5–29   Provocative Tests for Carpal Tunnel Syndrome

Provocative Tests	Description
Tinel's sign	Percussion of the median nerve at the wrist
Phalen's test	Hold the wrist at 90° of flexion for approximately one minute
Tourniquet test	Inflated BP cuff reproduction of symptoms at one minute
Carpal compression test	Hold thumb compression over the tunnel for 30 seconds
Reverse Phalen's test	Hold the wrist at 90° of extension for approximately one minute

- EDX Findings

TABLE 5–30   EDX Findings for Different Levels of Severity of Carpal Tunnel Syndrome

Severity	NCS	EMG
Mild	SNAP: Prolonged latency	
	CMAP: Normal	Normal
Moderate	SNAP: Plus a decreased amplitude	
	CMAP: Prolonged latency	Normal
Severe	SNAP: Absent	
	CMAP: Plus a decreased amplitude	Abnormal activity

- Special Studies

  Certain tests can be performed to further support the diagnosis of a median neuropathy. These include comparison studies of the median nerve to the ulnar or radial nerve. This can have an added benefit because each nerve can act as an internal control for the other since they have comparatively similar diameters, temperatures, and distances from stimulator to recording electrode.

- Treatment

  Interventions may include:

Rehabilitation
Indications: Mild symptoms (no weakness or atrophy, no denervation on EMG)
Orthotics: Hand splint 0–30° neutral to extension
Medications: NSAIDs or a steroid injection, diuretics, vitamin B6
Ergonomic modifications
Treat underlying medical disorders

Surgical
Indications: Muscle atrophy, severe pain, and conservative treatment failure

Prognosis
Poor outcome with conservative management may occur with:
- Symptoms greater than 10 months in duration
- Constant paresthesias
- Positive Phalen's Test in less than 10 seconds
- Weakness, atrophy
- Marked prolonged latency on NCS
- Abnormal spontaneous activity on EMG

Anomalous Innervation

- *Martin-Gruber Anastomosis*
  - **General**
    This is a median to ulnar nerve anasto-mosis. The ulnar nerve fibers travel with the AIN branch of the median nerve. It crosses over in the forearm to innervate the ADP, ADM, and most commonly the FDI muscle. This can occur in 15% to 20% of the population. (Figure 5–88)
  - **EDX Findings 📖 (Figure 5–89)**
    - 📖 An initial positive deflection of the CMAP (5–89A) can occur at the elbow, which is not seen at the wrist. This is due to the proximal stimulus branching to the ulnar muscles and reaching the recording electrode, via volume conduction, before the potential on the median nerve, as a result of the median nerve fibers being entrapped and slowed at the wrist.
    - 📖 An increased amplitude of the median nerve CMAP (5–89B) is seen at the elbow compared to the wrist. This is due to simultaneously stimu-lating the median and the ulnar nerve innervated muscles at the elbow. This can occur without a median nerve entrapment.
    - An artificially fast conduction velocity can be demonstrated. This is

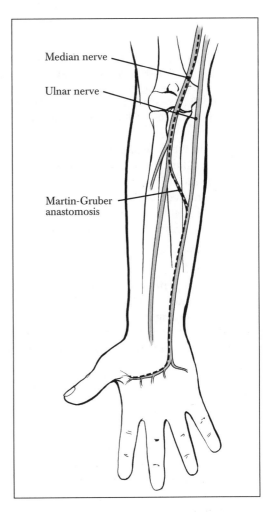

FIGURE 5–88. Martin-Gruber Anastomosis.

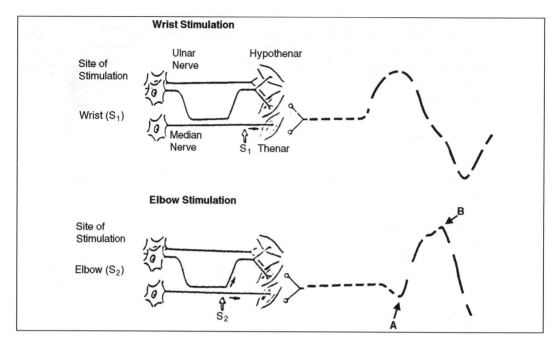

FIGURE 5–89. Martin-Gruber Anastomosis with CTS Electrodiagnostic Findings: **A:** Initial positive deflection of the CMAP is caused by response of ulnar muscles innervated by the median nerve which has gotten to the recording electrode earlier, since the aberrant portion of the median nerve is not entrapped. **B:** Increased amplitude of the median nerve CMAP is seen at the elbow (as opposed to the wrist). This is due to simultaneously stimulating the median and ulnar innervated muscles at the elbow.

a mathematical error due to using a normal proximal latency reading obtained by stimulating the branch to the ADM. This is subsequently calculated with the prolonged distal latency obtained by the entrapped median nerve, giving a falsely increased conduction velocity.

Example: Elbow latency (6.0 ms) – Wrist latency (4.5 ms) = 1.5 ms.

Forearm measurement (150 mm)/Forearm latency (1.5 ms) = 100 m/s

- *Riche-Cannieu Anastomosis*
  - **General**

    This is a connection of the deep branch of the ulnar nerve and recurrent branch of the median nerve in the hand. It causes an all ulnar hand.
  - **EDX Findings**

    A CMAP performed to the APB muscle is absent with median nerve stimulation but present with stimulation of the ulnar nerve.

ULNAR NERVE

Anatomy

- **Origin**

  These nerve fibers originate from the C8–T1 roots. They continue on to contribute to the lower trunk, medial cord, and finally form the ulnar branch. (Figure 5–90)

- **Course**

Arm

The nerve descends along the medial surface of the medial head of the triceps. It runs within a deep groove of thick fascia, the *Arcade of Struthers*. It continues posteriorly in a sulcus between the medial epicondyle and olecranon, called the *retrocondylar groove*.

Forearm

It then continues distally in the *Cubital Tunnel* to innervate the:
- Flexor carpi ulnaris (FCU)
- Flexor digitorum profundus (FDP)
- Palmar ulnar cutaneous nerve 📖
- Dorsal ulnar cutaneous nerve
- Dorsal digital nerves

Hand

Through *Guyon's Canal* it splits into three branches:
- **Superficial Sensory Branch**
- **Hypothenar Branch**
  - Opponens digiti quinti
  - Abductor digiti quinti
  - Flexor digiti quinti
- **Deep Motor Branch**
  - Palmaris brevis
  - 4 <u>D</u>orsal interossei—("DAB": <u>Ab</u>duction)
  - 3 <u>P</u>almar interossei—("PAD": <u>Ad</u>duction)
  - 2 Lumbricals
  - 1 Adductor pollicis
  - 1/2 Flexor pollicis brevis (deep head)

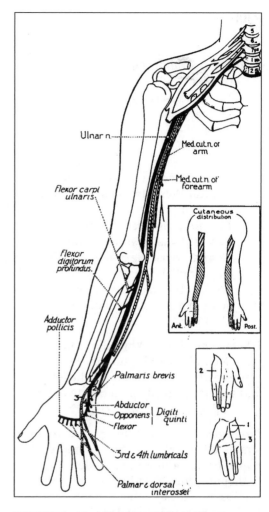

FIGURE 5–90. The Ulnar Nerve. (From Haymaker W., Woodhall B.: Peripheral Nerve Injuries: Principles of Diagnosis. Philadelphia, W.B. Saunders, 1953, with permission.)

The 1-1/2 Nerve
- **1-1/2 muscles of the thumb**
  1 Adductor pollicis
  1/2 Flexor pollicis brevis (deep head)
- **1-1/2 muscle of the forearm**
  1 Flexor carpi ulnaris
  1/2 Flexor digitorum profundus (fourth, fifth)
- **1-1/2 sensation of the fingers**
  fifth digit
  1/2 fourth digit

Injury

Arm

- *Arcade of Struthers (AOS)*
  - **General**
    This is a fascial band that connects the brachialis to the triceps brachii. (Figure 5–91)
  - **Etiology**
    The nerve can be injured by compression under the fascial band.
  - **Clinical Presentation and Muscles Involved**
    The patient may demonstrate involvement of all the ulnar nerve innervated muscles. Wrist flexion may result with a radial deviation (FCU weakness). Abnormal sensations may occur in all sensory branches of the ulnar nerve.

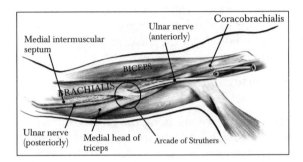

FIGURE 5–91. The Arcade of Struthers.

Ulnar Claw Hand: While the hand is at rest, an unopposed pull of the EDC causes partial finger flexion of the fourth and fifth PIP and DIP joint due to extension of the MCP. (Figure 5–92)

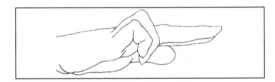

FIGURE 5–92. Ulnar Claw Hand.

Froment's Sign: 📖 This test demonstrates an inability to hold a piece of paper by the thumb and index finger with pure thumb adduction (adductor pollicis weakness). The patient substitutes the median innervated FPL muscle, causing flexion of the interphalangeal joint. (Figure 5–93)

Wartenberg's Sign: Inability to adduct the fifth digit. (Interossei weakness).

  - **EDX Findings**
    NCS
      SNAP: Abnormal dorsal ulnar cutaneous (DUC) and ulnar nerve findings
      CMAP: Abnormal
    EMG
      Abnormal activity in all the ulnar nerve innervated muscles
  - **Treatment**
    Interventions may include: Rehabilitation or surgical release of the AOS

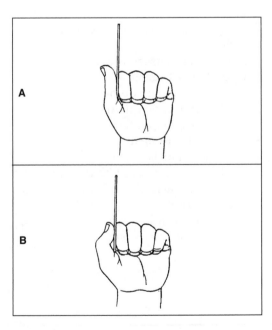

FIGURE 5–93. **A:** Normal. **B:** Froment's Sign.

Forearm

- *Tardy Ulnar Palsy*
  - **General**
    This is an ulnar neuropathy that can occur months to years after a distal humerus fracture.
  - **Etiology**
    The nerve can be injured secondary to a trauma that results in bone overgrowth or scar formation. Nerve traction can occur from an increased carrying angle due to a valgus deformity at the elbow.
  - **Clinical Presentation and Muscles Involved**
    The patient's muscle involvement and complaints are dependent on the site of injury. In most cases the patient may demonstrate involvement of all the ulnar nerve innervated muscles.
  - **EDX Findings**
    This is dependent on site of injury.
  - **Treatment**
    Interventions may include: Rehabilitation or surgical procedure.

- *Cubital Tunnel Syndrome*
  - **General**
    This is the most common site of elbow entrapment. It is bordered by the medial epicondyle and olecranon with an overlying aponeurotic band. NCS across the elbow should be performed at 90–110° of elbow flexion. (Figure 5–94)
  - **Etiology**
    The nerve can be injured from compression beneath the proximal edge of the FCU aponeurosis or arcuate ligament.
  - **Clinical Presentation and Muscles Involved**
    The muscles involved include all ulnar nerve innervated muscles with one exception, the FCU *may or may not* be involved. The patient may complain of symptoms similar to an injury at the Arcade of Struthers. A positive *Tinel's sign* may demonstrate paresthesias in the distribution of the ulnar nerve with percussion at the ulnar groove.

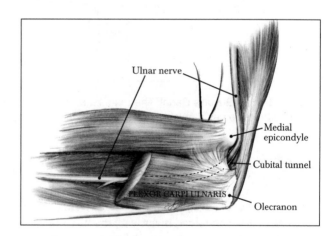

FIGURE 5–94. The Cubital Tunnel.

  - **EDX Findings**
    NCS
    SNAP: Abnormal findings in the dorsal ulnar cutaneous and ulnar nerve
    CMAP: Approximately 10 ms drop of conduction velocity across the elbow
    EMG
    Abnormal activity in the ulnar nerve innervated muscles
  - **Treatment**
    Interventions may include: Rehabilitation or surgical release

Hand

- *Guyon's Canal*
  - **General**
  Different branches of the ulnar nerve can be injured at the wrist. (Figure 5–95)

Classification: (Shea's System)

Type I	Involvement of the hypothenar and deep ulnar branch
Type II	Involvement of the deep ulnar branch
Type III	Involvement of the superficial ulnar sensory branch

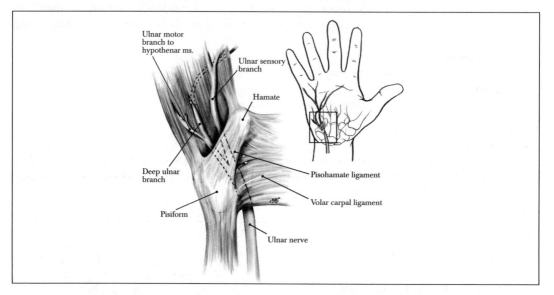

FIGURE 5–95. Guyon's Canal: The main ulnar nerve trunk is illustrated splitting into its superficial and deep branches as it enters Guyon's Canal (between the pisiform and hook of hamate bones).

  - **Etiology**
  The nerve can be injured by cycling activities (Cycler's Palsy), wrist ganglions, or rheumatoid arthritis
  - **Clinical Presentation and Muscle Involvement**
  The muscles involved include all the ulnar nerve innervated intrinsic muscles of the hand. (See side box.) The patient may complain of painless wasting of the FDI. A severe claw hand may occur (lumbrical weakness) while the FDP remains intact causing marked finger flexion.
  - **EDX Findings**
  NCS
    SNAP: DUC nerve is spared, ulnar nerve to the fifth digit is abnormal
    CMAP: Abnormal
  EMG
    Abnormal activity in the ulnar nerve innervates hand muscles
  - **Treatment**
  Interventions may include: Rehabilitation or surgical procedure.

Muscles Involved
4 dorsal interossei
3 palmar interossei
2 Lumbricals
1 Adductor pollicis
1/2 Flexor pollicis brevis

and the

Hypothenar muscle
Opponens digiti minimi
Abductor digiti minimi
Flexor digiti minimi

Note: Compression of the ulnar nerve at Guyon's canal may spare the hypothenar muscle

RADIAL NERVE

Anatomy

- **Origin**
  These ... from the C5–T1 ... to contribut... and lower trunk ... ally form the r... 5)

- **Cou...**

Arm

The nerve is ... or to the axillary artery. It descends between the long and medial heads of the triceps muscle toward the spiral groove.

Innervation above the spiral groove:
  – Triceps
  – Anconeus
  – Posterior cutaneous nerve
  – Lower lateral cutaneous nerve
  ⌑ Innervation below the spiral groove:
  – Brachioradialis (BR)
  – Extensor carpi radialis longus (ECRL)
  – Extensor carpi radialis brevis (ECRB)

Ten centimeters proximal to the lateral epicondyle of the humerus, the nerve pierces the lateral intermuscular septum and enters the anterior compartment of the arm. It continues distally between the brachioradialis and brachialis. ⌑ At the lateral epicondyle it then splits to a motor and sensory branch.

Elbow
- **Superficial radial nerve**
- **Posterior interosseus nerve (PIN)**
  – Supinator
  – Extensor digitorum communis (EDC)
  – Extensor digiti minimi (EDM)
  – Extensor carpi ulnaris (ECU)
  – Abductor pollicis longus (APL)
  – Extensor pollicis longus (EPL)
  – Extensor pollicis brevis (EPB)
  – Extensor indicis proprius (EIP)

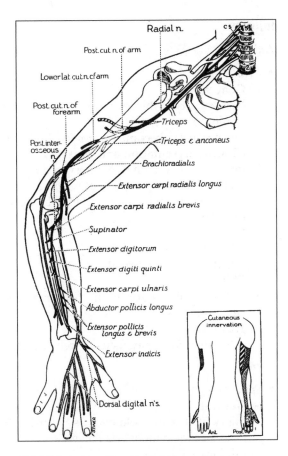

FIGURE 5–96. The Radial Nerve. (From Haymaker W., Woodhall B.: Peripheral Nerve Injuries: Principles of Diagnosis. Philadelphia, W.B. Saunders, 1953, with permission.)

Injuries

Axilla

- *Crutch Palsy*
  - **General**
  Nerve injury at this level can also involve the median, axillary, or suprascapular nerves.
  - **Etiology**
  The nerve can become compressed with improper crutch use.
  - **Clinical Presentation and Muscle Involvement**📖
  Involves all radial nerve innervated muscles.
  The patient may complain of weakness in all radial nerve innervated muscles, including the triceps brachii. Sensation may be decreased over the posterior arm and forearm.
  - **EDX Findings**
  NCS
      SNAP: +/- Abnormal
      CMAP: +/- Abnormal
  EMG
      Abnormal activity in all radial nerve innervated muscles
  - **Treatment**
  Interventions may focus on rehabilitation.

Arm

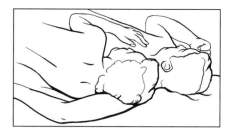

FIGURE 5–97. Mechanism of Honeymooner's Palsy

- *Spiral Groove*
  - **General**
  Injury at this site is known as Saturday Night Palsy or Honeymooner's Palsy.
  - **Etiology**
  This nerve injury can be due to an injection or by compression. Common mechanisms described are the arm being positioned over a sharp ledge, such as a chair back or from a person's head resting on the humerus. (Figure 5–97)
  - **Clinical Presentation and Muscle Involvement**
  Involves all radial nerve innervated muscles, except triceps brachii and anconeus.
  The patient complains of weakness of elbow flexion (BR weakness), supination (supinator weakness), wrist drop (ECRL, ECRB, ECU weakness), and finger extension (EDC weakness). There is preservation of elbow extension (triceps, anconeus). Sensory deficits may occur in the dorsal aspect of the hand and posterior arm.
  - **EDX Findings**
  NCS
      SNAP: ± Abnormal
      CMAP: ± Abnormal
  EMG
  Abnormal activity in all radial nerve innervated muscles below the Anconeus.
  - **Treatment**
  Interventions may focus on rehabilitation.

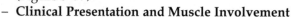

Differential Diagnosis of a Wrist Drop
Diffuse polyneuropathy: Lead
Mononeuropathy: PIN, radial nerve
Plexopathy: Posterior cord, upper trunk, middle trunk
Radiculopathy: C6 and C7
SCI/TBI/CVA, etc.

Forearm

- *Posterior Interosseus Nerve Syndrome*
  (Supinator Syndrome, Arcade of Frohse Syndrome)
  - **General**
  This is considered a *pure motor syndrome*
  - **Etiology**
  The nerve can be injured by compression of the nerve at the 📖 *Arcade of Frohse* of the supinator. (Figure 5–98) It can also be injured by a lipoma, ganglion cyst, synovitis from rheumatoid arthritis or a 📖 *Monteggia fracture.* This is a fracture of the proximal one-third of the ulna and dislocation of the radial head. It occurs secondary to a fall on the outstretched hand with the forearm locked in full pronation.
  - **Clinical Presentation and Muscle Involvement**
  Involves all the radial nerve innervated distal extensors: EDC, EIP, ECU, EPB, EPL, APL. The PIN syndrome spares supinator, brachioradialis, triceps, ECR-L, ECR-B, anconeus. The patient may complain of weakness in the distal extensors radial nerve innervated muscles. A pseudo claw-hand deformity may be demonstrated (finger extensor weakness). 📖 Radial deviation is noted with wrist extension (ECU weakness) and sensation is spared.

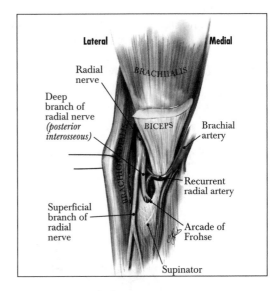

FIGURE 5–98. The Arcade of Frohse.

  - **EDX Findings**
  NCS
  SNAP: Normal
  CMAP: Abnormal findings in muscles innervated by the posterior interosseus nerve
  EMG
  Abnormal activity in the muscles innervated by the PIN, including the supinator
  - **Treatment**
  Interventions may include: Rehabilitation or surgical resection

- *Superficial Radial Neuropathy*
  - **General**
  This nerve injury is also known as *Cheiralgia Paresthetica* or *Wristwatch Syndrome.*
  - **Etiology**
  The nerve can be injured by compression at the wrist from a wristwatch, tight handcuffs, etc. (Figure 5–99)
  - **Clinical Presentation and Muscle Involvement**
  This is a pure sensory syndrome with no muscle involvement. The patient may complain solely of sensory abnormalities including numbness, burning, or tingling on the dorsal radial aspect of the hand. Discomfort may be exacerbated with palmar and ulnar wrist flexion or forced pronation.

- **EDX Findings**
  NCS
  SNAP: Abnormal
  CMAP: Normal
  EMG
  Normal
- **Treatment**
  Interventions may include: rehabilitation and removal of the compressive irritant.

MUSCULOCUTANEOUS NERVE

Anatomy

- **Origin**
  These nerve fibers originate from the C5, C6, and C7 roots. This continues on to contribute to the upper trunk and lateral cord to finally form the musculocutaneous branch. (Figure 5–100)

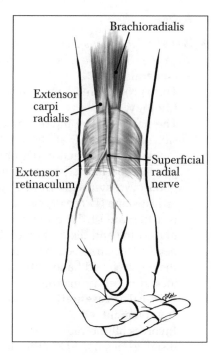

FIGURE 5–99. Superficial Radial Neuropathy Injury.

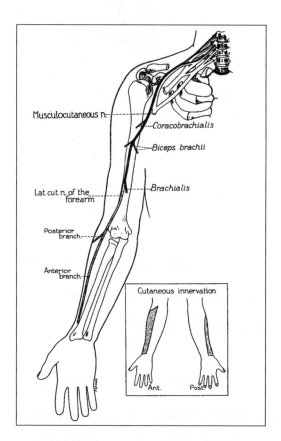

FIGURE 5–100. The Musculocutaneous Nerve. (From Haymaker W., Woodhall B. Peripheral Nerve Injuries: Principles of Diagnosis. Philadelphia, W.B. Saunders, 1953, with permission.)

- **Course**

Arm

The nerve passes along the medial aspect of the humerus and innervates the:
- Coracobrachialis
- Biceps brachii
- Brachialis

Forearm

It continues anterior to the antecubital fossa, lateral to the biceps tendon, to innervate the lateral forearm.
- Lateral antebrachial cutaneous nerve

Injury

- **Musculocutaneous Neuropathy**
  - **General**
    An injury to the distal portion is more common than to the proximal portion.
  - **Etiology**
    The nerve can be injured by entrapment proximally from the coracobrachialis or distally, where it runs superficially. It can also be injured by gunshot wounds, shoulder dislocation, and phlebotomy.
  - **Clinical Presentation and Muscle Involvement**
    Involves musculocutaneous nerve innervated muscles including biceps, brachialis, and spares the coracobrachialis
    The patient may complain of elbow flexion weakness (biceps, brachialis weakness) and abnormal sensation over the lateral forearm.
  - **EDX Findings**
    NCS
    SNAP: Abnormal findings in the lateral antebrachial cutaneous nerve
    CMAP: Abnormal findings to the Biceps Brachii
    EMG
    Abnormal activity in the brachialis and biceps brachii
  - **Treatment**
    Interventions may include: rehabilitation or surgical procedure.

AXILLARY NERVE

Anatomy

- **Origin**
These nerve fibers originate from the C5 and C6 roots. They continue on to contribute to the upper trunk and posterior cord to finally form the axillary branch. (Figure 5–101)

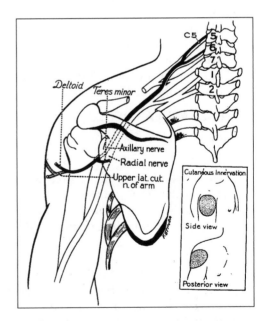

FIGURE 5–101. The Axillary Nerve. (From Haymaker W,. Woodhall B. Peripheral Nerve Injuries: Principles of Diagnosis. Philadelphia, W.B. Saunders, 1953, with permission.)

- **Course**

Axilla

The nerve passes inferior to the glenohumeral joint, through the quadrilateral space to the posterior aspect of the humerus. It innervates the:
- Teres minor
- Deltoid
- Upper lateral cutaneous nerve

Injury

- *Axillary Neuropathy*
  - **General**
    The nerve runs through the quadrangular space. This is bordered by the humerus, long head of the triceps brachii, teres minor, and teres major.
  - **Etiology**
    The nerve can be injured by traction or compression from a shoulder dislocation, humeral head fracture, or improper crutch use.
  - **Clinical Presentation**
    Involves all axillary nerve innervated muscles; deltoid and teres minor
    The patient may complain of weakness of shoulder flexion and abduction (deltoid weakness), and external rotation (teres minor weakness). There may also be lateral shoulder sensation abnormalities.
  - **EDX Findings**
    NCS
      SNAP: Not available
      CMAP: Abnormal
    EMG
      Abnormal activity in the axillary nerve innervated muscles
  - **Treatment**
    Interventions may include: rehabilitation or surgical decompression.

SUPRASCAPULAR NERVE

Anatomy

- **Origin**
  These nerve fibers originate from the C5 and C6 roots. They continue on to contribute to the upper trunk to finally form the suprascapular branch. (Figure 5–102)

- **Course**

Neck

It passes the posterior triangle of the neck and runs beneath the trapezius to the superior margin of the scapula. It runs through the suprascapular notch, which is covered by the transverse scapular ligament and branches to innervate the:
- 📖 Supraspinatus (SS)
  The nerve wraps around the spinoglenoid notch to innervate the:
- Infraspinatus (IS)

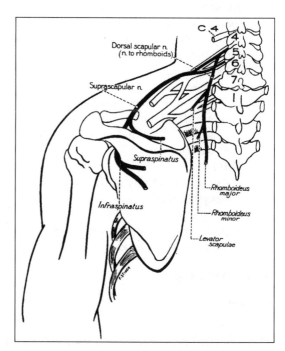

FIGURE 5–102. The Suprascapular Nerve. (From Haymaker W., Woodhall B. Peripheral Nerve Injuries: Principles of Diagnosis. Philadelphia, W.B. Saunders, 1953, with permission.)

Injury

📖

- *Suprascapular Neuropathy*
  - **General**
    This is the only peripheral nerve injury at the trunk level. (Figure 5–103)
  - **Etiology**
    The nerve can be injured from forced scapular protraction, penetrating wounds, improper crutch use, traction (as seen in volleyball players due to overhead serving) rotator-cuff rupture, Erb's palsy, spinoglenoid ganglions, hematoma, suprascapular or spinoglenoid notch entrapment.
  - **Clinical Presentation and Muscle Involvement**
    Involves both suprascapular nerve innervated muscle; both infraspinatus and supraspinatus.
    The patient may complain of weakness in abduction (SS weakness) and external rotation (IS weakness) of the glenohumeral joint. Atrophy occurs in the infraspinatus and supraspinatus with injury at the suprascapular notch. Atrophy of the infraspinatus alone may occur with injury at spinoglenoid notch.
  - **EDX Findings**
    NCS
    SNAP: Not available
    CMAP: Abnormal
    EMG
    Abnormal activity in the suprascapular nerve innervated muscles
  - **Treatment**
    Interventions may include: Rehabilitation or surgical release.

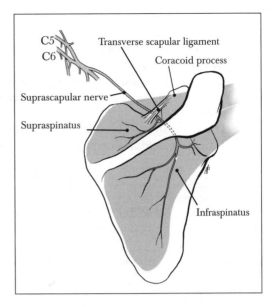

FIGURE 5–103. Suprascapular Nerve Injury Sites.

LONG THORACIC NERVE

Anatomy

- **Origin**
  These nerve fibers originate from the C5, C6 and C7 roots. (Figure 5–104)

- **Course**

Neck
The nerve runs distally along the thoracic wall to innervate the:
- Serratus anterior
- (SALT: <u>S</u>erratus <u>A</u>nterior <u>L</u>ong <u>T</u>horacic)

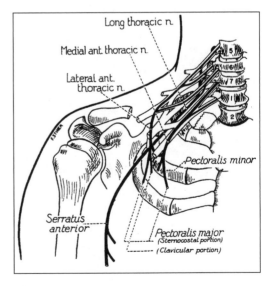

FIGURE 5–104. The Long Thoracic Nerve. (From Haymaker W., Woodhall B. Peripheral Nerve Injuries: Principles of Diagnosis. Philadelphia, W.B. Saunders, 1953, with permission.)

Injury

📖

- 📖 *Long Thoracic Neuropathy*
  - **General**
    There are two main types of shoulder winging that should be differentiated from each other: medial (long thoracic) and lateral (spinal accessory)
  - **Etiology**
    The nerve can be injured by traction from a fall, MVA, sports activities, or shoulder bags.
  - **Clinical Presentation and Muscle Involvement**

TABLE 5–31. Comparison of Long Thoracic Winging and Spinal Accessory Winging

Nerve	Innervation	Winging	Position of Scapula (medial border)	Abduction
Long Thoracic	Serratus anterior	Medial	Closer to midline	Decreases winging
Spinal Accessory	Trapezius	Lateral	Away from midline	Increases winging

  - **EDX Findings**
    NCS
      SNAP: Not available
      CMAP: Abnormal
    EMG
      Abnormal activity in the serratus anterior
  - **Treatment**
    Interventions may include: rehabilitation or surgical procedure.

■ LOWER LIMB MONONEUROPATHY

LATERAL FEMORAL CUTANEOUS NERVE

Anatomy

- **Origin**
  These nerve fibers originate from the L2 and L3 roots. They continue on to contribute to the posterior division of the lumbar plexus and finally the lateral femoral cutaneous nerve. (Figure 5–105)

- **Course**

Pelvis
The nerve continues down to pass over the iliacus toward the anterior iliac spine. It tunnels under the inguinal ligament to provide sensation for the lateral thigh.

Injury

- *Lateral Femoral Cutaneous Neuropathy*
  - **General**
    This nerve injury is known as meralgia paresthetica and is mainly a clinical diagnosis.
  - **Etiology**
    The nerve can be injured from compression by a repeated low-grade trauma, protuberant abdomen, pregnancy, or tight clothing. Diabetes, tumor, and infection can also affect the nerve in a nonspecific manner.
  - **Clinical Presentation and Muscle Involvement**
    This is a pure sensory syndrome with no muscle involvement.
    The patient may complain of sensory complaints at the lateral thigh including pain, numbness, burning or a dull ache. It may be exacerbated with hip extension and does not demonstrate motor abnormalities.
  - **EDX Findings**
    NCS
       SNAP: Abnormal findings in the lateral femoral cutaneous nerve
       CMAP: Not available
    EMG
       Not available
  - **Treatment**
    Interventions may include: Rehabilitation, NSAIDs, cortisone injections, surgical release, or the symptoms may be self-limited.

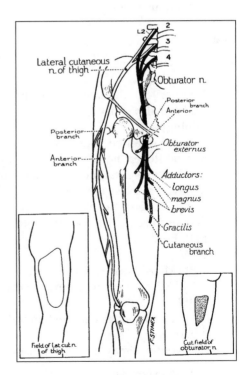

FIGURE 5–105. The Lateral Femoral Cutaneous Nerve. (From Haymaker W., Woodhall B. Peripheral Nerve Injuries: Principles of Diagnosis. Philadelphia, W.B. Saunders, 1953, with permission.)

FEMORAL NERVE

Anatomy

- **Origin**

  These nerve fibers originate from the L2, L3, and L4 roots. They continue on as the posterior division of the lumbar plexus and finally the femoral nerve. (Figure 5–106)

- **Course**

  The nerve runs through the psoas. It goes under the inguinal ligament, lateral to the femoral artery and travels through the femoral triangle to innervate the:
  – Iliacus
  – Pectineus
  – Sartorius
  – Rectus femoris
  – Vastus lateralis
  – Vastus intermedius
  – Vastus medialis
  – Saphenous nerve

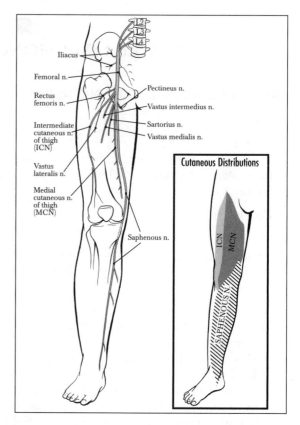

FIGURE 5–106. The Femoral Nerve.

Injury

- *Femoral Neuropathy*
  - **General**
    This nerve is the largest branch of the lumbar plexus
  - **Etiology**
    The nerve can be injured by a compressive lesion in the pelvis from trauma, fracture, retroperitoneal hematoma, tumor, or cardiac catheterization.
  - **Clinical Presentation and Muscle Involvement**
    Involved muscles include all femoral innervated muscles.
    The patient may complain of weakness of knee extension (quadriceps weakness) and decreased sensation over the anterior thigh and medial leg (saphenous nerve).
  - **EDX Findings**
    NCS
      SNAP: Abnormal findings from the saphenous nerve
      CMAP: Abnormal findings to the rectus femoris
    EMG
      Abnormal activity in the femoral nerve innervated muscles
  - **Treatment**
    Interventions may include: Rehabilitation or surgical procedure.

- *Diabetic Amyotrophy*
  - **General**
    This injury is the most common cause of a femoral neuropathy
  - **Etiology**
    The nerve can be injured from an abnormality of the vaso-nevorum due to diabetes mellitus. This amyotrophy has also been noted to occur after marked weight loss.

– **Clinical Presentation and Muscle Involvement** 📖
May have involvement of all femoral nerve innervated muscles.
The patient may complain of asymmetric thigh pain, knee extension weakness (quadriceps weakness), and atrophy. Loss of the patella reflex may also occur.
– **EDX Findings**
NCS
Variable findings
EMG
Variable findings
– **Treatment**
Interventions may include: Rehabilitation and control of blood sugar.

- *Saphenous Neuropathy*
  – **General**
  This nerve is the largest and longest branch of the femoral nerve. It supplies sensation to the medial aspect of the leg, and the medial malleolus and medial arch of the foot.
  – **Etiology**
  The nerve can be injured by entrapment in the subsartorial (Hunter's) canal or between the sartorius and gracilis. It can also be related to trauma from knee or vascular surgery.
  – **Clinical Presentation and Muscle Involvement**
  This is a pure sensory syndrome with no muscle involvement.
  The patient may complain of medial knee pain with abnormal sensation radiating distally along the medial aspect of the leg and foot.
  – **EDX Findings**
  NCS
  SNAP: Abnormal findings in the saphenous nerve
  CMAP: Not available
  EMG
  Not available
  – **Treatment**
  Interventions may include: Rehabilitation or surgical procedure.

OBTURATOR NERVE

Anatomy

- **Origin**
  These nerve fibers originate from the L2, 3, 4 roots. They continue on as the anterior portion of the lumbar plexus to finally form the obturator nerve. (Figure 5–107)

- **Course**

Leg
The nerve passes through the psoas major and obturator foramen to innervate the:
- Pectineus
- Adductor brevis
- Adductor longus
- Adductor magnus
- Obturator externus
- Gracilis
- Cutaneous branch

Injury

- *Obturator Neuropathy*
  - **General**
  This nerve injury can occur in conjunction with a femoral nerve injury
  - **Etiology**
  The nerve can be injured by compression from a pelvic fracture or hernia within the obturator foramen
  - **Clinical Presentation and Muscle Involvement**
  Can involve all muscles innervated by the obturator nerve.
  The patient may complain of hip adduction weakness (adductor brevis, adductor longus, adductor magnus weakness). There may also be a decrease in sensation along the medial aspect of the thigh.
  - **EDX Findings**
  NCS
    None
  EMG
    Abnormal activity in the obturator nerve innervated muscles
  - **Treatment**
  Intervention may include: Rehabilitation or surgical procedure.

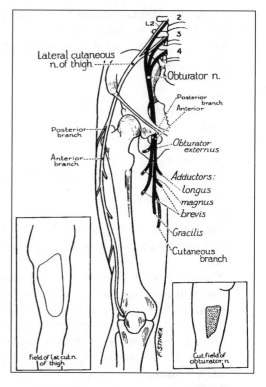

FIGURE 5–107. The Obturator Nerve. (From Haymaker W., Woodhall B. Peripheral Nerve Injuries: Principles of Diagnosis. Philadelphia, W.B. Saunders, 1953, with permission.)

SCIATIC NERVE

Anatomy

- **Origin**
  These nerve fibers originate from the L4, L5, S1, S2 and S3 roots. They continue on as the posterior division of the lumbosacral plexus running posteriorly in the leg to finally form the sciatic nerve. (Figure 5–108)

- **Course**

Pelvis

  The nerve exits the pelvis through ▢ the greater sciatic foramen, between the greater trochanter and ischial tuberosity. The sciatic nerve proper is made up of a tibial and peroneal portion, which travels as one unit to the mid-thigh area where it splits into its respective divisions.

  The peroneal portion innervates the: ▢
  - Short head of the biceps femoris (SHBF)
  The tibial portion innervates the: ▢
  - Long head of the biceps femoris (LHBF)
  - Semitendinosus
  - Semimembranosus
  - Adductor magnus

Injury

- *Sciatic Neuropathy*
  - **General**

    This is the largest nerve in the human body. The peroneal portion makes up the outer two-thirds of the nerve proper. It is anchored at the fibular head, rendering it more susceptible to injury.
  - **Etiology**

    The nerve can be injured by hip trauma, hip replacement, injection, hematoma, pelvic fracture, penetrating wounds, or a gravid uterus. ⊞ A *Piriformis Syndrome* can also occur. This is a compressive sciatic neuropathy at the pelvic outlet affecting mainly the peroneal portion of the nerve as it runs inferior or through this muscle. (Figure 5–109)
  - **Clinical Presentation and Muscle Involvement**

    Involves all muscles innervated by the sciatic nerve.

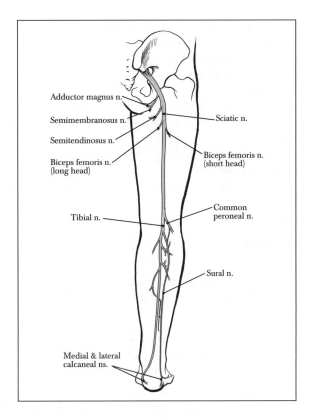

FIGURE 5–108. The Sciatic Nerve.

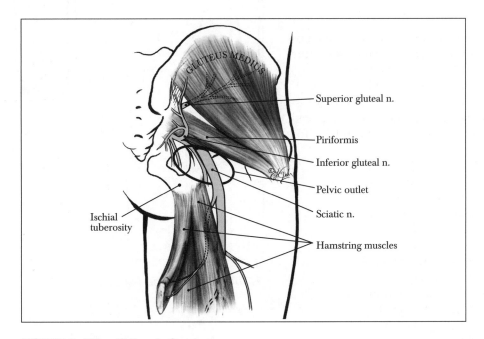

FIGURE 5–109. Piriformis Syndrome.

The patient's complaints depend on which portion of the nerve is more involved. It can present as weakness of knee flexion (hamstring weakness) and include muscles and cutaneous innervation of both the peroneal and tibial nerve.

- **EDX Findings**
  NCS
  SNAP: Abnormal findings in the superficial peroneal and sural nerve
  CMAP: Abnormal findings in the tibial and peroneal nerves
  EMG
  Abnormal activity in all sciatic nerve innervations, including the SHBF and LHBF.
- **Treatment**
  Interventions may include: Rehabilitation or surgical procedure.

TIBIAL NERVE

Anatomy

- **Origin**
  These nerve fibers originate from the L4, L5, S1, and S2 (S3) roots. They continue on as the sciatic nerve to finally form the tibial branch. (Figure 5–110)

- **Course**
  At the distal one-third of the thigh, the tibial portion of the nerve runs posterior to the knee and continues distally to innervate the:
  - Plantaris
  - Medial gastrocnemius
  - Lateral gastrocnemius
  - Popliteus
  - Soleus

At the Soleus it continues as the posterior tibial nerve and innervates the:
  - Tibialis posterior (TP)
  - Flexor digitorum longus (FDL)
  - Flexor hallucis longus (FHL)

The nerve runs under the flexor retinaculum and divides into three branches:

- **Medial Plantar Nerve**
  - Adductor hallucis
  - Flexor diiatorum brevis
  - Flexor hallucis brevis
  - Lumbrical
  - Sensory branch
- **Lateral Plantar Nerve**
  - Lumbricals
  - Abductor digiti minimi
  - Quadratus plantae
  - Sensory branch
- **Calcaneal Nerve**
  - Sensory branch

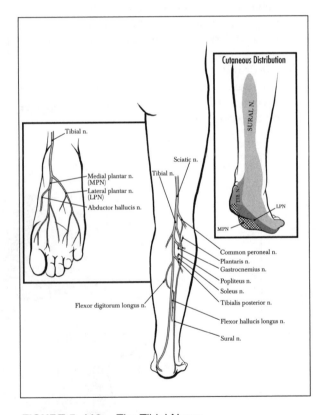

FIGURE 5–110. The Tibial Nerve.

Injury

- *Tibial Neuropathy*
  - **General**
  The most common tibial nerve injury occurs in *tarsal tunnel syndrome.* (Figure 5–111)

TABLE 5–32. Tunnel Contents 📖

Tom	**T**ibialis posterior
Dick	Flexor **d**igitorum longus
And	Tibial **a**rtery and vein
Harry	Flexor **h**allucis longus

  - **Etiology** 📖
  The posterior tibial nerve can be injured by compression under the flexor retinaculum.
  - **Clinical Presentation and Muscle Involvement**
  Involves all muscles that pass through the tarsal tunnel. (see Table 5–32)
  The patient may complain of symptoms related to intrinsic foot weakness. Perimalleolar pain, numbness, and paresthesias may extend to the toes and soles. It is reproduced by ankle inversion. A positive Tinel's sign may be elicited at the ankle. Heel sensation may be spared due to the calcaneal branch departing proximal to the tunnel.
  - **EDX Findings**
  NCS
    SNAP: Abnormal findings in the plantar nerves. Normal calcaneal nerve
    CMAP: Abnormal findings in the medial and lateral plantar nerves
  EMG
  Abnormal activity in the tibial nerve innervated muscles
  - **Treatment**
  Interventions may include: Rehabilitation or surgical release.

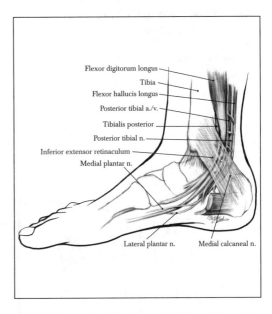

FIGURE 5–111. The Posterior Tarsal Tunnel.

PERONEAL NERVE

Anatomy

- **Origin**

  These nerve fibers originate from the L4–S2 roots. They continue on as the sciatic nerve to finally form the peroneal branch.

- **Course**

  In the distal posterior thigh, the peroneal portion of the sciatic nerve branches to form the common peroneal nerve. This travels through the popliteal fossa, winds around the fibular head, and splits into the deep and superficial portions. (Figures 5–112 and 5–113)

Superficial Peroneal Nerve innervates the:	**Deep Peroneal Nerve** innervates the:
• Peroneus longus • Peroneus brevis • Medial cutaneous nerve • Lateral cutaneous nerve	• Tibialis anterior (TA) • Extensor digitorum longus (EDL) • Extensor hallucis longus (EHL) • Peroneus tertius • Extensor digitorum brevis (EDB) • First dorsal interossei • Dorsal distal cutaneous nerve

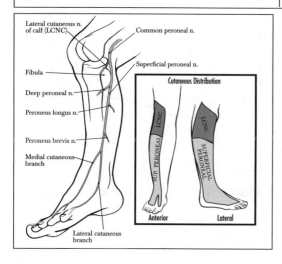

FIGURE 5–112. The Superficial Peroneal Nerve.

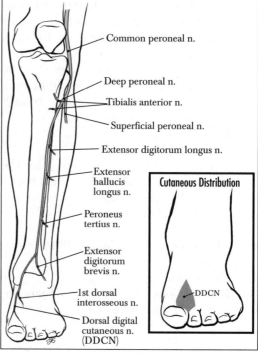

FIGURE 5–113. The Deep Peroneal Nerve.

ANOMALOUS INNERVATION

ACCESSORY PERONEAL NERVE

- **General**
  This nerve branches from the superficial peroneal nerve It travels behind the lateral malleolus to innervate all or some of the EDB. (Figure 5–114)
- **EDX Findings**
  Stimulation behind the lateral malleolus reveals a CMAP from the EDB. This muscle can remain spared regardless of a deep peroneal nerve injury.

Injury

- *Peroneal Neuropathy*
  - **General**
    The most common site of this nerve injury is at the fibular head. (Figure 5–115)
  - **Etiology**
    The muscles involved include all muscles supplied by the deep and superficial branch of the peroneal nerve (the short head of the biceps f. is spared). The nerve can be injured by compression from prolonged leg crossing, weight loss, poor positioning during surgery, poor cast application, prolonged squatting position (Strawberry pickers' palsy) and metabolic disorders, such as diabetes.
  - **Clinical Presentation**
    The patient may complain of weakness of the dorsiflexors (TA, EDL, EHL weakness), resulting in a *foot drop* and *steppage gait*. Weakness of only the dorsiflexors and ankle everters helps to clinically differentiate a peroneal nerve injury from an L5 radiculopathy. A radiculopathy will also involve the ankle invertors. Sensory loss may be noted over the distribution of the deep and superficial peroneal nerve.
  - **EDX Findings**
    NCS
    SNAP: Abnormal findings in the superficial peroneal nerve
    CMAP: Abnormal findings to the EDB
    EMG
    Abnormal activity in the muscles innervated by the superficial and deep peroneal nerves. The short head of the biceps femoris is spared.
  - **Treatment**
    Interventions may include: rehabilitation or surgical procedure.

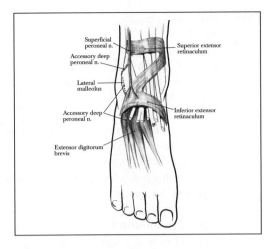

FIGURE 5–114. The Accessory Peroneal Nerve.

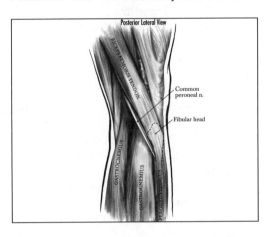

FIGURE 5–115. Peroneal Nerve Proximity to the Fibula Head.

Differential Diagnosis of Foot Drop
- Diffuse Polyneuropathy: Diabetes
- Mononeuropathy: Common Peroneal, Peroneal portion of the Sciatic
- Plexopathy
- Radiculopathy: L4–L5
- Cerebral Involvement : Tumor, CVA, AVM, SCI

Deep Peroneal Neuropathy

- **General**

  A common injury to this nerve is associated with an anterior tarsal tunnel syndrome. (Figure 5–116)

- **Etiology**

  The terminal portion of the deep peroneal nerve can be injured by compression, from trauma or high heeled shoes, as it passes under the extensor retinaculum.

- **Clinical Presentation**

  The patient may complain of foot weakness and atrophy (EDB weakness). There may also be numbness and paresthesias in the first and second web space. Pain may be located over the dorsum of the foot and relieved with motion.

- **EDX Findings**

  NCS

  SNAP: Abnormal findings to the first web space

  CMAP: Abnormal findings to the EDB

  EMG

  Abnormal activity in the EDB

- **Treatment**

  Interventions may include: rehabilitation or surgical resection.

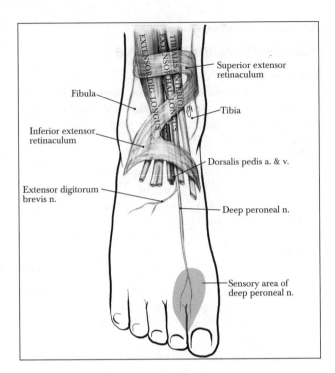

FIGURE 5–116. The Anterior Tarsal Tunnel.

- *Superficial Peroneal Neuropathy*
  - **General**

    After innervating the peroneus longus brevis, the nerve descends as a pure sensory nerve.

  - **Etiology**

    The nerve can be injured by compression from trauma, ankle sprain, muscle herniation, or a lipoma.

  - **Clinical Presentation and Muscle Involvement**

    Includes peroneal longus and peroneal brevis. Patient complains of loss of sensation in distribution of superior peroneal nerve.

  - **EDX Findings**

    NCS

    SNAP: Abnormal superficial peroneal nerve

    CMAP: Not available

    EMG

    Abnormal activity in the peroneal longus or brevis if the lesion is proximal

  - **Treatment**

    Interventions may include: rehabilitation or surgical release.

SURAL NERVE

Anatomy

- **Origin**
  These nerve fibers originate from branches of the tibial and common peroneal nerve. (Figure 5–117)

- **Course**
  Calf
  It passes from the proximal calf to the proximal ankle, posterior to the lateral malleolus. It supplies cutaneous innervation to the lateral calf and foot.

Injury

- *Sural Neuropathy*
  - **General**
    This is a pure sensory nerve.
  - **Etiology**
    The nerve can be injured by compression from tight socks, a Baker's cyst, or a laceration.
  - **Clinical Presentation and Muscle Involvement**
    This is a pure sensory injury; there is no muscle involvement. The patient may complain of abnormal sensations to the lateral calf and foot. A positive Tinel's sign may be elicited along the course of the nerve.
  - **EDX Findings**
    NCS
    SNAP: Abnormal findings in the sural nerve
    CMAP: Not applicable
    EMG
    Not applicable
  - **Treatment**
    Interventions may included: rehabilitation or surgical procedure.

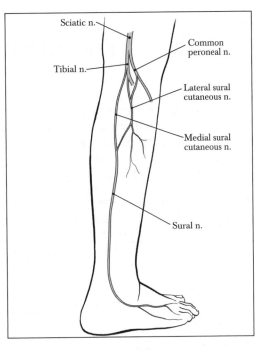

FIGURE 5–117. The Sural Nerve

■
PERIPHERAL NEUROPATHY

Definition

This pathology affects the myelin and/or axon of the peripheral nerves. If demyelination becomes extensive it can be accompanied by mild axonal damage. Determining a primary and predominating process is helpful in understanding the course of the disorder. The primary process can help determine etiology of a neuropathy, while the predominant process can help access prognosis. Two typical patterns have been described: diffuse and multifocal.

Pattern	Presentation
Diffuse	This essentially involves all nerves in a length-dependent fashion to a relatively equal extent.
Multifocal	This involves one or multiple nerves in an asymmetric or patchy distribution.

Etiology

There are several ways to classify peripheral neuropathies. Two systems are listed in Tables 5–33 and 5–34.

Clinical Presentation

The patient may describe a Classic Triad that presents more in the lower limbs than the upper limbs

- Sensory changes in a stocking/glove distribution
- Distal weakness
- Hypo/Areflexia

EDX Findings

The diagnostic criteria consists of evaluating at least three limbs. Abnormalities of SNAPs, CMAPs, and MUAPs are dependent on the type and timing of the pathology affecting a nerve.

Special Studies

Description: Small nerve fiber abnormalities and associated autonomic dysfunction may not be seen with conventional NCS and can require additional tests.

Autonomic Nerve Studies

- Sympathetic Skin Potentials
  This study is dependent on exocrine sweat glands and cutaneous innervations. Stimulation should be performed at irregular intervals, greater than 30 seconds, to avoid a process of habituation. The stimulus sources used are electrical, coughing, noises, breathing, or tactile. The normal latency is 1.5 seconds in the upper limbs and 2 seconds in the lower limbs.
- Sinus Arrhythmia
  This cardiovagal innervation study is dependent on the normal heart rate variations that occur with respiration via parasympathetic activity. Loss of this sinus arrhythmia represents a denervation process. The test consists of measuring the R-R ratio with an EKG machine attached to the amplifier of the EMG.
- Valsalva Ratio
  During a Valsalva maneuver the heart rate varies in response to changes in blood pressure and intrathoracic pressure via sympathetic and parasympathetic activity. Four phases are measured using a standard EMG machine. The findings measured in Phase 2 and Phase 4 are used for monitoring. Phase 2 should demonstrate a heart rate increase and Phase 4 should demonstrate a decrease in the normal population.

TABLE 5–33. Classification I

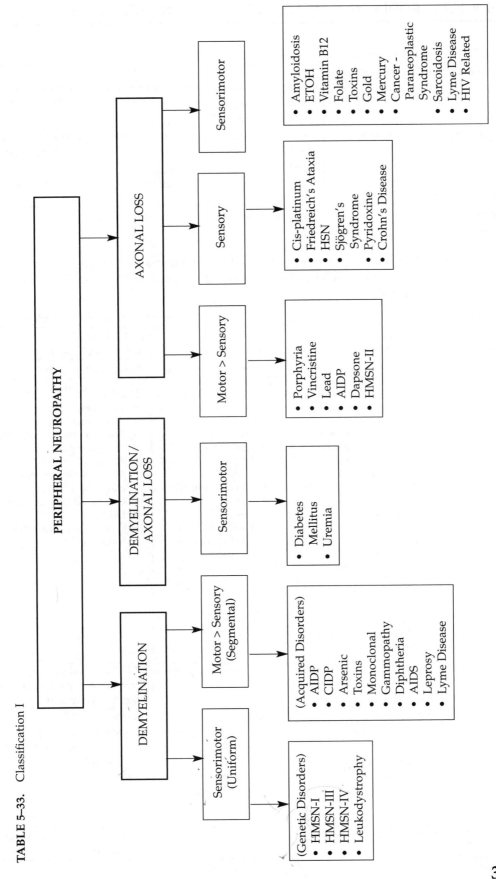

TABLE 5–34. Classification II

Diffuse Axonal Polyneuropathy	Toxins—Heavy metals; Drugs—Vincristine, alcohol; Deficiency—Vitamin B6 deficiency; Metabolic—Uremia, diabetes; paraneoplastic syndrome; Hereditary—HMSN II; Infectious—Leprosy, HIV
Multifocal Axonal Neuropathy	Microangiopathic—Vasculitis, diabetes; amyloidosis; paraneoplastic syndrome; Infectious—CMV; Metabolic—Porphyria; compression
Diffuse Demyelinating Polyneuropathy	Hereditary—HMSN-I; Deficiency—Hypothyroidism; Toxic—Amiodarone, Arsenic
Multifocal Demyelinating Neuropathy	Autoimmune—AIDP, CIDP; Compression

The following tables outline pertinent peripheral neuropatterns as they are defined by criteria in Classification I; please refer to Table 5–33 as an overview for Tables 5–35, 5–36, 5–37, 5–38, 5–39, 5–40 and 5–41.

TABLE 5–35. Uniform Demyelinating Mixed Sensorimotor Neuropathies: Common Disorders

Disease	HMSN I: Charcot Marie Tooth (CMT)	HMSN III: Déjérine Sottas	HMSN IV: Refsum's Disease
Etiology	Autosomal dominant	Autosomal recessive	Autosomal recessive
Onset	Early childhood	Birth–infancy	Approximate third decade
Clinical Presentation	• Slowly progressive • Sensory loss more apparent in the lower limbs than the upper limbs • Abnormal vibration and proprioception • Abnormal muscle stretch response (MSR) • Foot intrinsic atrophy: Pes cavus, hammer toes • Bilateral foot drop—steppage gait • Stork leg appearance • Hypertrophy of peripheral nerves (greater auricular nerve) • Roussy-Levy Syndrome: CMT associated with an essential tremor	• Severe progression • Sensory loss • Weakness • Abnormal MSR • Hypotonic/floppy baby • Delayed milestones • Ataxia • Pes cavus • Kyphoscoliosis • Nystagmus • Deafness	• Weakness • Abnormal MSR • Lower extremity wasting • Steppage gait • Ataxia • Retinitis pigmentosa (night blindness) • Cerebellar dysfunction • Deafness • Cardiac abnormalities • Cataract
Labs	Cerebrospinal Fluid (CSF): Increased Protein (N Bx): Onion bulb formation	CSF: Increased protein	CSF: Increased protein, N Bx: Onion bulb formation, Blood: High phytanic acid

EDX Findings	**NCS**
	  SNAP: Abnormal
	  CMAP: 📖 Abnormal, CV decreased 70%
	  No temporal dispersion
	EMG
	  Normal
		NCS
		  SNAP: Abnormal
		  CMAP: Abnormal,
		  *CV is < 6 m/s,
		  latency is 7x
		  slower than NL
		EMG
		  Normal
			NCS
			  SNAP: Abnormal
			  CMAP: Abnormal, CV is 10 m/s
			EMG
			  Normal

Treatment	Rehabilitation; orthotics	Rehabilitation	Rehabilitation; phytanic acid absent diet

N Bx = Nerve Biopay

TABLE 5-36. Segmental Demyelinating Motor and Sensory Neuropathies: Common Disorders

Disease	Acute Inflammatory Demyelinating Polyradiculopathy: (AIDP) Guillain-Barré Syndrome (GBS)	Chronic Inflammatory Demyelinating Polyradiculopathy: (CIDP)	Leprosy (Hansen's Disease)
Etiology	Possible viral attack on the myelin and Schwann cells	Possible immune mediated response	Mycobacterium Leprae Immune status dependent
Onset	1–4 weeks post illness, vaccination, or surgery	Any age, peaks at 50–60 years of age	
Clinical Presentation	• Male > Female • Ascending sensory abnormalities • Ascending symmetric weakness • Abnormal MSR • Possible respiratory and autonomic failure • Possibly bedridden within two days • CN involvement (Most common: CN VII affected, CN I and II unaffected, • Variants: Miller-Fisher Syndrome, Pure sensory	• Relapsing and remitting course • Sensory abnormalities • Symmetric weakness: proximal > distal • Abnormal MSR • Less cranial nerve involvement	• Most common world-wide neuropathy • Sensory abnormalities • Wrist drop • Foot drop • Facial palsy
Labs	CSF: Increased protein, few mononuclear cells	CSF: Increased protein	N Bx: Foamy histiocyte invasion
EDX Findings	**NCS** SNAP: Abnormal CMAP: Abnormal, temporal dispersion: Increased F wave: Abnormal—first sign **EMG** Normal ☐ **Poor Prognosis:** CMAP: Amplitude < 20% of normal, NCV <40% of normal F wave: Absent EMG: Abnormal Activity (Axonal Involvement)	**NCS** SNAP: Abnormal CMAP: Abnormal, TD: Increased F wave: Abnormal **EMG** Abnormal, if severe	**NCS** SNAP: Abnormal CMAP: Abnormal **EMG** Abnormal, if severe
Treatment	Rehabilitation. Plasmapheresis, IV Immunoglobulins. Steroids are ineffective, respiratory support.	Rehabilitation. High-dose steroids	Rehabilitation. Antileprosy treatment

TABLE 5-37. Axonal Motor > Sensory Neuropathies: Common Disorders

Disease	Porphyria	Toxins			AIDP Axonal	HMSN II CMT–II
		Lead	Vincristine Chemotherapy	Dapsone Leprosy treatment		
Etiology	Defect heme synthesis	Lead	Chemotherapy	Leprosy treatment	Same as demyelination	Autosomal dominant
Clinical Presentation	• Female > male • Lower limb pain • Limb weakness • Back and abdominal pain • Seizures • Mental status changes • Reaction to medication, i.e., barbiturates, sulfonamides	• Progressive onset of upper-limb weakness • Radial neuropathy: Wrist drop (adult, child) • Encephalopathy (Child) • Abdominal discomfort • Blue lines in the gums • Blindness • Epilepsy	• Lower limb paresthesias • Lower limb weakness • Abnormal MSR	• Ascending foot and hand neuropathy Side effects include: Methemoglobinemia	• Areflexia • Autonomic and cranial nerve involvement • Poorer prognosis than with pure demyelination • Associated with CMV and C jejuni infection	• Onset commonly in the 2nd decade • Weakness • Abnormal MSR • Less foot intrinsic involvement • Tremor • Ataxia
Labs	Urine: Deep red	Blood/Urine: Lead Basophilic stippling in RBCs, X-ray-lead lines			CSF: Increased protein	N Bx: No onion bulb formation
EDX Findings	NCS SNAP: Abnormal CMAP: Abnormal EMG Abnormal activity	NCS SNAP: Normal CMAP: Abnormal EMG Abnormal radial muscles	NCS SNAP: Abnormal CMAP: Abnormal EMG Abnormal	NCS SNAP: Normal CMAP: Abnormal EMG Abnormal activity	NCS SNAP: Abnormal CMAP: Abnormal EMG Abnormal activity	NCS SNAP: ± abnormal CMAP: Preserved CV EMG Abnormal activity in the paraspinal
Treatment	Rehabilitation	Rehabilitation: Penicillamine, EDTA	Rehabilitation	Rehabilitation	Rehabilitation	Rehabilitation

TABLE 5–38. Axonal Sensory Neuropathies: Common Disorders

Disease	Toxins	Friedreich's Ataxia	Sjögren's Syndrome	Toxins
Etiology	Cis-platinum	Autosomal Recessive	Autoimmune Disorder	Pyridoxine (B6)
Clinical Presentation	• Painful paresthesias in the hands and feet. • Abnormal sensation • Side Effects: – Nephrotoxicity – Ototoxicity – Myelosuppression – GI complaints	• Onset: 2–16 years old • Abnormal sensation • Weakness • Abnormal MSR • Ataxia: limb and trunk • Optic Atrophy • Kyphoscoliosis • Dysarthria • Pes cavus deformity • Cardiomyopathy • Wheel chair use by 16 years of age	• Dry eyes • Dry mouth • Keratoconjunctivitis Associated with Rheumatoid arthritis • Gland Involvement: – Parotid – Lacrimal – Salivary	• Abnormal Sensation • Gait disturbances • Positive Lhermitte's sign • This may occur with doses of B6 > 600 mg/day • Symptoms improve with drug withdrawal
Lab	N Bx: Abnormal large axons	N Bx: Abnormal large axons	N Bx: Abnormal large axons	N Bx: Abnormal large and small axons
EDX Findings	NCS SNAP: Abnormal CMAP: Normal EMG Normal	NCS SNAP: Abnormal CMAP: Normal EMG Abnormal activity	NCS SNAP: Abnormal CMAP: Normal EMG Abnormal	NCS SNAP: Abnormal CMAP: Normal EMG Abnormal
Treatment	Drug cessation	Rehabilitation	Rehabilitation	Stop vitamin B6

TABLE 5–39. Axonal Sensorimotor Neuropathies: Common Disorders

Disease	ETOH	Amyloidosis	Sarcoidosis
Etiology	Malnutrition or direct nerve injury	Amyloid deposition in DRG	Granulomatous disorder
Clinical Presentation	• Sensory abnormalities • Foot or wrist drop • Muscle spasms • Korsakoff's psychosis • Wernicke's encephalopathy • +/– associated with a myopathy	• Sensory abnormalities • Weight loss • Ankle edema • Hepatomegaly • Purpura • Nephrotic syndrome • Congestive heart failure	• Low birth weight • Fatigue • Bilateral hilar adenopathy • Uveitis • Cranial nerve involvement (CN VII most common)
Labs	N Bx.: Wallerian Degeneration	Tissue Bx: (+) birefringence with congo red staining	Blood: Increased ESR, N Bx: Sarcoid tubercles

EDX Findings	NCS
	  SNAP: Abnormal
	  CMAP: Abnormal
	EMG
	  Abnormal activity
		NCS
		  SNAP: Abnormal
		  CMAP: Abnormal
		EMG
		  Abnormal activity
			NCS
			  SNAP: Abnormal
			  CMAP: Abnormal
			EMG
			  Abnormal activity

Treatment	Vitamins, diet, stop alcohol consumption, orthotics	Rehabilitation	Rehabilitation

TABLE 5–40. Mixed Axonal And Demyelinating Neuropathies: Common Disorders

Disease	Diabetes Mellitus	Uremia
Clinical Presentation	• Sensory abnormalities • Variants: Polyneuropathy, mononeuropathy, autonomic disorders, or amyotrophy • Most common peripheral neuropathy in North America	• Occurs in 60% of patients with renal failure • Sensory abnormalities • Hypersensitivity to touch • Associated with restless leg syndrome
Labs	Blood: Elevated glucose, N Bx: Small and large fiber abnormalities	Blood: Increased nitrogen and urea., N Bx: Paranodal demyelination, axon loss

EDX Findings	**NCS**
	  SNAP: Abnormal
	  CMAP: Abnormal
	EMG
	  Abnormal activity
		NCS
		  SNAP: Abnormal
		  CMAP: Abnormal
		EMG
		  Abnormal activity

Treatment	Rehabilitation: Control blood sugar	Rehabilitation:. Dialysis, kidney transplant

TABLE 5–41. Other Neuropathies

HIV
Five Major Categories • 📖 Distal Symmetric Polyneuropathy • Inflammatory Demyelinating Polyneuropathy • Mononeuropathy Multiplex • Progressive Polyradiculopathy • Autonomic Neuropathy
Most commonly presents with demyelination and axonal loss.

NCS
  SNAP: Abnormal
  CMAP: Abnormal
EMG
Abnormal activity

Rehabilitation, Medications

■
NEUROMUSCULAR JUNCTION DISORDERS

Definition

These disorders hinder the production, release, or uptake of acetylcholine. A low safety factor causes the amplitude of the end plate potentials to fall below the threshold needed to generate a muscle fiber action potential. This occurs due to an alteration of quantal response or content. Myasthenia gravis is a disorder resulting in a decreased quantal response due to loss of acetylcholine receptors. This leads to reduced miniature end plate potential amplitudes, but their frequency remains normal. Lambert-Eaton Syndrome (Myasthenic Syndrome) is a disorder resulting in decreased quantal content leaving normal miniature end plate potential amplitudes but with decreased frequency.

TABLE 5–42   Neuromusclar Junction Disorders

	Myasthenia Gravis	Lambert-Eaton Syndrome (LEMS)	Botulism
Location	*Postsynaptic*	*Presynaptic*	*Presynaptic*
Etiology	• A disorder of neuromuscular transmission due to an autoimmune response against ACh receptors on the postsynaptic membrane • Associated with thymic disorder or thymic tumor	• A disorder of neuromuscular transmission due to an autoimmune response against the active sites on the presynaptic membrane • This decreases Ca^{++} entry into the cell, causing a decreased released of ACh into the synaptic cleft • Associated with small cell (oat cell) carcinoma of the lung	• A disorder of neuromuscular transmission caused by Clostridium Botulinum toxins blocking exocytosis of ACh from the nerve terminal • Associated with ingestion of contaminated raw meat, fish, canned vegetables, honey
Onset	Female > Male	Male < Female (>40 yrs)	Begins 2–7 days after ingestion
Clinical Presentation	• Proximal fatigue and weakness • Exacerbated with exercise, heat, or time of day (evening) • Normal MSR • 📖 Facial or bulbar symptoms: – Ptosis – Diplopia – Dysphagia – Dysarthria • Improved with rest • Edrophonium (Tensilon) Test: 2 mg dose followed by a 8 mg dose, improvement begins in 1 minute	• Proximal fatigue and weakness • Mainly affects the lower limbs (quadriceps) • Abnormal MSR • Exacerbated with rest • Improved with exercise • Viselike grip • Rarely involves the neck, facial, or bulbar muscles	• Bulbar symptoms are noted first: – Ptosis – Dysphagia, – Dysarthria • GI Symptoms: diarrhea, N/V • Widespread paralysis or flaccidity • Abnormal MSR • Respiratory and cardiac dysfunction *(continued)*

TABLE 5–42 *continued*

Location	Myasthenia Gravis *Postsynaptic*	Lambert-Eaton Syndrome *Presynaptic*	Botulism *Presynaptic*
Labs	Muscle Biopsy: Simplification of the postsynaptic membrane with loss of junctional folds and receptors. (Fig. 5–118) Blood: Anti ACh receptor antibodies	Muscle Biopsy: Overdevelopment of neuromuscular junction. (Figure 5–119) Decreased active zones are noted	Stool: Toxins noted. Blood: toxins noted

EDX Findings	**NCS**
	  SNAP: Normal
	  CMAP: Normal
	EMG
	  Unstable MUAP, drop-off occurs with sustained contraction (Figure 5–119)
	See special studies
		NCS
		  SNAP: Normal
		  CMAP: Low amplitude
		EMG
		  Unstable MUAP, drop-off occurs with sustained contraction
		See special studies
			NCS
			  SNAP: Normal
			  CMAP: Abnormal amplitude
			EMG
			Unstable MUAP
			See special studies

Treatment	• Thymectomy • Anticholinesterase drugs: Mestinon 30 mg q 4–6 hours • Corticosteroids • Immunosuppressive agents • Plasmapheresis • One-third improve spontaneously	• Treat malignancy • Corticosteroids • Immunosuppressive agents • Plasmapheresis • Guanidine—increases ACh quanta • Side effects: GI, bone marrow suppression, renal tubular necrosis	• Treat with trivalent ABE antitoxin • Recovery occurs from collateral sprouting

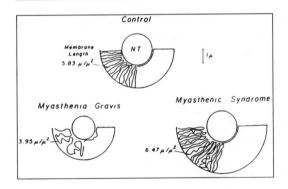

FIGURE 5–118. Postsynaptic Membrane Changes. MG—Simplification of the postsynaptic membrane. The NMJ demonstrates a reduction in the number of postsynaptic juntional folds. MS—Hypertrophy of postsynaptic membrane; the NMJs demonstate an increase in the complexity of the postsynaptic membrance architecture. (From Engel AG, Santa T. Histometric analysis of the ultrastructure of the neuromuscular junction in myasthenia gravis and the myasthenic syndrome. Ann N Y Acad Sci 1971;183:46-63, with permission.)

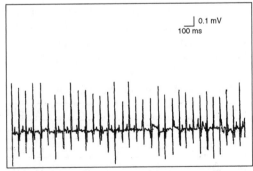

FIGURE 5–119. Unstable Motor Unit Action Potential. Same MUAP with varying amplitudes. This is seen in patients with MG (myasthenia gravis); amplitude variations are from NMJ blocking.

REPETITIVE NERVE STIMULATION (RNS)

Definition

These are studies in which a repeated supramaximal stimulation of a motor nerve is performed. A run of CMAPs are recorded for pathologic amplitude changes. Muscles should be evaluated in a proximal progression if an abnormality is suspected, but not demonstrated. Proper setup is essential to obtain the appropriate responses. (Figure 5–120)

TABLE 5–42   Muscle Evaluation for RNS

Progression	Muscles
First	ADM or APB
Second	Deltoid
Third	Trapezius
Fourth	Orbicularis oculi

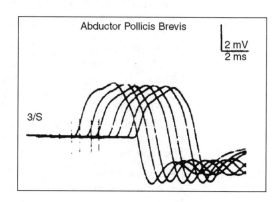

FIGURE 5–120.   Repetitive Nerve Stimulation: Normal Response.

Set-up
- Immobilize the electrode
- Immobilize the limb
- Stimulate at a supramaximal level
- Control limb temperature (~30° C)
- Minimize electrode gel
- Stop anticholinesterase inhibitors

Abnormality:

A greater than 10% decrease in amplitude from the first to fifth waveform is significant for pathology.

Low Rate Repetitive Stimulation (LRRS)

Description: This repetitive stimulation test is performed at a rate of 2–3 Hz. Each stimulus causes the endplate potential (EPP) amplitude to drop. If the safety factor is decreased the potential will fall below the threshold necessary for activation. This results in a decrease of the MUAP amplitude. (Figure 5–121)

TABLE 5–44   LRRS Amplitude Changes

Disorder	Amplitude Change
Myasthenia Gravis⌨	Greater than 10% decrement
Eaton-Lambert Syndrome	Greater than 10% decrement
Botulism	Greater then 10% decrement

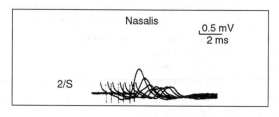

FIGURE 5–121.   LRRS Decremental Response.

Post Activation Facilitation (PAF)

After a decrement is noted with LRRS, a 10-second isometric contraction or tetany producing stimulation (50 Hz) should be performed. PAF demonstrates a repair in the CMAP's amplitude with an immediate follow-up LRRS because of an improvement in neuromuscular transmission.

Post Activation Exhaustion (PAE)

This response is seen as a CMAP amplitude decreases. It occurs with a LRRS performed every minute for 5 minutes after an initial 3-second isometric contraction. ▢ The greatest dropoff is between 2–4 minutes. This test should be used if a decrement does not present with the initial LRRS, but a diagnosis of a neuromuscular junction disorder is suspected. (Figure 5–122)

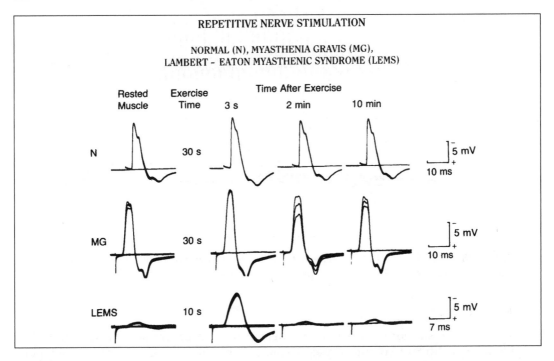

FIGURE 5–122. Postactivation Facilitation and Postactivation Exhaustion. Repetitive nerve stimulation studies in a normal subject (N) and patients with myasthenia gravis (MG) and Lambert-Eaton Myasthenic Syndrome (LEMS). Three successive M waves were elicited by repetitive nerve stimulation at a rate of 2 Hz. The three responses were superimposed. This method of display emphasizes a change in the configuration of successive responses, but does not permit identification of the order of the responses, In each superimposed display of three responses where the configuration did change, the highest amplitude response was the first response, and the lowest amplitude response was the third response. After testing the rested muscle, the muscle was forcefully contracted for 10 to 30 seconds (exercise time). The repetitive nerve stimulation was carried out again 3 s, 2 min, and 10 min after the exercise ended. The results illustrate facilitation and postactivation depression (exhaustion). (Reprinted with permission from Dumitru D. Electrodiagnostic Medicine. Philadelphia, Hanley & Belfus, 1995.)

High Rate Repetitive Stimulation (HRRS)

Description: This repetitive stimulation test is performed at a rate of 10–50 Hz. It causes an accumulation of calcium in the cell, which assists ACh release and repairs the waveforms. HRRS is uncomfortable and a maximal isometric contraction can serve as a substitute. (Figure 5–123).

TABLE 5–45 HRRS Amplitude Changes

Disorder	Amplitude Change
Myasthenia Gravis	Decrement demonstrated
Lambert-Eaton Syndrome	200%–300% Increment
Botulism	Mild increment

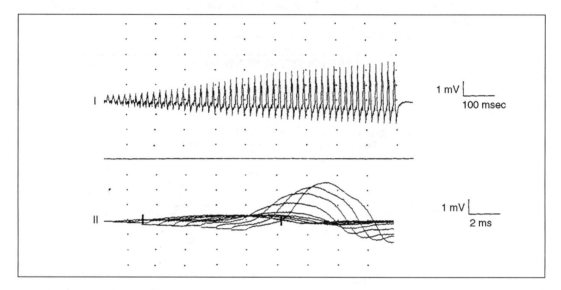

FIGURE 5–123. High Rate Repetitive Stimulation. **I:** Increment with 50 Hz stimulation. **II:** Increment with voluntary contraction (50Hz simulation/train of 50, Femoral/Rectus Femoris, 500% facilitation

Pseudofacilitation

Description: This is a normal reaction and demonstrates a progressive increase in CMAP amplitude with HRRS or voluntary muscle contraction. It represents a decrease in temporal dispersion and increased synchronicity of muscle fiber contraction. The waveforms produced maintain a constant area under the curve though the amplitude appears increased. (Figure 5–124)

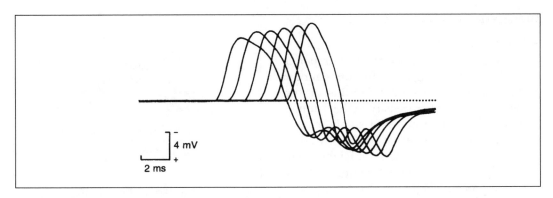

FIGURE 5–124. Pseudofacilitation. Repetitive Nerve Stimulation Study in a Normal Subject. The successive M waves were recorded with surface electrodes over the hypothenar eminence (abductor digiti quinti) during ulnar nerve stimulation at a rate of 30 Hz. Pseudofacilitation may occur in normal subjects with repetitive nerve stimulation at high (20–50 Hz) rates or after strong volitional contraction, and probably reflects a reduction in the temporal dispersion of the summation of a constant number of muscle fiber action potentials due to increases in the propagation velocity of action potentials of muscle cells with repeated activation. Pseudofacilitation should be distinguished from facilitation. The recording shows an incrementing response characterized by an increase in the amplitude of the successive M waves with a corresponding decrease in the duration of the M wave resulting in no change in the area of the negative phase of the successive M waves. (Reprinted with permission from Dumitru D. Electrodiagnostic Medicine. Philadelphia, Hanley & Belfus, 1995).

SINGLE FIBER EMG (SFEMG)

Definition

This is a study that monitors the parameters of single muscle fiber action potentials. It is useful if repetitive stimulation of at least three muscles is normal and an abnormal diagnosis is still suspected. Abnormalities can be associated with neuromuscular junction disorders, motor neuron disorders, and peripheral neuropathies.

📖 Parameters

- *Fiber Density (FD)*
  Description: This represents the number of single fibers belonging to the same motor unit within the recording radius of the electrode. The fiber density is determined by dividing the number of single muscle fibers action potentials at 20 sites by 20. A fiber density of 1.5 is normal. Higher than this represents a denervation and reinnervation process. (Figure 5–125)

- *Jitter*
  Description: During voluntary contraction a small variation exists between the interpotential discharges of two muscle fibers belonging to the same motor unit. This variation is normally 10–60 μ. It is typically considered abnormal if higher than this amount. (Figure 5–126)

- *Blocking*
  Description: This is an abnormality that occurs when a single muscle fiber action potential fails to appear. It occurs if the jitter becomes greater than 100 μ. 📖 It typically resolves in approximately 1–3 months, after reinnervation is completed.

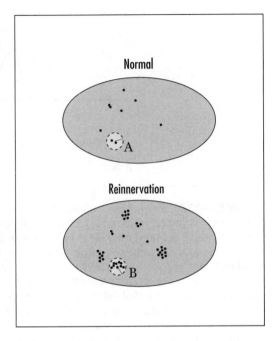

FIGURE 5–125. Increased Fiber Density. The dots represent single muscle fibers of one motor unit with the recording radius.
A. Normal muscle (Action Potentials from 1–2 fibers recorded)
B. Reinnervation (Action Potentials from many fibers recorded)

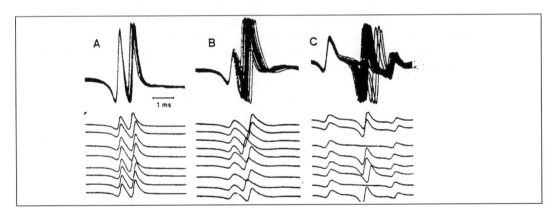

FIGURE 5–126. Single Fiber EMG Recordings. Top: Superimposed view. Bottom: Rastered view. **A:** Normal. **B:** Increased Jitter. **C:** Increased Jitter with blocking. (From Stalberg, E. Clinical electromyography in myasthenia gravis. J Neurol Neurosurg Psychiatry 43:622-633, 1980, BMJ Publishing, with permission.)

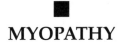

MYOPATHY

Definition

This is a skeletal muscle fiber disorder that can occur from a variety of etiologies. Important factors to consider in its diagnosis are: age of onset; developmental milestones; familial involvement; prodromal illness; and patient history. Please refer to the pediatric section for added information on this topic.

Etiology

TABLE 5–46 Etiology of Myopathies

Dystrophic	Congenital	Metabolic	Inflammatory	Endocrine	Toxic	Steroid

• Duchenne
• Becker
• Limb-girdle
  disorder
• Fascioscapulo-
  humeral
• Myotonic
	• Central core
	• Nemaline rod
	• Centronuclear
	• Fiber type
	  Disproportion
		• Acid maltase
		  deficiency
		• Myophosphorlyase
		  deficiency
		• Phosphofructo-
		  kinase deficiency
		• Hyperkalemic
		  periodic paralysis
		• Hypokalemic
		  periodic paralysis
			• Polymyositis
			  Dermatomyositis
			• Sarcoidosis
			• Viral
			• Bacterial
			• Parasitic
				• Thyroid
				  Parathyroid
				• Adrenal
				  Pituitary
					• Alcohol
					• Diuretic
					• Vincristine
					• Steroid
						• Cortico-
						  steroid use

Clinical Presentation

The patient may demonstrate muscle related changes presenting as: atrophy, hypertrophy, abnormal muscle stretch response, weakness, hypotonia, gait abnormalities, or myotonia. Myotonia is a painless delayed relaxation of skeletal muscles following a voluntary contraction. It is exacerbated by cold but relieved with exercise, dilantin, procainamide, and calcium channel blockers. Arthrogryposis, which is a fixed deformity of the extremities due to intrauterine hypomobility, may occur in newborns from myopathies, muscular dystrophies, or oligohydramnios. A hallmark sign of myopathy is the inability to generate a forceful contraction.

EDX Findings

NCS

SNAP: Normal

CMAP: Abnormal amplitude due to muscle fiber atrophy. Normal conduction velocity

EMG

Resting Activity: Abnormal activity (AA) depends on the type of disorder involved.

TABLE 5–47   Abnormal Spontaneous Activity in Myopathies

Fibrillations and Positive Sharp Waves	Complex Repetitive Discharge	Myotonic Discharge
• Polymyositis • Dermatomyositis • Inclusion body myopathy • Trichinosis • Toxic myopathies • Direct muscle trauma • Rhabdomyolysis • Acid maltase deficiency • Myotubular myopathy • Hyperkalemic periodic paralysis • Nemaline rod • Sarcoid myopathy • Muscular dystrophies	• Polymyositis • Dermatomyositis • Muscular dystrophies • Schwartz-Jampel syndrome • Inclusion body myopathy	• Myotonia congenita • Myotonic dystrophy • Paramyotonia congenita • Hyperkalemic periodic paralysis • Acid maltase deficiency • Hypothyroid myopathy • Myotubular myopathy • Chloroquine myopathy • Diazocholesterol intoxication • Polymyositis • Dermatomyositis

TABLE 5–48.   Recruitment: Early Onset with Minimal Effort.

Presentation	Possible Causes of MUAP Alterations
SDSA	These classic polyphasic potentials are due to loss of muscle fibers
LDLA	These polyphasic potenials are due to collateral sprouting
Unstable	These variable amplitude potentials are due to blocking of immature neuro-muscular junctions, which are formed at the beginning of collateral sprouting

Quantitative EMG

This study may provide a more detailed measurment of the MUAPs. It is a better indication of waveform duration, which is a sensitive parameter for diagnosing myopathies. The mean duration is calculated using 20 MUAPs and on a screen set with a trigger and delay line. This avoids superimposing MUAPs and falsely creating a polyphasic.

Repetative Stimulation

A normal or a decremental response can occur. This is due to the reduced safety factor found in regenerating immature neuromuscular junctions that form during recovery or reinnervation.

SFEMG

This can demonstrate increased jitter, fiber density, and blocking.

LABS

Muscle Biopsy

Type I Fiber Atrophy	Type II Fiber Atrophy
• Myotonic dystrophy • Nemaline myopathy • Fiber type disproportion	• Steroid myopathy • Myasthenia gravis • Deconditioning

The following tables outline pertinent myopathic patterns. Please refer to Table 5-46 as an overview for Tables 5–49, 5–50, 5–51, 5–52, 5–53, 5–54, 5–55.

Dystrophic Myopathies: Common Disorders

TABLE 5-49

Disorder	Duchenne Muscular Dystrophy (most common myopathy)	Becker Muscular Dystrophy	Myotonic Dystrophy (Steiner's) (second most common)	Fascioscapulohumeral Dystrophy FSH
Etiology	X-linked recessive (xp21), spontaneous	X-linked recessive	Autosomal dominant	Autosomal dominant
Onset	3–5 years old	Adulthood	Infant	Childhood-early adult
Course	Severely progressive (death by 20s)	Slowly progressive		Spreads to other muscles
Clinical Presentation	• Proximal muscle weakness (pelvic girdle) • Abnormal MSR • Increased lumbar lordosis • Ambulation difficulties: Toe walking (< 5 years), clumsy running (<7years) • Gower's sign: Difficulty rising from the floor due to hip and knee extensor weakness • Calf pseudohypertrophy with fat and fibrous tissue • Contractures: Iliotibial Band—First Achilles Tendon • Scoliosis, causing cardiomyopathy and restrictive lung disease • Possible mental retardation • Wheelchair by 12 years old • Extraocular muscles are spared	• Proximal weakness • Calf pseudohypertrophy • Cardiomyopathy • Less mental retardation than DMD	• Weakness: Distal > Proximal myotonia with sustained grip • Hatchet Face (wasting of the temporalis and masseter) • Frontal balding • Poor vision • Ptosis • Impotence • Hypertrichosis • Mental retardation • Cardiac abnormalities • Endocrine abnormalities • Congenital Myotonic Dystrophy: – "Shark mouth" appearance – Facial diplegia – Possible club foot	• Proximal muscle weakness • Facial droop • Weak eye closing • Weak forehead wrinkling • Arm atrophy with deltoid and forearm sparing (Popeye arm) • Cataracts (dry sclera) • Retinopathy • Lip protrusion • Transverse smile • Frontal balding • Testicular atrophy • Extraocular muscles are spared • #1 muscle to test in FSH is Tib. Ant. • Inability to whistle
Labs	Muscle Bx: No dystrophin, internal nuclei variation in fiber size. Blood: Increased CPK and Aldolase. ECG: Abnormal	Muscle Bx.: Decreased dystrophin (15%–85%), Increased CPK	Muscle Bx.: Type I fiber atrophy with type II hypertrophy. No dystrophin involvement	Muscle Bx.: Scattered fiber necrosis and regeneration. Inflammatory infiltrate may be noted
EDX Findings	NCS SNAP: Normal CMAP: +/- Decreased Amplitude EMG (AA is rare) ER, +/- SDSA MUAP	NCS SNAP: Normal CMAP: +/- Dec. Amplitude EMG (AA is rare), ER, SDSA MUAP	NCS SNAP: Normal CMAP: +/- Dec. Amplitude EMG (AA is rare), ER, SDSA MUAP, myotonia	NCS SNAP: Normal CMAP: Decreased amplitude in the involved muscles EMG AA, ER, SDSA MUAP
Treatment	Rehabilitation. Scoliosis surgery before the vital capacity is below 35%. (usually due to a curve of >30°)	Rehabilitation: Bracing, tendon lengthening, possible scoliosis surgery	Rehabilitation: bracing, medications: procainamide, dilantin, and quinine (PDQ). May need a pacemaker	Rehabilitation

AA: Abnormal Activity, ER: Early Recruitment

Congenital Myopathies: Common Disorders

TABLE 5–50

Disorder	Central Core Disease	Nemaline Rod Myopathy	Centronuclear Myotubular	Fiber Type Disproportion
Hereditary	Autosomal dominant	Autosomal dominant/recessive	X –linked recessive	Variable
Onset	Infancy	Infancy	Infancy	Infancy
Clinical Presentation	• Floppy infant/hypotonia • Proximal weakness • Congenital hip dislocation • Delayed milestones • ▣ Associated with malignant hyperthermia	• Floppy infant/hypotonia • Diffuse weakness • Facial involvement • Narrowed long face • High arched palate • Death: Respiratory failure • Foot drop EOM spared	• Floppy infant/hypotonia • Ptosis • Extra ocular muscle involvement • Facial diplegia • Dysphagia • Respiratory insufficiency	• Floppy infant/hypotonia • Hip contractures • Hip dislocations
Labs	Muscle biopsy: Central cores in Type I fibers. Absent mitochondria	Muscle biopsy: Rod shaped bodies on Gomori trichrome stain	Muscle biopsy: Central location of fiber nuclei, forming chains	Muscle biopsy: Numerous small Type I and normal to large Type II fibers
EDX Findings	**EMG** ER, SDSA MUAP	**EMG** ER, SDSA MUAP	**EMG** ▣ AA, ER, SDSA MUAP	**EMG** ER, SDSA MUAP
Treatment	Bracing	Rehabilitation, surgery	Rehabilitation, Antiseizure medication	Rehabilitation, bracing Inflammatory Myopathies: Common disorders

Inflammatory Myopathies

TABLE 5–51

Disorder	Polymyositis/Dermatomyositis	Inclusion Body Myositis
Etiology	Autoimmune, connective tissue disorder, infection, cancer	Unknown

Clinical Presentation	• Symmetrical proximal weakness: Hips followed by shoulders
	• Neck flexion weakness
	• Myalgias, dysphagia, dysphonia
	• No facial or ocular muscle weakness
	• Dermatimyositis: (includes)
	  – Periorbital violet rash and edema
	  – Gottron's sign: red-purple patches over the knuckles, elbows, knees
		• Asymmetric, slowly progressive, painless weakness in proximal and distal muscles
		• Associated with a polyneuropathy

Labs	Blood: Increased CPK, ESR, Aldolase, SGOT, SGPT, LDH, Muscle Biopsy Necrosis of the Type I and II fibers. Perifascicular atrophy	Blood: Increase in CK, Muscle BX: Rimmed or cytoplasmic/basophilic vacuoles. Eosinophilic inclusion bodies

EDX Findings	NCS
	  SNAP: Normal
	  CMAP: Normal
	EMG
	  📖 AA (most commonly in the paraspinals), ER, SDSA MUAP
		NCS
		  SNAP: +/-Abnormal
		  CMAP: +/-Abnormal
		EMG
		  AA, ER, +/-SDSA MUAP

Treatment	Rehabilitation: corticosteroids, cytotoxic agents, plasmapheresis, rest	Rehabilitation: this condition is refractory to steroid treatment

Metabolic Myopathies: Common Disorders

TABLE 5–52

Characteristics	McArdle's Disease (Type V)	Pompe's Disease (Type II)
Etiology	Autosomal recessive *Myophosphorylase deficiency*	Autosomal recessive *Acid maltase deficiency*
Onset	< 15 years of age.	Infant–adult
Clinical Presentation	• Exercise intolerance • Easy fatigability • Muscle stiffness • Cramping • Second-wind phenomenon: Brief rest improves symptoms • Strenuous exercise can precipitate myolysis. (Possibly cause renal failure and death)	• Hypotonia • Tongue enlargement • Cardiomegaly • Hepatomegaly • Respiratory insufficiency • Death by 2 years of age • A milder form may affect adults

EDX Findings	NCS
	  SNAP: Normal
	  CMAP: Normal
	EMG
	Electrical silence during attacks (contracture)
		NCS
		  SNAP: Normal
		  CMAP: Normal
		EMG
		  AA, ER, SDSA MUAP

Labs	Urine: Myoglobinuria; muscle biopsy: Excess glycogen, absent phosphorylase	Blood: Increase CK during the attacks, nerve biopsy vacuoles in Type I and II fibers
Treatment	Supportive	Supportive

Metabolic Myopathies
Periodic Paralysis: Common Disorders

TABLE 5–53

Characteristics	Hyperkalemic periodic paralysis	Hypokalemic periodic paralysis
Etiology	Autosomal dominant Multiple secondary causes	Autosomal dominant Multiple secondary causes
Onset	Childhood–second decade	Starts in early second decade
Clinical Presentation	• Proximal muscle weakness • Paresthesias of the lips and lower limbs • Myotonia • 🔲 Attacks last 10–60 minutes • May be aborted with exercise • Exacerbated with cold exposure and rest following exercise	• Weakness starts in the legs and spreads proximally • 🔲 Attacks last 12–24 hours • Myotonia seen in the eyelids • 🔲 Exacerbated with rest after exercise, stress, and a high carbohydrate diet

EDX Findings	NCS
	  SNAP: Normal
	  CMAP: Normal
	EMG
	  During an attack: ER, SDSA, MUAP, AA
		NCS
		  SNAP: Normal
		  CMAP: Normal
		EMG
		  During an attack: Electrical silence

Labs	Blood: High K+ during the attack	Blood: Low potassium; muscle biopsy normal
Treatment	Diet: High carbohydrate	Diet: K+ supplement

Myotonic Myopathies: Common Disorders

TABLE 5–54

Characteristics	Myotonia Congenita (Thompson's Disease) (Little Hercules)	Paramyotonia Congenita (Eulenburg)
Etiology	Autosomal dominant	Autosomal dominant
Onset	Birth–adulthood	Birth–adulthood
Clinical Presentation	• Severe spasms exacerbated by the cold • Improves with warmth and exercise • Muscle hypertrophy • Myotonia • No weakness	• Stiffness • Weakness • Fatigue • Myotonia • Exacerbated with cold and exercise
Labs	Blood: CK—normal	Muscle biopsy: Fiber size variation

EDX Findings	NCS
	  SNAP: Normal CMAP Normal
	EMG
	AA (myotonic discharges, no fibs, no pos. waves) normal recruitment, normal MUAP
		NCS
		  SNAP: Normal
		  CMAP: Decreased with cooling
		EMG
		Electric silence or AA with cooling.

Treatment	Medication: PDQ	Warm extremities

Steroid Myopathy

TABLE 5–55

Characteristics	Steroid
Etiology	Due to corticosteroid use
Onset	Weeks to years post use
Cinical Presentation	📖 Proximal muscle weakness
Labs	Muscle biopsy: Type II atrophy

EDX Findings	NCS
	  SNAP: Normal
	  CMAP: Normal
	EMG
	  Normal

Treatment	Rehabilitation: Stop steroids

■

MOTOR NEURON DISEASE

Definition
This is a disorder resulting from the progressive degeneration of the motor neurons in the spinal cord, brainstem, or motor cortex. It manifests as muscular weakness and atrophy with varying corticospinal tract signs. See Pediatric section for further information.

Etiology

TABLE 5–56   Motor Neuron Diseases

Lower Motor Neuron Lesion	Upper and Lower Motor Neuron Lesion	Upper Motor Neuron Lesion
Spinal muscle atrophy (SMA) Poliomyelitis/postpolio syndrome	Amyotrophic lateral sclerosis (ALS)	Primary lateral sclerosis

Clinical Presentation

LMN vs. UMN Signs

TABLE 5–57   Signs: LMN vs. UMN

Lower Motor Neuron	Upper Motor Neuron
Atrophy	Weakness
Flaccidity	Spasticity
Hyporeflexia	Hyperreflexia
Fasciculations	Up-going plantar response

EDX Findings

NCS
SNAP: Normal
CMAP: Normal early. Possible decreased amplitude or conduction velocity

EMG
Resting activity: Abnormal activity (AA) depends on the type of disorder involved
Recruitment: Decreased (DR)

TABLE 5–58   Abnormal Spontaneous Activity in Motor Neuron Disease

Fibrillations and Positive Sharp Waves	Fasciculations	Complex Repetitive Discharge
• SMA Type I • SMA Type II • SMA Type III • Amyotrophic Lateral Sclerosis (ALS) • Poliomyelitis	• ALS • Poliomyelitis • Postpolio syndrome	• SMA Type III

The following tables outline pertinent motor neuron disease patterns. Please refer to Table 5–56 as an overview for Tables 5–59 and 5–60.

TABLE 5–59　Motor Neuron Disease: SMA I, II, III

Characteristics	Spinal Muscle Atrophy Type I (Werdnig-Hoffman Disease)	Spinal Muscle Atrophy Type II (Chronic Werdnig-Hoffman)	Spinal Muscle Atrophy Type III (Kugelberg-Welander Disease)
Etiology	Autosomal recessive	Autosomal recessive	Autosomal recessive/dominant
Onset	3–6 months	2–12 months	2–15 years
Course	Death by 2–3 years of age	Death ~ by 10 years old	Normal life expectancy
	Worst prognosis	Wheelchair by 2–3 years of age	Wheelchair by 30 years of age
Progression	Rapid. Fatal (respiratory failure)	Slower. Fatal (respiratory failure)	Slowly
Clinical Presentation	• Floppy baby/hypotonia • Unable to reach milestones • Progressive weakness • Absent MSR • Difficulty feeding • Weak cry • Frog legged position • Tongue fasciculations • 📖 Facial muscle affected least • Extraocular muscles intact • Sphincter muscles are spared • Paradoxical breathing • 📖 Never sits independently	• Floppy baby/hypotonia • Gradual progressive limb weakness; upper > lower • Absent MSR • Face least affected • Kyphoscoliosis • Equinus deformity of the feet • ± Tongue fasciculations • Progressive pulmonary involvement • 📖 Independent sitting • 📖 Assistive devices for standing and walking	• Symmetric weakness: lower limb then upper limb • Abnormal MSR • 📖 ± Gowers' sign • 📖 ± calf pseudohypertrophy • ± Dysphagia • ± Dysarthria • Tongue fasciculations—late onset • Normal intelligence • 📖 Independent standing/walking
Labs	Blood: Increase CPK levels M. Bx.: Hyper/Atrophic fibers	Blood: Increase CPK levels M. Bx.: Hyper/Atrophic fibers	Blood: Increase CPK levels M. Bx.: Hyper/Atrophic fibers
EDX Findings	NCS 　SNAP: Normal 　CMAP: +/- Abnormal EMG 　AA, LDLA/SDSA MUAP, DR	NCS 　SNAP: Normal 　CMAP: +/- Abnormal EMG 　AA, SDSA MUAP, DR	NCS 　SNAP: Normal 　CMAP: Normal EMG 　AA, LDLA/SDSA MUAP, DR
Treatment	Supportive	Supportive. rehabilitation	Supportive

TABLE 5–60 Motor Neuron Disease: ALS, Polio, Postpoliomyelitis

Characteristics	Amyotrophic Lateral Sclerosis (Als)	Poliomyelitis	Postpoliomyelitis Syndrome
Pathology	Degeneration of the anterior horn cell	Degeneration of the anterior horn cell	Loss of the anterior horn cell
Etiology	Unknown	Picornavirus orally enters the body and spreads via lymphoid system leading to orphaned muscle fibers	Death of the motor neuron due to aging Burnout of motor unit from increased metabolic demand. (Figure 5–127)

Clinical Presentation	• Most commonly in men after the sixth decade
	• ⊡ First signs: asymmetric atrophy, weakness, fasciculations
	• ⊡ Dysphagia (oral, pharyngeal), dysarthria
	• Pseudobulbar signs (crying and laughing)
	• Bowel and bladder are spared
	• Sensation is spared
	• Extraocular muscles are spared
	• Upper and lower motor neuron signs
	• Prognosis: 50% die within 3 years, 30% live for 5 years, 10% live for 10 years
	• Wheelchair by 12–18 months
	• Predictors of survival:
	  – Age of onset (younger is better)
	  – Severity of onset
	  – Pulmonary function
		• Signs of infection: fever, malaise, sore throat, vomiting headache, back and neck pain and stiffness
		• Weakness
		• Absent MSR
		• Bulbar palsies: dysphasia, nasal voice
		• ⊡ Sensation is spared
		• Autonomic dysfunction can occur
		• **Prognosis**
		Disease can progress or remit
		25%: Severe disability
		25%: Mild disability
		50%: Complete recovery
		Mortality: 1%–4% chance in children. 10% chance in adults with bulbar and respiratory involvement
			Halstead-Ross Criteria
			1) History of a previous diagnosis
			2) Recovery of function
			3) Stability for approximately 15 years
			4) Return of symptoms
			5) No other medical problems to explain new symptoms:
			  • Weakness
			  • Atrophy
			  • Fatigue
			  • Arthralgia
			  • Myalgia
			  • Cold intolerance

EDX Findings	**NCS** SNAP: Normal CMAP: Normal **EMG** AA, DR, LDLA MUAP **LRRS** Increased decrement **SFEMG** ⊡ Increased jitter and fiber density **Protocol:** Abnormal activity in two muscles from two different nerve roots in three different body regions. **Body Regions:** Brain stem, Cervical, Thoracic, Lumbar	**NCS** SNAP: Normal CMAP: Normal **EMG** AA, DR, LDLA MUAP	**NCS** SNAP: Normal CMAP: Abnormal **EMG** AA, DR, GIANT MUAP **LRRS** Normal activity **SFEMG** Increased jitter, fiber density and Blocking Postpoliomyelitis syndrome electrophysiologically resembles old stable poliomyelitis. Its diagnosis is not based on EMG/NCS but on clinical presentation.
Treatment	Rehabilitation, prevent contractures, tracheostomy, respiratory therapy, riluzole (Rilutek®) antiglutamate slows disease progression, prolongs ventilator time	Rehabilitation, pain management, prevent contractures	Rehabilitation, assistive devices, energy conservation, psychological counseling, avoid fatigue

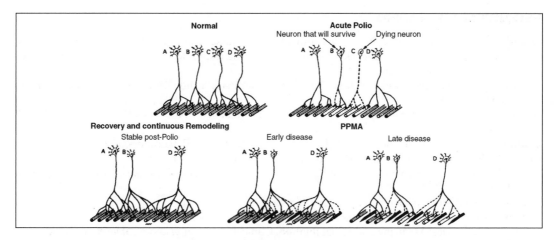

FIGURE 5–127. Post Poliomyelitis Progressive Muscular Dystrophy. (From Stalberg, E. Clinical electrophysiology in myasthenia gravis. J Neurol Neurosurg Psychiatry 43:622-33, 1980, with permission.)

▪

WEAKNESS: DIFFERENTIAL DIAGNOSIS

TABLE 5–61

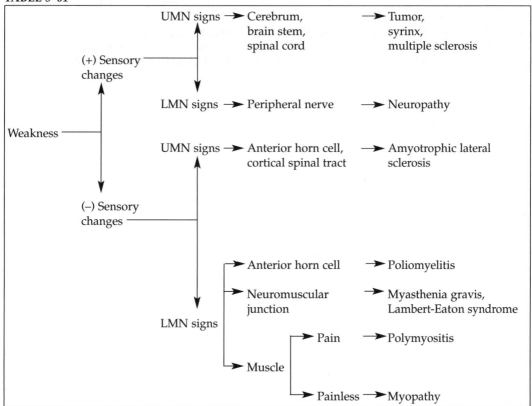

RECOMMENDED READING

AAEM's 1995 Course C: Finally, an Instrumentation Course You Can Understand. Dumitru D. Instrumentation: Parts, Pieces, and Function. Rochester, MN: American Association of Electrodiagnostic Medicine, 1995.

American Society for Surgery of the Hand. The Hand: Examination and Diagnosis. New York: Churchill Livingstone, 1990.

Andressen BL, Wertsch JJ, Stewart WA. Anterior tarsal tunnel syndrome. *Arch Phys Med Rehabil.* 1992 Nov. 73(11); 1112–7.

Braddom RL Physical Medicine and Rehabilitation. Philadelphia: W.B. Saunders, 1996.

Crouch JE. Functional Human Anatomy 4th ed. Philadelphia: Lea & Febiger, 1985.

DeLisa JA. Manual of Nerve Conduction Velocity and Clinical Neurophysiology 3rd ed. New York: Raven Press, 1994.

DeLisa JA. Rehabilitation Medicine. Philadelphia: Lippincott-Raven, 1998.

Dumitru D. Electrodiagnostic Medicine. Philadelphia: Hanley & Belfus, 1995.

Geiringer SR. Physical Medicine and Rehabilitation, Clinical Electrophysiology. *State of the Art Reviews.* June 13(2). Philadelphia: Hanley & Belfus, 1999.

Guyton AC. Textbook of Medical Physiology 8th ed. Philadelphia: W.B. Saunders, 1991.

Hoppenfeld S. Physical Examination of the Spine and Extremities. Norwalk: Appleton-Century-Crofts, 1976.

Johnson EW. Practical Electrography 2nd ed. Baltimore: Williams & Wilkins, 1988.

Johnson EW. Practical Electrography 3rd ed. Baltimore: Williams & Wilkins, 1997.

Kimura J. Electrodiagnosis in Diseases of Nerve and Muscle: Principles and Practices 2nd ed. Philadelphia: F.A. Davis, 1989.

Liveson JA. Peripheral neurology: Case Studies in Electrodiagnosis 2nd ed. Philadelphia: F.A. Davis, 1991.

McArdle WD, Katch FL, Katch VL. Exercise Physiology: Energy, Nutrition, and Human Performance 2nd ed. Philadelphia: Lea & Febiger.

Miller M. Review of Orthopaedics 2nd ed. Philadelphia: W.B. Saunders, 1996.

Pecina MM, Krmpotic-Nemanic J, Markiewitz AD. Tunnel Syndromes. Boston: CRC Press, 1991.

Sethi RK. Thompson LL. The Electromyographer's Handbook. Boston: Little, Brown and Company, 1989.

6

PROSTHETICS AND ORTHOTICS

Heikki Uustal, M.D. and Edgardo Baerga, M.D.

■

GAIT ANALYSIS

TERMINOLOGY:

Gait cycle (Figure 6–2, Table 6–3)

A single sequence of functions of one limb is called a gait cycle. It is essentially the functional unit of gait. The gait cycle has two basic components, the *swing phase* and the *stance phase*.
- Stance: phase in which the limb is in contact with the ground
- Swing: phase in which the foot is in the air for limb advancement.

A gait cycle is also referred to as a *stride*.

Stride (Stride length): Linear distance between corresponding successive points of contact of the same foot (e.g., distance measured from heel strike to heel strike of the same foot) (Figure 6–1)

Step (Step Length): Linear distance in the plane of progression between corresponding successive contact points of opposite feet (e.g., distance measured from heel strike of one foot to heel strike of the other foot). Normally, the step length is approximately 15–20 inches. (Figure 6–1)

 Each stride comprises two steps.

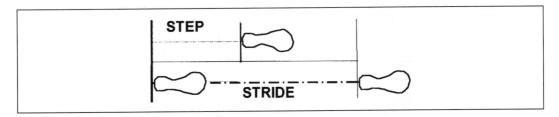

FIGURE 6–1. Step and Stride.

Stance phase can be subdivided into:
1. Initial contact
2. Loading response

3. Midstance
4. Terminal stance
5. Preswing

Remember: "I Like My Tea Pre-sweetened"

Swing phase subdivisions:
1. Initial swing
2. Midswing
3. Terminal swing

Remember: "In My Teapot"

Stance phase

Sub-phases/events
1. **Initial contact**—Instant the foot contacts the ground
2. **Loading response**—Time period from immediately following initial contact to the lift of the contralateral extremity from the ground, during which weight shift occurs
3. **Midstance**—Time interval from lift of the contralateral extremity from the ground to the point where the ankles of both extremities are aligned in the frontal (or coronal) plane
4. **Terminal stance**—Period from ankle alignment in the frontal plane to just prior to initial contact of the contralateral (swinging) extremity
5. **Preswing**—Time interval from initial contact of the contralateral extremity to just prior to lift of the ipsilateral extremity from the ground (unloading weight)

Swing phase

Subphases/events
1. **Initial swing**—Lift of the extremity from the ground to position of maximum knee flexion
2. **Mid swing**—Immediately following knee flexion to vertical tibia position
3. **Terminal swing**—Following vertical tibia position to just prior to initial contact

TABLE 6–1.   Gait Cycle Phases/Events

New terminology (Figure 6–2A)	Old (traditional) terminology (Figure 6–2 B)	
Initial contact	Heel (foot strike) strike	
Loading response	Foot flat	
Midstance	Midstance	STANCE PHASE
Terminal stance	Heel off	
Preswing	Toe off	
Initial swing	Acceleration	
Midswing	Midswing	SWING PHASE
Terminal swing	Deceleration	

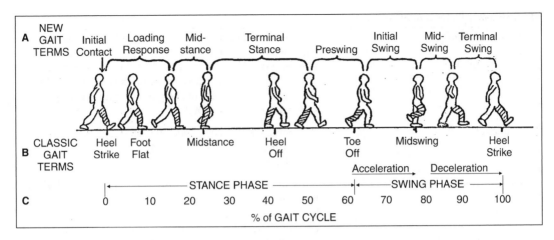

FIGURE 6–2. Gait Cycle: **A:** New Gait Terms. **B:** Classic Gait Terms. **C:** The normal distribution of time during the gait cycle at normal walking speed. (Illustration courtesy of Carson Schneck, M.D.)

- Normal step length = 38cm; normal base of support (distance between heels) = 6–10cm
- ▣ The normal distribution of time during the gait cycle at normal walking speed is *60% for stance phase* and *40% for swing phase*. Walking faster decreases the time spent in stance phase (increasing time spent in swing phase). (Figure 6–2 C)
- **Double-limb support:** period during which both feet are in contact with the floor. Both the beginning and the end of the stance phase are considered to be double-support period.
- **Single- limb support:** period starts when the opposite foot is lifted for the swing phase
- **Double-support** usually comprises *20%* of the normal gait cycle vs. *80%* of single-limb support. The amount of time spent during double-limb support decreases as the speed of walking increases. Walking is differentiated from running, because in the latter there is no double-support period.
- **Cadence:** Number of steps per unit of time.
- Comfortable walking speed = 80 m/min or 3 mph. Speed slows by either reducing the cadence or by decreasing step or stride length.
- **Center of gravity (COG)**—located 5 cm anterior to second sacral vertebra. The COG is displaced 5 cm (< 2 in.) horizontally and 5 cm vertically during an average adult male step.
- **Base of Support:** defined as the space outlined by the feet and any assistive device in contact with the ground. Falling is avoided if the COG remains positioned over the base of support.

▣ DETERMINANTS OF GAIT (SAUNDERS 1953) (TABLE 6–2)

These factors are applied in normal human gait to minimize the excursion of the body's center of gravity and help produce forward progression with the least expenditure of energy. The six determinants of gait are

1. Pelvic rotation
2. Pelvic tilt
3. Knee flexion in stance phase
4. Foot mechanisms
5. Knee mechanisms
6. Lateral displacement of the pelvis

TABLE 6–2. Determinants of Gait

1. Pelvic rotation	The pelvis rotates medially (anteriorly) on the swinging-leg side, lengthening the limb as it prepares it to accept weight. With 4° pelvic rotation in either direction during double support, the limbs are essentially lengthened in the would-be lowest point of the gait cycle (preventing a sudden drop of the COG).
2. Pelvic tilt	The pelvis on the side of the swinging leg (opposite to the weight-bearing leg) is lowered 4°–5°, which lowers COG at midstance
3. Knee flexion in stance	Early knee flexion ⇒ knee flexion at foot strike (15°). The bending of the knee reduces the vertical elevation of the body at midstance (would-be highest point in the gait cycle) by shortening the hip-to-ankle distance. This lowers the COG (by minimizing its vertical displacement) decreasing the energy expenditure. It also tends to absorb the shock of impact at heel strike by lengthening the contraction of the quadriceps.
4. Foot mechanisms (ankle flexion/ extension mechanisms)	At heel strike, ankle plantar flexion smoothes the curve of the falling pelvis. It is associated with controlled plantar flexion during the first part of stance.
5. Knee mechanisms	After midstance, the knee extends as the ankle plantar flexes and the foot supinates to restore the length to the leg and diminish the fall of the pelvis at opposite heel strike.
6. Lateral displacement of the pelvis	There is displacement toward the stance limb The net COG of the body must lie above the base of support (the stance foot).

Determinants 1–5 reduce displacement on the vertical plane.
Determinant 6 reduces displacement on the horizontal plane.

TABLE 6-3
Major Muscle Activity During Gait Cycle
The major muscle activity during each phase of the gait cycle varies dramatically with relation to whether the muscles are inactive, concentrically contracting, or eccentrically contracting.

CLASSIC GAIT TERMINOLOGY:	Heel Strike	Foot Flat	Midstance	Heel Off	Toe-Off	Acceleration	Midswing	Deceleration
Rancho Los Amigos Terms NEW TERMINOLOGY	INITIAL CONTACT	LOADING RESPONSE	MID STANCE	TERMINAL STANCE	PRE-SWING	INITIAL SWING	MID SWING	TERMINAL SWING
			STANCE PHASE 60%				SWING PHASE 40%	
% OF TOTAL PHASE	0-2%	0-10%	10-30%	30-50%	50-60%	60-73%	73-87%	87-100%
ILIOPSOAS	inactive	inactive	inactive	concentric	concentric	concentric	concentric	inactive
GLUTEUS MAXIMUS	eccentric	inactive	inactive	inactive	inactive	inactive	inactive	inactive
GLUTEUS MEDIUS	eccentric	eccentric	eccentric	eccentric	inactive	inactive	inactive	inactive
HAMSTRINGS	eccentric	eccentric	inactive	inactive	inactive	eccentric	eccentric	eccentric
QUADRICEPS	eccentric	eccentric	inactive	inactive	eccentric	eccentric	inactive	inactive
PRETIBIAL MUSCLES	eccentric	eccentric	inactive	inactive	inactive	concentric	concentric	concentric
CALF MUSCLES	inactive	inactive	eccentric	concentric	concentric	inactive	inactive	inactive

KEY:

INACTIVE   CONCENTRIC   ECCENTRIC

413

GAIT PATHOLOGY AND PROBABLE CAUSES (TABLE 6–4.)

TABLE 6–4

Gait Pathology	Probable Causes
1. Foot strike to foot flat – Foot slap	Moderately weak dorsiflexors
2. Foot strike through midstance – Genu recurvatum	Weak, short, or spastic quadriceps; compensated hamstring weakness; Achilles tendon contracture; plantarflexor spasticity
– Excessive foot supination	Compensated forefoot valgus deformity; pes cavus; short limb; uncompensated external rotation of tibia or femur
– Excessive trunk extension	Weak hip extensor or flexor; hip pain; decreased knee ROM
– Excessive trunk flexion	Weak gluteus maximus and quadriceps
3. Foot strike through toe off – Excessive knee flexion	Hamstring contracture; increased ankle dorsiflexion; weak plantar flexor; long limb; hip flexion contracture
– Excessive medial femur rotation	Tight medial hamstrings; anteverted femoral shaft; weakness of opposite muscle group
– Excessive lateral femur rotation	Tight hamstrings; retroverted femoral shaft; weakness of opposite muscle group
– Increased base of support	Abductor muscle contracture; instability; genu valgum; leg length discrepancy
– Decreased base of support	Adductor muscle contracture; genu varum
4. Foot flat through heel off –Excessive trunk lateral flexion 📖 (Trendelenburg gait)	Ipsilateral gluteus medius weakness; hip pain (see below)
–Pelvic drop	Contralateral gluteus medius weakness
–Waddling gait	Bilateral gluteus medius weakness
5. Midstance through toe off – Excessive foot pronation	Compensated forefoot or rearfoot varus deformity; uncompensated forefoot valgus deformity; pes planus; decreased ankle dorsiflexion; increased tibial varum; long limb; uncompensated internal rotation of tibia or femur; weak tibialis posterior
– Bouncing or exaggerated plantar flexion	Achilles tendon contracture; gastroc-soleus spasticity
– Insufficient push-off	Gastroc-soleus weakness; Achilles tendon rupture; metatarsalgia; hallus rigidus
– Inadequate hip extension	Hip flexor contracture; weak hip extensor
6. Swing phase – Steppage gait	Severely weak dorsiflexors; equinus deformity; plantarflexor spasticity
– Circumduction	Long limb; abductor muscle shortening or overuse
– Hip hiking	Long limb; weak hamstring; quadratus lumborum shortening

(Tan, 1998 p. 65)

📖 Trendelenburg gait (gluteus medius gait):

- When the hip abductor muscles (gluteus medius and minimus) are weak, the stabilizing effect of these muscles during gait is lost.
- E.g., Stand on right leg, if left hip drops, then it's a + right. Trendelenburg (the contralateral side drops because the ipsilateral hip abductors do not stabilize the pelvis to prevent the droop).
- When patient walks, if he swings his body to right to compensate for left hip drop, he will present a compensated Trendelenburg; the patient exhibits an excessive lateral lean in which the thorax is thrust laterally to keep the center of gravity over the stance leg.

Energy Expenditure During Ambulation:

Energy Expenditure of Different Levels of Amputation/Etiologies vs. Normal Controls During Ambulation (Tables 6–5 and 6–6)

TABLE 6–5   Energy Expenditure of Different Levels of Amputation

Level of Amputation	Increased Metabolic Cost Above Normal
Syme's	15%
Traumatic TT (BKA)	25%
Traumatic TF (AKA)	68%
Vascular TT (BKA)	40%
Vascular TF (AKA)	100%

TT= transtibial
TF= transfemoral

TABLE 6–6   Energy Expenditure of Traumatic Amputees

Level of Amputation (Correlates with traumatic amputee)	Increased Energy Expenditure above normal
BKA	20%–25% (Short BKA—40% Long BKA—10%)
BKA + BKA	41% (Gonzalez 1974)
AKA	60–70%
AKA + BKA	↑ 118% net cost (Traugh 1975)
AKA + AKA	>200% (260% Huang 1979)

(Traugh, 1975; Gonzalez, 1974; Tan, 1998; Huang, 1979)

Energy demands required to return to normal ambulatory functions are high
Even the healthiest amputees cannot achieve normal gait in terms of velocity, cadence, or energy consumption

📖 Wheelchair propulsion (Cerny et al 1980)

- Investigated the use of wheelchair as alternatives to ambulation in patients with paraplegia
- In the subjects studied, there was only 9% increase in energy expenditure (compared to ambulation in normal subjects)

📖 **Crutch Walking**
- Crutch walking: requires more energy than walking with a prosthesis
- Muscles that need strengthening in preparation for crutch walking:
  - Latissimus dorsi
  - Triceps
  - Biceps
  - Quads
  - Hip Extensors
  - Hip Abductors

■

PROSTHETICS

DEFINITION

Prosthesis—A prosthesis is an artificial substitute for a missing body part

UPPER-LIMB PROSTHETICS

Acquired upper-limb amputations

Most common causes
1. Trauma is the leading cause of acquired amputation in the upper extremity (approximately 75%), occurring primarily in men aged 15 to 45 years.
2. Cancer/tumors
3. Vascular complications of diseases

Standard levels of arm amputation and exceptions to their use.

In the upper extremity, the following are the preferred levels of amputation: (Figure 6–3)
1. Transphalangeal
2. Transmetacarpal
3. Transcarpal
4. Wrist disarticulation
5. Transradial (below elbow) amputation
6. Elbow disarticulation
7. Transhumeral (above elbow) amputation—6.5cm or more proximal to the elbow joint
8. Shoulder disarticulation
9. Forequarter amputation

Finger amputation (transphalangeal) can occur at the distal interphalangeal, proximal interphalangeal, and metacarpophalangeal levels

Transmetacarpal amputation and wrist amputation are seen less because they have decreased functional outcomes
- Multiple finger amputations, including thumb and partial hand amputation, and those through the wrist, need to be considered care-

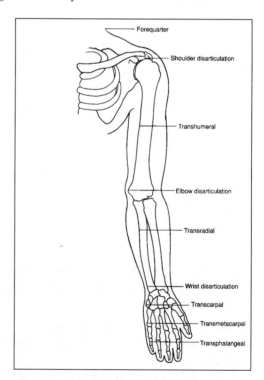

FIGURE 6–3. Levels for Amputation (new terminology). (From Braddom R.L. Physical Medicine and Rehabilitation, Philadelphia W.B. Saunders, 1996. Reproduced with permission.)

fully in view of the possible functional and cosmetic implications of prosthesis fitting and restoration. Inappropriate choice of amputation site can result in a prosthesis with disproportionate length or width

- Partial hand amputation should be carefully planned to ensure adequate residual sensation and movement. For these amputations a prosthesis may not be necessary. Surgical reconstruction may be a more appropriate choice of treatment to preserve or enhance function while maintaining sensation in the residual partial hand. There is little point in salvaging a partial hand if no metacarpals are present to provide pinch.

Wrist disarticulation

- A wrist disarticulation spares the distal radial ulnar articulation and thus preserves full forearm supination and pronation
- Socket designs for this level are tapered and flattened distally to form an oval that allows the amputee fully to use active supination and pronation, thus avoiding having to preposition the terminal device for functional activities
- A special thin wrist unit is used to minimize the overall length of the prosthesis because of the extremely long residual limb
- If cosmesis is of importance to the amputee, a long below elbow amputation may be a more appropriate amputation level.

Transradial / below-elbow (BE) amputation

- The transradial amputation is preferred in most cases
- It can be performed at three levels: (Figure 6–4)
  1. very short—residual limb length of less than 35%
  2. short—residual limb length of 35% to 55%
  3. long—residual limb length of 55% to 90%
- The long below-elbow residual limb retains from 60° to 120° degrees of supination and pronation, and the short below-the-elbow residual limb retains less than 60°.
- The long forearm residual limb is thus preferred when optimal body powered prosthetic restoration is the goal. It is the ideal level for the patient who is expected to perform physically demanding work.
- A residual limb length of 60% to 70% is preferred when optimal externally powered prosthetic restoration is the goal. This length typically permits good function and cosmesis.
- The short and very short transradial amputation level can complicate suspension and limit elbow flexion strength and elbow range of motion
- Transradial amputation is the most common level and allows a high level of functional recovery in the majority of cases.

Elbow disarticulation (Figure 6–4)

- The elbow disarticulation has some surgical and prosthetic advantages and disadvantages.
- Pros: The surgical technique permits reduction in surgery time and blood loss, provides improved prosthetic self-suspension (by permitting the use of a less encumbering socket), and reduces the rotation of the socket on the residual limb, as compared with the transhumeral level of amputation.
- Cons: Major disadvantages are the marginal cosmetic appearance caused by the necessary external elbow mechanism, as well as the current limitations in technology that impede the use of externally powered elbow mechanisms at this level of amputation. These drawbacks often outweigh the advantages in the long run.
- In the patient for whom bilateral transhumeral amputation is the alternative, the elbow disarticulation is the more desirable level when feasible in spite of the possible cosmetic problems.

Transhumeral/above-elbow (AE) amputation

- The transhumeral amputation can be performed at three levels: (Fig 6–4)
  1. humeral neck—Residual limb length of less than 30% [residual limb (humerus) length]
  2. short transhumeral—Residual limb length of 30% to 50%
  3. standard transhumeral—Residual limb length of 50% to 90%.
- Longer residual limb length (up to 90% of humeral length) will give best control and function with a prosthesis
- These three amputation levels in most cases require similar prosthetic components, which can be externally powered, body powered, passive, or have a combination of these
- In above-elbow amputations with residual limb lengths greater than 35%, usually the proximal trim line of the socket extends to within 1 cm to the acromion, and the socket is suspended by either a figure-eight or shoulder saddle and chest strap suspension systems.
- Sockets for residual limbs shorter than 35% should have the proximal trim line extend 2.5 cm. medially to the acromion.

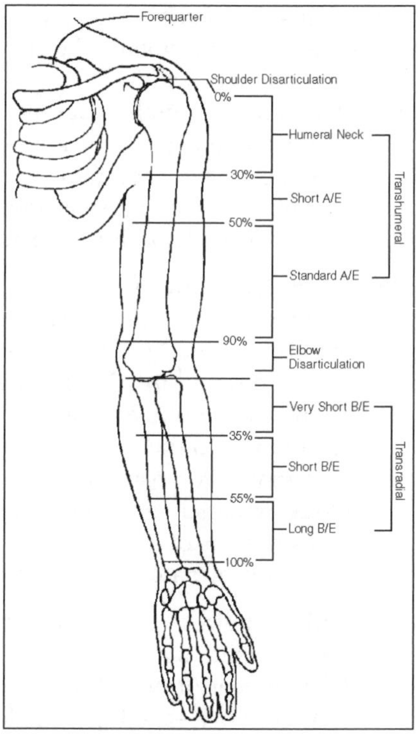

FIGURE 6–4. Levels of upper extremity amputation. (A/E = above elbow, B/E = below elbow)

Shoulder disarticulation and forequarter amputations (Figure 6–4)

- Fortunately, the shoulder disarticulation and forequarter amputations are seen with less frequency than amputations of other levels
- In most cases, they are made necessary as part of the surgical intervention to remove a malignant lesion
- Patients with these levels of amputation are the most difficult to fit with a functional prosthesis, due to the number of joints to be replaced and the problems related in maintaining secure suspension of the prosthesis
- For shoulder disarticulation and forequarter amputations, the socket extends onto the thorax to suspend and stabilize the prosthesis
- Prosthetic replacement in these cases is more successful in those who are young, healthy, and male
- Prosthetic components are similar to those of the transhumeral prosthesis, with the addition of the shoulder unit, which allows passive (active mechanisms used less often) positioning of the shoulder joint in flexion extension and adduction-abduction
- The joint may be provided with controls, in addition to the body-powered or externally-powered control mechanisms needed for the elbow, wrist, and hand
- Functional prosthetic use in the forequarter amputation is less successful because suspension is difficult to maintain. In some cases, a better option is to provide a passive, cosmetic prosthesis. Special consideration should be made for providing a shoulder cap to allow the patient to wear clothing more easily and improve cosmesis. The use of an ultralight passive prosthesis is usually well accepted in these patients.

Prosthetic Components for Transradial/Below-Elbow (BE) and Transhumeral/Above-Elbow (AE) Amputations

Prosthetic components include terminal devices, wrists, elbows, and shoulders

Terminal devices (TD)
- Most patients who suffer an upper-limb amputation and undergo prosthetic restoration require a terminal device for their prosthesis; they are used in all upper-limb prostheses for amputations at the wrist level and above
- TDs lack sensory feedback and have limited mobility and dexterity
- There are a variety of prosthetic terminal devices available and include *passive, body-powered*, and *externally powered* hooks and hands

1. Passive TDs
   - Lighter
   - Have no functional mechanisms and provide no grasp
     a. Passive hand
       ♦ Intended for cosmetic use only
     b. Flexible passive TDs
       ♦ Mitt-shaped TDs used to absorb shock and store and release energy during sports and other activities

2. Body-powered terminal devices (hooks or hands) can be *voluntary-opening* or *voluntary-closing* types
   - *Prosthetic hands* provide a three-jaw chuck pinch (three-jaw chuck involves grip with the thumb and index and middle fingers)
   - *Hooks* provide the equivalent of lateral or tip pinch (In the normal hand, lateral or key grip involves contact of the pulp of the thumb with the lateral aspect of the corresponding finger)
     a. Voluntary-opening (VO) terminal device
       ♦ 📖 Most common and practical type
       ♦ Device maintained in closed position by rubber bands or tension springs.
       ♦ The amputee uses cable-control harness powered by proximal muscles to open the terminal device against the force of the rubber bands or spring
       ♦ To grasp, patient releases the opened terminal device on an object; the rubber bands or spring provide the prehensile force
       ♦ The pinch force is determined by the number and type of rubber bands or springs (each rubber band provides about one pound of pinch force)
       ♦ To control the amount of prehensile force, the patient must generate a continued opening force
     b. Voluntary-closing (VC) terminal device
       ♦ More physiological function than voluntary opening
       ♦ Device is maintained in an open position and has to be closed voluntarily by pulling with the cable on the harness system to grasp an object
       ♦ To release, the patient releases the pull on the harness, and a spring in the terminal device opens it
       ♦ The maximum prehensile force is determined by the strength of the individual
       ♦ Disadvantage: prolonged prehension requires constant pull on the harness, heavier and less durable than voluntary opening units.

3. Externally powered (electric-powered) TDs
   - Are controlled by switches or myoelectric signals and are powered with energy provided from external batteries.

- – The electric-powered TD can be handlike (ie., Otto Bock system electric hands or Steeper electric hands) or nonhandlike in appearance (Otto Bock Greifer hand, Hosner NU-VA synergistic prehensor and Steeper powered gripper)

a. Myoelectric-controlled TDs
  - – Use surface electrodes placed on the muscles of the residual limb.
  - – Devices can have a *digital* or *proportional control* system
    - ♦ digital control system—on/off system
    - ♦ proportional control system—the stronger the muscle contraction producing the signal, the faster the action

b. Microswitch-controlled TDs—use either a push-button switch or a pull-switch to activate the TD

📖 **Prosthetic wrist units**
  - – Wrist units are used for attaching terminal devices to prostheses as well as providing pronation and supination to place the terminal device in its proper position.
  - – The rotation function is passive; the amputee rotates the terminal device in the wrist unit with his sound hand or by pushing against a part of the body or other surface to produce either pronation or supination. The wrist unit also permits interchange of the terminal devices.

- • Two types of wrists: friction or locking
  1. Friction wrists permit pronation and supination of the terminal device and hold it in a selected position by means of friction derived from a compressed rubber washer or from forces applied to the stud of the terminal device.
  2. Locking wrists permit manual rotation and then lock the terminal device in its fixed position.
  - – Advantage: The locking mechanism prevents inadvertent rotation of the TD in the wrist unit when a heavy object is grasped.
- • Two types of wrist-flexion units are also available: add-on and combination
  - – *Add-on* is worn between the wrist and the terminal device and allows manual positioning of the terminal device in either the straight or the flexed position.
  - – *Combination* type combines a friction wrist and a wrist-flexion component in one and provides for setting and locking in one position.
  - – Electric wrist rotator units are also available and are generally considered for bilateral upper-extremity amputees.

Transradial / Below-Elbow (BE) Amputation Prostheses

In addition to the components discussed above, a transradial amputee needs a socket, elbow-hinge, an upper arm cuff, and a harness and control system.

BE Sockets
  - – The socket must provide a comfortable but stable, total contact interface with the residual limb (avoiding inadvertent motion and precluding uncomfortable concentrations of pressure), efficient energy transfer from the residual limb to the prosthetic device, secure suspension and adequate appearance.
  - – To accomplish these goals, most sockets are double walled with the inner wall giving total contact fit and the outer wall matching the contour and the length of the contralateral forearm.
  - – Proximally, the socket extends posteriorly to the olecranon and anteriorly to the elbow crease. The shorter the residual limb, the closer is the trimline to the crease.

1. Split socket

   Split socket consists of a total-contact segment encasing the residual limb and connected by hinges to a separate forearm shell to which the wrist unit and the terminal device are attached. It is sometimes *used in patients who have very short stumps* so that the special elbow hinges can be used to increase available joint range of motion or to incorporate an elbow-lock mechanism in the prosthesis.

2. 📖 Muenster socket (self-suspended socket) (Figure 6–5)
   - An alternative to the split socket (for short transradial amputees) is the Muenster-type socket design. In this, the socket and forearm are set in a position of initial flexion and the socket encloses the olecranon and the epicondyle of the humerus. The intimate stump encapsulation, flexion attitude, and high trimlines provide excellent retention and security. Although there is *some limitation in the range of flexion-extension* this may be compensated by *preflexing.*
   - When this type of suspension is used, a figure nine harness can be used for control purposes only
   - With these prostheses the patient can operate his terminal device in common positions and still apply full torque about the elbow. Although these techniques yield less elbow flexion than the split socket, the reduction in force requirements and the ease of use more than compensate for this limitation.
   - Northwestern University socket is another example of a self-suspended socket design

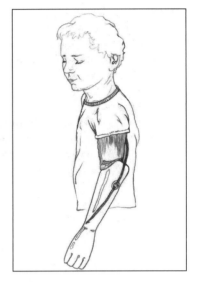

FIGURE 6–5. The Muenster Socket.

Elbow Hinges

Transradial amputation prosthesis hinges connect the socket to a cuff on the upper arm and are important for suspension and stability

Types:
   1. Flexible elbow hinge
      - Used primarily to suspend the forearm socket
      - Permits active pronation and supination of the forearm
      - Used where sufficient voluntary pronation and supination are available to make it desirable to maintain these functions: wrist-disarticulations and long transradial amputations
   2. Rigid elbow hinge
      - Used in short transradial amputations when normal elbow flexion is present but there is no voluntary pronation-supination and more stability is needed
      - *Types:*
        a. single axis
        b. polycentric
        c. Step-up design—used with split-socket prosthesis, in very short transradial amputation where flexion is limited. By virtue of a gear or double-pivot arrangement, these hinges permit the stump to drive the prosthetic forearm through an increased range of motion. Disadvantage is that it takes twice the force (energy cost doubles) to provide the same amount of flexion than is the case with no step-up design.
   3. Residual limb-activated locking elbow

Cuffs and Pads

Except in the Muenster socket, a half-cuff or a triceps pad, with appropriate elbow hinge, is used on the upper arm to connect the socket to the harness and help furnish socket suspension and stability. It also serves as an anchor for the cable control action point. The half-cuff is used in the majority of short transradial fittings. The triceps pad is used with long transradial, wrist-disarticulation, and transmetacarpal prostheses.

Transradial Harness Suspension and Control Systems

– The functions of the below-elbow harness: to suspend prosthesis from the shoulder so the socket is held firmly on the residual limb, utilize body motions as sources of power or force, and transmit this force via a cable system to operate the terminal device.
– Three types:
a. Figure-eight
b. Figure-nine
c. Chest-strap with shoulder saddle
1. 📖 **Figure-eight** (O-ring harness) (Figure 6–6)
– Most commonly used harness. The axilla loop, worn on the sound side, acts as a reaction point for the transmission of body force to the terminal device.

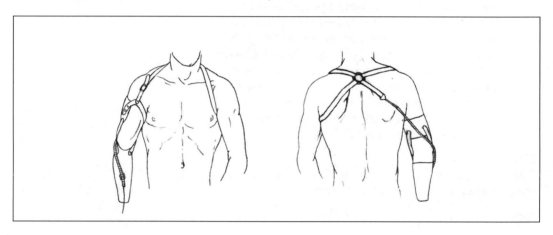

FIGURE 6–6. O-Ring Harness.

2. **Figure-nine**
– Figure-nine harness is often employed with a self-suspended transradial socket (e.g., Muenster socket) that requires a harness only for controlling the TD
– Consists of an axilla loop and a control attachment strap
– Pros: is lighter and provides a greater freedom and comfort by the elimination of the usual front support strap and triceps pad or cuff
3. **Chest-strap with shoulder saddle** (Figure 6–7)
– Chest-strap with shoulder saddle is used if the patient cannot tolerate the axilla loop. Also used with those who will be doing heavy lifting.

Control Systems

• The typical control system for transmission of power to the prosthesis consists of a flexible, stranded stainless-steel cable with appropriate terminal fittings or coupling units and a flexible tube or housing inside which the cable slides. The terminal fittings are used to attach one end of the cable to a harnessed body control point and the other end to a point of operation or control of the prosthesis. The housing acts as a channel or guide for the transmission offered by the cable.

- There are two types of control-cable systems:
  1. Bowden control cable system
  2. Dual-control (or fair-lead control) cable system

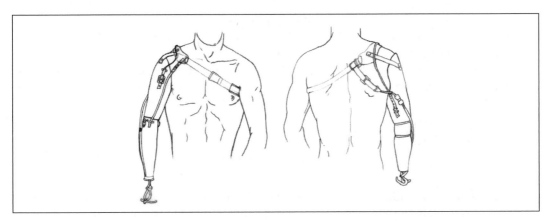

FIGURE 6–7. Shoulder Saddle Harness (modified) for Above Elbow Prosthesis.

1. Bowden Control Cable System
   - The Bowden control system is used in the transradial single-control cable system
   - The dual-control system is used in the transhumeral control–cable system and in the very short transradial split-socket prosthesis with stump-activated *locking* hinge
   - The Bowden control system consists of a continuous length of flexible housing through which the cable slides. The housing is fastened by a base plate and retainer to the forearm shell and by a housing cross-bar assembly to the cuff of the triceps pad; these housing retainers also serve as reaction points when force is applied to the cable. The Bowden system is required to transmit body power for a single purpose—*to operate the terminal device.*

2. The dual-control cable system consists of one cable with two functions:
   1. *Flex* the elbow unit when the elbow is unlocked
   2. *Operate* the terminal device when the elbow is locked
      - The cable is held in place and guided by separate lengths of housing. The pieces of housing are fastened with retainers at points where the cable must be supported or operated through an angle. Since the system must provide force for elbow flexion and operation of the terminal device, two fair-lead housings are necessary; the proximal lead, through which the cable slides when the elbow is flexed; and the distal lead, through which the cable also slides when the terminal device is operated.

Transhumeral/Above-Elbow (AE) Prostheses

- Transhumeral prostheses consist of a terminal device, wrist unit, forearm, elbow unit, an upper arm, a socket, and a harness and control-cable system.
- The terminal devices and wrist units are the same as those used for the transradial prostheses, but the sockets, elbow unit, and harness and control systems differ in several respects from those used in the transradial prostheses

- **AE Sockets**

As in transradial prostheses, the transhumeral socket is usually of double-wall construction, with the inner wall providing a snug, total-contact fit and the outer shell providing appropriate length and shape. The lateral socket wall extends to the acromion and the medial socket wall is flattened below the axilla to help prevent inadvertent socket rotation.

Elbow Units

- When an amputation occurs at or above the elbow joint, elbow function is supplied by the use of an elbow unit, which provides for elbow flexion and for locking in various degrees of flexion
- Elbow-locking systems are divided into two types:
  1. External (outside) locking elbow
  2. Internal locking elbow
- The former is used with elbow-disarticulations because there is not enough space for the internal locking mechanism, and the latter is used with transhumeral and shoulder prostheses

1. Internal elbow joint
   - Preferred because of greater mechanical durability
   - Used in level of amputation 4 cm or more proximal to the level of the epicondyles

2. External elbow joint
   - Used when the residual limb extends more distally than 4 cm to the level of the epicondyles to maintain the elbow joint center equal to that in the nonamputated side.
   - Both types of elbows are flexed by means of the control cable of the dual-control system and locked at the desired flexion angle by a separate elbow-lock control cable, which is attached at one end to the elbow mechanism and at the other end to the harness
   - The lock mechanism operates on the alternator principle, that is, locking and unlocking actions alternate with each control-cable cycle of tension and relaxation
   - For amputees who have difficulty flexing their prosthetic forearm, an accessory in the form of a spring-assist for elbow flexion may be provided for the use with the internal elbow.
   - In transhumeral and shoulder prostheses, passive humeral rotation is accomplished by means of a turntable between the elbow unit and the upper arm shell or socket. As in the case of a wrist unit, friction between the elbow unit and the turntable permits control of the rotation to maintain the desired plane of elbow operation.

Transhumeral Harness and Control Systems

- In addition to suspending the prosthesis from the shoulders, the transhumeral harness must transmit power to flex the prosthetic forearm, to lock and unlock the elbow unit, and to operate the terminal device.
- Harness in AE
  - 📖 The harness designs *most frequently used for transhumeral prosthesis* are modifications of the basic figure-8 and chest-strap patterns used with the transradial prosthesis.
- Control Cable System in AE
  - As previously mentioned, the *dual-control* (fair-lead control) cable system is used in the transhumeral prosthesis to transmit force for *two functions*:
    1. Elbow flexion and
    2. Terminal device operation
  - *Elbow locking and unlocking* are controlled by a second cable, the elbow-lock cable
  - When the elbow is extended and unlocked, flexing the shoulder (humeral flexion) (assisted by biscapular abduction) transmits force to the forearm lever loop *flexing the elbow* to the desired level
  - If the amputee wishes to use the terminal device at this point, first, he/she locks the elbow (by doing shoulder depression, extension and abduction—"down, back, out")
  - Then, the patient can operate the terminal device by continuation of the control motion ⇒ shoulder flexion and biscapular abduction
  - The same combination of shoulder movements done to lock the flexed elbow is needed to unlock the elbow (shoulder extension, depression, and abduction). Then, the elbow extends by gravity.

📖 Dual-control cable mechanism operation in the transhumeral amputee

TABLE 6-7

	1. Elbow flexion	2. Lock elbow (in desired degree of flexion)	3. TD operation (opening and closing)	4. Unlock elbow
Movements	Humeral flexion and biscapular abduction	Shoulder depression, abduction, extension (down, back, out)	Further humeral flexion and biscapular abduction	Shoulder depression, extension, and abduction (down, back, out)
Cable-mechanism used	Dual-control cable	Single-control cable (elbow-lock cable)	Dual-control cable	Single-control cable (elbow-lock cable)
				After desired TD function is accomplished, in order to extend the elbow, the patient has to unlock it. (elbow will passively extend by gravity)

Shoulder Prostheses

- All shoulder prostheses consist of a terminal device, a wrist unit, a forearm section, an elbow unit, humeral and shoulder sections, and a harness and cable-control system
- The terminal device, wrist unit, forearm section, and elbow unit are identical to those used in the transhumeral prosthesis
- The shoulder section includes a socket, which provides:
  - A comfortable, stable bearing on the residual shoulder elements and thorax, and
  - A means of utilizing whatever mobility remains in the shoulder girdle for control of the prosthesis
- Several components are available for the socket allowing ROM

ISSUES IN AMPUTEE CARE AND REHABILITATION

- There are three important considerations in a clinical decision from a medical standpoint for a prosthesis:
  1. Determination of amputation level
  2. Careful assessment of bilateral proximal muscle strength and ROM is critical when planning for prosthetic control mechanisms
  3. Evaluation of general health
- Generally, in upper extremity amputations, the general health is no different than in the regular population. The exception may be those with malignancies.
- It is also necessary to discover any condition that should be treated before being fitted with a prosthesis. Cognitive impairment and other neurologic problems can be a major roadblock to prosthetic training.

Diagnosis of specific residual limb conditions:

- As far as the residual limb is concerned, it appears that abnormalities, such as bone spurs, tender scars, skin rashes, neuromas, and other conditions are of low statistical importance. When present, many of these can be dealt with by suitable fitting modifications.

Other Rehabilitation Issues

Rehab Prescription
- Another important aspect of the initial management of the upper limb amputee is pre-prosthetic therapy with physical therapy and occupational therapy
- Preprosthetic therapy includes: stump shrinkage, muscle strength and ROM, postural problems, desensitization, scar mobilization, and home exercise program
- Exercises should be prescribed if there are any deficiencies. Forearm and humeral rotation are the motions most seriously affected. Among transhumeral amputations, 80% had limitations of humeral rotation. Among transradial amputations 80% had limitations of forearm rotation. If bone malformations limit ROM, physical therapy is of no help.

Vocational Issues
- The terminal device is extremely important to the amputee's vocational success. By far, the greatest occupational effect of amputation is on skilled and semiskilled laborers who are unable to continue their original occupations. This is a source of emotional maladjustment and of reduction in earning power. The prosthetic team should serve in an advisory capacity on any contemplated change in occupation because the patient may be able to return to his job with the prosthesis.

Emotional / Psych Issues
- Although there is no evidence to indicate that the amputee population varies from the general population with regard to emotional stability, psychological problems can act as a deterrent to rehabilitation. It is a waste of time and money to fit an amputee with a prosthesis, and then to accept failure because the amputee does not cooperate fully. There is always a period of adjustment to limb loss. Psychological counseling should be made available to all amputees to deal with grieving, anger, and depression.
- Personal factors also must be taken into consideration. One should consider age, sex, educational history, prosthetics history, and personal preference. In many cases the educational background completes the picture of the amputee and gives us a better idea of the prescription necessary. A large majority do not have personal preferences for the prosthesis, but if they exist, they must be explored. If these preferences cannot be accommadated, the reason must be explained to the amputee.

Prosthetic operation and training

- In the unilateral amputee, the prosthesis generally will be used to assist the remaining limb, allowing a portion of the lost function to be regained. The prosthetic device is still far from duplicating the lost part and the patient must be aware of its functional limitations
- The training period consists of an orientation to the prosthesis and its controls and use of the prosthesis, which initially emphasizes activities of daily living
- During the preprosthetic phase, the amputee was introduced to the prosthesis and learned something of its function. Now the introduction should be repeated and the patient should be specifically instructed in the correct terminology and function of each component part. This understanding will help the patient communicate with the prosthetist if something is wrong. General instruction about the care of the prosthesis should be covered at this time
- The next step for training is instruction for donning and doffing the prosthesis. After this initial instruction the patient is ready to begin learning the basic motions of operation. The therapist should take the amputee through each required motion so that he can see and feel the motion being performed. The patient then repeats the same motion independently.

Transradial Amputee Training
- For the transradial amputee, training is concentrated on operation of the terminal device
- Forearm and elbow control require no special training
- The basic motion for opening terminal device is forward flexion of the humerus with some assistance from biscapular abduction.
- The shoulder on amputated side should not flex excessively to give a smooth motion. The shoulder on the opposite side acts as a stabilizer
- Once the patient has learned the mechanics of the prosthesis and how to use it efficiently, he/she is ready for training in purposeful activity. The therapist should present different activities to help solve new problems that inevitably arise in the patient's life. Before attempting any activity, prepositioning of the terminal device is essential. Instruction and practice in this prepositioning is necessary. It will allow an amputee to approach an object correctly.
- Prehension is the final phase of control training before practice in daily activities is started. Drills in the approach, grasp, and release of various sizes of objects and different types of materials are used. The amputee is taught to grasp objects with adequate pressure control on the terminal device.
- Control training may be considered complete when the patient has maximal control of the terminal device in space.
- Once basic operations are learned, these techniques are applied to practice activities of daily living. The amputee should gain confidence in using the prosthesis in a wide range of activities that are meaningful and important. Initially the activities of most importance for the amputee are feeding and dressing.
- For the unilateral amputee this independence is not difficult to achieve. Because a prosthesis is not needed to achieve basic independence, activities chosen for him should require the use of two hands. Cutting food with a knife and fork or tying shoelaces are examples. As the patient attempts, performs, and succeeds in these activities, he becomes more willing to accept the use of the prosthesis and can rely on it. After training in feeding, dressing, and grooming is completed, progression to specialized activities such as communication skills, which involve use of the telephone or keyboard, can be made. Homemaking, vocational, and recreational interests should be encouraged, and the activities associated with these interests should be emphasized in the training process.

Elbow Disarticulation and Transhumeral Amputee Training
- The prosthetic training for the elbow disarticulation or transhumeral amputee follows the same general principles as for the transradial amputee
- Control training of this level of amputee is more difficult, since the amputee must now concentrate on locking the prosthetic elbow before being able to use the terminal device
- Training with dual control/elbow-locking transhumeral prosthesis should not be attempted prior to age three
- When the elbow is unlocked, the basic humeral control motion (humeral flexion) produces flexion of forearm section of the prosthesis (elbow flexion)
- Shoulder on the amputated side should not flex more than is necessary for smooth movement. The opposite shoulder acts as a stabilizer. This should be repeated by the amputee until the speed of the movement and the angle of flexion are smooth and controlled.
- Elbow extension (when elbow still unlocks) is achieved by slowly bringing the shoulder back to its starting position

Next control motion is for locking and unlocking the elbow
- This motion is a combination of shoulder depression extension, and abduction.
  - This motion should be practiced with the elbow extended until the lock clicks

- Once the locking and unlocking of the elbow can be accomplished smoothly with the elbow extended, the amputee can be taught to flex the elbow and maintain tension on the cable while the elbow lock is used
- To unlock the elbow, the amputee repeats this procedure, allowing the forearm to return smoothly to the starting position
- When the elbow is locked, additional humeral flexion will operate the terminal device (opening in VO terminal device, or closing in VC terminal device)
- For the terminal device to be operated closer to the body, rotation of the prosthetic forearm is necessary. To do this, the amputee is instructed to first flex the elbow to 90° and then manually rotate the turntable medially or laterally.

LOWER LIMB PROSTHETICS

Lower Limb Amputation

- Between 1989 and 1992 there were approximately 105,000 amputations of the lower extremity. 32% of those were toe amputations. (Seymour, 2002).

Age group (yrs.)	Most common cause of amputation
0–5	Congenital or deformity requiring amputation
5–15	Cancer
15–50	Trauma
50+	Vascular disease

Distribution of lower-extremity amputation and cause in survey by Kay and Newman of 5,830 new amputees:

Distribution (%)
Syme's 3
Transtibial 59
Knee disarticulation 1
Transfemoral 35
Hip disarticulation 2

Causes (%)
PVD and infection 70
Trauma 22
Tumor 5
Congenital deformity 3

(Kay and Newman, 1975).

Important definitions

📖 **Myodesis:** muscles and fasciae are sutured directly to bone through drill holes
- Residual limb is more structurally stable
- Contraindicated in severe dysvascularity in which the blood supply to the muscle may be compromised

📖 **Myoplasty:** opposing muscles are sutured to each other and to the periosteum at the end of the cut bone with minimal tension
- Generally takes less operating time
- May be procedure of choice in severe dysvascular residual limbs

Temporary Prosthesis

Temporary (preparatory) prosthesis is usually made prior to a definitive prosthesis, which is cosmetically finished

- Provides prosthetic fitting before the residual limb volume stabilizes
- Helps in shrinking and shaping of the residual limb
- Allows for early prosthetic training (gait and functional training), and fine tuning of the prosthetic alignment as the amputee's gait progresses
- May be used as a trial when there is uncertainty about a patient's potential success at using a prosthesis
- Usually used for 3 to 6 months postsurgery (until maximal stump shrinkage has been achieved)

Definitive Prosthesis:
- When shaping and shrinking process has ended and residual limb volume has stabilized, a definitive or permanent prosthesis is made.
- A definitive prosthesis will typically need to be replaced about every 3 to 5 years.

Levels of amputation in the lower limb: (Figure 6–8)

TABLE 6–8. Descriptions of Level of Amputation in the Lower Limb

Partial toe	Excision of any part of one or more toes
Toe disarticulation	Disarticulation at the MTP joint
Partial foot/ray resection	Resection of a portion of up to three metatarsals and digits
Transmetatarsal amputation (TMA)	Amputation through the midsection of all metatarsals
Lisfranc	Amputation at the tarso-metatarsal junction
Chopart	Midtarsal amputation—only talus and calcaneus remain
Syme's	Ankle disarticulation with attachment of heel pad to distal end of tibia; may include removal of malleoli and distal tibial/fibular flares
Long BKA (transtibial)	> 50% of tibial length
Short BKA (transtibial)	< 20% of tibial length
Knee disarticulation	Amputation through the knee joint, femur intact
Long AKA (transfemoral)	> 60% of femoral length
AK (transfemoral)	35%–60% of femoral length
Short AKA (transfemoral)	< 35% of femoral length
Hip disarticulation	Amputation through hip joint, pelvis intact
Hemipelvectomy	Resection of lower half of the pelvis
Hemicorporectomy	Amputation of both lower limbs and pelvis below L4, 5 level

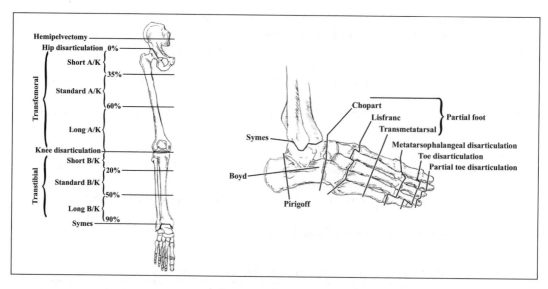

FIGURE 6–8. Levels of lower extremity amputations (A/K = above knee, B/K = below knee).

Indications, Advantages And Disadvantages Of Common Levels Of Amputation In Lower Extremities

Unsatisfactory levels for elective sites of leg:

1. **Distal two-fifths of tibia (below gastroc-soleus muscle)**
   The added length of the lever arm at this level is outweighed in importance by difficulties of good skin and soft tissue management, because the tibia and fibula are both subcutaneous. The conventional below-the-knee prosthesis is difficult to shape and contour in a cosmetic manner with amputations at this level. Modular limbs do not circumvent this cosmetic difficulty.

2. **Very short below knee amputation proximal to the tibial tubercle:**
   Knee extension strength is lost and the knee becomes valueless. The added length creates difficulties in prosthetic fit as compared to a knee disarticulation. Knee flexion contractures occur often. When active knee extension is present and the knee can be flexed through a range of 45° or more, the residual limb can be comfortably fit with an effective prosthesis if surgery is performed not less than 3 cm below the tibial tubercle. Above this level, most patients will be better served by a knee disarticulation.

3. **Very high above-knee amputation.**
   When transection is just a short distance below the lesser trochanter, the limb tends to develop excessive flexion and abduction at the hip joint. Socket fit may become a difficult problem. Releasing the contractive deformity through flexor and abductor muscle release at the hip can circumvent this. Many surgeons prefer to leave a short segment of femur rather than amputate at the hip disarticulation level.

Partial Toe Amputation, Toe Disarticulations, and Metatarsal Ray Resection
Performed for deformity resulting from trauma to the toes, loss of tissue, infection, gangrene due to frostbite, diabetes, arterial sclerosis, scleroderma, Buerger's disease, and similar conditions

1. By preserving the length of the foot, there is a better mechanical advantage
2. There is better gait pattern than a transmetatarsal amputation
3. Disadvantages in these type of amputations are mostly seen in the vascular patient, including arterial sclerosis and diabetes. One must be assured that the vascular supply to the rest of the foot be intact so as not have a continuous progression of amputations up to trans-tibial amputation.

Transmetatarsal Amputation (TMA) (Figure 6–9)

Also performed for deformity resulting from trauma to the toes, loss of tissue due to an infection, or gangrene due to frostbite, diabetes, arterial sclerosis, scleroderma, Buerger's disease, and similar conditions.

1. Gangrene must be limited to the toes and should not involve the web space. Infection should be controlled. The incision should not extend through hypo-aesthetic areas or through infected areas. The patient should be free of pain. Palpable foot pulses are not necessary, but there should be no dependent rubor. Venous filling should be less than 25 seconds.
2. Not indicated in cancers of the metatarsal bones because post surgically it would not be conclusive that all bony cancer would have been resected.
3. This is an important amputation through the foot because it preserves the attachment of the dorsiflexors and plantar flexors and their function. This continues to give the patient a good mechanical advantage with the foot.
4. For functional use, it is also a good level of amputation because these amputations can be fitted with sole stiffeners and toe fillers with minor apparent loss of function during stance and walking on level surfaces.

Other Foot Amputations (Figure 6–9)

1. ▢ **Lisfranc** amputation at the tarso-metatarsal junction
2. ▢ **Chopart** amputation is a midtarsal, talo-navicular, calcaneo-cuboid amputation. Only talus and calcaneus bones remain
3. **Pirogoff** is a vertical calcaneal amputation (in this amputation, the lower articular surfaces of the tibia/fibula are sawn through)
4. **Boyd** is a horizontal calcaneal amputation (all tarsals removed except calcaneus/talus)
- These amputations are not indicated in patients with ischemia or diabetes. They may be indicated, at times, in patients with trauma, although their outcomes are still poor.
- ▢ In both the Lisfranc and Chopart amputations, the remaining foot often develops a significant equinovarus deformity resulting in excessive anterior weight bearing with breakdown. Adequate dorsiflexor tendon implantation with Achilles tendon lengthening has been advocated to prevent this deformity.

▢ Syme's Amputation (Figure 6–9)

It is essentially an ankle disarticulation procedure with attachment of the distal heel pad to the end of the tibia; may include *removal* of the *malleoli* and/or distal *tibial/fibular* flares (transection of the tibia and fibula proximal to the flare of the tibial malleolus).

- **Indications:** Trauma above the foot, congenital anomalies, tumors, and deformities that necessitate amputation.
- **Disadvantages:** healthy plantar heel skin is necessary for weight bearing in this area. The patient also must have good perfusion in this area, thus making it a difficult procedure for the dysvascular patient.
- **Pros:** Functionally, this procedure represents an excellent level of amputation because:
  1. It maintains the length of the limb
  2. There is preservation of the heel pad, providing an excellent weight-bearing stump
  3. Immediate fitting of prosthesis is possible with excellent results
  4. Stump weight bearing is possible almost immediately after the procedure (~ within 24 hrs)
- **Cons:** ↓ cosmesis (bulbous, bulky residual limb); fitting for a prosthesis may be more difficult than for other amputation levels.

Foot and Ankle Amputations

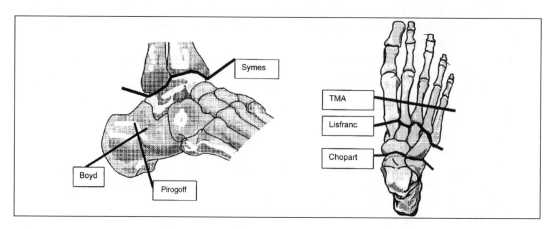

FIGURE 6–9. Foot and Ankle Amputations.

Transtibial Amputation / Below-Knee Amputation (BKA)
- When an amputation in the lower limb becomes necessary due to trauma, tumor, or disease, the importance of saving the knee joint cannot be overemphasized. Preservation of the knee joint means preservation of a near-normal life style with minimal physical limitations
- In the elderly amputee, saving the knee may well mean the difference between being able to walk or being confined to a wheelchair
- Studies performed to compare the energy requirements of below-the-knee amputees to above-the-knee amputees in walking have consistently shown significantly greater demands at the above-the-knee level
- The ability of performing a below-the-knee amputation as opposed to a higher-level amputation will be determined by tissue viability in cases of trauma and by principles of tumor surgery when dealing with neoplasm
- In the case of the dysvascular patient, below-the-knee amputation is not only feasible, it is the level of choice in most instances
- Reported healing rates for ischemic BKAs of 80% to 90%
- There is also general agreement in the literature that mortality is lower following below-the-knee than after above-the-knee amputations, because below-the-knee amputations have higher healing rates and better tissue viability and weight-bearing surface. BKAs also show decreased mortality and decreased energy expenditure.
- When the surgeon is performing a BKA, preserving length is critical as long as viable skin and muscle is available for distal coverage. The longer the below-the-knee stump, the greater will be its leverage, strength, and proprioceptive qualities, and the better the amputee will walk. The energy costs of walking will be less if a longer amputation stump is provided to the amputee. On the other hand, a very short below-the-knee stump is far superior to a knee disarticulation, and satisfactory fitting with a below-the-knee prosthesis can be accomplished at levels as high as the tibial tuberosity.
- If there is a severe flexion contracture (greater than 50°) and the limb is ischemic, knee disarticulation should be the procedure of choice, although a very short below-the-knee amputation may be fitted as a knee disarticulation with a bent-knee prosthesis.

Functional outcomes after a below-knee amputation:

Preoperatively the patient should be familiarized with the procedures and activities to be performed after the amputation. Instruction should be given in the following:

1. Proper bed and wheelchair positioning.
2. Exercises to be executed, as well as the rationale for such treatment.
3. If possible, the patient should be taught ambulation techniques with appropriate assistive devices.
4. The type of prosthetic device to be used postoperatively; in using a below-the-knee prosthesis, there is again much less energy expenditure and the patient's functional abilities should be greater than those of a patient with an above-the-knee amputation.
5. Prolonged sitting after the amputation should be avoided to prevent contractures. The increase of contractures will result in a decrease in the patient's functional ability.

Knee Disarticulation
- Advantages
  1. Less traumatic to tissue
  2. Blood loss is minimal
  3. A long, strong stump with excellent end-bearing quality is produced
  4. Prosthetic suspension is facilitated by the bulbous contour of the stump end
- Disadvantages
  1. Relatively long flaps are necessary and healing may be impaired in the dysvascular patient. A valid objection to the common use of this procedure in vascular disease is that a short below-the-knee amputation usually can be performed if sufficient soft tissue is available to cover a knee disarticulation. There is a fine line of distinction between sufficient viable skin for coverage of a short below-the-knee stump and sufficient viable skin for coverage of a knee disarticulation. A short below-the-knee stump that is otherwise unimpaired is functionally quite superior to knee disarticulation.
  2. Until relatively recently, another major disadvantage to knee disarticulation was the inability to provide the patient with a prosthesis that was functional and cosmetic. Recent advances in prosthetic knee mechanisms and socket design now permit swing-and-stance phase control and cosmesis that equal available above-the-knee prostheses.

Transfemoral Amputation/Above-Knee Amputations
1. This was the most common level of amputation in the past because it was easily accomplished in cases of peripheral vascular disease and could more easily assure satisfactory healing. Today, because of the understanding of the principles of site selections, potentials for rehabilitation, and improved fitting methods for amputation at lower levels, the AKA is done much less frequently, even in the presence of ischemia.
2. Approximately 85% of above-the-knee amputations are secondary to vascular disease.
3. Two-thirds of all major amputations performed for lower extremity peripheral vascular disease will heal and be functional at the below-the-knee level. Many studies indicate below-knee healing with prosthetic rehabilitation in 75% to 85% of patients.
4. There is increased healing rate in patients with BKA with vascular disease; therefore, this is preferred to the AKA. The AKA is thus only indicated in those cases where we expect to find poor tissue viability in knee disarticulation or BKA. It may also be indicated in large tumors of the tibia where the surgeon needs to go to the next level.

Hip Disarticulation and Hemipelvectomy Amputation
- *Hip disarticulation* is the surgical removal of the entire lower limb by transection through the hip joint.
- *Hemipelvectomy* is the surgical removal of the entire lower limb plus all or a major portion of the ileum.
- Ablative surgery of this magnitude is indicated most often to irradiate a malignant tumor of the bone or soft tissues above the thigh, hip, or pelvic region.

1. Indications are extensive trauma or uncontrolled infection, especially gas gangrene. On rare occasions, function and fit of a prosthesis to connect a congenital limb anomaly may be improved by surgical conversion to a hip disarticulation.
2. In spite of large functional deficits, it is still possible to fit prostheses for these levels of amputation.
- Hip disarticulation amputation produces a stump with an excellent weight-bearing characteristic. Lack of a femoral shaft acting as a lever arm on the prosthesis results in poor mediolateral trunk stability and the loss of voluntary control of hip flexion, knee stability, stride length, and alterations in cadence. Design of prosthesis must compensate for this missing function.
- In addition to all the functional deficits created by hip disarticulation, the hemipelvectomy amputee has also lost the excellent weight bearing of the ischial tuberosity, and the prosthesis must bear weight on the semi-solid abdominal viscera. Socket design for this amputation level must, therefore, produce weight forces on the abdominal viscera in a manner that is tolerable to the amputee and not injurious to the viscera. Many hemipelvectomy amputees reject the prosthesis because of the bulk and weight of the prosthesis and the energy expenditure required for ambulation when wearing it.

Postoperative Stump Management and Care

- When evaluating a patient after an amputation, the history should include reason for and date of amputation, dates of revisions, prior ambulatory status, self-care status, cardiopulmonary status, neurological status, peripheral vascular status, diabetic control, previous surgical procedures, residual limb pain, phantom sensation, and phantom pain.
- Physical examination should include an evaluation of vision and mental status, peripheral vascular status, surgical incision and drainage, skin lesions, residual limb skin mobility, edema and pitting, induration, tenderness, skin redundancy, graft and graft-donor sites, passive ROM, joint stability, sensation, and strength in all extremities.
- The ideal shapes for transtibial residual limb is *cylindrical*, whereas the ideal transfemoral residual limb is *conical*. Records should be kept of several circumferential measurements of the residual limb at specific distances from the greater trochanter for a transfemoral amputee or from the medial knee joint line for a transtibial amputee. The residual limb, soft tissue status, and bone length should also be assessed.
- One of the keys for success after an amputation is adequate wound healing. Evaluating and optimizing nutrition, anemia, diabetic control, and antibiotic use maximizes wound healing. Whirlpool treatment with debridement may be helpful for an infected wound, but not for an uninfected wound, because whirlpool causes residual limb edema. An open incision or wound should be covered with a Telfa® pad under the shrinkage device or prosthesis. A chronically draining sinus may be the result of a superficial abscess, a bone spur, or localized osteomyelitis. The opening should be probed to determine its depth, and plain films and bone scans should be obtained to determine bony involvement.

Other postoperative goals of preprosthetic management include:
1. Pain control
2. Preparation of residual limb for prosthetic fitting
3. Maintaining ROM, especially in the remaining proximal joints of the amputated extremity
4. Independent mobility
5. Independence in self-care and activities of daily living
6. Education about prosthetic fitting and care
7. Support for adaptations to the changes resulting from the amputation.

- In the postop program, muscle strengthening should be emphasized. In the Syme's amputee, BKA, knee disarticulation or AKA, strengthening of the gluteus medius and gluteus maximus muscles should be accomplished in addition to strengthening any residual hamstring or quadriceps muscles, and strengthening of the upper extremities.

Residual Limb Management

- A postoperative plaster or fiberglass rigid dressing prevents edema, protects from trauma, and decreases postoperative pain. Postoperative edema occurs within a few minutes, so immediate replacement of the dressing is necessary. Once they are removed for inspection or suture removal, rigid dressings must be replaced within minutes to prevent recurrence of edema.
  1. *The removable rigid dressing (RRD)* for the transtibial amputee consists of a plaster or fiberglass cast suspended by a stocking and supracondylar cuff, and is adjusted by adding or removing socks to maintain compression. Provides good edema control with the advantage of allowing daily inspection.
  2. When a rigid dressing is not being used, one may wrap cotton elastic bandages around the residual limb. Elastic bandages are the least effective shrinkage devices, because patients fail to master the wrapping technique, which requires a reapplication many times a day. Poorly applied elastic bandages also can cause circumferential constriction with distal edema. Double length four-inch bandages should be used for the transtibial limb and double length six-inch bandages for the transfemoral limb.
  3. Elastic shrinker socks are easy to apply and provide uniform compression, but are more expensive than elastic bandages. They should fit snugly and reach the groin in the transfemoral amputee. They also may cause skin damage with constriction if not properly fitted and maintained.
- The amputee *should wear a shrinkage device 24-hours a day except for bathing.* A shrinkage device for the nonprosthesis candidate helps control pain and edema and facilitates healing. The shrinkage device can be discontinued after fitting the definitive prosthesis if the amputee wears the prosthesis regularly. It can be used at night if overnight edema occurs.
- *Contractures* are easy to prevent but difficult to correct.
  - The amputee must not lie on an overly soft mattress, use a pillow under the back or thigh, or have the head of the bed elevated. Standing with the transfemoral residual limb resting on a crutch should be avoided. All these practices can lead to hip flexion contractures.
  - The amputee must not place a pillow between the legs, since this creates a hip abduction contracture
  - A transtibial amputee must not lie with the residual limb hanging over the edge of the bed, with a pillow placed under the knee, or with the knees flexed, and, must not sit for a long period of time in order to avoid knee flexion contractures. The transtibial amputee should sit with the knee extended on a board under the wheelchair cushion with a towel wrapped over the board.
  - Crutch walking with or without prosthesis promotes good ROM and, when feasible, is preferred over wheelchair mobility
  - Amputees should lie prone for 15 minutes three times a day to prevent hip flexion contractures. The amputee who cannot lie prone should lie supine and actively extend the residual limb while flexing the contralateral leg.

After suture removal, the residual limb should be cleansed daily with bland soap and warm water. The limb should be patted completely dry before the application of any shrinkage devise. Gentle massage decreases sensitivity to pressure, and deep friction massage perpendicular to the scar prevents scar adhesions. Be sure that the residual limb scar has mobility in all directions. One may use a thin layer of emollient to decrease the friction from massage, but discourage the use of thick creams. For very dry skin, a thin emollient can be applied in the evening for absorption overnight. Shaving of the residual limb should be discouraged.

Prosthesis Prescription and Component Parts By Site at Amputation

Partial Foot Amputations

- Small-toe amputations do not affect ambulation and usually require no replacement
- Partial foot prostheses are used to restore foot function (particularly walking) and fore-foot contour.
- Amputation of the great toe reduces push-off force, thus requiring a resilient toe filler and also a molded insole with arch support to maintain the alignment of the amputated foot.
- Partial foot amputations involving the forefoot, such as ray resections and trans-metatarsal amputations, generally require only shoe fillers or shoe modifications. The shoe modifications required may include a stiff sole, the addition of a spring steel shank extending to the metatarsal heads, a rocker sole and/or padding of the tongue of the shoe to help hold the hind foot firmly in the shoe.
- Transtarsal amputations, such as Chopart, Lisfranc, and Boyd, are not the most desirable levels of elective amputation, but they will have better functional results if there is an active balanced dorsiflexion and plantar flexion with normal skin and heel pad present. The best prosthetic option for a hindfoot amputation is the use of a custom prosthetic foot with a self-suspending split socket, which allows a regular low quarter shoe to be worn. A posterior leaf spring ankle–foot orthosis is another alternative.

🕮 Syme Amputation

- In the Syme amputation, preservation of the articular cartilage covered by the heel pad allows direct end bearing on this residual limb.
- The patient can stand easily and walk on the end of the residual limb without wearing a prosthesis for short household distances.
- Prosthesis: Canadian Syme socket (either posterior or medial opening).
  - ♦ Both require removal of a portion of the socket wall to get bulbous stump in
  - ♦ Major disadvantage: poor cosmesis.
- Newer socket designs that incorporate an expandable air suspension chamber inside the socket or a thin removable expandable inner socket liner provide a more cosmetically acceptable prosthetic design.
  - Pros: thinner, tighter, and stronger prosthetic socket (there is no need to remove a section from the socket wall maintaining the structural integrity of the prosthesis)
- 🕮 Prosthetic feet available: for Syme's Amputation
  - ♦ Syme solid ankle cushion heel (SACH)
  - ♦ Syme SAFE (stationary ankle flexible endoskeleton)
  - ♦ Seattle Syme foot
  - ♦ Syme flex foot
  - ♦ Carbon copy Syme foot
  - ♦ No STEN (stored energy) available for Syme's amputees

Transtibial (TT) Amputation/Below the Knee Amputation

- The components in a BKA prosthesis include the socket, the shank, the suspension, and the prosthetic foot.

Socket for BKA

🕮 Patellar tendon bearing (PTB) socket

- The standard socket used for the average below-the-knee amputee is the total contact patellar tendon bearing (PTB) socket

- PTB socket is a custom-molded plastic socket that distributes weight through convex buildups (bulges) over pressure-tolerant areas; it provides concavities (relief areas) on pressure-sensitive areas
- Characterized by bar in anterior wall designed to apply pressure on patellar tendon.
- The trimline extends anteriorly to the midpatellar level, may extend medially and laterally to the femoral condyles, and extends posteriorly to below the level of the PTB bar
- Despite name, pressure should be equally distributed over pressure-tolerant areas, with more weight bearing in the area of the patellar tendon and the tibial flare and reduced weight bearing over the bony prominences, such as the tibial crest, distal end of the tibia, and head of the fibula. (Figure 6–10)

📖 PRESSURE-TOLERANT AREAS (Figure 6–10 a,b,c)
  1. Patellar tendon
  2. Pretibial muscles
  3. Popliteal fossa—Gastroc-soleus muscles (via gastrocnemius depression)
  4. Lateral shaft of fibula
  5. Medial tibial flare

PRESSURE-SENSITIVE AREAS—(RELIEF AREAS) (Figure 6–10 d,e,f)
  1. Tibial crest, tubercle, and condyles
  2. Fibular head
  3. Distal tibia and fibula
  4. Hamstring tendons

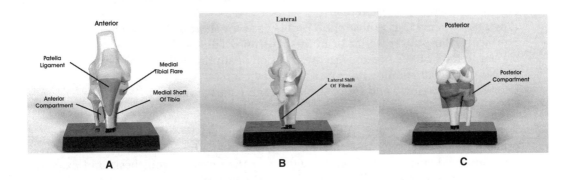

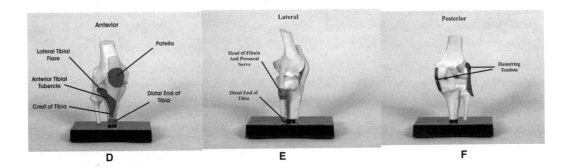

FIGURE 6–10. **A,B,C:** indicate pressure-tolerant areas in a patella tendon bearing (PTB) socket. **D,E,F:** indicate pressure relief areas in a patella tendon bearing (PTB) socket.

- The socket is aligned on the shank on slight flexion (about 5°) to enhance loading of the patellar ligament, prevent genu recurvatum, resist the tendency of the stump to slide down the socket and to place quadriceps muscle in a more efficient and mechanically advantageous position, facilitating its contraction
- The alignment of the socket also includes a slight lateral tilt to reduce pressure on the fibular head
- A liner can be added to the socket to protect fragile or insensate skin, to reduce shear forces, provide a more comfortable socket for tender residual limbs, or accommodate for growth
- Liners can be made of closed-cell thermal plastic foams, rubber covered with leather, or silicone gels. Custom silicone liners without the suspension pin have been particularly helpful in managing shear problems that can occur with residual limbs covered with split thickness skin grafts.

Some Commonly Used Suspension Systems for BKA:

A. Supracondylar cuff suspension socket
- Consists of a cuff or strap that wraps circumferentially around the thigh, fitted immediately above the femoral epicondyles
- May be used with or without a fork strap and waist-belt suspension

B. Brim suspension
- **Supracondylar brim suspension**/supracondylar wedge (PTB-SC)
- PTB socket with medial and lateral walls extending above the femoral epicondyles for suspension.
- Instead of removable medial brim or wedge, a compressible foam wedge build-up may be incorporated into the soft liner
- Provides extra mediolateral support and is used for short residual limbs
- **Supracondylar-Suprapatellar Brim Suspension** (PTB-SC/SP)
- Similar to the PTB-SC socket with the addition of suprapatellar trimlines
- The suprapatellar trimline improves the suspension
- Used for short stumps and for controlling genu recurvatum

C. Rubber or neoprene sleeve
- Sleeves made of neoprene, rubber, latex, or other elastic materials may be used as primary suspension system or in combination with another suspension mechanism
- Provides good suspension, fitting snugly over the proximal prosthesis and extending several inches up onto the thigh over the prosthetic sock
- Should not be used as a primary form of suspension with standard PTB sockets in very short residual limbs, in patients with decreased mediolateral knee stability or when hyperextension control is required
- Increased perspiration may be a problem

D. Silicone suction suspension
- Design includes a silicone insert or liner with an attached distal pin or ring that locks into the bottom of the plastic laminated socket
- Provides excellent suspension for amputees with greater suspension demands, e.g., athletes, and for those with short residual limbs, and excellent skin protection for the scarred residual limb
- Expensive

E. Thigh corset
- Connects a leather thigh (femoral) corset to a PTB prosthesis through metal joints and side bars to decrease distal residual limb weight bearing by 40% to 60%

– Used when the patellar tendon cannot tolerate weight bearing or when knee joint is unstable or painful

Prosthetic Feet (see also Table 6–9 and Figure 6–12)

1. **Solid ankle cushioned-heel (SACH) foot**—most commonly used prosthetic foot
   a. Durable, lightweight, inexpensive, and easily interchanged to accommodate shoes of different heel height
   b. Compressible heel and wooden keel in this design allow it to simulate the motions of the ankle in normal walking without actual ankle movement occurring
   c. Accommodates partially for uneven terrain, but this foot is best suited for flat, level surfaces.

2. **Single axis foot**—permits movement of the foot ankle complex in one plane.
   a. Movement occurs in the plantar flexion dorsiflexion axis. The movement is controlled by the use of adjustable internal rubber bumpers that provide resistance to dorsiflexion and plantar flexion.
   b. This foot is heavier than the SACH foot, and the internal components need periodic adjustment or replacement
   c. Typically used for more proximal amputations that require additional knee control or stability. Can relieve pressure on distal tibia for BKA.

3. **Multi-axis prosthetic foot**—for the amputee who is involved in athletic activities or who walks on uneven terrain
   a. Some controlled movement in the normal anatomic planes of the ankle dorsiflexion, plantar flexion, inversion, eversion, and rotation
   b. A number of different foot designs are available to provide this motion
   c. Some of the feet accomplish this movement without the use of mechanically moving parts. They rely on the inherent flexibility of the materials and design of the foot. Other multi-axis feet use mechanical systems
   d. The additional mechanical components necessary for the movement of these feet add to their overall weight and may require frequent maintenance, especially in the very active amputee
   e. For the active amputee, however, the improved balance, coordination, and function provided by these feet outweigh the disadvantages of increased weight and more frequent maintenance.

4. **Flexible keel prosthetic foot**

5. **Energy storing/dynamic response prosthetic foot**
   • Major advances in lower-extremity component design continue in the development in dynamic-response prosthetic feet such as the Flex foot, the spring-light foot, Seattle foot, Endolite foot, and the Carbon copy II and III feet. The design of these feet incorporates the use of resilient, flexible, energy-storing materials. Energy is stored in the foot at the time of heel strike, as the weight of the body compresses or flexes the resilient material within the foot and is returned to the amputee at the time of push off. Resiliency of these feet makes them particularly suitable for amputees involved in activities that require running and jumping. Many amputees report they believe they are more functional with a prosthesis with a dynamic response foot. It has been assumed, thus, that these prosthetic designs make ambulation more efficient and require less energy consumption. The flex foot and spring-light foot have the added advantages of reducing energy expenditure because they are lightweight.

TABLE 6–9. 📖 Prosthetic Feet

Foot unit	Main use	Advantages	Disadvantages
Rigid keel			
• **SACH** (solid ankle cushion heel) • Wooden keel • Compressible heel	• General use • Kids-durable • If ambulation needs are limited	• Inexpensive • Light (lightest foot) • Durable • Reliable	• Energy consuming • Rigid • Best on flat surface
Single-axis foot			
• Movement in one plane (DF and PF)	To enhance knee stability • AKA who needs greater knee stability (goes to flat foot quick before knee buckles; knee goes back into extension (gives stability in early stance)	• Adds stability to prosthetic knees	• Increased weight (70% heavier than SACH) • Increased cost • Increased maintenance
Multi-axis foot			
• College-park • Endolite Multiplex • Otto Bock "Greissinger" • Allow PF, DF, inversion, eversion and rotation	• Used for ambulation on uneven surfaces • Absorbs some of the torsional forces created in ambulation	• Multidirectional motion • Permits some rotation • Accommodates uneven surfaces • Relieves stress on skin and prosthesis	• Relatively bulky • Heavy • Expensive • Increased maintenance • Greater latitude of movement may create instability in patients with ↓ coordination
Flexible keel			
• **SAFE** (stationary ankle flexible endoskeleton)	• Used for ambulation as uneven surfaces	• Flexible keel • Multidirectional motion • Moisture and grit resistant • Accommodates uneven surfaces • Absorbs rotary torques • Smooth roll-over	• Heavy • Increased cost • Not cosmetic • Does not offer inversion/eversion • Increased maintenance
• Otto Bock dynamic foot	• Similar to SAFE	• Elastic keel • Conforms to uneven ground	• Similar to SAFE
• **STEN** (Stored Energy)	• Used when smooth roll-over needed	• Elastic keel • Moderate cost • Accommodates numerous shoe styles • Mediolateral stability similar to SACH	• Moderate-heavy weight

Foot unit	Main use	Advantages	Disadvantages
Energy-storing foot/Dynamic Response			
• **Seattle** foot – Consists of a cantilevered plastic C or U-shaped keel, which acts as a compressed spring	• Jogging, general sports, conserves energy	• Energy storing • Smooth roll-over	• High cost • No SACH heel makes it difficult to change compressibility of heel
• **Carbon copy II** – consists of a solid-ankle rigid posterior bolt block made of reinforced nylon/Kevlar® and combined with two flexible deflection plates	• Jogging, general sports, conserves energy	• Light weight • Energy storing • Smooth roll-over • Very stable mediolaterally	• High cost • Not as much spring as flex and Seattle foot
• **Quantum** – Lightweight, non-articulated, energy-storing foot – Two deflection plates (anterior and posterior)	• Similar to Carbon Copy II	• Light weight • Energy storing	• High cost
• 📖 **Flex-foot** – Pylon and foot incorporated into one unit – The flex-foot keel extends to the bottom of the transtibial socket (and in AKA, to the level of the knee unit) – **Flex-walk** is a version of the Flex-foot, which is shorter, attaching to the shank at the ankle level	• Running, jumping, vigorous sports, conserves energy	• Very light • Most energy storing • Most stable mediolaterally • Lowest inertia	• Very high cost • Alignment can be cumbersome

Ankle Units
- Seattle ankle
- Endolite Multiplex Ankle: component of the Endolite foot-ankle system, which is a multi-axis foot, can be used separately in conjunction with a different foot , i.e., with Seattle lite foot
- Ankle requires increased maintenance

Knee Disarticulation
- The socket in a knee disarticulation is usually a modified quadrilateral socket with some ischial weight bearing, and a soft socket liner with supracondylar buildups to provide suspension. Proximal socket trimlines prevent socket rotation on the limb, though ischial weight bearing is not an absolute requirement, as the femoral condyle provides suspension. The problem with prosthetic fitting of a knee disarticulation is that the prosthetic knee's center of rotation needs to go through the distal residual limb. Fitting a knee unit distal to the residual limb has caused problems in the past, but the four-bar polycentric knee has helped to solve the problem. *The polycentric knee, unlike the single-axis knee, has an instantaneous center of rotation that changes, and is proximal and posterior to the knee unit itself. This allows greater knee stability, a more symmetrical gait, and equal knee length when sitting.*

Transfemoral (TF) amputation/Above-knee amputation (AKA)

Sockets for AKA
- The initial design developed specifically for the AKA socket was the total contact quadrilateral socket. This design replaced the plug fit socket as the standard for above-the-knee prosthesis. In the past, the quadrilateral socket was the only socket design used for above-the-knee prosthesis. Now, more recent socket designs are being used; these are the *ischial containment socket* with narrow mediolateral configuration, and the above-knee frame socket with a flexible liner known is the ISNY.
- Ischial containment, narrow mediolateral design, also known as normal shape normal alignment (NSNA) or contoured adducted trochanter-controlled alignment method (CAT-CAM) was developed to provide for a more normal anatomic alignment of the femur and for the prosthesis. It also stabilizes the relationship between the pelvis and proximal femur because the ischial tuberosity is controlled inside the socket, rather than just sitting on top of the posterior brim as the tuberosity does in the quadrilateral socket. To control the pelvis, the trim line of the socket brim is brought more proximally than that of the quadrilateral socket. A higher trim line results in better control of the residual limb, especially for short above-the-knee amputations.

📖 *Transfemoral (TF) amputation/Above-knee amputation socket design (Figure 6–11)*
1. Quadrilateral transfemoral socket (Figure 6–11 a,b)
2. Narrow mediolateral (narrow ML) socket/Ischial containment (IC) socket/ Contoured adducted Trochanteric–Controlled Alignment Method (CAT-CAM) socket (Figure 6–11 c,d)

1. Quadrilateral Transfemoral Socket (Quad) Socket (Figure 6–11 a,b)
- Narrow antero-posteriorly and relatively wide mediolaterally
- Posterior socket has a flat, horizontal shelf on which the ischial tuberosity and the gluteal muscles rest
- 📖 It has a prominent bulge over the Scarpa's triangle for wide pressure distribution

- There are reliefs for the adductor longus, hamstring, greater trochanter, gluteus maximus and rectus femoris
- Ischial tuberosity sits on top of the post brim of quad socket
- Use with hip joint and pelvic band because of lack of stability, especially in geriatric patients
- Low trimline

Disadvantages of the quad socket
- ↑ discomfort while seated from either the anterior proximal brim or from the rigid posterior socket wall
- ↑ skin irritation at ischium and pubis from the proximal brim
- Tenderness on anterior distal femur
- ↓ stability compared to narrow mediolateral socket
- More lateral lurch when walking
- Poor cosmesis with gapping of lateral socket wall during stance
- Poor control of the residual femur allowing lateral shift of the socket.

2. Narrow Mediolateral (M-L)/Ischial Containment (IC)/CAT-CAM Socket (Figure 6–11 c,d)
- Developed as the normal shape normal alignment (NSNA) socket by Long; also developed as the contoured adducted trochanteric-controlled alignment method (CAT-CAM) by Sabolich
- Mediolateral dimension is narrower than the anteroposterior measurement
- Narrow mediolateral design was developed to provide a more normal anatomic alignment of the femur inside the socket
- The ischial tuberosity is contained inside the socket, providing a bony lock between the ischium and greater trochanter
- Weight bearing is concentrated in the medial aspect of the ischium and the ischial ramus

▢ Advantages
- It stabilizes the relationship between the pelvis and proximal femur since the ischial tuberosity is controlled inside the socket rather than on top like in the quad socket
- Narrow M-L design is intended to keep the femur in adduction; keeping the femur in adduction during the stance phase permits the hip adductors to be in a more stretched and efficient position.
- More energy efficient ambulation at high speed
- ↑ comfort in groin area compared to quad socket (in which weight bearing is done primarily on the ischial tuberosity)
- There is less lateral thrust of prosthesis at midstance
- Higher trimline results in better control of the residual limb especially for short stump AKA
- Able to accommodate smaller residual limb

Disadvantages
- More expensive and difficult to fabricate than the quad socket
- Wider anterior to posterior dimension at level of ischial ramus leads to increased movement in anterior/posterior plane

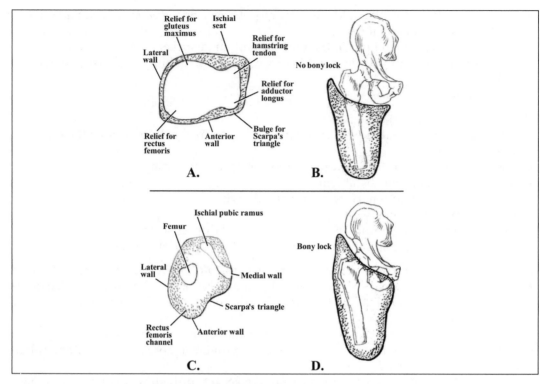

FIGURE 6–11. Transfemoral Amputation/Above Knee Amputation Socket Design. **A,B:** Quadrilateral Transfemoral Socket. **C,D:** Ischial Containment Transfemoral Socket.

Suspension of AKA Prosthesis (Figure 6–12)

A. Suction Socket:
- Suction suspension sockets are provided with a one-way valve at the distal end of the socket wall that allows air to escape but not to enter to ensure proper fitting
- A pull sock is used over the residual limb; the sock is passed through the valve hole and is used to assist in pulling the limb into the socket
- the amputee usually dons a total suction prosthesis while standing
- Suction socket use requires stable residual limb volume (size)
- if volume ↑, it will prevent fit
- if volume ↓, result is loss of suction
  Total suction socket: worn without socks on residual limb. It provides the best suspension biomechanically but requires minimal volume fluctuation, good hand strength and dexterity, good balance, and good skin integrity.
  Partial suction socket: It uses a socket with a suction valve but it is worn with socks, which reduces the airtight suction fit
  Provides less suspension than the total suction socket, requiring auxiliary suspension, (e.g., Silesian belt or TES belt)

B. Silesian Belt:
- Can be worn as primary form of suspension or if suction is not adequate.
- Standard Silesian belt attaches to the posterolateral area of the socket wall (near the greater trochanter) and passes around the back and over the opposite iliac crest where it achieves more of its suspension. It then attaches to the proximal anterior wall at the midline.
- Provides good control of rotation

C. *Total Elastic Suspension (TES) Belt:*
- The TES belt is a neoprene belt attached to the prosthesis and pulled around the waist
- Comfortable; enhances the rotational control of the prosthesis

D. *Pelvic Band and Belt with Hip Joint:*
- Pelvic band is closely contoured about the anterior iliac crest on the side of the amputation to discourage rotation of the prosthesis on the residual limb during ambulation
- Belt use over bypass graft surgery sites and in pregnant women is contraindicated.

Knee units (Figure 6–12, Table 6–10)
- All knee units, except for the hydraulic stance control units, attempt to keep the knee flexion and extension fixed at one angle throughout the stance phase.
- Provide stability during walking, particularly during early knee stance, to prevent knee from buckling, and allow the knee to bend when the patient sits and, in most cases, during swing phase (to allow easy clearance of the toes).
- Most are single axis; some are multi-axis

1. *Conventional single-axis knees*
   a. Light, durable, and inexpensive
   b. Rely on alignment for stability and work best at one speed
   c. Excessive heel rise in the early swing phase, as well as terminal swing impact in the late swing phase, may occur at faster cadences
   d. Amputee must prevent knee buckling by activating hip extensors
   e. The debilitated amputee or amputee with a short residual limb cannot adequately contract the hip extensors, and requires a knee that is set posterior to the trochanter knee angle line. This alignment has a disadvantage of causing difficulty in flexion of the knee for the swing phase that causes increased energy expenditure compared to other units.

2. *Manual locking knee*
   a. Maximum stability for the debilitated or elderly amputee
   b. Worst gait efficiency and increased energy consumption

3. *Stance control knee*
   a. Weight-activated stance-controlled knee or safety knee may provide a stable stance for up to 20 degrees of flexion by producing friction when the weight increases during stance
   b. Design is for amputees with weak hip extensors or for geriatric amputees
   c. Stance control is not automatic, and the amputee must be able to initiate and maintain control of the knee

4. *Four-bar polycentric* works well for patients with very long residual limbs, as well as for those with poor stability due to short residual limbs, poor balance, or weak hip extensors. Fluid control can be added and some polycentric knees can be manually locked.

5. *Hydraulic and pneumatic control knee* units are cadence responsive through cadence dependence resistance.
   a. Pneumatic units are air-filled and are lighter in weight, but they cannot support the heavier or more athletic amputee as well as the hydraulic units can
   b. Hydraulic/fluid-controlled knees (oil) are helpful for the active amputee who varies cadence and who can tolerate the extra weight and expense.
   c. 📖 Most fluid-controlled knees control the knee velocity during swing phase only, although hydraulic stance-controlled knees give gradually yielding resistance to knee flexion during the late stance phase as well.

– When weight is applied to the slightly flexed knee, the unit allows a slow yielding action instead of a precipitous collapse. This permits the young, agile amputee to descend ramps and stairs in a step-over-step manner.

d. The Endolite pneumatic intelligent prosthesis has a computer-controlled valve that adjusts knee swing phase speed based on cadence.

e. The hydro cadence knee is unique in that it also hydraulically controls ankle dorsiflexion and plantarflexion.

TABLE 6–10. ▭ Knee Units

Constant friction knee (single axis with constant friction unit)	Advantages	Disadvantages
• Friction mechanisms are devices used in swing control knee to dampen the pendular action of the prosthetic knee during swing phase, to decrease the incidence of high heel rise in early swing and decrease terminal impact in late swing • Single walking speed • May be used in kids • No stance control; a screw used to adjust the friction to determine how fast or slow the knee swings	• Inexpensive • Reliable	• Low stability (at mid-stance the single axis has the lowest zone of stability) • Fixed cadence • Too much friction prevents knee from flexing • Too little friction causes the knee to swing too easily; patient needs to vault
Stance control knee/safety knee/weight activated friction brake		

• Single axis knee with stance control
• Stance control acts as a brake system
• Indications:
  1. Geriatrics
  2. Short residual limb
  3. General disability
  4. Uneven surfaces
  5. Amputees with weak hip extensors
	• Improved knee stability	• Slightly increased weight
		• Increased cost
		• Increased maintenance
		• Must unload fully to flex
		▭ Cannot use in bilateral AKA (knees won't bend with loading) → cannot bend both knees at the same time (patient cannot sit down)
		• ▭ Activities that require knee motion under weight-bearing, such as step-over-step stair descent, are incompatible with this knee

Polycentric/Four-bar knee		
• No stance control, but inherently stable • Short knee unit ⇒ can be used in knee disarticulation and long residual limb	• Excellent knee stability • Improved cosmesis in knee disarticulation and long residual limb patients	• Greater weight, cost, maintenance • Although durable, needs maintenance every 3 to 6 months

Constant friction knee (single axis with constant friction unit)	Advantages	Disadvantages
Manual locking knee		

• Knee of last resort used in:
  1. Blind
  2. Stroke patient with amputation
• Commonly uses a spring-loaded pin that automatically locks the knee when the amputee stands or extends the knee
• Knee is kept extended throughout the entire gait cycle to ↑ stability
	• Ultimate knee stability :	• Abnormal gait
		• Awkward sitting
		Cannot use in bilateral AKA, because, like the stance control knee, patients cannot sit. Knees lock on loading, therefore, cannot bend both knees at the same time to sit down

📖 Fluid-controlled knee units		

1. Hydraulic (oil)
2. Pneumatic (air)
  • Cadence-responsive knee units through cadence-dependent resistance
  • 📖 Allows for either swing phase, or swing and stance phase control
  • Indications:
    1. For patients who vary cadence frequency
    2. Active walkers
    3. Ambulation in uneven terrain:
	• Variable cadence
	• Smoothest gait
	• Stable; will not lock unless at full extension
	• Pneumatic units are lighter but hydraulic units tolerate more weight (can support the heavier and more athletic amputee)
	• Can unlock for some activities (e.g., biking) :
		• Greatest weight
		• Increased cost
		• Increased maintenance

Socket Design—Transtibial and Transfemoral Amputations

Flexible Socket
• Provide softer, thermoplastic material for weight transmission
• Sits in rigid frame
  Advantages
   – Comfort
   – Better sense of outer objects through socket
   – Often translucent or transparent
   – Feels cooler
   – Rapidly fabricated and modified
   – Suction suspension if desired
  Disadvantages
   – Expensive
   – Imprecise fit secondary to linear shrinkage of thermoplastic material

Silicone Gel Liner/Suction Suspension
- Properties similar to human adipose tissue
  Advantages
  – Able to distribute shear forces generated at socket interface
  – Assists vascular inflow by creating a negative pressure
  – Can provide suction suspension
  Disadvantages
  – Not always tolerated, excessive sweating
  – Need constant volume to ensure suction fit
  – Expensive
Laminated socket
  Advantages
  – Cheaper
  – Durable
  Disadvantages
  – Less comfortable
  – Less total contact
  – Not easily modified

There are a variety of prosthetic options for the transfemoral amputee as illustrated in Figure 6–12.

Hip Disarticulation/Hemipelvectomy

Amputees with less than five centimeters of residual femur usually are fitted as hip disarticulation level amputees.
- Canadian hip disarticulation prosthesis is the standard prosthesis for a hip disarticulation
  – Socket of this prosthesis encloses the hemipelvis on the side of the amputation and extends around the hemipelvis of the nonamputated side, leaving an opening for the nonamputated lower extremity.
  – There is a flexible anterior wall with an opening that allows the prosthesis to be donned. Weight bearing is on the ischial tuberosity of the amputated side
  – Endoskeletal prosthetic components are preferred for this level of amputation to reduce the overall weight. The endoskeletal hip joint has an extension assist as does the knee unit, which usually is a constant friction knee
  – Endoskeletal components may be made from aluminum, titanium, or carbon graphite composite
  – Single axis foot or SACH foot with a soft heel used most. The newer lightweight foot-ankle combination may be even a better option. The prosthesis for a hemipelvectomy resembles that for the hip disarticulation socket except in the interior configuration of the socket. In the hemipelvectomy, most of the weight bearing is by the soft tissues of the amputated side, with some of the weight bearing by the sacrum on the opposite ischial tuberosity.

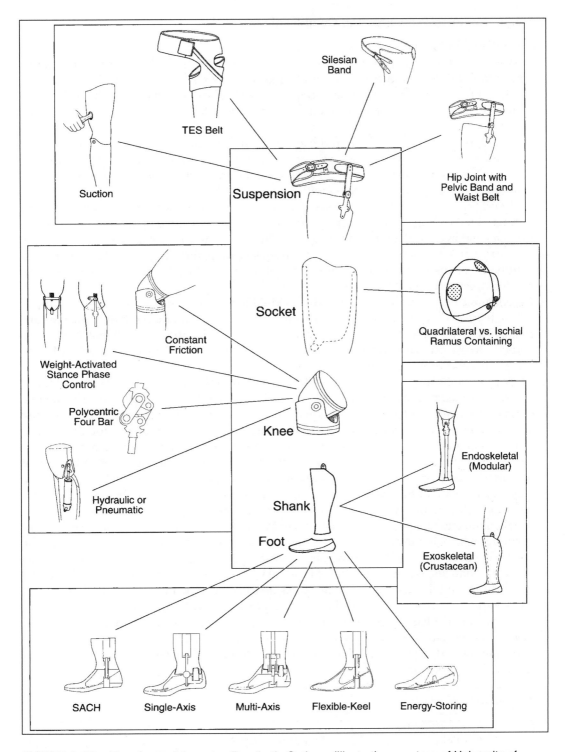

FIGURE 6–12. Transfemoral Amputee Prosthetic Options. (Illustration courtesy of University of Texas Health Science Center at San Antonio).

Common Amputee Problems And Complications

Dermatologic problems

Numerous skin problems can occur on the amputee's residual limb including folliculitis, allergic dermatitis, hyperhidrosis, and fungal infections. Skin lesions of the residual limb can expand rapidly, so early intervention is required, particularly for diabetic patients. Careful daily inspection of the residual limb should be done as well as daily residual limb and socket washing.

1. *Folliculitis* is a common problem in the amputee. It is a hair root infection resulting from poor hygiene, sweating, poor socket fit, or postioning. It is important to clean the area with antiseptic cleanser, to keep it dry, and to consider administration of oral antibiotics.

2. *Boils* and *abscesses* should be treated with limited prosthetic use.

3. *Epidermoid cysts* occur when sebaceous glands are plugged by keratin and usually are not apparent until months or years after a prosthesis is worn. They grow up to five centimeters in diameter and may break to discharge purulent fluid. They may require incision and drainage.

4. *Tinea corporis and tinea cruris* mainly results from sweating, they may be confirmed through culture or microscopy and are treated by topical or oral fungicides, as well as by good residual limb and socket hygiene.

5. *Hyperhidrosis* (excessive sweating) of the residual limb is a common problem after amputation. Increased sweating on the residual limb may cause skin maceration, which in turn predisposes the skin to infection by bacteria and fungi and injury by outside forces. Hyperhidrosis can be controlled with antiperspirants (e.g., Drysol® or Certain-Dry®); astringents and rubbing alcohol should be avoided as they dry the skin excessively.

6. *Allergic dermatitis* may arise from the detergents used to wash the limb socks, from lotions and topical medications, or from agents used in the prosthetic manufacture. The allergic dermatitis should resolve with cessation of contact with the offending agent. Eczema may appear acutely with small blisters and later with scaling and erythema. Topical corticosteroids should be applied and the offending agent should be identified and removed.

- 📖 "Choked stump" syndrome: Brawny edema, induration, and discoloration of the skin of the distal stump in a circular shape (with well-circumscribed margins) may indicate choking. The skin of the distal residual limb becomes darkened due to hemosiderin accumulation. This occurs when the residual limb becomes larger (typically from excessive weight gain) and no longer fits in the total contact socket. The prosthetic socket will be tight circumferentially in the proximal region and there is lack of good distal contact between the residual limb and the socket. The proximal constriction results in obstruction of the venous outflow, producing edema of the distal residual limb. If a gap exists between the skin of the distal stump and the distal socket wall, pressure causes edema fluid to accumulate.

- 📖 *Verrucous hyperplasia* is a wartlike skin overgrowth, usually of the residual distal limb, resulting from inadequate socket wall contact with subsequent edema formation. *A chronic choke syndrome* may lead to verrucous hyperplasia of the distal residual limb skin.

- Relieving the proximal constriction and reestablishing total contact within the socket can reverse these processes.

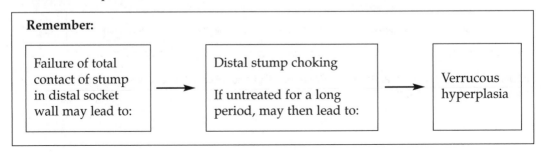

Remember:

| Failure of total contact of stump in distal socket wall may lead to: | → | Distal stump choking

If untreated for a long period, may then lead to: | → | Verrucous hyperplasia |

Bone Problems

- If the periosteum is incorrectly stripped during surgery or if it was stripped during trauma, *bone spurs* may arise, causing pressure on the skin and pain. Socket modifications generally take care of the problem. However, in some cases, surgery may be needed.
- Bone pain may also result from a hypermobile fibula that is left longer than the tibia. If a balanced myodesis was not performed in a transfemoral amputation, the femur may extrude through the muscle and present subcutaneously. If prosthetic adjustments, such as a flexible socket, are inadequate for the extruded femur, then surgical intervention might be needed.
- Bone overgrowth: In children, when amputation of a long bone through its diaphysis is done before bone maturity, there might be continued bone growth and lengthening due to endosteal and periosteal growth, with the skin not growing as much. This leads to a pointed bone end that pushes through the skin. Skin traction is the preferred mechanism to avoid stump shortening, but surgery may be required.

Pain

Pain in the amputee patient can be broken down into both incisional pain on the residual limb and phantom pain and phantom sensation.

1. Increased pain

Incisional pain should subside with healing, although shear forces on adherent scars or bone spurs can be painful. Deep massage helps prevent scar adhesions. Local pain may be due to an unprotected neuroma (nerve ending left "exposed" during surgery) that is being pressed upon. Neuroma exposed to pressure may give great pain and may require revision if unresponsive to conservative treatment.

- Remember that not all residual limb pain is a result of a problem within the amputation site or due to a poorly fitting prosthesis
  - The amputee may experience intermittent claudication pain in parts of the residual limb. Patients with herniated discs may feel referred pain in a specific segmental distribution even after those body parts have been removed
  - After *tumor* amputation, local recurrence of tumor might also be an explanation for a painful residual limb

2. Phantom sensation

All people with an acquired amputation will experience some form of phantom sensation. It is a normal occurrence after amputation of a limb. Phantom sensation is awareness of a nonpainful sensation in the amputated part (distal to the site of amputation). Phantom sensation usually diminishes with time but can persist throughout the amputee's life.

3. Phantom pain

- Awareness of pain in the portion of the extremity that has been amputated. It may accompany the phantom sensation, localizing in the phantom limb rather than in the residual limb.
- The pain has been described as cramping, aching, burning, and, occasionally lancinating
- Etiology: phantom pain appears to be related to *neuron deafferentation hyperexcitability*.
- It may be diffuse throughout the entire limb or may be localized to a single nerve distribution.
- Studies have suggested that 50% to 85% of amputees experience some phantom limb pain.
- Recent data does not suggest a predisposition for phantom limb pain among traumatic amputees, elderly amputees, or those with pain in the amputated limb before amputation. There appears to be no correlation between phantom pain and amount of time after amputation or use of prosthesis.

- Phantom pain usually diminishes with time and chronic phantom pain is rare. The occurrence of phantom pain generally is considered to be a significant long-term problem in only 5% or less of the total amputee population.
- If pain persists longer than 6 months, prognosis for spontaneous recovery is poor.
- 📖 Phantom pain does not occur in congenital amputation.

Treatment
- Physical interventions/ physical modalities: usually offer temporary relief. Relief is probably mediated by the gate control mechansim.
  - Acupuncture
  - Transcutaneous electrical stimulation (TENS)
  - Vibration
  - Ultrasound
- Medical intervention (Neuropharmacologic intervention)
  - Tricyclic antidepressants
  - Anticonvulsants
  - Calcitonin
  - Capsaicin
  - Propanol
  - Mexiletine—Na$^+$ channels
- Psychological intervention:
  - Hypnosis
  - Biofeedback
  - Cognitive therapy
  - Behavioral
  - Support groups
  - Relaxation therapy
  - Voluntary control of the phantom limb (mental imaging)
- Procedures and surgical intervention:
  - Usually less favorable, with poor long-term success
  - Severe cases may need nerve blocks, steroid injections, or epidural blocks
  - Regional guanethidine or reserpine blocks have been tried with little success
  - Sympathectomy and other neurosurgical procedures

Common Causes of Prosthetic Gait Abnormalities by the Level of Amputation

1. **Partial Foot Amputee:** The average patient with a partial foot amputation will require little gait training, unless other parts of the body are involved.
2. **Syme's amputee:** the patient has usually walked in a plaster cast with a rubber heel or artificial foot prior to delivery of the definitive prosthesis. Minimal training is required during the cast period, except for occasional use of crutches or a pick-up walker at the outset.
   a. Gait speed is typically decreased 32%
   b. Oxygen consumption increased 13% per distance walked in the vascular Syme's amputee with prosthesis, compared with normal subjects without vascular disease.
3. 📖 **Transtibial Amputee:** Gait deviations (Table 6–11)
   Excessive knee flexion
   Excessive knee extension
   Excessive varus moment at the knee during stance phase and excessive lateral thrust
   Excessive valgus moment at the knee during stance

TABLE 6–11. Transtibial Amputee Gait Deviations: Flexion/Extension

Excessive knee flexion (↑ Knee flexion at moment of initial contact)	Excessive knee extension (recurvatum) (↑ Knee extension at moment of initial contact)
• ↑ ankle dorsiflexion	↑ ankle plantar flexion
• Excessive anterior displacement of the socket over the foot • Moving *socket* anteriorly in relation to the *foot*	Moving *socket* posteriorly in relation to the *foot*
• Excessive posterior displacement of the foot in relation to the socket • Moving *foot* posteriorly in relation to the *socket*	Moving *foot* anteriorly in relation to the *socket*
• Too hard heel cushion (or plantar-flexion bumper)	Too soft heel cushion (or plantar-flexion bumper)
• Knee flexion contracture	Quads weakness (Excessive knee extension used as a stabilizing technique)
	Distal anterior tibial discomfort
	Habit

Excessive varus moment at knee during stance phase/Excessive lateral thrust
• Foot too inset (excessive medial placement of prosthetic foot in relation to socket)
• Abducted socket
• Patient may complain of pressure on medio-proximal or disto-lateral aspect of residual limb

Excessive valgus moment at knee during stance phase
• Foot too outset (excessive lateral placement of prosthetic foot in relation to socket)
• Adducted socket
• Patient may complain of pressure on proximo-lateral or disto-medial aspect of residual limb

An overview of the transtibial amputee is reviewed in Table 6–12, including problems, causes, and solutions.

TABLE 6–12. Gait Analysis of the Transtibial Amputee

Problem	Cause	Solution
Delayed, abrupt, and limited knee flexion after heel-strike	Heel wedge is too soft, foot is too far anterior	Stiffen heel wedge, move foot posterior
Extended knee throughout stance phase	Too much plantar flexion	Dorsiflex foot
Toe stays off the floor after heel-strike	Heel wedge too stiff, foot too anterior, too much dorsiflexion	Soften heel wedge, move foot posterior, plantar flex foot
"Hill-climbing" sensation toward end of stance phase	Foot too anterior, too much plantar flexion	Move foot posterior, dorsiflex foot
High pressure against patella throughout most of stance phase, heel is off floor when patient stands	Foot too planter-flexed	Dorsiflex foot
Knee too forcefully and rapidly flexed after heel strike, high pressure against anterio-distal tibia at heel-strike and/or prolonged discomfort at this point	Heel wedge too stiff, foot too far posterior, foot too dorsiflexed	Soften heel, move foot anterior, plantar flex foot
Hips level, but prosthesis seems short	Foot too far posterior, foot too dorsiflexed	Move foot anterior, plantar flex foot
Drop-off at end of stance phase	Foot too far posterior	Move foot anterior

(continued)

TABLE 6–12. (*Continued*)

Problem	Cause	Solution
Toe off of floor as patient stands or knee flexed too much	Foot too dorsiflexed	Plantar flex foot
Valgus moment at knee (knock-knee) during stance phase, excessive pressure on disto-medial limb and proximo-lateral surface of knee	Foot too outset	Inset foot
Excessive varus moment at knee (bow-legged) during stance phase (a varus moment at the knee should occur in stance phase but should never be excessive), the disto-lateral residual limb is painful	Mediolateral dimension of socket too large, foot too inset	Fit of socket should be checked, outset foot

4. ▢ TRANSFEMORAL AMPUTEE : GAIT DEVIATIONS (Table 6–13)
a. Lateral Trunk Bending
b. Abducted Gait
c. Circumduction
d. Vaulting
e. Whips (Swing Phase) Medial and Lateral
f. Foot Rotation at Heel Strike
g. Foot Slap
h. Uneven Heel Rise
i. Terminal Impact
j. Uneven Step Length
k. Exaggerated Lordosis
l. Instability of Prosthetic Knee During Stance
m. Drop-off at End of Stance Phase

TABLE 6–13. Gait Analysis of the Transfemoral Amputee

Problem and Characteristics	Prosthetic Causes	Amputee Causes
a. Lateral bending of trunk: excessive bending occurs laterally from midline, generally to prosthetic side	• Prosthesis may be too short • Improperly shaped lateral wall may fail to provide adequate support for femur • High medial wall may cause amputee to lean away to minimize discomfort • Prosthesis aligned in abduction may cause wide-based gait, resulting in this defect	• Amputee may not have adequate balance • Amputee may have hip abduction contracture • Residual limb may be oversensitive and painful • Very short residual limb may fail to provide a sufficient lever arm for pelvis • Defect may be due to habit pattern
b. Abducted gait: very wide-based gait with prosthesis held away from midline at all times	• Prosthesis may be too long • Too much adduction may have been built into prosthesis • High medial wall may cause amputee to hold prosthesis away to avoid ramus pressure • Improperly shaped lateral wall can fail to provide adequate support for femur • Pelvic band may be positioned too far away from patient's body	• Patient may have hip abduction contracture • Defect may be due to habit pattern

(continued)

TABLE 6–13. (*Continued*)

Problem and Characteristics	Prosthetic Causes	Amputee Causes
c. Circumducted gait: prosthesis swings laterally in wide area during swing phase	• Prosthesis may be too long • Prosthesis may have too much alignment stability or friction in knee, making it difficult to bend knee in swing-through	• Amputee may have abduction contracture of residual limb • Patient may lack confidence for flexing prosthetic knee because of muscle weakness or fear of stubbing toe • Defect may be due to habit pattern
d. Vaulting: rising on toe of sound foot permits amputee to swing prosthesis through with little knee flexion	• Prosthesis may be too long • Socket suspension may be inadequate • Excessive stability in alignment or some limitation of knee flexion, such as knee lock or strong extension aid, may cause this deficit	• Vaulting is fairly frequent habit pattern • Fear of stubbing toe may cause this defect • Residual limb discomfort may be a factor
e. Medial or lateral whips: whips best observed when patient walks away from observer; a medial whip is present when heel travels medially on initial flexion at beginning of swing phase; a lateral whip exists when heel moves laterally	• Lateral whips may result from excessive internal rotation of prosthetic knee • Medial whips may result form excessive external rotation of knee • Socket may fit too tightly, thus reflecting residual limb rotation • Excessive valgus or "knock" in prosthetic knee may contribute to this defect • Badly aligned toe break in a conventional foot may cause twisting on toe-off	• None
f. Foot rotation at heel strike: As heel contacts the ground, the foot rotates laterally, sometimes with vibrating motion	• Too hard heel cushion or plantar flexion bumper	• None
g. Foot slap: the foot plantar flexes too rapidly and strikes the floor with a slap	• Plantar flexion bumper is too soft, offering insufficient resistance to foot motion as weight is transferred to the prosthesis	• None
h. Uneven heel rise: prosthetic heel rises quite markedly and rapidly when knee is flexed at beginning of swing phase	• Knee joint may have insufficient friction • Extension aid may be inadequate	• Amputee may be using more power than necessary to force knee into flexion
i. Terminal swing impact: rapid forward movement of shin piece allows knee to reach maximum extension with too much force before heel-strike	• Knee friction is insufficient • Knee extension aid may be too strong	• Amputee may try to assure himself or herself that knee is in full extension by deliberately and forcibly extending the residual limb

(*continued*)

TABLE 6–13. (Continued)

Problem and Characteristics	Prosthetic Causes	Amputee Causes
j. Uneven step length: the length of the step taken with the prosthesis differs from that of the sound leg	• Insufficient socket flexion • Insufficient friction at the prosthetic knee or too loose an extension aid	• Pain or insecurity causing amputee to transfer weight quickly from the prosthesis to the sound leg • Hip flexion contracture
k. Exaggerated lordosis: the lumbar lordosis is exaggerated when the prosthesis is in stance phase, and the trunk may lean posteriorly	• Insufficient socket flexion • Insufficient support from the anterior socket brim	• Hip flexion contracture • Weak hip extensors • Weak abdominal muscles
l. Instability of the prosthetic knee creating a danger of falling	• Knee joint may be too far ahead of trochanter-knee-ankle (TKA) line • Insufficient initial flexion may have been built into socket • Plantar flexion resistance may be too great, causing knee to buckle at heel-strike • Failure to limit dorsiflexion can lead to incomplete knee control	• Amputee may have hip extensor weakness • Severe hip flexion contracture may cause instability
m. Drop-off at end of stance phase; downward movement of trunk as body moves forward over prosthesis	• Limitation of dorsiflexion of prosthetic foot is inadequate • Heel of SACH-type foot may be too short, or toe break of a conventional foot may be too far posterior • Socket may have been placed too far anterior in relation to foot	• None

(Braddom, 1996)

5. HIP DISARTICULATION:

During the course of gait training, various prosthetic gait deviations may become obvious. *Knee instability* in the stance phase (caused by increased knee flexion moment) may be due to improper alignment of the prosthesis so that the weight-bearing line passes posterior to the knee axis of motion, the plantar flexion bumper of the articulated foot or the heel cushion of the SACH being too firm, or the hip bumper contacting the socket too soon. In contrast, difficulty in flexing the knee will occur if the knee axis of motion is placed too far posterior to the weight-bearing line. Excessive knee flexion in the swing phase occurs if the extension aid is too weak or the friction in the knee bolt is inadequate. Medial or lateral width of the shank and foot section during swing phase is due to excessive external or internal rotation of the knee bolt. Circumduction of the prosthesis during swing phase or vaulting on the sound side may be due to excessive length of the prosthesis, inadequate suspension, or excessive knee stability.

Pediatric/Juvenile Amputees

Prosthetic management of the juvenile amputee

• *Prosthetic Training:* Training is different from that for adults. The child's level of development and attention span must be considered when planning training sessions. Prosthetic training frequently must be included as part of play activities. Parents are taught how to assist their child in attaining skills necessary to use the prosthesis successfully. Parent acceptance of the prosthesis is a prerequisite to the child's acceptance.

- *Congenital Limb Deficiency:* Adults always lose a limb, whereas some children are born with a limb deficiency. In such children, there is no period of psychological adjustment or sense of loss. The prosthesis is perceived as an aid rather than a replacement and will be discarded if it is not helpful.

- *Prosthetic Fitting:* Table 6–14 gives an overview of the key components for proper pediatric prosthetic fitting.

TABLE 6–14. Pediatric Prosthetic Fitting

Level of pediatric amputation	Age for prosthetic fitting	Developmental milestones	Prosthetic prescription
Transradial	6 months	Child can sit and reaches across midline for bimanual manipulation of objects	Body-power—passive mitt terminal device, plastic laminate, self-suspending socket
	9 months		External-power—cookie-crusher, single-site control
	18 months		Go to two-state control
Transhumeral	6 months	Same as transradial	Body-power—passive mitt and elbow, activate elbow at 18 months
	24 months		External-power—variety village elbow with two-state control
Transtibial	9–12 months	Child pulls to stand	PTB, plastic laminate, supra-condylar strap, SACH foot, pediatric dynamic responsive feet now available for use
Transfemoral	9–12 months	Child pulls to stand	Narrow mediolaterally, ischial containment with no knee unit, suspension with Silesian bandage, add knee unit at 18 months

(DeLisa, 1998)

- *Prosthetic Adjustments/Replacements:* pediatric amputees require frequent prosthetic adjustment and replacements. This is due to normal growth and more rigorous use of the device. It can be expected that a socket or prosthesis will have to be replaced yearly in the first 5 years of life, every 18 months for ages 5 to 12, and every 2 years until the age of 21.

Prosthetic replacement frequency in the pediatric amputee	
First 5 years of age	Yearly
Ages 5–12	Every 18 months
Ages 12–21	Every 2 years

- To address growth problems, multilayered sockets (onion sockets) for body powered devices can be used. Length allows removal of one layer at a time to accommodate growth. A socket made this way can increase life span of the prosthesis 6–18 months. Length adjustment is also important.
- This can be adjusted by adding material to the wrist or elbow sites. Harnesses and cables need to be adjusted for length and replaced more frequently.

- *Bony Overgrowth:*
  - Much more common in *acquired amputations in children* than in adults
  - Bone usually grows faster than the overlying skin and soft tissue in the distal end of amputated long bones (residual limb)

- Formation of bursa may occur over the sharp end and at times the bone may actually protrude through the skin.
- Overgrowth is seen most frequently in the humerus, fibula, tibia, and femur, in that order.
- Overgrowth been reported in congenital limb deficiencies, but very rarely
- This may require surgical revision several times before skeletal maturity. Different techniques are available, including capping the end of the involved long bone with a cartilage epiphysis to eliminate the overgrowth

- *Parental Counseling and Support:* This is key because the acceptance of the prosthesis by the child is often dependent on the acceptance by the parents.

■

ASSISTIVE DEVICES—AMBULATION AIDS

CANES

When properly used canes will:
1. Increase base of support
2. Decrease loading and demand on the lower limbs
3. Provide additional sensor information
4. Assist acceleration/deceleration during locomotion

Prescribed in various disabilities to:
1. Improve balance
2. Decrease pain
3. Reduce weight-bearing forces of injured structures
4. Compensate for weak muscles
5. Scan the immediate environment

Components
- Handle
- Adjusting knob for handle
- Shaft
- Adjusting mechanism for height
- Rubber tip

C-handle or crook top cane

Advantages: inexpensive
Disadvantages: uncomfortable, difficult to grasp (i.e., RA patient), weight-bearing line falls behind the shaft of the cane reducing support, not adjustable

Adjustable metal cane

Advantages: inexpensive, adjustable
Disadvantages: same as above

Functional grip cane

Advantages: handle fits the grip, conforms to natural angle of hand. and is more centered over the shaft of the cane, provides more support
Disadvantages: more expensive

Wide-based or quadruped cane

Advantages: more support
Disadvantage: heavy, awkward appearance, WBQC does not fit on stairs

> **Difference Between Crutch and a Cane?**
> - Cane has one point of contact with the body
> - Crutch has 2 points of contact with the body

Cane Measurement/Prescription

20° elbow flexion or height of greater trochanter

CRUTCHES

Axillary Crutches

Components
- Padded axillary piece (on top)
- Two upright shafts
- Handpiece (in middle)
- Extension piece
- Rubber tip

Advantages: inexpensive, adjustable, easier to use
Disadvantages: need good strength and ROM in upper limbs, ties up hands. Increased cardiac/ metabolic demand

Forearm Crutches/Lofstrand crutches

Components
- Forearm cuff with narrow anterior opening
- Forearm piece bent posteriorly and adjustable (extends to 2 inches below elbow)
- Molded handpiece
- Single aluminum tubular shaft
- Rubber tip

Advantages: lightweight, easily adjustable, freedom for hand activities
Disadvantages: needs more strength, requires more skill, and better trunk balance

Platform Crutches

Advantages: Do not need weight bearing through wrist and hand (i.e., fractures, arthritis of wrist or hand. or weakness triceps or grasp)
Disadvantages: awkward, heavy

📖 WALKERS

Indications

1. Bilateral weakness and/or incoordination of the lower limbs or whole body, whenever a firm, free standing aid is appropriate (i.e., multiple sclerosis or Parkinsonism) to ↑ balance
2. To relieve weight bearing either fully or partially on a lower extremity (allow the upper extremities to transfer body weight to the floor)
3. Unilateral weakness or amputation of the lower limb where general weakness makes the greater support offered by the frame necessary (i.e., osteoarthritis or fractured femur)
4. General support to aid mobility and confidence (i.e., after prolonged bedrest and sickness in the elderly)

Advantages

Provide a wider base of support
More stable base of support
Provide a sense of security for patients fearful of ambulation

Disadvantages

More conspicuous in appearance
Interfere with development of a smooth reciprocal gait pattern (e.g., ↓ step length with step-to-gait pattern)
Interfere with stair negotiation / difficult to maneuver through doorways or bathrooms

Types

- Lightweight walking frame
- Folding walking frame
- Rolling walking frame
- Forearm resting walking frame
- Hemi-walking frame

■

SHOES AND LOWER LIMB ORTHOSES

SHOE COMPONENTS (Figure 6–13)

A shoe consists of the *upper*, the *sole*, and, in most cases, an added *heel*.

Upper—part of shoe above the sole
- The shoe upper is made of a flexible material—leather, woven fabrics, or synthetic materials such as urethane or vinyl
- In the oxford style shoe, the *upper* consists of three basic parts:
  - Vamp (one piece)—anterior part covering the instep and toes
  - Quarters (two pieces sewn together)—the pieces that make up the posterior part; laterally, the quarter is cut lower to avoid infringing on the lateral malleolus
  - High quarter—referred to as high top, offers mediolateral stability
- Tongue—strip of leather lying under the laces
- Throat—opening at the base of the tongue, entrance to shoe
  - The more anteriorly the throat is located, the more room for internal modification (extra depth shoes also allow more room for shoe orthotics)
- Toe Box—anterior part of the vamp, protects toes from trauma

Sole—bottom part of the shoe; consists of three layers: insole, outsole and the filler between them
- Outsole—part that touches the ground; may be made of leather, rubber, crepe, plastic, wood, or other materials
- Insole—may be made of thin leather or man-made material; part closest to foot
- The filler is usually made of cork dust and latex
- Leather soles—indicated if shoe modifications are needed or attachment to metal AFO
- Rubber soles—modifications are more difficult
- Ball—widest part of sole, at the metatarsal heads
  Can be modified internally or externally to help alleviate forefoot pain

- Shank—narrowest part of sole, between heel and ball,
  - Usually reinforced with metal, leather, fiberboard, or other firm material (to provide additional support for the shoe in the region corresponding to the arch of the foot)
  - Can be reinforced with metal for attachment of metal Ankle Foot orthosis (AFO)
- External heel seat—the posterior part of sole to which heel is attached

Heel—attached to outer sole

- The heel height varies from a negative heel that is lower than the forefoot position to 2–3 inches high.
- Purpose of heel
  - Acts as a shock absorber and prevents shoe from wearing out
  - Shifts weight to the forefoot
- Materials—leather, wood, plastic, rubber, or metal
- Heel block—part attached to heel seat, made of firm material
- Breast—anterior part of heel; height of heel is measured in 1/8 inches at the breast
- Types of heels
  - Flat heel—broad base, measures 0.75 to 1.25 inches in height
  - Thomas heel—flat with medial extension to support weak foot arch
  - Military heel—slightly narrower base, measures 1.25 to 1.375 inches
  - Cuban heel—still narrower base, higher heel
  - Spring heel—placed under outer sole, eliminates breast, only 0.125 inches
- Many athletic shoes eliminate the heel because one can run faster this way
- Height may be a factor in clinical conditions
  - Shortening of gastrocnemius
  - Low back pain
  - High heels make ankle and foot more unstable (remember, articular surface of talus is narrower posteriorly ⇒ this is the area of contact when ankle is plantarflexed)
- Heel counter—reinforces the shoe, stabilizing the foot by supporting and controlling the calcaneus
  - Usually extends anteriorly to the heel breast
  - May extend further in specially made shoes
- Collar—band of leather stitched to the top of the quarters,
  - Sometimes used to reduce postioning
  - Can also prevent shoe from falling off
- Lace Stay—portion containing the eyelets for laces
  - Usually part of the vamp
  - Can be part of the quarters

BASIC OXFORD (LOW-QUARTER) SHOE TYPES (FIGURE 6–13)

- Bal or Balmoral: front-laced shoe in which the lace stays meet in front and are stitched to the vamp.
- Blucher: front-laced shoe in which the quarters (specifically, the lace stays) are not attached (stitched) distally to the vamp and remain loose and fully open, thus leaving more room for the entering foot.

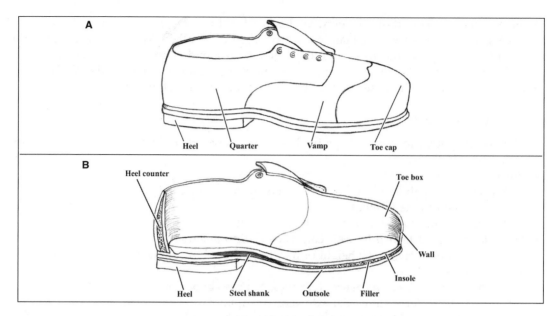

FIGURE 6–13. Oxford Shoe component parts. **A:** External view. **B:** Longitudinal section.

SHOE MODIFICATIONS

Internal modifications
- **Heel cushion-relief/excavation:** is a soft pad with excavation under painful part of heel (e.g., a calcaneal spur)
- **Inner sole excavation/relief:** is a soft pad with excavation under one or more painful bony prominence (usually metatarsal heads). The excavation is usually filled with compressible material
- **Scaphoid pads/arch cookies/navicular pad:** a rubber, cork, or plastic foam wedge used to provide medial longitudinal arch support
- **Metatarsal pads:** dome shaped pads glued to the inner sole with the apex under the metatarsal shafts. It relieves pressure from the metatarsal heads by transferring the load to the metatarsal shafts
- **Internal heel wedges:** can be applied medially and promote hindfoot inversion (eg, in flexible pes planus) or laterally, and promote hindfoot eversion and relive pressure on the cuboid (e.g., in flexible pes varus.) It also increases total plantar-bearing area and can be used in fixed pes varus
- **Toe crest:** used to relieve pressure at the distal end and plantar surface of the toes (typically for hammer toes).

Foot orthoses (inserts or inlays)
- **Univ. of California Biomechanics Lab orthosis (UCBL):** custom-molded orthosis used to realign flexible flat foot; it encompasses the heel and hindfoot, providing very effective longitudinal arch support.
- **Heel cup:** provides calcaneal support; used to prevent lateral calcaneal shift (calcaneal valgus) in the flexible flat foot.
- **Longitudinal arch insert:** can be applied medially or laterally.
- **Plastazote full-contact insoles:** custom molded, made of various densities and thickness. Accommodating many foot problems/deformities, these insoles provide almost immediate comfort for plantar outgrowths.

- Other available foot orthoses include: sesamoid inserts, metatarsal inserts, Levy balancer, the Mayer, Morton's toe extension

External Modifications

Sole modifications
- 📖 **Rocker bar:** this is a convex strip placed across the sole just posterior to the metatarsal heads. It is longer than the metatarsal bar.
  - It can be used to relieve metatarsal pain (by relieving pressure), quicken the gait cycle (by assisting rollover during stance), assist dorsiflexion or decrease demand on weak plantar flexors (push off).
  - It can include entire heel and sole to become rocker-bottom shoe
- **Metatarsal bar:** This is a simple bar placed in the sole just posterior to the metatarsal heads; it relieves pressure from the metatarsal heads by transferring load to the metatarsal shafts during stance.
- **Sole wedge:** lateral sole wedge promotes forefoot eversion; medial wedge promotes forefoot inversion
- **Toe wedge:** medial toe wedge is used to encourage toeing-in and is commonly used with a medial heel wedge. Lateral toe wedge (pigeon-toe wedge) is used to assist the foot to toe out
- **Sole flare:** provides greater stability by widening the base of support of the shoe; a medial flare resists eversion, while a lateral flare resists inversion of the foot
- **Shank filler:** can be applied medially to support medial longitudinal arch or it can be applied laterally to support lateral longitudinal arch
- **Steel shank:** is inserted between the inner and outer soles to prevent motion of the anterior sole (bending of the sole) and thus reduce stress on metatarsals/phalanges. It is commonly used with the rocker bar to assist rollover.

Heel Modifications
- **Heel wedge:** can be placed either medially (to rotate hindfoot into inversion) or laterally (to rotate hindfoot into eversion).
- **Heel flare:** applied either medially (to resist hindfoot eversion) or laterally (to resist hindfoot inversion).
- **Heel extension:** can project anteriorly either medially (Thomas heel) or laterally (reverse Thomas heel). The Thomas heel provides support to the medial longitudinal arch; the reverse Thomas heel provides support to the lateral longitudinal arch.
- **Cushioned Heel ("SACH" heel):** is a heel with the posterior portion replaced by a rubberized, compressible material to absorb shock at heel (foot) strike. Cushioned heel with shift weight line (line of gravity) anterior to the knee joint at initial contact causing an extension moment of the knee (thus stabilizing knee).
- **Heel lift:** is used to compensate for fixed pes equinus deformity or for a leg length discrepancy of more than one fourth to one half inch (or if symptomatic).

ORTHOTIC AND SHOE MODIFICATIONS PRESCRIPTION

Insensitive and Dysvascular Foot

Causes
  - Peripheral nerve or spinal-cord injury
  - Myelodysplasias
  - Stroke
  - Neuropathies
  - Peripheral vascular disease
  - Chronic venous insufficiency

Careful Evaluation
- Assessment of skin condition
- Distribution of plantar pressure during standing and walking
- Thickness of fat pads. calluses, and scarring on the plantar surfaces

Sensory-impaired feet with no soft tissue or skeletal deformity need carefully fitted shoes that accommodate area of concentrated pressure
- Microcellular rubber insole will distribute stress over larger area
- Extra-depth shoe need: may be needed

Feet scarred on plantar surface need:
- Insoles
  - Molded polyethylene foam backed by microcellular rubber
  - Soft-grade and medium-grade Plastazote® may also be used
- Extra-depth shoes

Bone Deformity on Plantar Aspect
- Soft molded insole of polyethylene foam recommended
- Areas of relief under bony prominences
- Metatarsal bar attached to flexible sole will relieve stress at metatarsal heads
- When sole is rigid, rocker bar may be fitted

Preventative Foot Care
- Regardless of cause, patient must follow daily foot care and inspection program
- Patient may not be aware that footwear is too tight or breakdown is occurring
- Daily foot examination
- Detect areas of tissue trauma
- Particular attention to metatarsal heads
- May need mirror
- Handicapped patient may need assistance
- Skin may lack normal perspiration moisture
- Leads to scaling and fissuring
- Daily foot soaks followed by application of emollient may be needed

Arthritic Foot

General
- Foot involved in 90% of patients with RA
- Metatarsophalangeal (MTP) joints often affected early
- Tenosynovitis, rheumatoid nodules, and inflamed bursae are common
- Atrophy of fat pads occurs
- Advanced—hallux valgus, clawing of toes, spread of forefoot, and rigid flat foot

Shoe Prescription and Modifications
- Wide shoe with soft upper recommended to avoid mediolateral tarsal compression MTPs
- Flexible sole
- Soft heel counter—useful in patients with heel pain due to nodules or bursae
- Extra-depth—for clawing of the toes, avoids pressure on dorsum
- Soft toe box—to adjust for deformities
- Metatarsal pad—relief of pressure on painful metatarsal heads
- Full molded insole—may be preferable to metatarsal pad that can move
- Redistribute weight over entire weight-bearing surface
- As with insensitive foot, can be heat-moldable or nonmoldable material
- External modification with metatarsal bar may reduce pressure over MTP region

Custom-made Shoe
- Severely deformed foot will require a custom-made shoe
- Made according to plaster cast of foot
- Leather should be used for the upper; sole can be leather or rubber
- Other options include sandals with soft molded insole and straps adjusted to avoid pressure areas
- High heels are heavy and not suitable
- May also require modification of closure as hands may be involved

Painful Foot

Heel Spurs and Plantar Fasciitis
- Insert of soft rubber or soft-grade polyethylene foam (Plastazote®) under heel
- Decrease in amount of weight-bearing
- Other methods - Univ. of Calif. Biomechanics Laboratory (UCBL) shoe insert
  - ◆ UCBL is a plastic shell made by laminating layers of nylon and fiberglass
  - ◆ UCBL cast is made from negative taken with leg ext rotated, forefoot pronated
  - ◆ UCBL holds foot in a position that relieves tension on plantar fascia
  - ◆ Inverts heel with forces against navicular bone

Foot Problems Associated with Running
Factors
- Training errors—most common cause (too much, too far, or too fast)
- Poor training surface
- Poor flexibility
- Inadequate warming-up
- Biomechanical abnormalities
- Poor footwear
- Growth and development

Sports Shoes
- All provide cushioning, stability, and surface traction
- Varied designs to meet specific demands of individual or sport
- Remember—check shoe

Pronated Foot
Most common biomechanical problem with runners
Associated problems
- Tibial stress syndrome
- Patellofemoral syndrome
- Posterior tibial tendinitis
- Achilles tendinitis
- Plantar fasciitis

Shoe Modifications
- Board and straight-last construction
- Motion control heel counter
- Medial support
- High-density insole medially
- Wider flared heel

Soft or Semirigid Orthosis
- Remove shoe insole
- Replace with commercial support according to shoe size
- For permanent use—made according to plaster cast of the foot
- Usually flexible orthosis of leather or semi-rigid polyethylene

▪

ORTHOTICS

Orthosis, or brace, is an external device applied to body parts to provide or more different functions, including:

1. Reduction in pain/comfort
2. Prevent or correct deformity
3. Support/stability
4. Improvement in function
5. Augment weak muscles (assist motion)
6. Control spastic muscles
7. Limit ROM (restriction of motion)
8. Unload diseased or damaged joints
9. A kinesthetic reminder (orthosis provides sensory/visual feedback that reminds the patient to adopt a more corrective or appropriate position, or to avoid some activities/movements)

Biomechanical principles of prescription, selection of materials, fit, and fabrication.

Biomechanics- Application of force and counterforce. ⇒ Three point principle

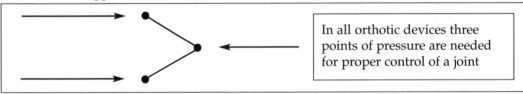

In all orthotic devices three points of pressure are needed for proper control of a joint

Center of gravity (COG)—while standing, the COG is in the midline just in front of the second sacral vertebra.

Line of gravity (weight line)—line passing through the center of gravity to the center of the Earth.

- Passes behind the cervical vertebrae, in front of the thoracic vertebrae, and behind the lumbar vertebrae.
- Hip
  - Line of gravity is slightly behind (posterior to) the hip joint
  - Tends to hyperextend the hip joint
- Knee
  - Line of gravity is in front of (anterior to) the knee joint
  - Hyperextends the knee
- Ankle
  - Line of gravity passes one or two inches anterior to the ankle joint
  - Tends to dorsiflex the ankle; this activity is resisted by the soleus and gastrocnemius muscles

When selecting appropriate materials for orthotic devices, their strength, durability, flexibility, and weight need to be considered carefully

The orthotic design should be simple, inconspicuous, comfortable, and as cosmetic as possible

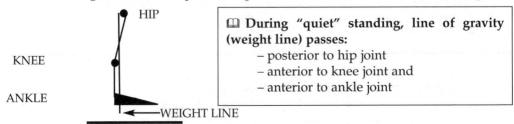

HIP

KNEE

ANKLE

WEIGHT LINE

📖 **During "quiet" standing, line of gravity (weight line) passes:**
- posterior to hip joint
- anterior to knee joint and
- anterior to ankle joint

Materials Used in Fabrication of Orthotics

Metals

a. Steel—major advantage is low cost, abundance, and ease. It is fatigue resistant, provides high strength and rigidity. Main disadvantage is its weight and need for expensive alloys to prevent corrosion.

b. Aluminum—corrosion resistant and provides high strength. It is used when light weight is a major consideration. However, it has lower endurance limit under repeated dynamic loading conditions than does steel.

c. Titanium alloys—strength comparable to steel, but only 60% of the density. More resistant to corrosion than aluminum alloys or steel. They have limited use because of limited availability and high cost.

d. Magnesium alloys—very light weight. Useful when bulk instead of strength is important.

- Leather—Most commonly used as covering for braces and straps, covering for pelvic bands, and various types of molded applications such as the girdle for the Milwaukee braces.
- Rubber—tough resiliency, shock-absorbing qualities. It can be used in padding for various assistive devices, seals in hydraulic mechanisms, and padding in body jackets and limb orthoses.
- Plastics

📖 *Thermoplastics*—soften (and become moldable) when heated and harden when cooled so they can be molded and remolded by heating.

Low Temperature Thermoplastics:
- Can be molded at temperatures just above body temperature (< 80°C or <180°F), hence they may be shaped directly to the body without the need for a cast
- Cannot be used effectively when high stress is anticipated, as in spasticity or in many lower extremity applications. Main use is in upper limb orthotics, where rapid provision of an assistive or protective orthosis is often desirable.
- E.g., Orthoplast®, Aquaplast®, Bioplastics®, Glassona®, Hexcelite®, Kay-splint®, Lightcast®, Polysar®, Warm-N-Form®

High-Temperature Thermoplastics—used to manufacture permanent orthotic devices using the vacuum-forming techniques.
- Major types: acrylic, polyethylene, polypropylene, polycarbonate, ABS (acrylonitrile-butadiene-styrene), vinyl polymers, and copolymers

Thermosetting Plastics—develop a permanent shape when heat and pressure are applied and maintain a memory. More difficult to use than the thermoplastics and generally cause more body irritation and allergic reactions. Examples: polyesters, epoxies, polyurethane foam

LOWER LIMB ORTHOTIC PRESCRIPTION (AFO, KAFO, HKAFO)

Ankle-Foot Orthosis (AFO)—Commonly prescribed for weakness affecting the ankle and subtalar joints. These can be made of plastic, metal, or a hybrid of both.

Plastic AFO

Plastic ankle foot orthoses are either prefabricated out of thermal plastic or custom molded over a model of the patient's limb taken from a casting. Generally they would encompass the posterior calf area with anterior Velcro® strap closure continuing down posteriorly by the ankle and extending down the plantar surface of the foot to assist in dorsiflexion and limit plantar flexion. The design of the trim lines and the design of the foot plate will help determine the structural support and rigidity of the device. The following includes typical designs:

1. **Posterior Leaf Spring–PLS** design is the most flexible plastic AFO with a very thin plastic band behind the ankle allowing the patient to overpower the brace during the push-off or plantar flexion phase and yet allowing dorsiflexion position of the foot during swing phase. This design is typically used for flaccid foot drop.

2. **Semi-rigid plastic AFO** with trim lines just behind the malleoli will allow for increase of support and provide both dorsiflexion positioning of the foot and mediolateral stability of the ankle. Much less motion is allowed with this brace design and the patient cannot easily propel during push-off. This design is most commonly used for patients that have foot drop with some extensor tone and/or with mediolateral instability of the ankle.

3. **Rigid or solid plastic AFO** used most commonly for patients that have the highest levels of spasticity or tone when complete immobilization of the ankle is necessary. In this case the plastic trim line may be at the malleoli or anterior to the malleoli with no motion allowed at the tibiotalar or subtalar joint. The standard plastic AFO would typically have a foot plate extending through the metatarsal heads, but if the toes are also spastic and claw into a flex position, then a full foot plate should also be incorporated into this type of solid plastic AFO. Inhibitory foot plate designs are commonly used, which may put the toes into extension to help reduce tone throughout the entire limb. This brace design is typically used for patients with the highest levels of spasticity, early to moderate Charcot joint, and for postoperative immobilization of the foot or ankle.

Plastic vs. Metal AFO

Plastic design AFOs are most desirable due to their light weight, intimate fit, cosmetic appeal, and lack of attachment to the shoe. However, in some cases, the selection of plastic materials may be inappropriate due to risk of excessive pressure or skin breakdown on the leg or foot. Commonly patients with insensate foot due to peripheral neuropathy or peripheral nerve injury should be considered candidates for metal AFOs rather than plastic. Also patients with fluctuating edema that is not managed with compression stockings should be considered most appropriate for metal AFOs rather than plastic AFOs.

AFOs with Hinged Ankle Joint

1. **Paralysis of Dorsiflexion, Plantarflexion, Inversion, Eversion**

   Most mechanical ankle joints prevent mediolateral instability and either control or assist dorsiflexion and plantar flexion by means of stops or assists (springs)

   a. Plantar flexion control:
   - May use *plantar flexion stop*-angulation of the top of the stirrup posteriorly that restricts plantarflexion but allows unlimited dorsiflexion. Substitutes for paralyzed foot dorsiflexors during swing phase. Prevents rapid foot flat after *heel strike* and maintains the ground reaction force posterior to the knee joint.

   b. Dorsiflexion control
   - May use dorsiflexion stop-anterior angulation that allows full plantar flexion while limiting dorsiflexion. Substitutes for paralyzed gastroc-soleus muscles during push-off. Allows center of gravity and the ground reaction force to move forward to the metatarsal head area, and creates a moment arm in front of (anterior to) the knee, which promotes knee extension and stability.

   c. Dorsiflexion—assist spring joint (Klenzak joint)
   - Uses coils located posteriorly that are compressed following heel (or foot) strike (in stance phase). At heel strike, the springs also yield slightly into plantar flexion and

help prevent inadvertent knee flexion. During swing phase, the spring rebounds to aid dorsiflexion.

d. Dorsiflexion/plantar flexion assist joint
 – Has an anterior spring that is compressed at midstance and as it recoils, it helps to plantarflex the ankle into push-off. It is used in flail ankle.

e. Bi-channel adjustable ankle lock (BICAAL) joint
 – Has anterior and posterior receptacles with springs that can be compressed to assist motion. The springs can be replaced by pins to alter the alignment of the joint and thus convert it into adjustable stops.

2. **Prevention and Correction of Deformities**
3. **Reduction of Weight Bearing**

- *Patellar Tendon Bearing (PTB) Orthosis*
 – For reduction of weight transmission through the mid or distal tibia, ankle and foot.
 – E.g., healing of os calcis fracture, postoperative ankle fusion, heel with refractory pain, delayed unions or nonunions of fractures or fusions, avascular necrosis of the talar body, DJD of the talar or ankle joint, osteomyelitis of the os calcis, and diabetic ulceration/Charcot joint.
 – Supports weight on the patellar tendon or tibial flares with the load being transmitted to the shoe via the metal uprights.
 – To bypass the lateral aspect of the foot in patients with Charcot joints
 – May have plastic bivalve design or calf corset if the patient has fluctuating edema.
 – Because little or no ankle motion is allowed, a cushion heel or a rocker bottom is added to provide smoother gait pattern.

- *Ischial Weight-Bearing Orthosis*
 – Quadrilateral brim or an ischial (Thomas) ring to relieve weight from the femur or knee.

- *Patten—Bottom Orthosis*
 – Uses uprights with no ankle joint that terminate in a floor pad distal to the shoe so the foot is freely suspended in midair. A shoe lift is needed in the opposite side to equalize leg length.

- *Fracture Orthosis*
 – Stabilize the fracture site and help promote callus formation by allowing weight bearing and joint movement after initial rest period to allow pain and edema to subside. Minimize joint stiffness and reduce complications such as nonunions. Circumferential compression of the soft tissue can be used to prevent undue bony motion at the fracture site

4. **Reduce the energy cost of ambulation—e.g., in patients with spastic diplegia (CP), LMN weakness (poliomyelitis), and spastic hemiplegia (stroke)**

Knee-Ankle/Foot-Orthosis (KAFO)

Represents extensions of the AFO proximally to control knee motion and alignment:
1. Control genu recurvatum, genu valgum and varum. Used with free-motion knee joints. *Free-motion knee joint* or polycentric knee joint provides unlimited flexion and extension but usually has a stop to prevent hyperextension. For patients with genu recurvatum but with enough strength to control the knee in stance and ambulation.
2. To provide skeletal support following surgery or nonunion fracture
3. Knee-flexion contractures. Locked knee joints are usually used for these applications. Adjustable knee lock:
 – Serrated adjustable keen joint permits locking in almost any degree of flexion
 – Useful in a patient with a knee flexion contracture which its diminishing with treatment

4. Locked knee joints—to prevent knee buckling. To be able to lock the joint, the patient must be able to fully extend the knee, either actively or passively. Contraindicated in patients with knee contracture (use an adjustable knee lock instead)

- Drop-ring locks—rings drop over the joints in extension, locking them. They are designed to either drop by gravity, or with assistance from the patient.

- Pawl lock with bail release—engages when knee is fully extended, but easier to release because of the semicircular lever (bail) attached posteriorly, which unlocks the joint with an upward pull on the bail (either manually or by backing up to sit down on a chair).
  – Disadvantages: The bail is bulky and can be accidentally released is if hits a rigid object.

- Trick knee allows 0–25 degree of measurement while in the locked position to normalize gait. Free knee when unlocked.

- Offset knee joint—hinge is placed posterior to the knee joint so the patient's weight line falls anterior to the offset joint, stabilizing the knee during early stance on level surfaces. It is free to flex during swing phase, and allows sitting without the need to manipulate the lock. Should not be used in patients with knee- or hip-flexion contracture, or with plantar flexion stop at the ankle. The patient must be careful when walking on a ramp as the knee may flex inadvertently.

Hip-Knee-Ankle-Foot Orthosis (HKAFO)

- Hip joint and pelvic band attached to the lateral upright of a KAFO converts it to a HKAFO.
- Indications
  1. Hip flexion/extension instability
  2. Hip adduction/abduction weakness
  3. Hip internal rotation/external rotation instability

📖 **Scott-Craig orthosis (Scott-Craig long leg brace):** (Figure 6–14)
  – Bilateral KAFO designed for standing and ambulation in adults with paraplegia. It provides the paraplegic patient who has a complete neurological level at L1 or higher with a more functional and comfortable gait.
  – It eliminates unnecessary hardware to reduce weight and facilitate donning/doffing (eliminates the lower thigh and calf band)
    📖 Consists of:
    1. Sole plate extending to the metatarsal heads with a crossbar added to the metatarsal heads area for mediolateral stabilization.
    2. Ankle joint set at 10° of dorsiflexion
    3. Anterior rigid tibial band (patellar tendon strap)
    4. Offset knee joint with bail lock
    5. Proximal posterior thigh band

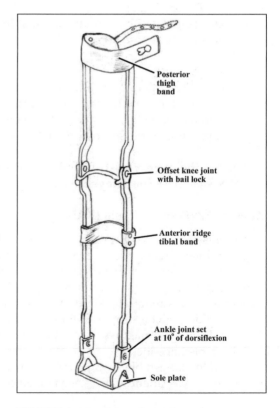

Posterior thigh band

Offset knee joint with bail lock

Anterior ridge tibial band

Ankle joint set at 10° of dorsiflexion

Sole plate

FIGURE 6–14. Scott-Craig Orthosis.

📖 *Unsupported standing* is possible with Scott-Craig orthosis.

With the ankles and knees locked, hip stabilization can be achieved by leaning the trunk backwards so that the COG of the trunk rests posterior to the hip joint, resulting in tightening of the anterior hip capsule, the "Y" ligament. In adults, the "Y" ligament (iliofemoral ligament, ligament of Bigelow) is usually strong/stable enough to provide hip-pelvic stability when using a KAFO without pelvic bands.

📖 Paraplegic patients can ambulate with Scott-Craig orthoses and crutches or walker using a swing-to or swing-through pattern gait

📖 Reciprocal Gait Orthosis (RGO)

- One special design of HKAFO is the *reciprocal gait orthosis*. RGO is used for upper lumbar paralysis in which active hip flexion is preserved
- RGO consists of bilateral HKAFO with offset knee joints, knee drop locks, posterior plastic AFO, thigh pieces, custom molded pelvic girdle, hip joints, and a thoracic extension with Velcro® straps, in addition to the control mechanism
- Several designs are available, including cord and pulley design (early versions), gear-box cable, single cable, dual-cable, and isocentric RGO (latest design). In the *isocentric RGO (IRGO)*, the cord is substituted by a pelvic band attached to the posterior surface of the molded thoracic section (Figure 6–15)
  - Advantages of the IRGO include less bulky appearance (no protruding cables in the back), and it may be more cost efficient than cable RGO (no energy loss due to cable friction)

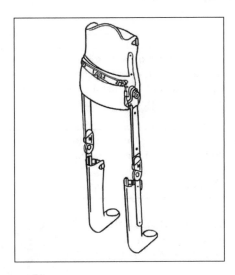

FIGURE 6–15. Isocentric Type RGO.

- In all RGOs, the hip joints are coupled together with cables (or to the pivoting pelvic band in the IRGO), which provides mechanical assistance to hip extension while preventing simultaneous bilateral hip flexion
- As a step is initiated and hip flexion takes place on one side, the cable coupling induces hip extension on the opposite side, producing a reciprocal walking pattern
- Forward stepping is achieved by active hip flexion, lower abdominal muscles, and/or trunk extension
- Using two crutches and an RGO, paraplegics can ambulate with a four-point gait. A walker or walkerette may also be used.

Knee Orthoses

Flexible Knee Orthosis
- Made from an elastic material or rubber
- May include hinged metal knee joints, patellar pads, adjustable straps to change tension, and anterior cutout to relieve pressure on the patella when the knee is flexed
- Function:
  - Provide comfort for patients with osteoarthritis, minor knee sprains, and mild edema
  - Proprioceptive feedback / kinesthetic reminder
  - Minimal mechanical support
  - Can retain body heat
  - Stabilize patellar tracking with patello-femoral dysfunction

Knee orthoses (KOs): Rehabilitative, Functional, and Prophylactic
- Generally prescribed to prevent genu recurvatum and to provide mediolateral stability. Prophylactic KOs, theoretically, are designed to prevent injury to the knee or at least to reduce the degree to which the knee is injured in athletic activities.
- KOs may be used during sports and other physical activities to provide functional support for unstable knees or during rehabilitation after injury or surgery of the knee. The use of KOs for the prevention of knee injuries in sports is controversial.
- Numerous designs of KOs available; most consist of two uprights, free or adjustable knee joints, and thigh and calf cuffs

Knee Orthoses—Force Systems

To limit flexion
1. Anteriorly directed force on posterior proximal thigh
2. Posteriorly directed force on anterior surface of the knee (either directly over the patella or a combination of support just proximal and just distal to the patella)
3. Anteriorly directed force on posterior aspect of the calf

To limit extension (genu recurvatum)
1. Two bands placed anterior to the knee axis (one superior and one inferior to the knee)
2. One band placed posterior to the knee joint in the popliteal area Use only top left portion
3. It also has an additional thigh band with longer uprights to obtain better leverage at the knee joint

Examples of KOs
- Swedish knee cage (Figure 6–16): Prefabricated brace that controls minor to moderate knee hyperextension/genu recurvatum due to ligamentous or capsular laxity
  - Available in nonarticulated and articulated forms
  - The articulated version prevents hyperextension but permits full flexion of the knee, using a three-point pressure system with two anterior straps and one posterior strap held in position by a metal frame medially and laterally (see earlier table).
- Lenox-Hill derotation orthosis (Figure 6–17): knee orthosis designed for control of knee axial rotation (in addition to anterio-posterior and mediolateral planes control).
  - Used in prevention and management of sports injuries to the knee (e.g., ACL injuries).

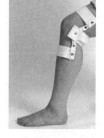

FIGURE 6–16.
Swedish Knee Cage.

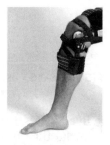

FIGURE 6–17.
Lenox Hill Orthosis.

■

UPPER LIMB ORTHOTICS

STATIC UPPER-LIMB ORTHOSES

- **Indications**
  1. Immobilize, stabilize, and support a joint in a desired position
  2. Protect weak muscles from overstretch
  3. Prevent contractures
  4. Support structures following surgical repair
  5. Facilitate the healing of soft tissue injuries and fractures

- **Complications associated with use of static orthoses**
  1. Skin breakdown
  2. Contractures
  3. Infection

Wrist, Hand, and Finger Static Orthoses

Positional orthoses

📖 *Opponens orthoses* (Figure 6–18): primarily used to immobilize the thumb to promote tissue healing and/or protection or for positioning of the weak thumb in opposition to other fingers to facilitate three-jaw-chuck pinch
  – Stabilization of the first MCP joint
Basic Opponens orthoses:
  – Thumb orthoses that consist of a dorsal and a palmar bar encircling the midpalm, with a thumb abduction bar projecting from the palmar bar.
  – Examples: short opponens splints, C-bar splints, cone splints, static thumb splints

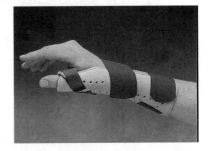

FIGURE 6–18. Basic Opponens Splint. Photo courtesy of North Coast Medical, Inc., Morgan Hill, CA.

Opponens orthoses with wrist control attachments
  – Similar to basic opponens orthosis with a forearm bar and proximal and distal crossbars for wrist control
  – 📖 Ex: *long opponens splints (Figiure 6–19) and thumb spica splints*
  – In addition to the benefits already mentioned for opponens orthoses (stabilizes first MCP), forearm bar maintains wrist in extension and prevent radial and ulnar deviation deformities

Opponens orthoses with lumbrical bar
  – Finger orthosis that prevents metacarpal phalangeal joint hyperextension but allows full MCP flexion
  – Prevents claw hand deformity (in addition to the benefits already mentioned for opponens orthoses)

FIGURE 6–19. Long Opponens Splint (forearm, wrist, thumb). Photo courtesy of North Coast Medical, Inc., Morgan Hill, CA.

Opponens orthoses with finger extension assist assembly
  – Similar to basic opponens orthoses plus finger orthosis that assist proximal interphalangeal and distal interphalangeal extension

– Used for interphalangeal flex contracture, boutonnière deformity, or postsurgical release of Dupuytren's contracture.

Utensil holders/ universal cuff (splints)/ ADL splints:
– Consist of a handcuff with palmar pocket onto which a utensil can be inserted.

Protective orthoses: used to protect wrist, hand, and/or fingers from potential deformity or damage by restricting active function / limiting motion

Digital stabilizers

Finger stabilizers/static finger orthoses (FOs):

Interphalangeal stabilizers (DIP, PIP, and DIP+PIP gutter splints, static finger splints, stax or stack splints, egg-shell finger casts, etc.)
- FOs used to restrict motions at the PIP and DIP
- Generally, IPs maintained in full extension to keep the collateral ligaments stretched and to prevent IP flex contracture (unless condition dictates otherwise)
- Used to promote healing (e.g., phalanx fx, PIP/DIP dislocation, etc.) and to provide prolonged finger stretch (e.g., burns and contractures)

Ring stabilizers (Figure 6–20)
- Swan neck ring—FO that prevents hyperextension of the PIP joint (via three point pressure system) but allows full IP flexion
- Boutonnière ring—FO that immobilizes the PIP in extension (prevents flexion) through a three point pressure system.

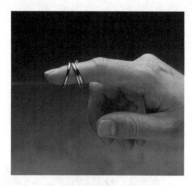 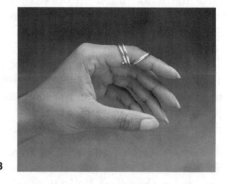

A   **B**

FIGURE 6–20. Ring Stabilizers: **A.** Swan Neck splint. **B.** Boutonnière splint. Photo courtesy of North Coast Medical, Inc., Morgan Hill, CA.

METACARPOPHALANGEAL ULNAR-DEVIATION RESTRICTION ORTHOSIS: (FIGURE 6–21)
- FO used to limit ulnar deviation of the MCP with unrestricted (if possible) MCP flex/extension in arthritic patients with ulnar deviation at the MCPs.

Thumb stabilizers

THUMB CARPOMETACARPAL STABILIZERS/THUMB POSTS
- Thumb orthosis that stabilizes the first CMC and MCP joints in neutral position to protect the thumb form inadvertent motion.

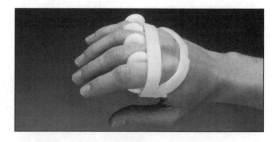

FIGURE 6–21. Ulnar Deviation Correction Splint. Photo courtesy of North Coast Medical, Inc., Morgan Hill, CA.

Thumb-web space stabilizers/thenar web spacers/c-bar splint (Figure 6–22)

- FO that consists of a rigid C-shaped splint held firmly in the thumb and index finger web space.
- Function: increases or maintains the thenar space and prevents web-space contractures
- Uses: Burns, postsurgical revision of scar, web-space contractures

Wrist-hand-finger stabilizers

Resting hand splints:

- Static wrist-hand finger orthosis (WHFOs) used to immobilize the wrist, fingers, and thumb

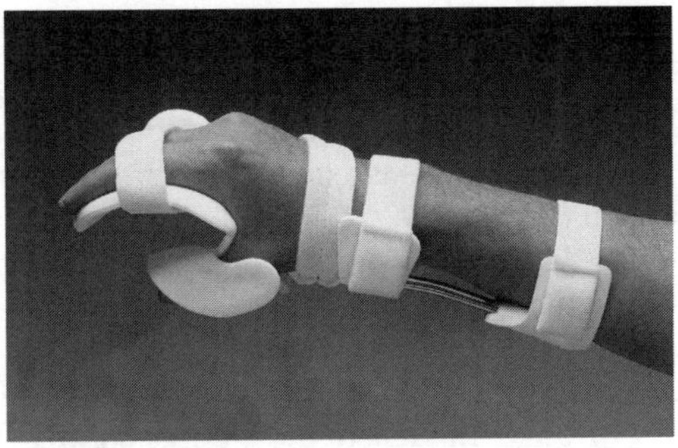

FIGURE 6–22. C Bar Splint (Thenar Web Spacer). Photo courtesy of North Coast Medical, Inc., Morgan Hill, CA.

- Usually applied to the volar surface (can be dorsally applied or circumferential)
- Extend from the fingertips to two-thirds of the distal forearm
- Hand usually placed with wrist in neutral to slight extension and the digits in an intrinsic plus position (MCPs flexed 70–90°, IPs in full extension, thumb CMC in palmar abd and thumb MCP/IP in full extension
- Immobilization in this position preferred because metacarpophalangeal joint and Interphalangeal collateral ligaments are kept stretched, minimizing future joint capsule contractures
- In addition, it provides functional thumb position for opposition and three-jaw chuck pinch.

Wrist-hand stabilizers

Volar wrist-hand stabilizers/wrist cock-up splint

- Wrist-hand orthosis (WHO) extending from distal two-thirds inch of forearm to about one-quarter proximal to the distal palmar crease to allow full metacarpophalangeal flexion while maintaining the functional position of the wrist and hand
- Uses include resting wrist and hand in acute arthritis (RA), wrist sprain/contusion, flexor/extensor tendinitis, carpal tunnel syndrome, postsurgical wrist extensor tendon repair, wrist fusion, and skin grafting, contractures prevention, reduce pain, reduce spasticity, prevent ulnar/radial deviation wrist/hand (e.g., RA)

Dorsal wrist-hand stabilizers

- WHO are used to provide the same functions of the volar WHO as well as greater stabilization because of rigid dorsal hand section
- More difficult to fabricate and fit than the volar WHO

DYNAMIC (FUNCTIONAL) ORTHOSES: UPPER LIMB

Elbow orthoses—assist in flexion or extension

- Dynamic elbow splints, static progressive elbow splints, turnbuckle elbow splints—gently elongate the soft tissues over a long period to attempt to reverse joint malalignment (contractures, burns, and late phase of fracture). They are not used in spastic muscles as they may further increase tone.
  a. **Dorsal elbow-extension mobilization orthosis**—extend the elbow as well as provide mediolateral elbow stability and rotational forearm stability
  b. **Dorsal elbow-flexion mobilization orthosis**—flex the elbow and provide mediolateral stability and rotational forearm stability

Forearm orthoses

Forearm mobilization (corrective) orthosis—dynamic supination/pronation splints
Used to increase supination or pronation in forearm rotational contracture, or to increase passive or active-assisted ROM in upper trunk brachial plexus lesions, or Erb's palsy, and spinal cord injury

- 📖 **Balanced forearm orthosis (BFO)** (Figure 6–23)

  • Shoulder-elbow-wrist-hand orthosis (SEWHO) that consists of a forearm trough (attached by a hinge joint to a ball-bearing swivel mechanism) and a mount (which can be mounted on the WC, on a table or working surface, or onto the body jacket)

  • Helps support the forearm and arm against gravity and allows patients with weak shoulder and elbow muscles to move the arm horizontally and flex the elbow to bring the hand to the mouth (e.g., patients with spinal cord injury, Guillain-Barré Syndrome, polio, muscular dystrophy, and brachial plexus injury)

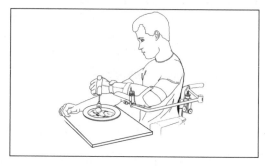

FIGURE 6–23. Balanced Forearm Orthosis.

Requirements
- Some residual muscle strength (MMT at least poor or grade 2) and coordination of elbow flexion (can be used for C5 quad)
- Adequate trunk stability and balance
- Adequate endurance in a sitting position
- Preserved ROM of the shoulder and elbow joints

Other uses: they also may be used in spastic patients to allow them to self-feed by dampening muscle tone through a friction device

Wrist Orthoses

1. Wrist control orthosis
Promotes slight extension of the wrist or prevent wrist flexion, thus assisting weak grasp (via tenodesis effect)
a. Volar wrist-flexion control orthosis (cock-up splints)
   - Wrist-hand orthoses (WHOs) in which the palmar section is extended (usually 20°. They are used to tighten finger flexors (via tenodesis effect) and prevent wrist flexion contracture in patients with radial neuropathy.
b. Wire wrist-extension assist orthosis (Oppenheimer splint)
   - Prefabricated from spring steel wire and padded steel bands to assist wrist extension by tensing the steel wire, thus aiding finger flexion through tenodesis effect

📖 **Wrist-driven prehension orthosis (tenodesis orthosis, flexor hinge splint) (Figure 6–24)**

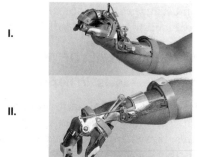

FIGURE 6–24. Wrist driven prehension orthosis. I. Wrist extension: three jaw chuck II. Wrist flexion: release

Used in C6 complete tetraplegia (in which no muscles to flex or extend fingers remain innervated but wrist extension, through the extensor carpi radialis muscle, is intact) to provide prehension trough tenodesis action and maintain flexibility of the hand, wrist, and elbow.
- Wrist extensors should be 3+ or better to use body-powered tenodesis
- May interfere with manual WC propulsion.
- Rarely accepted by C7 and C8 tetraplegics who prefer to use their residual motor power or utensil holders.

RIC tenodesis splint (Figure 6–25)
- 📖 Orthosis made of low-temperature thermoplastics in three separate pieces (wristlet, short opponens, and dorsal plate over index and middle finger)
- Easily and quickly fabricated; made as a training and evaluation splint for patients; light weight.
- Uses a cord/string running from the wrist piece, across the palm and up between the index and ring fingers. The string is lax when the wrist is flexed and tightens with wrist extension, bringing the fingers close to the immobilized thumb, accomplishing three-jaw chuck prehension.

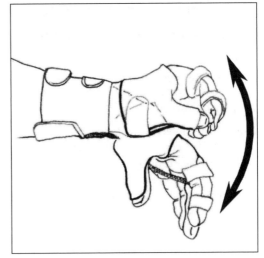

FIGURE 6–25. Rehabilitation Institute of Chicago Tenodesis Splint.

Finger Orthoses

Thumb mobilization orthoses
a. Thumb extension-mobilization orthosis—dynamic thumb IP extension splints. Use: thumb IP flexion contracture.
b. Thumb flexion-mobilization orthosis—dynamic IP flexion splints
   Use: Thumb IP flexion contractures.
c. Thumb abduction-mobilization orthosis—dynamic thumb abduction splint.
   Use: Thumb-adduction contracture.

2. Finger mobilization orthosis
a. *Interphalangeal extension-mobilization orthoses*—passively extend the PIP joints
   - **Uses**: Finger IP flexion contracture, Boutonnière deformity, and postsurgical release of Dupuytren's contracture
   - *Examples*: Dynamic IP extension splints, reverse finger knuckle benders, Capener splints, safety-pin splints, spring coil assist, eggshell finger extension casts, buddy splints
b. *Interphalangeal flexion mobilization orthoses*—passively flex PIP joints
   - *Use:* Finger IP extension contracture
   - *Examples:* Dynamic IP flexion splints, finger-knuckle benders, fingernail book orthoses, buddy splints

Metacarpophalangeal (MCP) mobilization orthoses
a. MCP- extension mobilization orthoses—
   - *Uses:* extend MCP joints in MCP-flexion contractures, burns, and post ORIF of metacarpal fracture, patients with weak finger extension (e.g., radial nerve lesion and brachial plexus lesion).
   - *Examples:* Reverse MCP knuckle benders, dynamic MCP extension splints with dorsal outrigger, MCP extension assists; radial nerve splints

b. MCP-flexion mobilization orthoses
- *Uses:* used to flex MCP joints in MCP collateral ligament contractures, extensor tendon shortening, median/ulnar lesion, claw hand, postcapsulotomy, post ORIF of metacarpal fracture.
- *Examples:* MCP knuckle benders, dynamic MCP flexion splints with volar outrigger and fingernail hooks, MCP flexion assists

TONE-REDUCING ORTHOSIS (FIGURE 6–26)

Theoretical basis for tone-reducing orthosis

- Inhibition of reflexes
- Pressure over muscle insertions
- Active and static prolonged stretch
- Orthokinetics

Inhibition of reflexes
- A reflex consists of a motor act that is elicited by some specific sensory input
- Primitive reflexes appear at birth and become integrated once more complicated movements emerge
- When the CNS is damaged, primitive reflexes reemerge and again dominate motor activity

Examples:
Toe grasp (plantar grasp) reflex
- Triggered: pressure over ball of foot
- Response: marked increased tone in toe flexion and ankle plantar flexion (PF)
- AFO design reportedly reduces stimulus pressure
- Inversion and eversion reflexes
  - Inversion triggered: pressure to medial border of foot over first metatarsal head
  - Eversion triggered: pressure to lateral border of foot over fifth metatarsal head
  - AFO design reduces abnormal tone by stimulating antagonist reflex

Pressure over muscle insertion
- Farber reported in 1974 that continuous firm pressure at point of insertion reduces tone
- AFO design: pressure on either side of tendo-calcaneus and insertion gastroc-soleus muscle group

Active and static prolonged stretch
- Decrease reflex tone by providing mechanical stabilization of the joint and altering properties of the muscle spindle
- AFO designs that provide total ankle-foot contact (Figure 6–27)

Orthokinetics
- Originally developed in 1927 by Julius Fuchs, an orthopedic surgeon
- Focuses on physical effects to materials placed over muscle bellies
- Passive field materials (those that are cool, rigid, and smooth) produce inhibitory effect
- Active field materials (those, warm, expansive, and textured) produce facilitatory effect
- AFO design
  - Active field stimulation (e.g., foam) over anterior tibialis to encourage dorsiflexion
  - Passive field inhibition over gastrocnemius to reduce spastic plantar flexion
  - Dual orthokinetic concepts interrelated and applied simultaneously

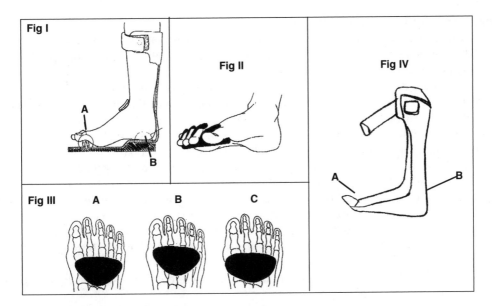

FIGURE 6–26. Tone Reducing Orthoses: **Fig I:** Side view of tone inhibitory orthosis. **A:** Spastic inhibitory bar. **B:** Internal heel. **Fig II:** The neurophysiological AFO is designed to provide total surface contact. The toe separators are made of Plastazote® and facilitate toe extension. **Fig III:** Strategies using metatarsal pad placement. **A.** Proximal to metatarsal heads. **B.** Under metatarsal heads. **C.** Medial extension to induce inversion reflex. **Fig IV:** Medial view of orthosis design to incorporate tone inhibitory characteristics of plaster casting. **A.** Toe hyperextension plate. **B.** Tendon pressure over gastroc-soleus insertion

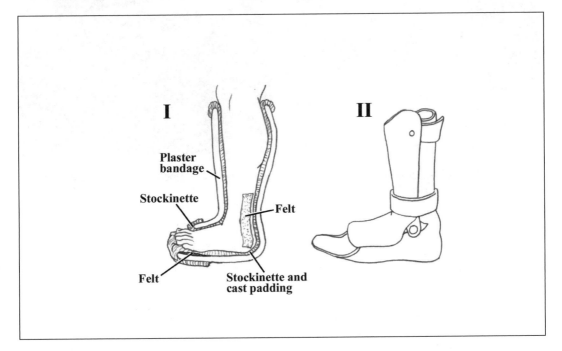

FIGURE 6–27. Fig I: Cross-section of inhibitory cast that provided heel and forefoot alignment on neutral as well as total surface contact. Fig II: Bi-valved Chattanooga articulating orthosis provides uniform contact of inhibitory cast as well as adjustable ankle joint to maintain consistent static force.

Upper Extremity Tone-Reduction Orthoses (Figure 6–28)

- They can be either hand-based wrist-hand orthoses (e.g., hand-cone splints) or forearm-based wrist-hand-finger orthoses (e.g., antispasticity ball splints and Snook splints).
- They can be volar based, dorsal based, or circumferential
- Typically worn two hours on and two hours off throughout the day
- Forearm based splints usually are more effective because of the extension positioning of the extrinsic finger flexors
- Rationales of efficacy of tone-reduction orthoses include:
  - Reflex-inhibiting positioning—NDT technique approach (Bobath)
  - Firm pressure into volar surface (palm)—Rood (sensorimotor) approach
  - Dorsal-based splints (eg, Snook): facilitation of muscle contraction by direct contact—it is theorized that stimulation of extensor surface might produce extensor muscle contraction and balance muscle tone and/or avoid increase flexor tone.
- Functions: flexor tone reduction, prevent skin breakdown/maceration of palm by fingernails, increase passive range of motion via low-load, prolonged stretch (serial static splinting)
- Indications: spasticity—upper motor neuron lesions (cerebral vascular accident, HI, multiple sclerosis, cerebral palsey)

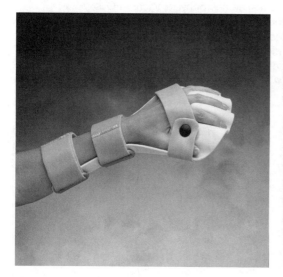 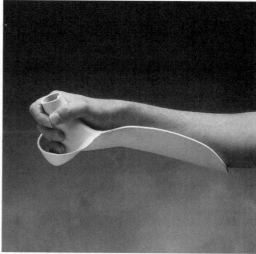

FIGURE 6–28. **A.** Anti-spasticity "Ball" Splint. **B.** Hand Cone Splint. Photo courtesy of North Coast Medical, Inc., Morgan Hill, CA.

■
SPINAL ORTHOSES

CERVICAL ORTHOSES (CO)/CERVICO-THORACIC ORTHOSES (CTO)

Soft cervical collar: (Figure 6–29a)

- Made of polyethylene foam or sponge rubber
    1. Provides no significant control of motion of the cervical spine but does provides a kinesthetic reminder (through sensory feedback) to limit motion
    2. Retains body heat (which may help reduce muscle spasm and aid in healing of soft tissue injuries
    3. Provides comfort (may be due in part to 1 and 2)
    Uses: soft tissue injuries of the neck (i.e., whiplash injury)

Hard cervical collars

- Prefabricated orthoses that provide more restriction to cervical flexion, extension, rotation, and lateral bending than the soft collar.
    1. **Thomas collar**
    – Made of firm plastic with superior and inferior padding that wrap around the neck and is secured with Velcro.
    – Uses: soft tissue injuries
    2. **Philadelphia collar** (Figure 6–29b)
    – Provides total contact in the cervical spine and a mild degree of motion control
    – Made of Plastazote®, has rigid anterior and posterior Kydex® plastic reinforcements, and is secured by Velcro® closures
    – It encompasses the lower jaw and the occiput and extends to the proximal thorax
    – Indications: soft tissue injuries, and stable bony or ligamentous injuries. Also used when patients are weaned of more restrictive orthoses to limit sudden strain on the neck after prolonged immobilization.

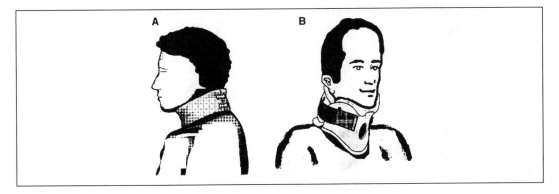

FIGURE 6–29. A: Soft cervical collar. **B:** Hard (Philadelphia) cervical collar.

3. **Miami–J collar, Newport, Malibu collars**—variants of the Philadelphia collar
- Provide better control
- More expensive

📖 Sterno-occipital mandibular immobilizer (SOMI) (Figure 6–30):

- Cervicothoracic orthosis with chest piece connected by uprights (going from anterior to posterior) to occipital plate. Therefore, it can easily be applied to a supine patient.
- Has removable mandibular piece so patient can eat, wash, or shave while lying supine
- Indications: cervical arthritis, postsurgical fusions, and stable cervical fractures

Poster-type cervicothoracic orthoses

- Two- or four-poster orthoses (Figure 6–31a,b)
- Provides cervical spine control through mandibular and occipital components connected to sternal and thoracic components by two or four (sometimes three) posters
- Provides good control of flex/extension; lateral bending and rotation are not well controlled.

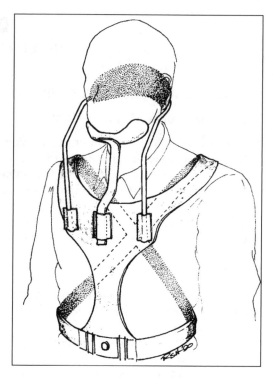

FIGURE 6–30. Sterno-occipital mandibular immobilization orthosis (SOMI). (From Braddom R.L. Physical Medicine and Rehabilitation. Philadelphia: W. B. Saunders; 1996. Reproduced with permission.)

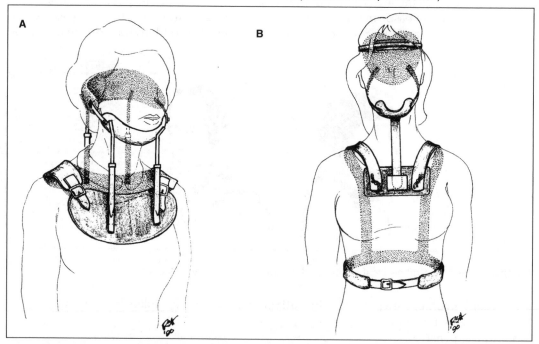

FIGURE 6–31. A: Four poster collar. **B:** Two poster orthosis (From Braddom R.L. Physical Medicine and Rehabilitation. Philadelphia: W. B. Saunders; 1996. Reproduced with permission.)

- Can hold head in extension or flexion by adjusting the length of anterior or posterior posters
- Cooler than cervical collars but bulkier
- Indications: mid or low (with extension) stable cervical fractures and arthritis

Yale cervico-thoracic orthosis

- Is similar to an extended Philadelphia collar reinforced with rigid plastic struts extending down onto the anterior and posterior thorax with strapping beneath the axilla
- The occipital piece can extend higher than the original Philadelphia collar

🕮 Minerva cervico-thoracic orthosis / Thermoplastic Minerva body jacket (TMBJ) (Figure 6–32)

- The Minerva CTO encloses the entire posterior skull, includes a band around the forehead, and extends downward to the inferior costal margin
- Forehead band provides good control of all cervical motions
- Advantages: lighter weight than the halo vest; no pins (no "invasive" supports), which carry risks of infection and slippage (as compared to the halo vest)
- Disadvantages: less restriction of motion compared to halo vest
- 🕮 Indications: Management of unstable cervical spine (although halo vest use is usually preferred for maximum motion control)
    - May be the preferred orthosis (over halo) in the management. of cervical spine instability in preschool age children due to ↑ comfort, ↓ weight, and because it allows early mobilization of the patient for rehabilitation, in addition to providing the necessary stability

Halo vest CTO (Figure 6–33)

- 🕮 Provides the best control of motion (all planes) in the cervical spine of all the cervical/cervico-thoracic orthoses
- Consists of a rigid halo secured to the skull with four external fixation pins
- The halo supports four posters attached to the anterior and posterior part of the vest (thoracic component)

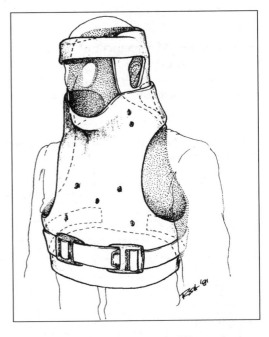

FIGURE 6–32. Thermoplastic Minerva body jacket. (From Braddom R.L. Physical Medicine and Rehabilitation. Philadelphia: W. B. Saunders; 1996. Reproduced with permission.)

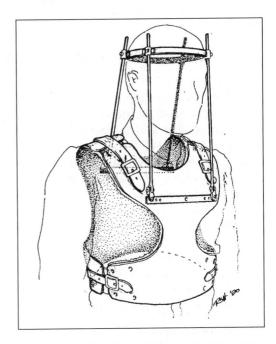

FIGURE 6–33. Halo Vest (From Braddom R.L. Physical Medicine and Rehabilitation. Philadelphia: W. B. Saunders; 1996. Reproduced with permission.)

- Indications: Management of unstable fractures of the cervical spine (especially high cervical fractures)
- Complications: pin-loosening, slippage, pin-site infection, pressure ulcers
  - Less commonly: reduced vital capacity, neck pain, brain abscess, and psychological trauma

TABLE 6–15. Normal Cervical Motion from Occiput to First Thoracic Vertebra and the Effect of Cervical Orthoses

	Mean of Normal Motion (%)		
	Flexion/Extension	**Lateral Bending**	**Rotation**
Normal*	100.0	100.0	100.0
Soft collar*	74.2	92.3	82.6
Philadelphia collar*	28.9	66.4	43.7
SOMI brace*	27.7	65.6	33.6
Four-poster brace*	20.6	45.9	27.1
Yale cervicothoracic brace*	12.8	50.5	18.2
Halo device*	4.0	4.0	1.0
Halo device†	11.7	8.4	2.4
Minerva body jacket‡	14.0	15.5	0

* Johnson RM, Hart DL, Simmons EF, et al: Cervical orthoses: a study comparing their effectiveness in restricting cervical motion in normal subjects. *J Bone Joint Surg* (AM) 1977; 59:332.
† Lysell E: Motion in the cervical spine, thesis. *Acta Orthop Scand Suppl* 1969; 123.
‡Maiman D, Millington P, Novak S, et al. The effects of the thermoplastic Minerva body jacket on the cervical spine motion. *Neurology* 1989; 25:363–68.
Braddom, 1996

THORACOLUMBOSACRAL ORTHOSES (TLSO)/LUMBOSACRAL ORTHOSES (LSO)

- 📖 In general, TLSOs extend from the sacrum to above the inferior angle of the scapulae and are used to support and stabilize the trunk (e.g., truncal paralysis, postspinal fusion, and postscoliotic surgery) and to prevent progression of moderate scoliosis (20–45°) until patient reaches skeletal maturity
- Except for the TLS flexion-control orthoses, TLSOs can increase intra-abdominal pressure (which in turn ↓ load on spine/intervertebral discs by transmission of the load to the surrounding soft tissues)
- They also cause an increase in O_2 consumption/energy expenditure
- During ambulation, with axial rotation between the pelvis and the shoulders, there may be increased motion at the unrestrained segments cephalad (rostral) and caudal to the orthosis, in addition to increased energy consumption of ambulation

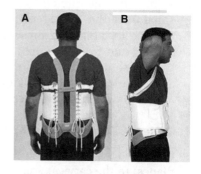

FIGURE 6–34. Taylor Brace: TLSO flexion-extension control orthosis. **A:** posterior view. **B:** lateral view.

Taylor brace (Figure 6–34)
- Flexion/extension control TLSO that consists of two posterior paraspinal bars attached inferiorly to a pelvic band; an interscapular band stabilizes the paraspinal bars and serves as attachment for the axillary straps.

- The orthosis also includes a corset or anterior, full-front abdominal support, which increases intracavitary pressure.

Knight-Taylor brace (Figure 6–35)

- Consists of a Taylor style TLSO with lateral bands and a thoracic band to restrict lateral bending.
- Indications: can be used for postsurgical or nonsurgical management of stable thoracic or lumbar fracture.

TLS spine flexion-control orthoses

📖 Jewett brace (Figure 6–36)
- Flexion control TLSO consisting of a sternal pad, suprapubic pad, and anterolateral pads connected by oblique lateral uprights counteracted by a dorsolumbar pad as well.
- The suprapubic band may be substituted by a boomerang band, which applies force on the iliac crests (used in females to avoid direct pressure on the bladder).

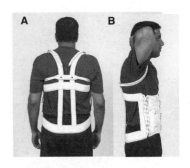

FIGURE 6–35. Knight Taylor Brace. **A:** posterior view. **B:** lateral view.

Indications:

1. 📖 Used to permit the upright position, while preventing flexion after compression fracture of the thoracolumbar spine
   - Use in the treatment of compression fractures in osteoporotic elderly patients is controversial because it can place excessive hyperextension forces on the lower lumbar vertebrae, which can induce posterior element fractures or exacerbate a degenerative arthritis condition.
2. Thoracolumbar Scheuermann's disease; used (although with limited efficacy) in thoracic osteoporotic kyphosis
   - Cruciform anterior spinal hyperextension (CASH) TLSO (Figure 6–37)
   - It has anteriorly, a cross-shaped vertical and horizontal metal uprights. It has sternal, pubic, posterior, and anterolateral pads. The vertical upright joins the sternal and pubic pad. The horizontal uprights connect the posterior thoracolumbar pad and the anterolateral pads.
   - Indications: similar to Jewett

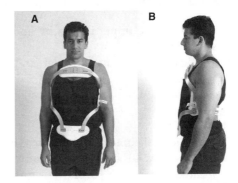

FIGURE 6–36. Jewett Hyperextension Orthosis. **A:** posterior view. **B:** lateral view

Milwaukee brace: (Figure 6–38)

- 📖 Cervico-thoracic-lumbo-sacral orthosis (CTLSO) used for *scoliosis*; consists of a rigid plastic pelvic girdle connected to a

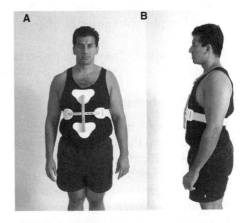

FIGURE 6–37. CASH (Cruciform Anterior Spinal Hyperextension Orthosis) TLSO. **A:** anterior view. **B:** lateral view.

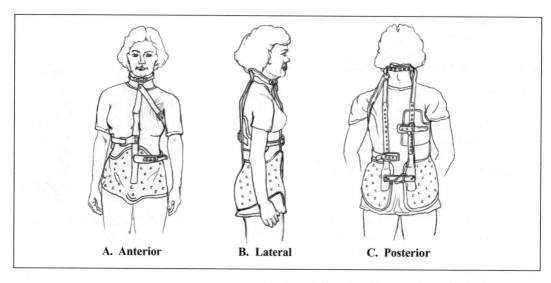

FIGURE 6–38. Milwaukee-style CTLSO. **A:** Anterior view. **B:** Lateral view. **C:** Posterior view.

neck ring over the upper thorax by one anterior, broad aluminum bar and two posterior paraspinal bars.

- The cervical ring has mandibular and occipital bars, which rest 20–30mm inferior to occiput and mandible
- Pads strapped to the bars apply a transverse load to the ribs and spine to correct scoliotic curvatures
- Indications:
  - Idiopathic or flexible congenital scoliosis
    - Curves 25 to 40° have traditionally been treated with this orthosis if the curve apex is located superior to T8, shows signs of progression, and growth remains
  - Thoracic Scheuermann's disease kyphosis

Corsets/flexible spinal orthoses

- Made of fabric/canvas with pouches for vertical stays
- A number of different types of corsets are available including LS, TLS, TL, sacroiliac, lumbar
- They are the most frequently prescribed orthotic for low back pain
- The efficacy of corsets remains controversial

Lumbar and lumbosacral corsets

- The most commonly prescribed LS support is the LS corset
- They surround the torso and hips, and they border the xiphoid or lower ribs, pubic symphysis, inferior angle of the scapula, and gluteal fold
- Indications: low back pain, muscle strain
- Special designs used for: pregnancy, abdominal ptosis, pendulous abdomen
- Pros: kinesthetic reminder, support abdomen, reduce load on LS spine, reduce excessive lumbar lordosis, decrease lateral bending (29%)
- Cons: may result in weakening of the muscles that support the trunk

RECOMMENDED READING

Berger N, Fishman S. (eds). *Lower Limb Prosthetics*. New York University Health Sciences Bookstore: New York, Prosthetics-Orthotics Publications, 1997.

Braddom, Randall L. *Physical Medicine and Rehabilitation*. Philadelphia: W.B. Saunders, 1996; 334–336, 1194–1196.

DeLisa JA, Gans BA. *Rehabilitation Medicine: Principles and Practice*, 3rd ed. Philadelphia: Lippincott-Raven, 1998; 167–187, 635–696.

DeLisa JA. *Gait Analysis in the Science of Rehabilitation. Rehabilitation Research and Development Service*. Department of Veterans Affairs–Veterans Health Administration. Monograph 002, 1998.

Downey JA, Myers SJ, Gonzalez EG, Lieberman JS. *The Physiological basis of Rehabilitation Medicine*. Boston: Butterworth-Heinemann, 1994.

Kottke FJ, Lehmann JF, eds. *Krusen's Handbook of PM & R*, 4th ed. Philadelphia: W. B. Saunders; 1990, 967–975.

O'Young B. Young MA, Stiens SA. *Physical Medicine and Rehibilitation Secrets*. Philadelphia: Hanley & Belfus, 1997.

New York University Medical Center Post-Graduate Medical School. *Prosthetics and Orthotics: Upper Limb Prosthetics*. New York: New York University Medical Center, 1986.

Reford JB (ed). *Orthotics: Clinical Practice and Rehabilitation Technology*. New York; Churchill Livingstone, 1995.

REFERENCES

Cerny, D, Waters R, Hislop H, Perry J. Walking and wheelchair energetics in persons with paraplegia. *Phys Ther* 1980, 60(9): 1133–1139.

Gonzalez EG, Corcoran PJ, Reyes RL. Energy expenditure in below-knee amputees: correlation with stump length. *Arch Phys Med Rehabil* 1974, 55:111–119.

Huang CT, Jackson JR, Moore NB, Fine PR, Kuhlemeier KV, Traugh GH, Saunders PT. Amputation: energy cost of ambulation. *Arch Phys Med Rehabil*. 1979; 60(1): 18–24.

Kay HW, Newman JD. Relative medicine of new amputations: Statistical comparisons of 6,000 new amputees. *Orthot Prosthet*. 1975; 29: 3–16.

Saunders JB. Dec M, Inman, UT, and Eberhart, HD The major determinants of normal and pathological gait. *J Bone Joint Surg*. 1953; 35A: 543–58.

Seymour R. *Prosthetics and Orthotics, Lower Limb and Spinal*. Philadelphia: Lippincott, Williams & Wilkins; 2002.

Tan JC. *Practical Manual of Physical Medicine and Rehabilitation: Diagnostics, Therapeutics, and Basic Problems*. St. Louis: Mosby, 1998.

Traugh GH, Corcoran PJ, Reyes RL. Energy expenditure of ambulation in patients with above-knee amputations. *Arch Phys Med Rehabil* 1975; 56: 67–71.

7

SPINAL CORD INJURIES

Steven Kirshblum, M.D., Priscila Gonzalez, M.D.,
Sara Cuccurullo, M.D., and Lisa Luciano, D.O.

■

EPIDEMIOLOGY OF SPINAL CORD INJURY (SCI)

In USA: 30–60 new injuries per million pop. /year
📖 **Incidence (new cases):** 10,000 new cases of SCI/year
📖 **Prevalence (total # of existing cases):** 200,000–250,000 cases
Gender: 82% male vs. 18% female
Age: 📖 Average age at injury: 31.7 years of age
   📖 Patients injured after 1990 had an average age at time of injury of 34.8 years
   56% of SCIs occur among persons in the 16–30 year age group
   Children 15 years of age or younger account for only 4.5% of SCI cases
   Persons older than 60 years of age account for 10% of SCI cases
   Falls are the most common cause of SCI in the elderly
   Motor vehicle accidents (MVAs) are the second most common cause of SCIs in the elderly
Causes: MVAs: 44%
   Violence (most are gunshot): 24%
   Falls: 22%
   Sports (most are diving): 8%
   Other: 2%
Time of Injury: Season: Summer (highest incidence in July)
   Day: Weekends (usually Saturday)
   Time: Night
Characteristics of Injury: Tetraplegia: C5 is most common level of injury
   Paraplegia: T12 is most common level of injury
Type of injury: Tetraplegia: 51.9%
   Paraplegia: 46.27%
   Incomplete tetraplegia: 29.6%
   Complete paraplegia: 28.1%
   Incomplete paraplegia: 21.5%
   Complete tetraplegia: 18.5%
   Complete or substantial recovery by time of discharge: 0.7%
   Persons for whom this information is not available: 0.7%

Demographics:

There is a close association between risk of SCI and a number of indications of social class, all of which have profound implications for rehabilitation:

- SCI patients have fewer years of education than their uninjured counterparts
- SCI patients are more likely to be unemployed than non-SCI pts.
- SCI patients are more likely to be single (i.e. never married, separated, divorced)

 Note: Postinjury marriages (injured and then married) survive better than preinjury marriages (injured after marriage)

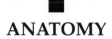

ANATOMY

The vertebral column (Figure 7–1) consists of:

7	cervical
12	thoracic
5	lumbar
5	sacral
4	coccyx

Spinal Cord:

Located in upper two-thirds of the vertebral column

The terminal portion of the cord is the conus medullaris, which becomes cauda equina (horse's tail) at approximately the L2 vertebrae

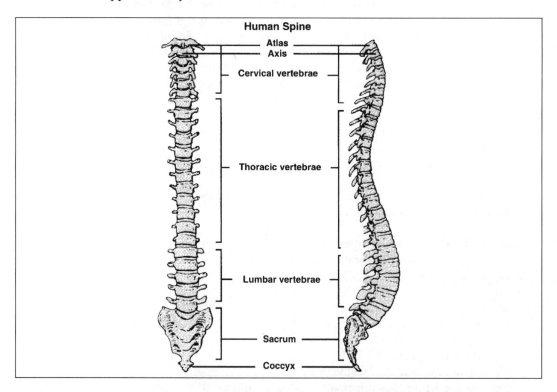

FIGURE 7–1. Human Vertebral Column. (From Nesathurai S. The Rehabilitation of People With Spinal Cord Injury: A House Officer's Guide. © Boston Medical Center for the New England Regional Spinal Cord Injury Center. Boston, MA: Arbuckle Academic Publishers, with permission).

The spinal cord has an inner core of gray matter, surrounded by white matter. The white matter consists of nerve fibers, neuroglia, and blood vessels. The nerve fibers form spinal tracts, which are divided into ascending, descending, and intersegmental tracts. The location and function of various tracts are shown below (Figure 7–2).

LONG TRACTS IN THE SPINAL CORD			
Key	Tract	Location	Function
▨	Fasciculus gracile: dorsal columns (posterior)	Medial dorsal column	Proprioception from the leg Light touch Vibration
Same as above	Fasciculus cuneate: dorsal columns (posterior)	Lateral dorsal column	Proprioception from the arm Light touch Vibration
▨	Spinocerebellar	Superficial lateral column	Muscular position and tone, unconscious proprioception
▨	Lateral spinothalamic	Ventrolateral column	Pain and thermal sensation
	Ventral spinothalamic	Ventral column	Tactile sensation of crude touch and pressure
▨	Lateral corticospinal tract (pyramidal)	Deep lateral column	Motor: Medial (cervical)-Lateral (sacral) C ⟶ S (motor neuron distribution)
▨	Anterior corticospinal tract	Medial ventral column	Motor: Neck and trunk movements

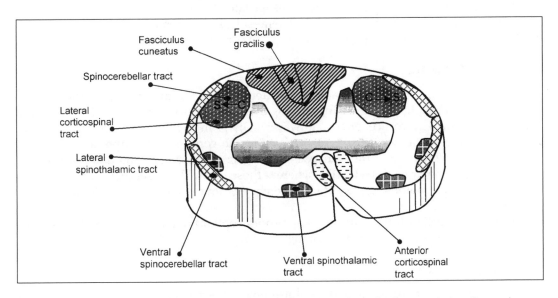

FIGURE 7–2. Transverse section of the spinal cord (use key above for long tracts location and function).

MAJOR ASCENDING AND DESCENDING PATHWAYS IN THE SPINAL CORD (A SCHEMATIC VIEW)

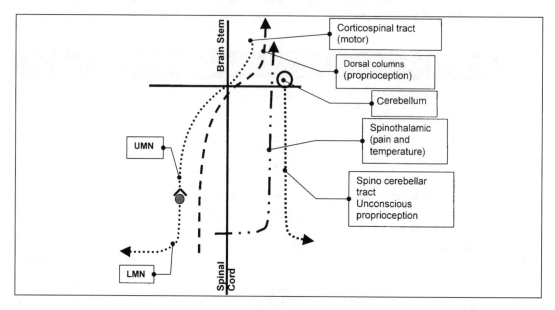

FIGURE 7–3. A Schematic View: The major long tracts in the spinal cord (ascending and descending arrows depict direction).

Note where tracts cross in relation to brain stem (Figure 7–3)
- Corticospinal tract crosses at brain stem to contralateral side, then descends
- Spinocerebellar tract does not cross; remains ipsilateral as it descends
- Spinothalamic tract crosses low to contralateral side, then ascends
- Dorsal columns ascends, crosses at brain stem to contralateral side

Descending Pathways

- The corticospinal tract (motor pathways) extends from the motor area of the cerebral cortex down through the brainstem, crossing over at the junction between the spinal cord and brainstem. The corticospinal pathway synapses in the anterior horn (motor grey matter) of the spinal cord just prior to leaving the cord. This is important for motor neurons above the level of this synapse [connecting anterior horn and anterior horn are termed upper motor neurons (UMN) whereas those below this level (peripheral neurons) are termed lower motor neurons (LMN)]. Cerebral lesions result in contralateral defects in general.
- The spinocerebellar tract (unconscious proprioception) remains ipsilateral. Cerebral lesions produce ipsilateral malfunctioning.

Ascending Pathways

- Spinothalamic tract (pain and temperature) enters the spinal cord, crosses over to the opposite half of the cord almost immediately (actually within 1–2 spinal cord vertebral segments), ascends to the thalamus on the opposite side, and then moves on the cerebral cortex. A lesion of the spinothalamic tract will result in loss of pain-temperature sensation contralaterally below the level of the lesion.

- Dorsal columns (proprioception vibration) initially remains on the same side of the spinal cord that it enters, crossing over at the junction between the spinal cord and brainstem. The synaptic areas just prior to this crossing are nucleus cuneatus and nucleus gracilis. Their corresponding spinal cord pathways are termed fasciculus gracilis and fasciculus cuneatus. Fasciculus gracilis and fasciculus cuneatus are collectively termed posterior (dorsal) columns. A lesion of the posterior columns results in the loss of proprioception and vibration ipsilaterally below the level of the lesion.

Blood Supply of the Spinal Cord (Figure 7–4)

- Posterior Spinal Arteries arise directly or indirectly from the vertebral arteries, run inferiorly along the sides of the spinal cord, and provide blood to the posterior third of the spinal cord
- Anterior Spinal Arteries arise from the vertebral arteries, uniting to form a single artery, which runs within the anterior median fissure. They supply blood flow to the anterior two-thirds of the spinal cord
- Radicular Arteries reinforce the posterior and anterior spinal arteries. These are branches of local arteries (deep cervical, intercostal, and lumbar arteries). They enter the vertebral canal through the intervertebral foramina
- The artery of Adamkiewicz or the arteria radicularis magna is the name given to the lumbar radicular artery. It is larger and arises from an intersegmental branch of the descending aorta in the lower thoracic or upper lumbar vertebral levels (between T10 and L3) and anastomoses with the anterior spinal artery in the lower thoracic region. The lower thoracic region is referred to as the watershed area. It is the major source of blood to the lower anterior two-thirds of the spinal cord
- The Veins of the Spinal Cord drain mainly into the internal venous plexus

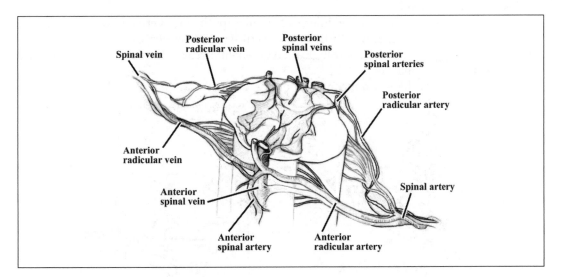

FIGURE 7–4. Arterial and venous supply to the spinal cord. (transverse section).

■
SPINAL PATHOLOGY

TYPES OF CERVICAL SPINAL CORD INJURY: PATHOLOGY

Compression Fractures—slight flexion of the neck with axial loading (Figure 7–5)
(Bohlmann, 1979)

- C5 is the most common compression fracture of the cervical spine
- Force ruptures the plates of the vertebra, and shatters the body. Wedge shaped appearing vertebra on X-ray.
- May involve injury to the nerve root and/or cord itself
- Fragments may project into spinal canal
- Stable ligaments remain intact

Flexion-Rotation Injuries

Unilateral facet joint dislocations (Figure 7–6)
- Vertebral body < 50% displaced on X-ray
- Unstable (if the posterior ligament is disrupted)
- Narrowing of the spinal canal and neural foramen
- C5–C6 most common level

FIGURE 7–5. Cervical compression fracture.

- Also note that flexion and rotation injuries may disrupt the intervertebral disc, facet joints, and interspinous ligaments with little or no fracture of the vertebrae
- Approximately 75% have no neurological involvement because the narrowing is not sufficient to affect the spinal cord
- If injury results, it is likely an incomplete injury

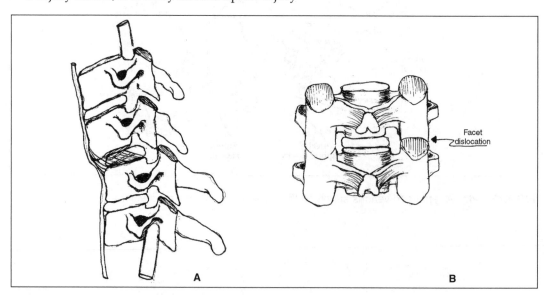

FIGURE 7–6. Unilateral facet joint dislocation. **A:** lateral view. Note: there is less than 50% anterior dislocation of the vertebral body. **B:** posterior view.

Flexion Injuries
Bilateral facet joint dislocations (Figure 7–7)

- Vertebral body > 50% displaced on X-ray
- Both facets dislocate
- Unstable; secondary to tearing of the ligaments
- Most common level is C5–C6 because of increased movement in this area
- More than 50% anterior dislocation of the vertebral body causes significant narrowing of the spinal canal
- Spinal cord is greatly compromised
- 85% suffer neurologic injuries
- Likely to be a complete injury

Hyperextension Injuries (Figure 7–8)

- Can be caused by acceleration-deceleration injuries such as MVA
- Soft tissue injury may not be seen in radiologic studies
- Stable; anterior longitudinal ligament is disrupted
- Spinal cord may be involved
- Can be seen in hyperextension of the C-spine and appear as Central Cord syndrome. This most commonly occurs in older persons with degenerative changes in the neck.
- Clinically: UE motor more involved than LE. Bowel, bladder, and sexual dysfunction occur to various degrees.
- C4–C5 is the most common level

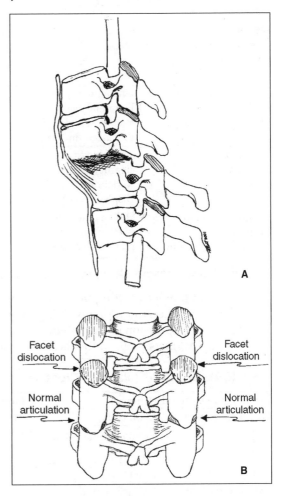

Facet dislocation

Facet dislocation

Normal articulation

Normal articulation

FIGURE 7–7. Bilateral facet joint dislocation. **A:** lateral view. Note: there is greater Than 50% anterior dislocation of the vertebral body. **B:** posterior view.

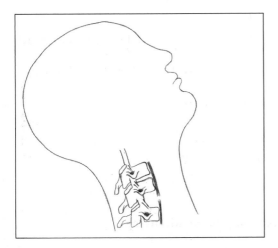

FIGURE 7–8. Cervical spine hyperextension injury.

TABLE 7-1. Spinal Cord and Pathology Associated with Mechanism of Injury

Types of Spinal Injury: Pathology			
Mechanism of Injury	Stability	Possible Resultant Injury	Most Common Level
Compression Axial loading (i.e., diving)	Stable Ligaments remain intact	Crush fracture w/ fragmentation of vertebral body and projection of bony spicules into canal	C5
Flexion Rotation Injury Unilateral dislocation	Unstable (if posterior ligament disrupted) Vertebral body <50% displaced on Xray	Spinal cord not severely compromised; likely to be incomplete injury	C5–C6
Flexion Bilateral dislocation	Unstable (if post ligament disrupted) Vertebral body <50% displaced on X-ray	Ant. dislocation of C-spine with compression of spinal cord; spinal cord greatly compromised; likely to be complete injury	C5–C6
Hyper Extension Injury Central Cord syndrome	Stable; Anterior longitudinal ligament may be disrupted	Hyperextension of C-spine clinically: UE weaker than LE; likely to be incomplete injury	C4 C5

📖 Spinal Compression 2° to metastatic disease

Majority of tumors affecting the SC are metastatic in origin
95% are extradural in origin involving the vertebral bodies
Results in compression of the anterior aspect of the spinal cord
70% of spinal mets occur in the thoracic spine

CERVICAL BRACING (also see Prosthetics & Orthotics Chapter)

Removable Cervical Orthoses:		Nonremovable Cervical Orthoses:
Least restrictive: ↓ Most restrictive:	Soft collar	Halo is the most restrictive cervical orthosis of all cervical orthoses.
	Philadelphia collar	
	SOMI brace	
	Four poster	
	Minerva brace	

📖 Cervical Bracing

The Minerva brace is the most restrictive removable brace, followed by the four poster, then SOMI.
Philly collar is less restrictive, and soft collar is the least restrictive of the listed braces.
Halo is the most restrictive, but not removable.
See P & O section for more in-depth discussion of spinal bracing.

COMPLETE vs. INCOMPLETE LESIONS

📖 Complete lesions are most commonly secondary to the following
1. Bilateral cervical facet dislocations
2. Thoracolumbar flexion-rotation injuries
3. Transcanal gunshot wounds

📖 Incomplete injuries are most commonly secondary to the following
1. Cervical spondylosis—falls
2. Unilateral facet joint dislocations
3. Noncanal penetrating gunshot/stab injuries

OTHER FRACTURES OF THE SPINE

Cervical Region:

Jefferson Fracture: (Figure 7–9)
- Burst fracture of the C1 ring
- Mechanism: axial loading causing fractures of anterior and posterior parts of the atlas
- If the patient survives, there are usually no neurologic findings with treatment

Hangman Fracture: (Figure 7–10)
- C2 burst fracture
- Body is separated from its posterior element, decompresses cord (No SCI)
- If the patient survives, there are only transient neurologic findings with appropriate Tx

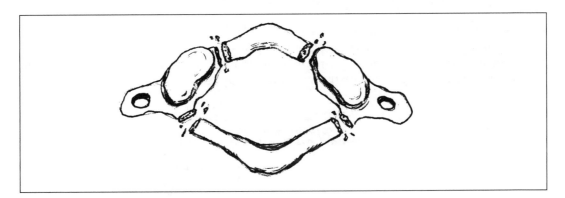

FIGURE 7–9.   Jefferson fracture (Superior view).

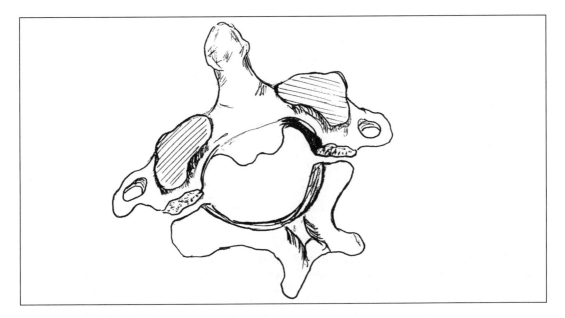

FIGURE 7–10.   Hangman fracture. (Superior posterior view).

Odontoid Fracture (Figure 7–11, 7–12)

- C2 odontoid is fractured off at its base
- Commonly results from trauma
- Patient usually survives
- Usually only transient neurologic signs with appropriate Tx

Thoraco Lumbar Region

📖 **Chance Fracture (Figure 7–13)**

- Most commonly seen in patients wearing lap seat belts
- Transverse fracture of lumbar spine through body and pedicles, posterior elements
- Chance fractures are seldom associated with neurologic compromise unless a significant amount of translation is noted on the lateral radiographs

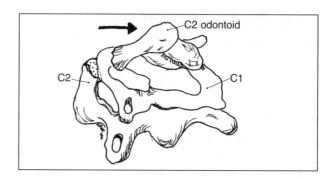

FIGURE 7–11. Odontoid fracture. Illustration by Heather Platt, 2001.

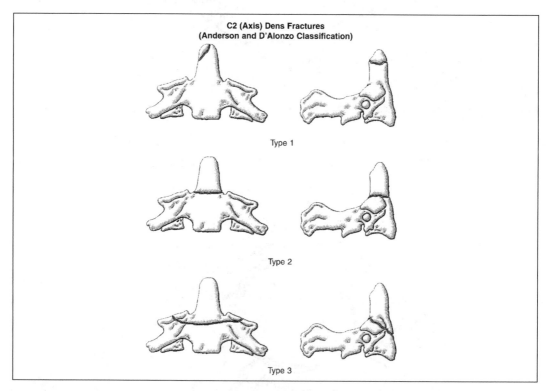

FIGURE 7–12. **Type 1:** Oblique fracture through upper part of the dens; treatment is with rigid cervical orthosis such as Philadelphia collar. **Type 2:** Fracture at the junction of the odontoid process and the vertebral body; if displacement is less than 5 mm and angulated less than 15 degrees, then halo is appropriate; otherwise operative treatment with C1 to C2 fusion or screw fixation. **Type 3:** Fracture extends down through vertebral body; treatment is with halo. (From Nesathurai S. The Rehabilitation of People With Spinal Cord Injury: A House Officer's Guide. © Boston Medical Center for the New England Regional Spinal Cord Injury Center. Boston, MA: Arbuckle Academic Publishers, with permission).

▢ Vertebral Body Compression Fracture (anterior wedge fracture) (Figure 7–14)

- Mechanism: most common injuries caused by axial compression with or without flexion: vertebrae body height is reduced—may cause thoracic kyphosis (Dowager hump)
- Spontaneous vertebral compression fractures are stable injuries—ligaments remain intact

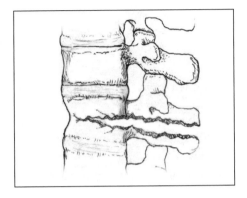

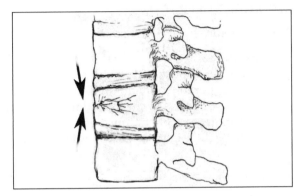

FIGURE 7–13. Chance Fracture.

FIGURE 7–14. Vertebral Body Compression Fracture.

SCIWORA – SPINAL CORD INJURY WITHOUT RADIOLOGIC ABNORMALITY

This condition is commonly seen in young children and older adults

Children

- **Mechanism of injury in children include**
  Traction in a breech delivery
  Violent hyperextension or flexion
- **Predisposing factors in children include**
  Large head-to-neck size ratio
  Elasticity of the fibrocartilaginous spine
  Horizontal orientation of the planes of the cervical facet joints

Older Adults

- **Mechanism of injury in the elderly includes**
  A fall forward and a blow on the head causing an acute central cord syndrome; the ligamentum flavum may bulge forward into the central canal and narrow the sagittal diameter as much as 50%
- Note: Delayed onset or paralysis may occur due to vascular mechanism or edema accumulation at the injury site, although this is uncommon
- Essential history in a person with head or neck pain includes identifying any neurological symptoms
- Flexion/Extension films should be done cautiously only after static neck films have been cleared by a radiologist and only if there are no neurologic symptoms or severe pain present
- Empiric use of a 24-hour cervical collar with repeat films at resolution of cervical spasm is warranted

■
CLASSIFICATION OF SCI

IMPORTANT DEFINITIONS

Types of Injuries

Tetraplegia
- Replaces quadriplegia
- Impairment or loss of motor and/or sensory function in the cervical segments of SC due to damage of neural elements within spinal canal
- Results in impairment of function in arms, trunk, legs, pelvic organs
- Does not include brachial plexus lesions or injury to peripheral nerves outside neural canal

Paraplegia
- Impairment or loss of motor and/or sensory function in thoracic, lumbar, or sacral segments of SC
- Trunk, legs, pelvic organs may be involved, arm function spared
- Refers to cauda equina and conus medullaris injuries, but not to lumbosacral plexus lesions or injury to peripheral nerves outside the neural canal

Other Definitions

Dermatome
Area of skin innervated by the sensory axons within each segmental nerve (root)

Myotome
Collection of muscle fibers innervated by the motor axons within each segmental nerve(root)

UPPER MOTOR NEURON INJURY vs. LOWER MOTOR NEURON INJURY

Upper Motor Neuron Injury	Lower Motor Neuron Injury
Supply: Begins in the prefrontal motor cortex, travels through the internal capsule and brainstem, and projects into the spinal cord	Supply: Begins with the anterior horn cells of the spinal cord and includes the peripheral nerves
Upper Motor Neuron Findings	**Lower Motor Neuron Findings**
Increased muscle stretch reflexes Babinski response Detrusor sphincter dyssynergia (depending on level of lesions)	Hyporeflexia Flaccid weakness Significant muscle wasting

Note: Lesions of the upper lumbar vertebral bodies can present with a mixture of upper and lower neuron findings

NEUROLOGIC LEVEL, SENSORY LEVEL, AND MOTOR LEVEL OF INJURY:
(Hoppenfeld, 1977)

Lesions are classified according to a *neurologic, motor, and sensory level of injury*. They are further divided into complete and incomplete lesions.

1. 📖 Sensory level of injury

- Most caudal segment of the SC with normal (2/2) sensory function on both sides of the body for pinprick, and light touch
- For the sensory examination there are 28 key sensory *dermatomes*, each tested separately for *light touch* (with a cotton tip applicator) and *pinprick* (with a safety pin)

Scores:	0	Absent
	1	Impaired
	2	Normal

The face is used as the normal control point.
For pinprick testing: The patient must be able to differentiate the sharp and dull edge of a safety pin.

Scores:	0	Not able to differentiate between the sharp and dull edge
	1	The pin is not felt as sharp as on the face, but able to differentiate sharp from dull
	2	Pin is felt as sharp as on the face

For light touch, a cotton tip applicator is compared to the face sensation

Scores:	2	Normal—same as on face
	1	Impaired—less than on the face
	0	Absent

📖 It is very important to test the S4/S5 dermatome for light touch and pinprick

2. 📖 Motor level of injury

- Most caudal key muscle group that is graded three-fifths or greater with the segments above graded five-fifths in strength.
- A possible score of 100 can be obtained when adding the muscle scores of the key muscle groups (25 points per extremity).

There are 10 key myotomes on the left and right side of the body:

Myotome	Index Muscle	Action
C5	Biceps brachialis	Elbow flexors
C6	Extensor carpi radialis	Wrist extensors
C7	Triceps	Elbow extensors
C8	Flexor digitorum profundus	Finger flexors (FDP of middle finger)
T1	Abductor digiti minimi	Small finger abductor
L2	Iliopsoas	Hip flexors
L3	Quadriceps	Knee extensors
L4	Tibialis anterior	Ankle dorsiflexors
L5	Extensor hallucis longus	Long toe extensors
S1	Gastrocnemius	Ankle plantarflexors

Manual Muscle Testing Grading System
0   No movement
1   Palpable movement or visible contraction
2   Active movement through full range of motion with gravity eliminated
3   Active movement through full range of motion against gravity
4   Active movement against moderate resistance through full range of motion
5   Normal strength based on age, sex, and body habitus

3. Neurologic level of injury

- Most caudal segment of the spinal cord with both normal sensory and motor function on both sides of the body, determined by the sensory and motor levels
- Since the level may be different from side to side, it is recommended to record each side separately

4. Skeletal level of injury

- Level where the greatest vertebral damage is noted by radiographic evaluation

COMPLETE VS. INCOMPLETE LESIONS

Complete injury (Waters 1991)

- Absence of sensory and motor function in the lowest sacral segment
- The term *Zone of Partial Preservation* is only used with *complete lesions*
- Refers to the dermatomes and myotomes *caudal* to the neurological level of injury that remain partially innervated

Incomplete injury

- Partial preservation of sensory and/or motor functions below the neurological level, which includes the lowest sacral segment. Sacral sensation and motor function are assessed.
- ▣ *Sacral Sparing* —voluntary anal sphincter contraction or sensory function (light touch, pinprick at the S4–S5 dermatome, or anal sensation on rectal examination) in the lowest sacral segments.
- Due to preservation of the periphery of the SC
- Indicates incomplete injury
- Sacral sparing indicates the possibility of SC recovery, with possible partial or complete return of motor power
- There is also the possibility of return of bowel and bladder function
- The concept of sacral sparing in the incomplete SCI is important because it represents at least partial structural continuity of the white matter long tracts (i.e., corticospinal and spinothalamic tracts). Sacral sparing is evidenced by perianal sensations (S4–S5 dermatome), and rectal motor function. Sacral sparing represents continued function of the lower sacral motor neurons in the conus medullaris and their connections via the spinal cord to the cerebral cortex.

ASIA IMPAIRMENT SCALE: CLASSIFIES COMPLETE AND INCOMPLETE INJURIES:

A = **Complete:** No motor or sensory function is preserved in the sacral segments
B = **Incomplete:** Sensory but not motor function is preserved below the neurological level and includes sacral segments
C = **Incomplete:** Motor function preserved below the neurological level; more than half the key muscles below the neurological level have a muscle grade less than 3
D = **Incomplete:** Motor function preserved below the neurological level; at least half the key muscles below the neurological level have a muscle grade of 3 or more
E = **Normal:** Motor and sensory function

Assigning an ASIA Level (Figure 7–15)

1. Examine 10 index muscles bilaterally
2. Examine 28 dermatomes for pinprick and light touch
3. Complete rectal exam to assess sensation and volitional sphincteric contraction
4. Determine left and right motor levels

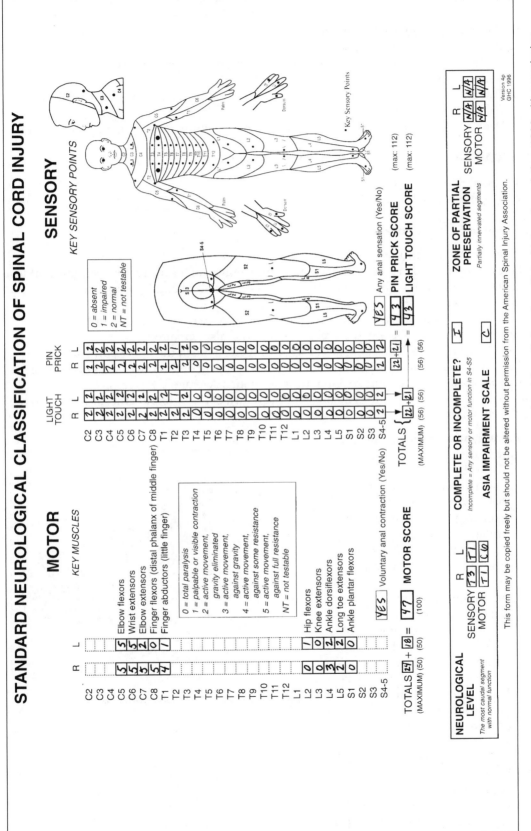

FIGURE 7-15. ASIA Scoring of hypothetical patient with a C6 motor incomplete injury. © American Spinal Injury Association, 1996 with permission.

5. Determine left and right sensory levels
6. 📖 Assign final motor and sensory levels
7. Determine neurological level, which is the most caudal segment with normal motor and sensory function
8. Categorize injury as complete or incomplete by ASIA impairment scale (A,B,C,D,E)
9. Calculate motor and sensory score
10. Determine zone of partial preservation if complete injury ("A" on impairment scale)

CLINICAL EFFECTS OF SCI: DIVIDED INTO TWO STAGES

1. Spinal Shock–Areflexia
2. Heightened Reflex Activity

1. Stage of Spinal Shock

- Reflex arc is not functioning
- Loss of motor function is accompanied by atonic paralysis of the bladder, bowel, gastric atony
- All the muscles below the level of the lesion become flaccid and hyporeflexic
- Loss of sensation below the level of the lesion
- Temporary loss or depression of all spinal reflex activity below the level of the lesion
- Autonomic function below the level of the lesion is also impaired
- Temporary loss of piloerection, sweating, vasomotor tone in the lower parts of the body
- Believed to be due to a sudden and abrupt interruption of descending excitatory influences

Duration: Lasts from 24 hours to 3 months after injury. Average is 3 weeks.

Minimal reflex activity is noted usually with the return of the bulbocavernosus reflex and the anal wink reflex

Bulbocavernosus reflex (male ♂):
(Figure 7–16)

- The bulbocavernosus reflex arc is a simple sensory-motor pathway that can function without using ascending or descending white-matter, long-tract axons.
- Usually the first reflex to return after spinal shock is over. If the level of the reflex arc is both physiologically and anatomically intact, the reflex will function in spite of complete spinal cord disruption at a higher level.
- Indicates that reflex innervation of bowel and bladder is intact
- Performed by squeezing the penis and noting stimulation of anal sphincter contraction
- At this time the bladder can be expected to contract on a reflex basis (although clinically this rarely occurs)
- Bowel will empty as a result of reflex induced by fecal bulb or rectal suppository stimulation

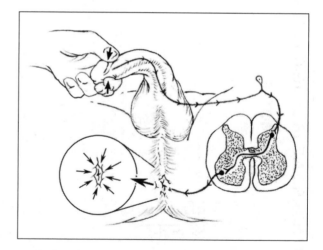

FIGURE 7–16. The bulbocavernosus reflex.

Perianal Sphincter Reflex (anal wink)
- Perianal stimulation causes contraction of the anal sphincter
- Indicates that reflex innervation of the bowel and bladder is intact

2. Stage of Increased Reflex Activity

- As the spine recovers from shock, the reflex arc functions without inhibitory or regulatory impulses from the brain, creating local spasticity and clonus
- Reflexes become stronger, and come to include additional and more proximal muscles
- Pattern of higher flexion is noted
- Dorsiflexion of the big toe (Babinski sign)
- Fanning of the toes
- Achilles reflex returns, then patellar
- Bladder starts to present contractions at irregular intervals with release of urine
- Reflex defecation

ASIA NEUROLOGICAL EXAMINATION TWO COMPONENTS—SENSORY AND MOTOR

Localizing Level of Injury and Asia Classification (Asia, 1996), (Mayard and Bracken, 1997)

ASIA Key Sensory Levels (Figure 7–17)

C2:	Occipital protuberance
C3:	Supraclavicular fossa
C4:	Superior AC Joint
C5:	Lateral side of the antecubital fossa
C6:	Thumb (and index finger)
C7:	Middle finger
C8:	Little finger
T1:	Medial ulnar side of antecubital epicondyle
T2:	Apex of axilla
T3:	Third intercostal space (IS)
T4:	Nipple line – fourth IS
T5:	Fifth intercostal space - fifth IS
T6:	Xiphoid – sixth IS
T7:	Seventh intercostal space – seventh IS
T8:	Eighth intercostal space – eigth IS
T9:	Midway between T8 and T10 – ninth IS
T10:	Umbilicus – tenth IS
T11:	Eleventh intercostal space – eleventh IS
T12:	Inguinal ligament at midpoint
L1:	Half the distance between T12 and L2
L2:	Midanterior thigh
L3:	Medial fem condyle
L4:	Medial malleolus
L5:	Dorsum of foot at third MTP joint
S1:	Lateral heel
S2:	Popliteal fossa in the midline
S3:	Ischial tuberosity
S4 and S5:	Perianal area (taken as one level)

ASIA Key Motor Levels

C1–C4:	Use sensory level and diaphragm to localize lowest neurological level
C5:	Elbow flexors
C6:	Wrist extensors
C7:	Elbow extensors
C8:	Finger flexors (FDP of middle finger)
T1:	ABD digiti minimi (small finger abductor)
T2–L1:	Use sensory level
L2:	Hip flexors
L3:	Knee extensors
L4:	DF ankle dorsiflexors
L5:	Long toe extensors
S1:	Plantar flexors

Reflexes

S1S2:	Gastrocnemius (ankle jerk)
L3L4:	Quadriceps (knee jerk)
C5C6:	Biceps, brachioradialis
C7C8:	Triceps, finger flexors
L5:	Medial hamstring

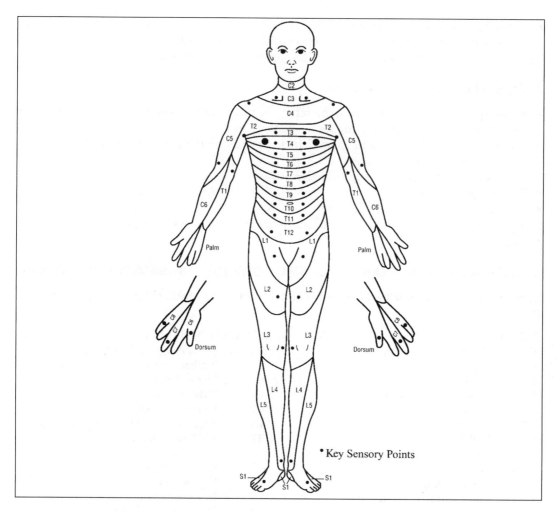

FIGURE 7–17. ASIA key sensory levels. © American Spinal Injury Association, 1996, with permission.

INCOMPLETE SPINAL CORD INJURY SYNDROMES

📖 **Central cord syndrome** (Figure 7–18) This is the most common syndrome.

- Results from an injury involving the center of the spinal cord
- It is predominantly a white matter peripheral injury
- Intramedullary hemorrhage is not common
- It may occur at any age, but is more common in older patients
- Produces sacral sensory sparing, greater motor weakness in the upper limbs than the lower limbs. Anatomy of the corticospinal tracts is such that the cervical distribution is medial and sacral distribution is more lateral. Since the center of the SC is injured, upper extremities are more affected than lower extremities.
- Patients may also have bladder dysfunction, most commonly urinary retention
- Variations in sensory loss below the level of the lesion

Recovery: Lower extremities recover first and to a greater extent. This is followed by improvement in bladder function, then proximal upper extremity, and finally intrinsic hand function. (Roth et al., 1990)

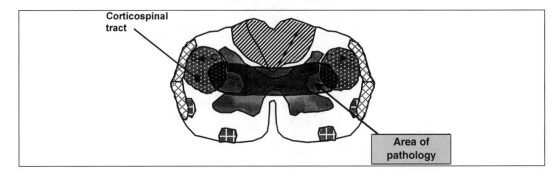

FIGURE 7–18. Central Cord Syndrome. (Transverse section of the spinal cord—refer to Figure 7–2 for anatomical landmarks).

📖 **Brown-Sequard Syndrome:** (Figure 7–19, 7–20) Constitutes 2%-4% of all traumatic SCI

- Results from a lesion that causes spinal hemisection
- (Ipsilateral) focal injury to the spinal cord causes deficits distal to the site of the lesion. Because tracts cross at different locations, deficits affect different sides, i.e.
- Ipsilateral—motor and proprioception deficits
- Contralateral—pain and temperature deficits
- Associated with stabbing and gunshot wounds
- Patients have ipsilateral motor and proprioceptive loss, and contralateral loss of pain and temperature

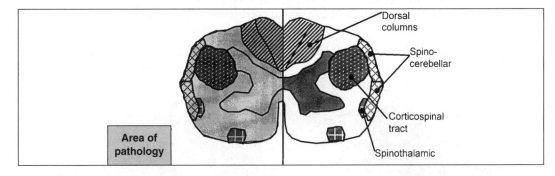

FIGURE 7–19. Brown-Sequard Syndrome. (Transverse section of the spinal cord—refer to Figure 7–2 for anatomical landmarks).

Result
Ipsilateral:
Motor and proprioceptive deficits (right sided)

Contralateral:
Pain and temperature deficits (left sided)

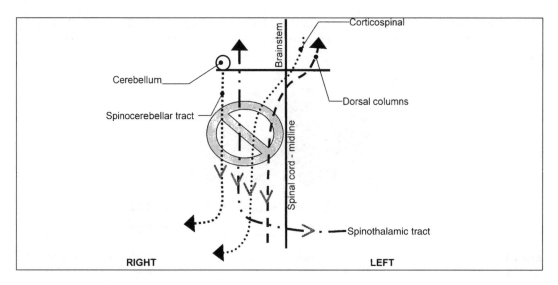

FIGURE 7–20. Brown-Sequard syndrome lesion: depicts point of injury, i.e. right-sided gunshot or knife wound. Follow tracts distal from the point of injury. Result is ipsilateral motor and proprioceptive deficits (right-sided) contralateral pain and temperature deficits (left-sided).

📖 Anterior Cord Syndrome: (Figure 7–21)

Caused by:

A lesion involving the anterior two thirds of the spinal cord preserving the posterior columns, such as:

Anterior spinal artery lesions, direct injury to the anterior spinal cord, bone fragments or a retropulsed disc

Polyarteritis nodosa, angioplasty, aortic and cardiac surgery, and embolism, can result in injury to the anterior two-thirds of the spinal cord (Ditunno, 1992)

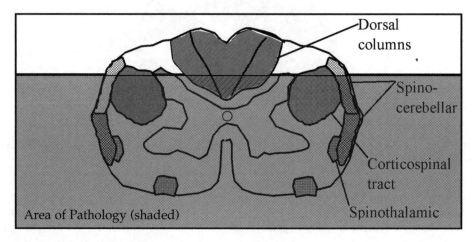

FIGURE 7–21. Anterior cord syndrome. (transverse section of the spinal cord—refer to Figure 7–2 for anatomic landmarks).

Result:
Variable loss of motor function (corticospinal tract) and sensitivity to pain and temperature, pinprick sensation, (spinothalamic tract) with preservation of proprioception and light touch

Recovery:
There is only 10%–20% chance of muscle recovery in most cases. (Kirshblum, 1998)
Of those who recover, coordination and muscle power is poor.

Posterior Cord Syndrome (Figure 7–22)

- Least frequent syndrome
- Injury to the posterior columns results in proprioceptive loss (dorsal columns)
- Pain, temperature, touch are preserved. Motor function is preserved to varying degrees.

Conus Medullaris Syndrome

- Injury to the sacral cord (conus) and lumbar nerve roots within the spinal canal, usually results in areflexic bladder and bowel, and lower limbs (in low-level lesions) i.e., lesions at B in Figure 7–23.
- If it is a high conus lesion, bulbocavernous reflex and micturition may be present, i.e., lesions at A in Figure 7–23.

Cauda Equina Syndrome:

- Injury to the lumbosacral nerve roots within the neural canal, results in areflexic bladder, bowel, lower limbs, i.e., lesions at C in Figure 7–23.
- Bulbocavernous reflex absent

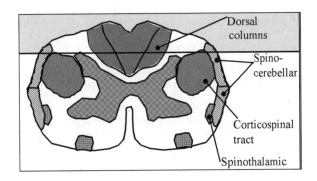

FIGURE 7–22. Posterior cord syndrome. (transverse section of the spinal cord—refer to Figure 7–2 for anatomical landmarks).

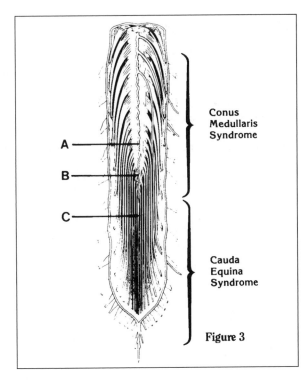

Figure 3

FIGURE 7–23. Distal spinal cord: Conus Medullaris Syndrome. **A:** high lesion. **B:** low lesion. Cauda Equina Syndrome: **C:** Lesion of the lumbosacral nerve roots. © American Spinal Injury Association, 1996, with permission.

Table 7-2 Conus Medularis vs. Cauda Equina Syndrome

CONUS MEDULLARIS L1–L2 vertebral level Injury to Sacral Cord (S1–S5)	CAUDA EQUINA SYNDROME L2–sacrum vertebral level Injury to Lumbosacral Nerve Roots
Location: L1–L2 vertebral level injury of sacral cord (S1–S5) and lumbar roots	**Location:** L2–sacrum vertebral level Injury to lumbosacral nerve roots
Causes: • L1 fracture • Tumors, gliomas • Vascular injury • Spina bifida, tethering of the cord	**Causes:** • L2 or below fracture • Sacral fractures • Fracture of pelvic ring • Can be associated with spondylosis

Resultant Signs and Symptoms:
 	
1. Normal motor function of lower extremities unless S1–S2 motor involvement (since only involves S1–S5)
 	
   Areflexic lower extremities
   If lumbar root involvement results in a lower motor neuron lesion (LMN)
 	
2. Saddle distribution sensory loss (touch is spared)
 	
3. No pain
 	
4. Symmetric abnormalities
 	
5. Severe bowel, bladder, sexual dysfunction
   Areflexic bowel
   Areflexic bladder
 	
6. If it is a high conus lesion, bulbocavernosus reflex may be present
	Resultant Signs and Symptoms:
	
	1. Flaccid paralysis of lower extremities of involved Lumbosacral nerve roots
	
	   Areflexic LE—results in a LMN Lesion
	
	2. Sensory loss in root distribution
	
	3. Pain
	
	4. Abnormalities predominate on one side (asymmetric)
	
	5. High cauda equina lesions (lumbar roots) Spare bowel and bladder
	   Lower lesions (S3–S5) can involve bowel and bladder and sexual dysfunction
	
	6. Bulbocavernosus reflex is absent (in low cauda equina [sacral] lesions)

EMG: Normal EMG (except for external sphincter or S1, S2 involvement)	**EMG:** Findings show multiple root level involvement Px: Good

TABLE 7-3. Functional Potential Outcomes for Cervical SCI (Complete) Patients (Kirshblum, 1998)

	C3–C4	📖 C5	📖 C6	C7	C8–T1
Feeding	May be able with adapted equipment	*BFO Independent with equiptment after set up	Independent with equipment	Independent	Independent
Grooming	Dependent	Independent with equipment after set up	Independent with equipment	Independent with equipment	Independent
UE Dressing	Dependent	Requires assistance	Independent	Independent	Independent
LE Dressing	Dependent	Dependent	Requires assistance	May be independent with equipment	Independent
Bathing	Dependent	Dependent	Independent with equipment	Independent	Independent
Bed Mobility	Dependent	Requires assistance	Independent with equipment	Independent	Independent
Weight Shifts	Independent with power Dependent in manual	Requires assistance	Independent	Independent	Independent
Transfers	Dependent	Requires assistance	Possible independent with transfer board	Independent with or without board except floor transfer	Independent
W/C Propulsion	Independent with power Dependent in manual	Independent with power Short distances in manual with lugs or plastic rims on level surfaces	Independent manual with plastic rims on level surfaces	Independent except curbs	Independent
Driving	Unable	Unable	Specially adapted van	Car with hand controls or adapted van	Car with hand controls or adapted van
Bowel and Bladder	Dependent	Dependent	Independent—bowel assists–bladder	Independent	Independent

📖 THE HIGHEST COMPLETE SCI LEVEL THAT CAN LIVE INDEPENDENTLY WITHOUT THE AID OF AN ATTENDANT IS A C6 COMPLETE TETRAPLEGIA.

- This patient would have to be *extremely motivated*
- Feeding is accomplished with a universal cuff for utensils
- Transfers require stabilization of elbow extension with forces transmitted from shoulder musculature through a closed kinetic chain
- Bowel care is performed using a suppository insertion wand or other apparatus for digital stimulation
- Outcome studies of a subset of patients with motor and sensory complete C6 SCI revealed the following percentage of patients were independent for key self-care tasks:

  Feeding—16%
  Upper body dressing—13%
  Lower body dressing—3%
  Grooming—19%
  Bathing—9%
  Bowel Care—3%
  Transfers—6%
  Wheelchair propulsion—88%

📖 C7 level is the *usual* level for achieving independence.

■

MEDICAL COMPLICATIONS OF SCI

📖
> **Important Levels to Remember:**
> T6 and above: Individuals with SCI are considered to be at risk for
>   1. Autonomic Dysreflexia
>   2. Orthostatic Hypotension
> T8: If lesion above T8, patient cannot regulate and maintain normal body temperature (Note: an easy way to remember this level is to spell the word ***temp eight ture***.)
> Central temperature regulation in the brain is located in the hypothalamus.

ORTHOSTATIC HYPOTENSION (see Table 7-4) (Corbett, 1971)

State of transient reflex depression

Cause: Lack of sympathetic outflow, triggered by tilt of patient > 60 degrees

Lesion T6 or above
T1–L2 responsible for:
    Tachycardia, vasoconstriction and increased arterial pressure
    Heart and blood vessels supplied by T1–T7

Mechanism

- Upright position causes decrease in blood pressure (BP)
- Carotid body baroreceptors sense decrease in BP, which would usually increase sympathetic outflow.

- However brainstem is unable to send a message through the SC to cause sympathetic outflow and allow vasoconstriction of splanchnic bed to increase BP

Resultant Symptoms

1. Hypotension—loss of sympathetic tone (decreased systemic venous resistance, dilation of venous vessels) (decreased preload to the heart)
2. ▢ Tachycardia—Carotid body responds to hypotension, no increase in sympathetic outflow, however, they can still inhibit parasympathetics, but the increase in heart rate is not sufficient enough to counterbalance decrease BP
3. Patient can lose consciousness

▢ Treatment

1. Reposition—Trendelenburg/daily tilt table/recliner wheelchair
2. Elastic Stocking/Abdominal Binder/Ace wrap LE
3. Add Salt/Meds:
   Salt Tablets 1 gram QID
   Florinef® (mineralocorticoid): 0.05–0.1 mg QD
   Ephedrine (alpha agonist): 20–30 mg QD–QID
   Use caution: The same patient is at risk for autonomic dysreflexia
4. Fluid resuscitation: monitor for neurogenic pulmonary edema
5. Orthostasis lessens with time due to the development of spinal postural reflexes. This causes vasoconstriction due to improved autoregulation of cerebrovascular circulation in the presence of perfusion pressure

▢ AUTONOMIC DYSREFLEXIA (see Table 7-4) (Braddom, 1991) (Lindan, 1980)

Onset: After spinal shock, usually within first 6 months–1 year
Incidence: 48%–85%
Cause: Noxious stimulus below the level of the lesion causing massive imbalanced sympathetic discharge, i.e., too much sympathetic outflow
Most commonly caused by distended, full bladder
Lesion: SCI patients with lesions T6 or above (complete lesions)
Mechanism: Syndrome of massive imbalanced reflex sympathetic discharge in patients with SCI above the splanchnic outflow
This is secondary to the loss of descending sympathetic control and hypersensitivity of receptors below the level of the lesion
**Potential
Symptoms:** Noxious stimuli—Increases sympathetic reflex spinal release
Regional vasoconstriction (especially GI tract)
Increases peripheral vascular resistance—increases cardiac output, increases BP
Carotid body responds to HTN causing reflex bradycardia by the dorsal motor nucleus of the vagus nerve
Symptoms: Headache, Flushing
Piloerection
Sweating above level of SCI
Blurry vision (pupillary dilation)
Nasal Congestion
Note: The brainstem is unable to send message through SCI to decrease sympathetic outflow and allow vasodilation of splanchnic bed to decrease BP

Most common causes:

- Bladder—blocked catheter
- Bowel—fecal impaction
- Pressure ulcers
- Ingrown toenails
- Urinary tract infections
- Bladder stones
- Gastric ulcers
- Labor
- Abdominal emergency
- Fractures
- Orgasm
- Epididymitis
- Cholecystitis

Treatment:

- Sit patient up
- Remove TEDS/Abdominal binder
- Identify and remove noxious stimulus
- Nitroglycerine—to control BP—1/150 sublingual or topical paste, which can be removed once noxious stimulus corrected
- Procardia®: 10 mg chew and swallow
- Hydralazine: 10–20 mg IM/IV
- Clonidine: 0.3–0.4 mg
- ICU - Nipride

Prevent Recurrence:

- Dibenzyline: 20–40 mg/day alpha blocker
- Minipress®: 0.5–1 TID alpha blocker
- Clonidine: 0.2 mg BID

Potential Complications of Autonomic Dysreflexia: If hypertensive episodes are not treated, complications can lead to: Retinal Hemorrhage, CVA, SAH, Seizure, Death

Autonomic Dysreflexia predisposes patient to atrial fibrillation by altering normal pattern of repolarization of the atria, making the heart susceptible to reentrant-type arrhythmias.

TABLE 7-4 Orthostatic Hypertension vs. Autonomic Dysreflexia

📖 Orthostatic Hypotension	📖 Autonomic Dysreflexia (AD)
Trigger: Tilt patient > 60 degrees	**Trigger:** Noxious stimulus: especially full bladder below level of lesion
Due to: Lack of sympathetic outflow **Lesion:** T6 or above	**Due to:** Too much sympathetic outflow, loss of descending control, hypersensitivity **Onset:** status post spinal shock usually within first six months **Lesion:** T6 or above
Symptoms: Hypotension due to being positioned in the upright position 📖 Tachycardia: carotid body responds to hypotension Patient loses consciousness	**Symptoms:** Hypertension due to noxious stimulus. Bradycardia: carotid body responds to hypertension HA flushing Piloerection Sweating above level SCI Blurred vision, pupillary dilation Nasal congestion
Note: Upright position causes decrease in BP, carotid body Baroreceptors sense decrease BP, but brainstem is unable to send message through SC to cause sympathetic outflow and cause vasoconstriction of splanchnic bed to increase BP	**Note:** Noxious stimulus causes massive sympathetic output Carotid body senses increased BP, but brainstem is unable to send message through SC to cause decreased sympathetic outflow and allow for vasodilation of splanchnic bed to bring BP down

Tx:
1. Reposition: Trendelenburg
2. Elastic stockings
3. Abdominal binders
4. Increase salt
5. Fluid resuscitation: monitor neurogenic pulmonary edema
 	
Meds:
Florinef® (Mineralocorticoid)
Salt Tablets
Ephedrine (Alpha Agonist)
	Tx:
	1. Sit patient up
	2. Remove noxious stimulus (look for bladder distension, fecal impaction, etc.)
	3. Treat hypertension
	  • Consider temporary treatment with nitrates (transderm), hydralazine (parenteral), morphine (parenteral), captopril (oral), labetalol (oral or IV)
	  • Decide need for intensive care and IV agents such as nitroglycerine, nitroprusside, spinal anesthesia
	It is estimated that 48%–85% of patients with high level SCI have symptoms of autonomic dysreflexia.
	Can lead to:
	
	1. Retinal Hemorrhage
	2. CVA
	3. SAH, seizure, death
	
	AD may predispose patient to A. fib. by altering the normal. pattern of repolarization of the atria, making the heart susceptible to reentrant-type arrhythmias.

BLADDER DYSFUNCTION

Neuroanatomy and Neurophysiology of Voiding

Central Pathways

- *Corticopontine Mesencephalic Nuclei*–Frontal Lobe
  Inhibits parasympathetic sacral micturition center
  Allows bladder storage
- *Pontine Mesencephalic*
  Coordinates bladder contraction and opening of sphincter
- 📖 *Pelvic and Pudendal Nuclei*–Sacral Micturition
  Integrates stimuli from cephalic centers
  Mediates the parasympathetic S2–S4 sacral micturition reflex
- *Motor Cortex to Pudendal Nucleus*
  Voluntary control (contraction/inhibition) of the external urethral sphincter

Peripheral Pathways (Figure 7–25)

- 📖 *Parasympathetic Efferents*–S2–S4
  Travel through the pelvic nerve to parasympathetic receptors
  Allows contraction of the bladder and emptying
- 📖 *Sympathetic Efferents*–T11–L2
  Travel through hypogastric plexi to sympathetic receptors
  (Alpha 1 + Beta 2 adrenergics)
  Urine Storage
- *Somatic Efferents*–S2–S4
  Travel through pudendal nerve to innervate striated muscle of external urethral sphincter
  Prevents urine leakage or emptying
- *Afferent Fiber*
  Travel through pudendal and pelvic nerve through the hypogastric plexi to thoraco-lumbar SC
  Origin — detrusor muscle stretch receptors
    external anal and urethral sphincter
    perineum and genitalia
    When bladder becomes distended, afferent nerve becomes activated for parasympathetic stimulation, resulting in emptying of bladder

📖 Neurologic Innervation of the Bladder (Bladder Receptors) (Figure 7–24)

- Cholinergic Muscarinic–M2
  Located in the bladder wall, trigone, bladder neck, urethra
- Beta 2 Adrenergic
  Concentrated in the body of the bladder, neck
- Alpha adrenergic
  Located on the base of the bladder (neck and proximal urethra)
  (Note: Bladder wall does not have baroreceptors)

> **Note:**
> Alpha Adrenergic receptors respond to the appearance of norepinephrine with contraction
>
> Beta adrenergic receptors respond to the appearance of norepinephrine with relaxation

Urethral Sphincter

Internal Sphincter:
- Innervated by T11–T12 sympathetic nerve
- Contracts sphincter for storage
- Smooth muscle

External Sphincter
- Innervated by S2–S4 pudendal nerve
- Prevents leakage or emptying
- Skeletal muscle, voluntary control

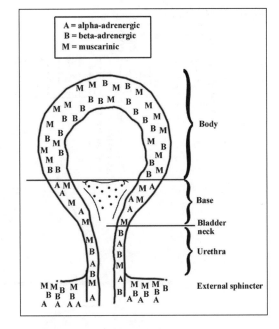

FIGURE 7–24. Bladder and proximal urethra distribution of autonomic receptors.

Storage

Sympathetic (Figure 7–25)
encouraged during fight, flight

T11–L2 sympathetic efferents
- Travel through the hypogastric nerve
- Causes the sphincter to contract and body to relax
- Urine is stored

📖 *Alpha1 Receptors Adrenergic*
- NE causes contraction of neck of bladder and prevents leakage
- Closes internal urethral sphincter and detrusor outlet, promoting storage

📖 *B2 Receptors Adrenergic*
- Located in body of bladder
- Activation causes relaxation of body of bladder to allow expansion
- Inhibitory when activated

Emptying

Parasympathetic (Figure 7–25)
encouraged during relaxation

Muscarinic (M2) cholinergic receptors are located in:
- The bladder wall
- Trigone
- Bladder Neck
- Urethra

Stimulation of pelvic nerve (parasympathetic)
- Allows contraction of bladder + therefore, emptying!

B2 Receptors Adrenergic
- Relaxation of the bladder neck on the initiation of voiding

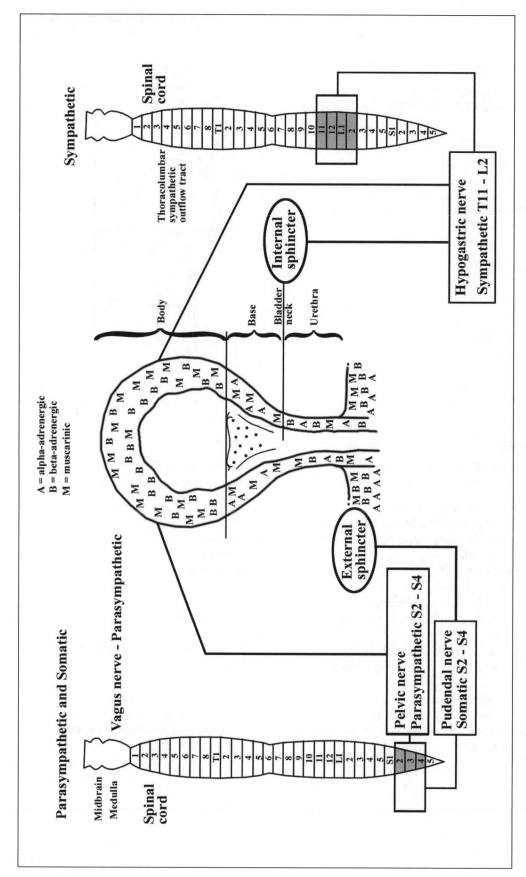

FIGURE 7-25. Neurologic innervation of the bladder.

Evaluation of Urinary Function: Cystometrogram and Pelvic Floor EMG

During cystometry: sensation, capacity, and the presence of involuntary detrusor activity are evaluated. A typical urodynamic study is depicted in Figure 7–26

- Sensations evaluated include:
  First sensation of bladder filling—occurs at approximately 50% of bladder capacity
  First urge to void—proprioceptive sensation
  Strong urge to void—proprioceptive sensation
- Accepted normal bladder capacity is 300–600ml
  Functional bladder capacity = voided volume + residual urine volume

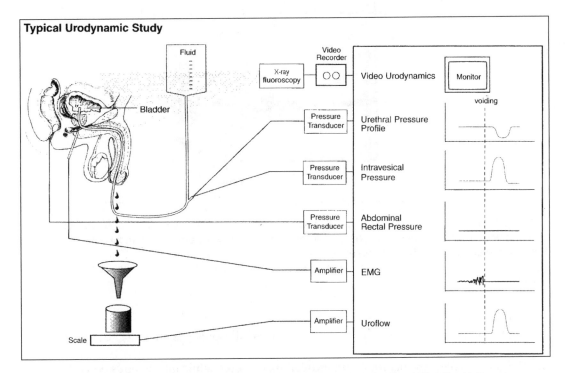

Typical Urodynamic Study

FIGURE 7–26. Instrumentation for urodynamic studies is not standardized. The illustration above uses radio-opaque fluid. Some physicians, however, prefer to use carbon dioxide. Normal bladder function can be divided into storage and voiding phases. The first sensation of bladder filling is between 100 cc and 200 cc. The patient experiences bladder fullness between 300 cc and 400 cc and the sense of urgency between 400 cc and 500 cc. Intravesical pressure does not increase significantly during the storage phase due to the vascoelasticity of the vesical wall. During the voiding phase, sphincter activity stops and the bladder contracts. During normal voiding, the EMG signal will be silent, intravesical pressure will increase, and urethral pressure will decrease. Fluoroscopy will qualitatively assess bladder contraction and document any potential vesioureteral reflux. (From Nesathurai S. The Rehabilitation of People With Spinal Cord Injury: A House Officers Guide. © Boston Medical Center for the New England Regional Spinal Cord Injury Center. Boston, MA: Arbuckle Academic Publishers, with permission).

Normal Detrusor Contraction
Detrusor Pressure cm H$_2$O and
EMG Pelvic Floor (Fig. 7-27)

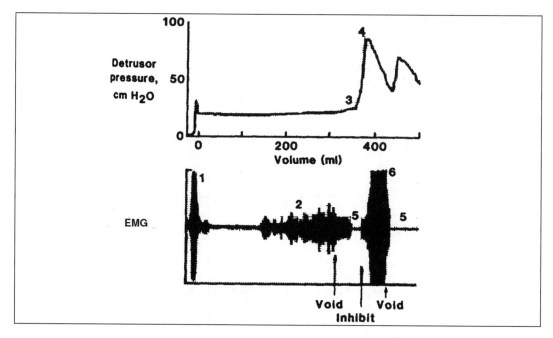

FIGURE 7–27. Normal Cystometrogram/Pelvic Floor EMG. 1. Bulbocavernosus reflex. 2. Contraction of pelvic floor muscles during later phase of filling (progressively increasing electrical activity) 3. Functional bladder capacity. 4. Detrusor contraction that occurs during voiding. 5. Electrical silence (abrupt) which occurs during voiding. 6. Electrical activity of pelvic floor muscles that occurs during voluntary inhibition.

Genitourinary Function and Management

During the acute period after injury, the bladder usually presents *areflexic*, i.e., spinal shock phase.

May initially manage the bladder with indwelling catheter, while intravenous body fluids are administered. An intermittent catheterization program should be established soon after, with fluid restriction of approx. 100 cc/hr.

📖 Volumes should always be monitored and maintained below 400–500 cc to avoid:
  – Vesicoureteral reflu*x*—caused by bladder hypertrophy and loss of the vesicoureteral angle (see previous page). This is normally prevented by the anatomy of the ureter, which penetrates the bladder obliquely through the trigone and courses several centimeters into the bladder epithelium.
  – Overflow incontinence
  – Hydro-ureter

Urodynamic studies should be performed to assess:

The bladder neck, the external sphincter, and the detrusor

  Note: Bladder dysfunction is closely related to the level of injury, i.e., lower motor neuron vs. upper motor neuron.

TABLE 7-5 Lower Motor Neuron Bladder vs. Upper Motor Neuron Bladder

LMN Bladder Failure to Empty (Fig. 7-28)	UMN Bladder Failure to Store (Fig. 7-29)
Causes: • Spinal Shock: when reflex arc is not functioning due to initial trauma • Conus Medullaris Syndrome • Cauda Equina Syndrome • Tabes Dorsalis, Pernicious Anemia, Syringomyelia • Multiple Sclerosis	**Causes:** • SCI: when reflex arc returns after initial trauma to cord passes • CVA • Multiple Sclerosis
Lesion: Complete destruction of Sacral Micturition Center (S2–S4) at S2 or below Lesion involving exclusively the peripheral innervation of the bladder	**LESION:** Above Sacral Micturition Center (above S2)
Can Result in:	**Can Result in:**
Big Hypotonic Bladder (flaccid, areflexic bladder),*Tight Competent Sphincter* Results in: **Failure to Empty** TX: • Intermittent Catheter • Crede maneuver (suprapubic pressure) • Valsalva maneuver • Drugs to induce urination Urecholine: stimulate cholinergic receptors Minipress®: block alpha adrenergic receptors Dibenzyline: block alpha adrenergic receptors Hytrin®: block alpha adrenergic receptors Cardura®: block alpha adrenergic receptors	*Small Hyperreflexic, Overactive, Little Bladder* Results in: **Failure to Store** (Incontinence) TX: Ditropan: direct smooth muscle relaxer Pro-Banthine®, Detrol®: anticholinergic Tofranil®, ephedrine: stimulates alpha, beta receptors to allow storage

LMN Bladder (Figure 7–28)
Failure To Empty
Cystometrogram and EMG

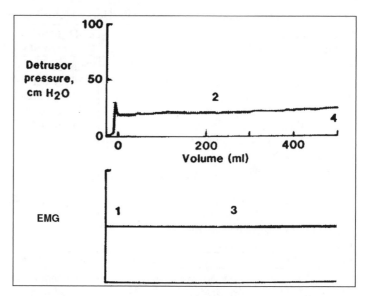

Note:
- Internal sphincter may have increased tension and prevent voiding

These patients usually only void by:
- *Overflow voiding* when bladder can no longer expand

FIGURE 7–28. Cystometrogram and EMG in a patient with complete lower motor neuron bladder dysfunction. 1. Absent bulbocavernosus reflex. 2. Major detrusor contractions are absent. 3. No pelvic floor muscle activity (external urethral sphincter). 4. Large bladder capacity.

UMN Bladder (Figure 7–29)
Failure to Store
Cystometrogram and EMG

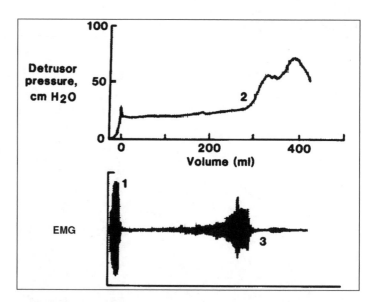

Due to upper motor neuron lesion, there is *no* suppression of micturition center, therefore, patient voids prematurely

FIGURE 7–29. Cystometrogram and EMG in a patient with complete uninhibited neurogenic bladder dysfunction. 1. Brisk bulbocavernosus reflex. 2. Spontaneous detrusor contraction at reduced bladder capacity. 3. Silence of pelvic floor muscles (external urethral sphincter).

Combination Type Bladder
(Figures 7–30, 7-31)

Many patients (as many as 85%) with SCI develop Detrusor Sphincter Dyssynergia (DSD)

Causes:
- Central Cord Syndrome
- MS
- Progression of SCI (UMN Lesion)

Lesion:
Neurologic injuries between the sacral (S2–S4) and pontine micturition center

Resultant Scenario:
Tight little bladder (Detrusor hyperreflexia)
Tight sphincter (Sphincter hyperactivity)

Result:
Failure to void

Risk if Not Treated:
- Infected urine travels up towards kidneys (Figure 7–30)
- Note: These patients frequently have frequency and urgency, but lack of coordination between bladder and sphincter. This prevents complete bladder emptying.
- Result: Increased residual volumes, urine becomes infected, patient then tries high-pressure voiding against closed sphincter, this sends infected urine up to kidneys

Treatment:
1. Anticholinergic Meds – to expand the detrusor to prevent infected urine from going up to the kidneys (intact sphincter is good for continence)
2. Intermittent catheterization
3. Antimuscarinic drugs (i.e., anticholinergic) to cause bladder relaxation
4. Alpha blocker—to open bladder neck
5. Sphincterotomy

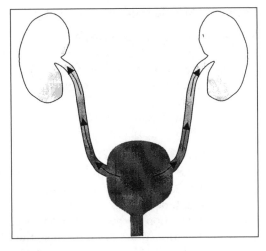

FIGURE 7–30. Reflux of infected urine backs up towards kidneys.

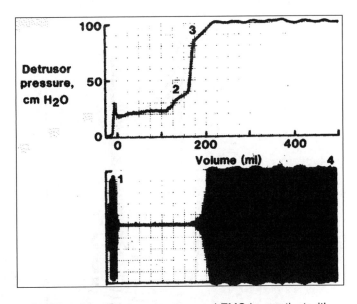

FIGURE 7–31. Cystometrogram and EMG in a patient with complete upper motor neuron bladder dysfunction shows: 1. Brisk bulbocavernosus reflex. 2. Bladder capacity is reduced. 3. High intravesical pressure during detrusor contraction. 4. Detrusor/external urethral sphincter dyssynergia with marked electrical activity of the pelvic floor muscles during detrusor contraction.

The normal bladder mechanism that prevents vesicoureteral reflux is described below:

Normal Anatomy (Figure 7–32A)
- The one-way valve mechanism can remain competent only as long as the oblique course of the ureter within the bladder wall is maintained
- During relaxation of the bladder, when urine is being stored, the ureter pumps urine into the bladder
- During bladder contraction the valve shuts closed. As a result urine cannot reenter the ureter and, therefore, the bladder is emptied with no reflux of urine into the ureters. (Figure A)

Bladder Wall Hypertrophy (Figure 7–32B)
- When bladder hypertrophy causes the course of the distal ureter to become progressively perpendicular to the inner surface of the bladder, the vesicoureteral function becomes incompetent, permitting vesicoureteral reflux
- During relaxation of the bladder, the ureter pumps urine into the bladder
- During bladder contraction, because the distal ureter becomes perpendicular to the inner surface of the bladder, the valve cannot close. Urine is forced up the ureter to the kidney and hydronephrosis can result. (Figure B)
- Reflux is further complicated by acute or chronic pyelonephritis with progressive renal failure.

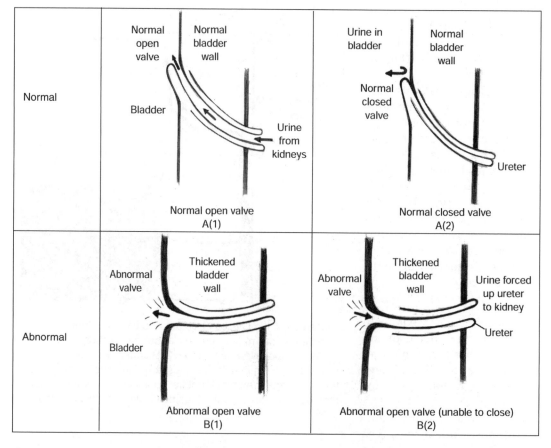

FIGURE 7–32. Vesicoureteral Junction. **A(1):** Normal Open Valve: The muscle of the ureter "milks" urine through the valve into the bladder. **(2):** Normal Closed Valve: When the bladder contracts, the valve is pressed shut. The normal valve prevents urine from flowing back into the ureter.
B(1): Abnormal Open Valve: The abnormal valve still allows urine to pass through the ureter into the bladder. **(2):** Abnormal Valve: The abnormal valve is unable to close. When the bladder contracts, urine is pushed back into the ureter and kidney.

📖 Intermittent Catheterization (IC)

IC has reduced many of the associated complications of the indwelling catheter, which include epididymitis, penoscrotal abscess, fistula formation, renal and bladder calculi, and malignancy. IC has been shown to reduce the incidence of urinary tract infection.
Pathophysiology of Urinary Tract Infections (UTI):
UTIs are generally caused by the endogenous flora of the host overcoming the competing normal flora and host defense mechanism. The presence of the UTI is affected by:

– The virulence of the invading microorganism
– The condition of the urine as the culture medium
– The host defense mechanisms

In general:
An acidic concentrated urine inhibits microbial growth. UTIs are prevented by the washout effort of large volumes of urine. The large flow of fluid impedes the adherence of microorganisms and dilutes the concentration of microorganisms.

Management of UTIs

Asymptomatic UTIs
📖 In SCI patients on an intermittent catheterization (IC) program recurrent asymptomatic bacteriuria (with less than 50 WBC per high power field) is generally not treated to avoid the development of resistant organisms.

(The exception to this is evidence of vesicoureteral reflux, hydronephrosis, or growth of urea splitting organisms.)

In general, asymptomatic UTI in individuals with indwelling catheters should not be treated.

Symptomatic UTIs
Symptomatic bacteriuria with fever leukocytosis or increased spasticity is treated and the catheterization is increased to reduce bacterial concentration and remove the urine that serves as a culture medium for bacterial growth. (A Foley may be necessary if volumes are too large for an IC program)

Most Common Urinary Tract Complications in Neurogenic Bladder

• Irregular, thickened bladder wall and small diverticuli—earliest changes
• Vesicoureteral reflux: 10%–30% of poorly managed bladders, leads to pyelonephritis, renal stones
• Hydronephrosis and hydroureters caused by outlet obstruction
• Overdistended areflexic bladder
• Bladder infections can lead to marked reduction in compliance of bladder

Prevention
All of these complications can be prevented by adequately draining the bladder at a pressure below 40 cm H_2O, either by intermittent catheterization along with the use of anticholinergic drugs or by timely surgical relief of the outflow obstruction

Prophylactic Treatment of UTIs in SCI patients
– Prophylactic antibiotic role is not fully established, but it is still used
    (i.e., Macrodantin® (nitrofurantoin))
– Vitamin C supplementation, cranberry juice, methenamine salts—overall used as acidifying agents

SEXUAL DYSFUNCTION

Physiology of Normal Sexual Act

Male Sexual Act (Bors, 1960)

Male erectile and ejaculatory function are complex physiologic activities that require interaction between vascular, nervous, and endocrine systems.
Erections are controlled by parasympathetic nervous system
Ejaculations are controlled by sympathetic nervous system

Erection:
Controlled by a reflex arc that is mediated in the sacral spinal cord
A reflex involves an afferent and an efferent limb

The Afferent Limb:
- Consists of somatic afferent fibers from the genital region that travel through the pudendal nerve into the sacral spinal cord

The Efferent Limb:
- Involves parasympathetic fibers that originate in the sacral spinal cord. These fibers travel through the cauda equina and exit via S2–S4 nerve roots.
- Postganglionic parasympathetic fibers secrete nitric oxide, which causes :
  - Relaxation of smooth muscle of the corpus cavernosum
  - Increases blood flow to the penile arteries—vascular sinusoids of the penis become engorged with blood
  - The result is an erection
  - This reflex is modulated by higher brainstem, subcortical, and cortical centers.

Ejaculation:
- Signals the culmination of the male sexual act, and is primarily controlled by the sympathetic nervous system
- Similar to sympathetic innervation to the bladder—these fibers originate in the thoracolumbar spinal cord (T11–L2), then travel through the hypogastric plexus to supply the vas deferens, seminal vesical, and ejaculatory ducts

Female Sexual Act
- Sexual excitation is the result of psychogenic and physical stimulation
- Stimulation of the genital region, including clitoris, labia majora, and labia minora, causes afferent signals to travel via the pudendal nerve into the S2–S4 segment of the spinal cord
- These fibers interact with the efferent parasympathetic fibers that project through the pelvic nerve
- The result is:
  - Dilation of arteries to perineal muscles and tightening of the introitus
  - Bartholin's glands secrete mucus, which aids in vaginal lubrication
- Female orgasm is characterized by the rhythmic contraction of the pelvic structures. Female orgasm also results in cervical dilation, which may aid in sperm transport and fertility.

Erectile Dysfunction

Men with SCI may obtain reflexogenic or psychogenic erections

Reflexogenic Erections
- Can occur independently of conscious awareness and supraspinal input (mediated by paraspinal division of ANS through sacral roots S2–S4)
- Are secondary to manual stimulation of the genital region (however, once stimulation has been removed, the erection may no longer be sustained)

Psychogenic Erections
- Involve supraspinal (above SC) effects, that are the result of erotic stimuli that result in cortical modulation of the sacral reflex arc
- Erection is mediated by central origin and psychological activated center

In general, erections are more likely with incomplete lesions (both UMN and LMN) than complete lesions. Many times, men with SCI can only maintain an erection while the penis is stimulated and the quality of the erection is insufficient for sexual satisfaction. As such, the erection must be augmented or induced.

Methods to Induce Erections
- Oral Therapy – Sildenafil, i.e., Viagra®
- Intracavernosal injection therapy – i.e. papaverine, alprostadil, phentolamine
- Penile vacuum device
- Transurethral devices – i.e., alprostadil
- Penile implants

Ejaculatory Dysfunction

In men with SCI, the ability to ejaculate is less than the ability to obtain an erection
The rate of ejaculation varies depending on the location and nature of the neurologic injury:
- Complete UMN lesions: ejaculation rate is estimated at 2%
- Incomplete UMN lesions: ejaculation rate is estimated at 32%
- Complete LMN lesions: ejaculation rate is estimated at 18%
- Incomplete LMN lesions: ejaculation rate is estimated at 70%

📖 Most SCI males are unable to ejaculate.
If they do, they are usually incomplete LMN lesions

Methods to Induce Ejaculation
- Intrathecal neostigmine
- Subcutaneous physostigmine
- Direct aspiration of sperm from vas deferens
- Vibratory stimulation – can be used at home
  - Increased incidence of autonomic dysreflexia
  - Males inseminate females with syringe
- Electroejaculation: most popular in USA
  - In incomplete lesion: very painful
  - If sensation is intact, patient cannot tolerate pain leading to heart rate and BP increase, and *autonomic dysreflexia* is a problem.

– Equipment used has been modified and it is possible to obtain the ejaculate through low-intensity constant repeatable current
– Patients need medical supervision
– Hospitals or office-based procedure: to evaluate through anoscopy before and after procedure to assess for injury to rectal mucosa
– Pretreat with Nifedipine (has lowered risk of autonomic dysreflexia)

Direct Stimulation of Hypogastric Nerve
– Ejaculate is obtained through the use of an implanted hypogastric nerve stimulator
– Surgical procedure—not appropriate for patients with intact pelvic pain sensitivity, since hypogastric nerve stimulation causes severe pain.

Sexual function might not return for 6–24 months. 80% experience return within 1 years of injury, 5% in 2 years

Infertility in Males With SCI (Linsenmeyer and Perkash, 1991)

Fertility in many paraplegic and tetraplegic men after SCI is severely impaired. Two major causes are (already discussed), *ejaculatory dysfunction* and *poor semen quality*

Poor semen quality is secondary to
• Stasis of prostatic fluid
• Testicular hyperthermia
• Recurrent UTI
• Abnormal testicular histology
• Changes in hypothalamic-pituitary-testicular axis
• Possible sperm antibodies
• Type of bladder management
• Chronic—Long-term use of various medications

Stasis of prostatic fluid
• Decreases sperm motility
• Studies have shown that in patients who did not have spontaneous ejaculations, there was an improvement in semen quality after 2–4 electroejaculations

Testicular Hyperthermia
Studies have shown higher deep scrotal temperatures (average = 0.9°C higher) in men with paraplegia who were seated when compared to noninjured control subjects who were seated. Men with SCI often sit with their legs close together, in contrast to nonimpaired men.

Sperm Counts and Motility Indices
• Sperm counts are lower in men who were having prostatic inflammation compared to those who were not
• Leukocytes (WBC > 10^6) in the spermatic fluid reduced total sperm count 41%, sperm velocity 12%, and total motile sperm 66%
• The single worst predictive factor for immobility to penetrate an ovum was leukocyte concentration in the semen
• Postinfective changes may affect fertility, such as atrophy of the testicles or obstruction of epididymal ducts.

Most Common Finding Noted on Biopsy is Atrophy of the Seminiferous Tubules
No investigations have found a significant correlation among biopsy finding, level of injury, length of injury, hormonal changes, or number of UTIs

Testosterone
Appears to remain normal or slightly above or below normal

Antisperm Antibodies
- Inhibit cervical mucous penetration
- Despite studies, immunologic-mediated infertility remains controversial
- Infertility due to antibodies is often not an absolute condition; additional time may be required but pregnancy can occur
- Two factors associated with antibody formation include: obstruction of the genital tract and UTIs

Female Infertility

Immediately postinjury 44%–58% of women suffer from temporary amenorrhea.
Menstruation returns within six months post injury.
Most women with SCI are fertile.

Birth Control
Can be problematic for SCI women:
- Condoms—provide protection
- Diaphragm—need adequate hand dexterity
- Oral Contraceptives—associated with increased risk of thromboembolism
- IUD—can increase risk of pelvic inflammatory disease, which may lead to autonomic dysreflexia

Pregnancy
The likelihood of pregnancy after spinal cord injury is unchanged, since fertility is unimpaired.
Pregnant women with SCI have an increased risk of:
- UTIs
- Leg edema
- Autonomic dysreflexia
- Constipation
- Thromboembolism
- Premature birth

Uterine innervation arises from T10–T12 level
Patients with lesions above T10 may not be able to perceive uterine contractions.
Pre-eclampsia may be difficult to differentiate from autonomic dysreflexia.
Autonomic dysreflexia may be the only clinical manifestation of labor.

GASTROINTESTINAL COMPLICATIONS AND BOWEL MANAGEMENT

Innervation of Bowel—Review of Anatomy and Neuroregulatory Control (Figure 7–33)

- The colon is a closed tube bound proximally by the ileocecal valve and distally by the anal sphincter
- The colon is composed of smooth muscle oriented in an inner circular and outer longitudinal layer
- The lower colon and anorectal region receive innervation by the sympathetic, parasympathetic, and somatic pathways
- In addition, the intrinsic enteric nervous system (ENS), composed of the Auerbach's (myenteric) plexus and the Meissner's (submucosal) plexus, coordinates the function of each segment of the bowel
- Auerbach's plexus is primarily motor; Meissner's plexus is primarily sensory. Both these plexi lie between the walls of smooth muscle mentioned earlier.
- The parasympathetic and sympathetic nervous systems modulate the activity of the ENS, which in turn inhibits the inherent automaticity of the bowel's smooth muscle

The Parasympathetic Nervous System
- Increases upper GI tract motility
- Enhances colonic motility
- Stimulation is provided by the action of the vagus nerve, which innervates proximal to mid. transverse colon, and by the splanchnic nerves (pelvic nerve), which originate from the S2–S4 region, which innervate the descending colon and rectal region

The Sympathetic Nervous System
- Stimulation inhibits colonic contractions, and relaxes the internal anal sphincter favoring the function of storage
- Innervation projects through the hypogastric nerve via superior mesenteric, inferior mesenteric, and celiac ganglia

The Somatic Nervous System
- Increases external anal sphincter tone to promote continence
- The external sphincter (EAS) consists of a circular band of striated muscle that is part of the pelvic floor

Anal Region

The Internal Anal Sphincter
- Composed of smooth muscle under the influence of the sympathetic system (T11–L2)
- Surrounds the anus proximally.
- In patients without SCI the sphincter normally relaxes with filling of the rectum.

The External Anal Sphincter
- Composed of skeletal muscle
- Helps to maintain continence by increasing its tone
- It acts under volitional control, learned by maturation, and reflex activity.
- It is innervated by the pudendal nerve (roots S2–S4). Higher cortical centers and the pontine defecation center send stimulus for EAS relaxation, allowing defecation.

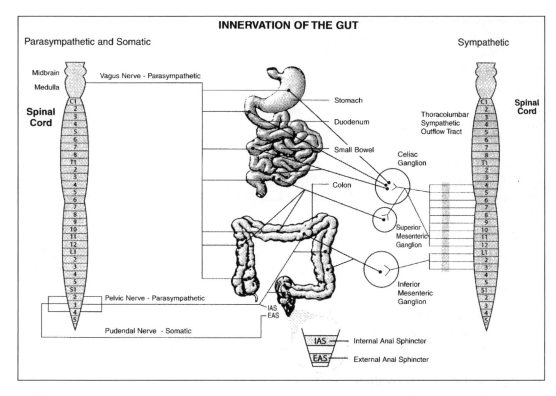

INNERVATION OF THE GUT

Parasympathetic and Somatic

Sympathetic

FIGURE 7–33. Innervation of the Gut. (From Nesathurai S. The Rehabilitation of People with Spinal Cord Injury: A House Officer's Guide. © Boston Medical Center for the New England Regional Spinal Cord Injury Center. Boston, MA: Arbuckle Academic Publishers, with permission).

Storage and Defecation in the Neurologically Intact Individual

Storage
- The internal anal sphincter, is sympathetically activated (T11–L2) allowing for relaxation This occurs with filling of the rectum in patients without SCI
- External anal sphincter (EAS) tone increases, secondary to spinal cord reflexes and modulated action of higher cortical regions, maintaining continence

Defecation
- Rectosigmoid distention causes reflex internal anal sphincter relaxation
- Volitional cortical activity sends signal to pontine defecation center. Volitional contraction of the levator ani muscle occurs, opening the proximal canal, relaxing the external anal sphincter and puborectalis muscles
- Reflexive rectal propulsive contractions take place resulting in expulsion of the stool bolus

Defecation in the Spinal Cord Injured Patient

Upper Motor Neuron Lesions (Hyperreflexic Bowel)
- Cortical control is disrupted, with decreased ability to sense the urge to defecate
- EAS cannot be voluntarily relaxed and pelvic floor muscles become spastic. However, nerve connections between the spinal cord and colon, as well as the myenteric (Auerbach's) plexus remain intact and the stool can be propelled by reflex activity.

Lower Motor Neuron Lesions (Areflexic Bowel)
- Spinal shock or lesion below conus medullaris
- Reflex defecation is absent

• Myenteric (Auerbach's) plexus coordinates the movement of stool, but movement is slow
• Overall, constipation may result (most common result)
Note: Attenuated or absent external anal sphincter contractions may result in fecal smearing or fecal incontinence

📖 In SCI the GI system can be affected by loss of sympathetic and parasympathetic input at the transverse and descending colon, resulting in decreased fecal movement. In SCI, fecal impaction and constipation is the most common complication during recovery.
To help with defecation, the physician may take advantage of two reflexes:

📖 *The Gastrocolic Reflex*
Increased colonic activity occurs in the first 30 to 60 minutes after a meal (usually within 15 minutes). Therefore, place the SCI patient on the commode within one hour subsequent to a meal.

📖 *The Anorectal Reflex (Rectocolic Reflex)*
Occurs when the rectal contents stretch the bowel wall reflexively, relaxing the internal anal sphincter. Suppositories and digestive stimulation cause the bowel wall to stretch and take advantage of this reflex.
Note this reflex
Can be manipulated by digital stimulation of the rectum.
Digital stimulation is accomplished by gently inserting a lubricated finger into the rectum, and slowly moving the digit in a clockwise manner.

Management of Bowel Dysfunction in SCI

Acute Phase

📖 **Gastric Atony and Ileus**
• After a significant SCI, the patient is at high risk for the development of gastric *Atony* and *Ileus*, which may cause vomiting and aspiration
• Stomach decompression by nasogastric tube should be considered in all acutely SCI patients.
• The ileus onset can be delayed for 24–48 hrs.
• The ileus usually lasts from 3–4 days up to 7 days.

Gastric Atony and Ileus (or Adynamic Ileus) occurs in 63% of patients with SCI
• Results from spinal shock and reflex depression.

   Management
   – NG suction to prevent GI dilation and respiratory compromise
   – IV fluids
   – Abdominal Massage—TENS to stimulate peristalsis of gut
   – Injections of neostigmine methylsulfate (Prostigmine) 3–5 hrs.
   – As soon as bowel sounds appear, start clear liquid diet
   – If persists—may use Reglan

Chronic Phase
• **Colonic distention:** problems with small bowel motility and gastric emptying
• **Pseudo obstruction:** no evidence of obstruction on radiographic studies.
• Abdominal distention, nausea, vomiting, constipation.
• **Secondary causes:** electrolyte imbalance and medications (narcotics, anticholinergics)

Management
- NG suction
- Remove offending agent
- If cecum is dilated >12 cm., surgical decompression or colonoscopy

Constipation

Long-Term Management
- Defecation done using bedside commode (sitting facilitates emptying)
- Maintain adequate fluid intake, medications that decrease bowel motility such as narcotics, tricyclic agents, and anticholinergics should be minimized

Diet: high fiber

Meds

Bulk Cathartics: promotes evacuation by retaining or pulling H_2O into colon
- Metamucil®: dietary fiber increase

Irritants
- Castor oil, irritates bowel—AVOID castor oil

Fecal Softener
- Colace®: increases fluid accumulation in GI tract, AVOID Peri-Colace®—causes cramping

Oral Stimulants
- Senokot®: stimulates peristalsis by acting on Auerbach's plexus

Suppositories: placed high against rectal wall
- Glycerine: draws water into stool/stretches rectal wall
- Dulcolax®: stimulates peristalsis. Stimulates sensory nerve endings

Bowel Program

Initially Aims for Bowel Movement Daily

Surgical Intervention—Bowel diversion done when incontinence becomes a problem

Bowel Program consists of:
- Glycerin supp. (or Dulcolax®)
- Encourage patient to have BM at same time QD
- Use Gastrocolic Reflex—Q1hr post breakfast or dinner

If meds. are used, start with:
1. Dulcolax® Q daily after meal - dinner or breakfast
2. Stool softener (Colace®): 100 mg. TID
3. Senokot®: PO q daily at noon

(Spasticity of external anal sphincter may signify interference with bowel care) complications of neurogenic bowel:

Fecal Incontinence: Skin breakdown, ulcerations, UTI

Fecal Impaction: Autonomic hyperreflexia

Must use Lidocaine® Gel during digital extraction

📖 Anticholinergic meds used for failure-to-store bladder can cause severe constipation

Bowel dysfunction affects the patient's community integration—socially, vocationally and psychologically

Other Gastrointestinal Complications

Gastroesophageal reflux
- Avoid prolonged recumbency; elevate the head of the bed
- Avoid smoking
- Avoid medications: Ca^+ channel blockers, Valium®, nitrates, anticholinergics

Treatment:
Provide antacids for mild to moderate symptoms:
H_2 antagonists, Metoclopramide 10 mg tid, Omeprazole 20 mg QD

Gastroesophageal bleeding
- Most frequently secondary to perforating and bleeding ulcers
- Stress ulcers secondary to interruption of sympathetic vasoconstrictors (vasodilatation and mucosal hemorrhage)
- Steroid use
- Increased gastric secretion

Treatment:
Provide prophylaxis with:
- Antacids
- H_2 blockers—Cimetidine, Ranitidine, Famotidine
- Sucralfate—stimulates local prostaglandin synthesis

Endoscopy is the diagnostic method of choice
With active GI bleeding—maintain BP, correct coagulation deficits, consult GI/Surgical service

Cholecystitis
- Most common cause of emergency abdominal surgery in SCI patients
- Increased risk: 3x > in SCI
- Possible causes: abnormal gallbladder motility in lesions above T10, abnormal biliary secretion, abnormal enterohepatic circulation

Treatment:
Observe, May opt for surgical removal or dissolution

Pancreatitis
- Most common in the first month post injury.
- May be related to steroid use—increased viscosity of pancreatic secretions
- May suspect when adynamic ileus doesn't improve.

Evaluate
- Radiographs
- CT
- Ultrasonogram
- Labs: amylase, lipase

📖 Superior Mesenteric Artery (SMA) Syndrome
Condition in which the third portion of the duodenum is intermittently compressed by overlying SMA resulting in GI obstruction (Figure 7–34) (Roth, 1991)

Predisposing factors include:
- Rapid weight loss (decrease in protective fatty layer)
- Prolonged supine position
- Spinal orthosis
- Flaccid abdominal wall causes hyperextension of the back

Exacerbated by:
- Supine positioning
- Tetraplegic patient with abdominal and cervical orthosis

Symptoms:
- Postprandial nausea and vomiting
- Bloating
- Abdominal pain

Diagnosis:
UGI Series: demonstrates abrupt duodenal obstruction to barium flow

Treatment:

Conservative
- Eat small, frequent meals in an upright position
- Lie in the left lateral decubitus position after eating
- Metoclopramide (Reglan®): stimulates motility of UGI tract

Rarely requires surgery
- If conservative treatment fails, surgical duodenojejunostomy (DJ ostomy)

Remember:
Any condition that decreases the normal distance between the SMA and aorta (weight loss, supine position, halo, flaccid abdominal wall) may result in compression of the duodenum described as the nutcracker effect

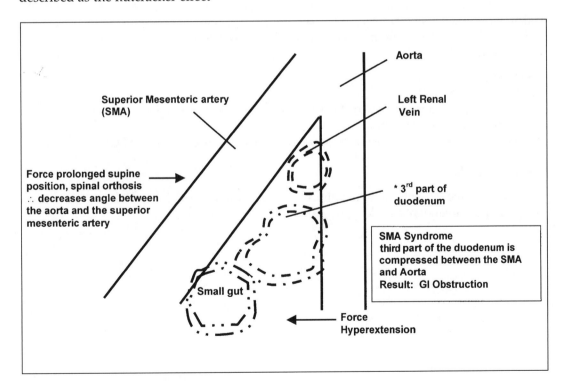

FIGURE 7–34. Lateral view through duodenum and left renal vein.

📖 METABOLIC COMPLICATIONS

Hypercalciuria

Immobilization, decreased weight bearing promotes bone resorption.
Patients become hypercalciuric—this may continue for 18 months.
Vitamin D, parathyroid hormone are not involved in the process.

Hypercalcemia

Patients with hypercalciuria can, in rare cases, develop hypercalcemia
Symptoms: nausea, vomiting, dehydration, decreased renal function, decreased mental status, abdominal discomfort, anorexia, malaise
Symptoms of hypercalcemia can be remembered with the mnemonic *stones, bones, and abdominal groans.*
Patients are most commonly young tetraplegic males.

Treatment: (Merli, 1984)
- Hydration—IV normal saline solution, furosemide
- Mobilize the patient: tilt table, weight bearing activities
- Decrease GI absorption of calcium: give steroids, decrease vitamin D
- Didronel®, Calcitonin

Osteoporosis

Secondary to disuse—localizes below the level of the lesion
Calcium excretion also increased (increased bone resorption)
Approx. 22% bone loss 3 months post injury (Claus-Walker, 1975)
Increased risk of fracture

Treatment
- Weight bearing
- FES cycling—demonstrated to decrease the rate of bone resorption in acute SCI, effect remains after discontinuation
- Pharmacologic agents have not been proven to reduce osteoporosis in SCI.

Hyperglycemia

Up to 70% of the patients show insulin resistance, with abnormal response to glucose load.
Rarely require treatment (Duckworth, 1983)

MUSCULOSKELETAL COMPLICATIONS

📖 Upper Extremity Problems

Shoulder is the most commonly affected joint. Frequently secondary to weight bearing and overuse.

Causes
- Impingement syndrome
- Overuse
- DJD
- Rotator cuff tear/bicipital tendinitis
- Subacromial bursitis
- Capsulitis
- Myofascial pain
- Disuse
- Cervical radiculopathy

Diagnosis
- Consider possible causes such as heterotopic ossification, syrinx
- Perform complete physical exam, including functional assessment, ROM, flexibility, and sensation

Treatment
- Rest, pharmacotherapy for pain treatment
- Compensatory techniques to be used for daily function
- Treat the condition
- Educate the patient regarding posture, weight bearing

Compression neuropathies
Have been noted to increase with the length of time from injury.
27% incidence of carpal tunnel syndrome in SCI patients seen 1–10 years post-injury
54% incidence of carpal tunnel syndrome in SCI patients seen 11–30 years post-injury
90% incidence of carpal tunnel syndrome in SCI patients seen more than 31 years post-injury
(Ditunno, 1992)

PULMONARY COMPLICATIONS OF SCI AND MANAGEMENT

Incidence

Respiratory complications occur in 50% of patients. During the first month post injury, if the initial rehabilitation period is included, the incidence increased to 67% of SCI patients. Atelectasis/pneumonia have an onset within the first 24 days post injury

Pulmonary complications are more common in high cervical injuries (C1—C4)
The *most frequent complications* are pneumonia, atelectasis, and ventilatory failure.
In low cervical (C5—C8) and thoracic (T11—T12) complications are equally frequent.
Thoracic injuries present with: *pleural effusion, atelectasis, pneumothorax, hemothorax, or both.*
(Fishburn, 1990; Jackson, 1994; Langis, 1992)

Pulmonary Dysfunction: Occurs for several reasons following SCI

1. Paralysis of some or all respiratory muscles to varying degrees
2. Loss of ability to cough secondary to varying levels of abdominal muscle paralysis
3. Injury to chest—e.g. rib fracture
4. Pulmonary injury—e.g. lung contusion

Predisposing Factors for Pulmonary Complications Include
Older Age
Obesity—restrictive respiratory deficits
Hx—COPD
Hx—Smoking

📖 *Pneumonia is the leading cause of death among long-term SCI patients.*
Patients tend to retain secretions in the lower lung fields due to:
• Difficulty in achieving postural drainage positions during the acute SCI period
• Altered ventilatory pattern after SCI (reduced airflow to lower lobes leads to atelectasis)
• Decreased ability to clear secretions independently, decreased effective cough

Left-sided respiratory complications are more common among hospitalized SCI patients. This is due to the following:
– The left mainstem bronchus takes off as a 40°–50° angle from vertical, making routine suctioning more difficult.
– In addition to this, there is a tendency to retain secretions in the lower fields.

Respiratory function may be affected to different degrees depending on the level of injury.

Pulmonary Compromise Related to Level of Injury

• Head trauma: May knock out respiratory drive
• Lesions above C3 (and incomplete lesions initially):
  – Initially they require ventilatory support
  – Later they will fall into two groups
  1. No damage to phrenic nucleus
  2. Damage to phrenic nucleus

No Damage to Phrenic Nucleus	Damage to Phrenic Nucleus
• C3,4,5	• C3,4,5
• Determined by EMG of phrenic nerve	• Determined by EMG of phrenic nerve
• Can stimulate phrenic nerve nucleus therefore, the patient will benefit from phrenic pacing (i.e., C1,2, and incomplete lesions)	• Cannot stimulate phrenic nerve nucleus, therefore, will not benefit from phrenic pacing (i.e., lesions of phrenic nucleus causing irreparable damage*) *Continue to require ventilatory support* *Note: Intercostal nerve grafts are being attempted

EMG of diaphragm is necessary to rule out damage to phrenic nerve nucleus

- C3: Respiratory failure secondary to disruption of diaphragmatic innervation, requiring mechanical ventilation
- C4: Generally the highest level of injury at which spontaneous ventilation can be sustained
- Injuries above C8: Loss of all abdominal and intercostal muscles, impairment of inspiration and expiration
- T1 through T5: Intercostal volitional function is lost
- T5 through T12: Progressive loss of abdominal motor function, impairing forceful expiration or cough
- Injuries below T12: Few complications if there is lung injury (e.g. trauma) otherwise, no respiratory dysfunction

Phrenic Pacing (Lee, 1989)

- Phrenic pacing has reduced the need for mechanical ventilation in tetraplegic patients with respiratory failure since its introduction in 1972
- The technique involves the electrical stimulation of intact phrenic nerves via surgically implanted electrodes to contract the diaphragm
- Induces artificial ventilation through electric stimulation of the phrenic nerve, which causes the diaphragm to contract
- Used successfully in patients with COPD, central hypoventilation, and high tetraplegia
- Treatment option in patients with respiratory paralysis after cervical injury above the origin of the phrenic neurons
- Option in patients who do not have significant impairment of the phrenic nerves, lungs, or diaphragm

📖 Contraindications to Phrenic Pacing
- Denervated diaphragm (determined in EMG)
- Denervated—nonviable anterior horn cells C3, C4, C5
- Placement of phrenic pacer prior to 6 months post injury is contraindicated
  From 0–6 months–the chest is too FLAIL and flaccid
  You need some rigidity of chest wall to allow pacer to work
- Significant lung impairment

Major Complications of Phrenic Pacemaker

📖 Signs of Failure of Pacemaker
1. Sharp chest pain
2. SOB—Shortness of Breath
3. Absence of breath
4. Erratic pacing
5. Must maintain adequate ventilation via manual resuscitation bag

📖 Causes of Phrenic Pacing Failure
1. Diaphragmatic failure—due to overly aggressive pacing schedule
2. Infection of lung and/or phrenic nerve
3. Meds: including sedatives, tranquilizers, and narcotics
4. Upper airway obstruction—tracheal aspiration
5. Phrenic nerve damage from overstimulation or surgery

📖 Benefits of Phrenic Pacing
- Increased arterial oxygenation despite decreased alveolar ventilation
- Longer survival in patients with SCI
- Increased daily function secondary to conditioning of the diaphragm from nocturnal pacing

Physiology of Lung:

Inspiratory Muscles	**Expiratory Muscles**
• Accessory muscles • Diaphragm—main respiratory muscle, main muscle during quiet breathing (75% of volume change) Contracts at inspiration, relaxes at expiration • External intercostals	• Abdominal muscles—primarily active during forceful expiration and in producing cough (contract); push the relaxed diaphgram toward the chest cavity • Internal intercostals

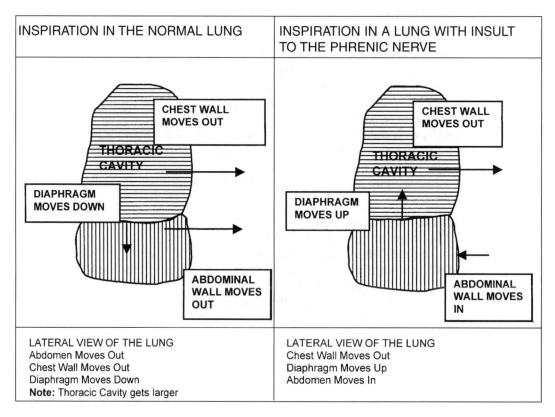

FIGURE 7–35. Inspiration in the Normal Lung and in a Lung with Insult to Phrenic Nerve

Pulmonary Function In SCI—Restrictive Respiratory Changes (Langis, 1992)

- *Forced Vital Capacity* (FVC) during the acute phase of cervical injury is noted to decrease 24%–31% when compared to the normal values secondary to paradoxical respirations
- With development of intercostal and abdominal spasticity *FVC can improve to 50–60%* of predicted normal value
- Tetraplegics develop *restrictive lung patterns*
  All volumes shrink (except residual volume)
  If VC < 1 liter: consider ventilation mechanically
  If VC < 600: must have ventilation mechanically
  If VC > 1.5 get off ventilator
- Signs of impending respiratory failure
  Increased respiratory rate with decreased tidal volume
  Decreased FVC < 15 cc/Kg body weight
  Decreased inspiratory force <20 mm H_2O
  Neurological level C3 or higher
  Patient can't count to 15 slowly

Mechanically ventilate when:
VC < 1 liter
📖 ABG show increasing PCO_2 or decreasing PO_2 levels
- PO_2 < 50
- PCO_2 > 50
Severe atelectasis

Prevention of Respiratory Complications
- Use of incentive spirometer
- Monitor CO_2 levels with ABGs
- Monitor vital capacity
- Cough assist—placing the hands on each side of the pts. upper abdomen and applying intermittent pressure, coordinated with the initiation of cough by the patient—helps produce forceful cough
- Suctioning—remember—tracheal suctioning may cause increased vagal tone with SA node suppression and brady-arrhythmia, leading to cardiac arrest (only suction as you withdraw catheter)
- Chest physical therapy—(see pulmonary chapter)
- Strengthening of pectoralis major muscle, clavicular portion, in tetraplegic patients
- Glossopharyngeal breathing—stroking maneuver to force air into the lungs by the use of the lips, soft palate, mouth, tongue, pharynx, and larynx, followed by passive exhalation.
- Pneumobelt—helps with exhalation. Inflatable, compresses the abdominal wall, diaphragm rises, and active respiration is produced.

HETEROTOPIC OSSIFICATION

Definition
Formation of mature lamellar bone indistinguishable from normal bone in soft tissues, most frequently deposited around a joint
As bone matures it becomes encapsulated, not connected to periosteum

Causes
- Possibly due to alteration in neuronal control over the differentiation of mesenchymal cells into osteoblasts which form new bone *or*
- A decrease in tissue oxygenation or induces changes in multipotential connective tissue cells in which new bone forms in planes between connective tissue layers
- No definitive explanation established.

Incidence: Heterotopic Ossification (HO) has been reported to occur in 16%–53% of patients following SCI.
Clinically significant HO: (resulting in significant limitation of joint range) affects 10%–20% of SCI patients.
Occurs below the level of neurological injury (only in the area of paralysis, unless other factors are present such as TBI or burn)
⌺ Most common joints involved in SCI (in orderof occurrence): hip/knee/shoulder/elbow

⌺ Onset
1–4 months status post injury most common, but can present after first 6 months

Symptoms: Early clinical findings include heat and soft tissue swelling
Swelling progresses to more localized and firm area over several days, may present as ROM in joint decreases
- Heat
- Localized soft tissue swelling—may look like DVT
- Decreased ROM of a joint
- Joint erythema/joint effusion
- Low grade fever

Risk Factors
- Spasticity
- Completeness of injuries
- Trauma or prior surgery to joint
- Age
- Pressure ulcer in proximity of joint

Diagnosis: Can be seen one week from onset in static bone scan or/triple phase bone scan precedes X-ray by at least 7–10 days
Plain film detects HO in 7–10 days after clinical signs are observed
Bone Scan returns to normal as HO matures in 6–18 months post injury
Serum Alkaline Phosphatase: Increases at 2 weeks—exceeds normal levels at 3 weeks—peaks at 10 weeks—returns to normal after HO matures
Not specific for HO

Treatment:
- ⌺ Didronel® (etidronate disodium): 20 mg/Kg/day for 2 weeks then 10 mg/Kg/day for 10 weeks
Does not change overall incidence, but less HO is laid down overall
- Indocin®—Not commonly used in acute SCI

- ROM—Maintain function while HO matures—The goal is to maintain functional range. The affected joint should be gently moved through functional range—vigorous force should not be used as this may lead to further ectopic bone formation
- Surgery—Used when HO severely limits ROM impairing function—should only be planned after bone is mature: 12–18 months post injury. Bone scan must be back to baseline and alkaline phosphatase should be back to normal

Complications
Peripheral nerve entrapment
Decreased ROM/loss of function/ankylosing
HO overlying a bony prominence will directly predispose to pressure ulcer/skin breakdown secondary to poor positioning

DEEP VENOUS THROMBOEMBOLISM (DVT)/ PULMONARY EMBOLISM (PE) IN SCI

Deep Venous Thrombosis (DVT)

Predisposing Factors
Virchow's Triad: Venous stasis/intimal injury/hypercoagulability
LE fractures
Obesity
Hx of previous DVT
DM
Arterial vascular disease
Immobility
Malignancy

Incidence
Ranges 47%–100%
 – Varies Widely depending on the method of detection and number of cases evaluated in the study
More common in neurologically complete patients
More common in tetraplegic patients
10 times more frequent in plegic leg
20% of calf vein thrombi extend proximally

Onset
Most common during first 2 weeks after SCI
Greatest incidence decreases after 8–12 weeks post SCI

Diagnosis
Venogram is the Gold Standard
Venous Doppler is used as a screening test for lower extremity DVTs
Impedance Plethysmography—accurate in assessment of DVTs above the calf
Sensitivity—95%, Specificity—98%
Used to look for occlusions in the thigh, place cuff around the thigh and listen for flow

Complications: 📖 Pulmonary Embolism (PE) leading cause of death in acute LCI

Pulmonary Embolism (Fluter, 1993; Goldhaber, 1998)

Symptoms
Pleuritic chest pain
Dyspnea

Fever, hemoptysis
Tachycardia
Hypoxemia

Physical Examination
1. Increased S2 sound: severe pulmonary HTN → cor pulmonale. → Right heart failure
2. Dullness at bases of lungs

Incidence
1%–7% of SCI patients (Hull)

Diagnosis (PE)
EKG: R. Axis Deviation
Right Bundle Branch Block (RBBB):—if massive PE
ABG:—decreased PO_2 (PO_2 drops severely)
Chest X-ray:
   wedge shaped opacity
   fluid
   vascularity
Perfusion lung scan: VQ mismatched
📖 *Gold Standard:* Pulmonary arteriogram

Treatment (PE)
O_2
Heparin
Vasopressor to treat shock

Surgical Treatment
Embolectomy

Other Complications of DVT

- **Postphlebitic syndrome (late complication of DVT)**
  - distal venous hypertension (residual obstruction of outflow—incompetent valve)
  - swelling
  - exercise induced pain
  - pigmentation
  - ulceration
  - long standing autonomic dysreflexia

Prophylaxis Treatment and Prevention of DVT

Prophylaxis for DVT (Merli, 1988)
- External intermittent pneumatic compression devices
  - increases LE venous return
  - decreases stasis and stimulates fibrinolysis
  - if delays > 72 hours—need to do duplex prior to initiation
- Enoxaparin—low molecular weight heparin (LMWH)
  - Dose 30 mg SQ BID
  - *Best intervention to prevent DVT if no contraindications*
  - Not used in patients with active bleeding, TBI or coagulopathy
- Thigh-high graded compression stockings (TEDS)—alone, not prophylaxis
- Coumadin®
- Minidose subcutaneous unfractionated Heparin
- Greenfield filter (may be indicated in selected cases, high risk, or failed prophylaxis)

Treatment DVT:
- Heparin—if not contraindicated
  - standard: 5,000 units IV bolus; followed by a constant infusion of 1,000 units/ (25,000 units in 250 cc D5W at 10 cc/hr)
  - maintain PTT 1.5-2 times normal
  - at least 5–10 days of anticoagulant prior to mobilization
- Warfarin started once PTT therapeutic (approximately three days after Heparin started); takes 5 days to load; target INR 3.0

  Coumadin for 3 months in case with DVT

  Coumadin for 3–6 months in case w/PE

  (Note: Heparin can be discontinued once coumadin is 1/2 times normal for 48 hrs.)
- No ROM in involved extremity. With small popliteal clots, patients may transfer to bedside chair in 1–2 days. If clot is in proximal veins or with PE, immobilization 5–10 days.
- If anticoagulation is contraindicated, then an IVC filter is necessary

Prevention:
- Recommended that patients receive both a method of mechanical prophylaxis as well as anticoagulant prophylaxis
- Pneumatic compression stockings or device should be applied to the legs of all patients during the first two weeks following injury

  If this is delayed for more than 72 hours after injury, test to exclude the presence of clots should be performed
- Anticoagulant prophylaxis—LMW heparin or adjusted unfractionated heparin should be initiated within 72 hours after injury if there is no hemorrhage or risk of bleeding

  LMWH: 30 SQ BID

▢ Functional Electrical Stimulation (FES) in SCI has two general uses

- As exercise to avoid complications of muscle inactivity
- As a means of producing extremity motion for functional activities

  ▢ *FES can be used to*
  - Provide a cardiovascular conditioning program
  - Increase muscle bulk strength and endurance
  - Attempt to decrease risk of DVT
  - Produce extremity motion for standing and ambulation

■

▢ PAIN IN THE SCI PATIENT

Incidence of chronic pain in SCI population is estimated between 20%–50%

Pain may be musculoskeletal, neuropathic, or visceral

MUSCULOSKELETAL PAIN

Upper Extremity Pain: common in the SCI patient

Patients with SCI load joints that do not normally bear weight (shoulder, elbow, wrist)

This predisposes them to painful UE conditions

These conditions include
- Carpal tunnel syndrome (which is present in up to 90% of SCI pts. at 31 years post injury)
- Rotator cuff tendonitis
- Rotator cuff tears
- Subacromial bursitis

- Cervical radiculopathy
- Lateral epicondylitis
- Medial epicondylitis
- Myofascial pain

Less common causes of UE discomfort include
- Syringomyelia
- Heterotopic ossification
- Angina
- Aortic dissection
- Pancoast tumor

📖 **Syringomyelia: posttraumatic cystic myelopathy (Dworkin, 1985; Umbach and Halpern, 1991; Williams, 1992)**
- The pathogenesis of posttraumatic syringomyelia is not entirely understood. Cavitation of the spinal cord usually occurs at the level of the initial injury. Cavity formation may be secondary to liquefaction of the spinal cord or from central hematoma present at the initial injury. The lesion usually progresses in a cephalad direction. As the lesion progresses and compromises more nerve fibers, symptoms may become more apparent.
- Occurs in .3%–3.2% of the SCI population and is the most common cause of progressive myelopathy after SCI.
- It can occur 2–34 months post injury, and even much later
- It may present as pain and numbness; motor weakness is often associated with sensory loss
- It occurs more frequently with thoracic and lumbar regions
- Extension of the cavity can be upward or downward (normally cephalad)
- MRI is the most accurate diagnostic technique
- Treatment is surgical and drainage can be accomplished with a shunt to the subarachnoid space or peritoneum. Motor weakness and pain have a good prognosis with surgical treatments.

Charcot Spine

Charcot Joints: A destructive arthropathy of joints, with impaired pain perception or position sense. Loss of sensation of deep pain or of proprioception affects the joints normal protective reflexes, often allowing trauma (especially repeated minor episodes) and small periarticular fractures to pass unrecognized.

Charcot Spine: Spinal trauma and analgesia below the level of injury makes SCI patients particularly prone to insensate joint destruction. Joints themselves can be a source of pain that triggers autonomic dysreflexia or a nidus of infection after hematogenous spread.

NEUROPATHIC PAIN

Neuropathic pain may be of central or peripheral origin. Patients will complain of a burning or shooting pain. The discomfort may involve the abdomen, rectum, or lower extremity. It may exacerbated by other noxious stimuli, including urinary tract infections, renal stone, HO, etc. Neuropathic pain is more common with incomplete lesions.
Neuropathic pain requires complete assessment.

VISCERAL PAIN

Evaluation of acute abdominal pathology in SCI patients with potentially impaired sensation can be very difficult. The typical clinical features may be absent. Pain, when present, may be atypical in quality and location. Increased spasticity and a general feeling of unwellness may be the only manifestations of a surgical emergency.

Spasticity

Spasticity presents as an abnormality of muscle tone and is common in SCI individuals. It becomes clinically apparent as spinal shock resolves. (See chapter on Spasticity.)

▪

PRESSURE ULCERS

25%–40% of SCI patients develop pressure ulcers at some time during their life. Pressure ulcers are classified according to the extent of tissue damage.

📖 SHEA CLASSIFICATION I–IV

I	Superficial epidermis and dermal layers
II	Extends to adipose tissue
III	Full thickness skin defect down to and including muscle
IV	Destruction down to bone and or joint structures

GRADE-DANIEL CLASSIFICATION (FIGURE 7–36)

Less commonly used classification:

Levels of ulceration	1	2	3	4	5
	Skin erythema or induration	Superficial ulceration advances into dermis	Extends into subcutaneous fat	Extends through muscle down to bone	Ulcer extends into bone/jt capsule, or body cavity

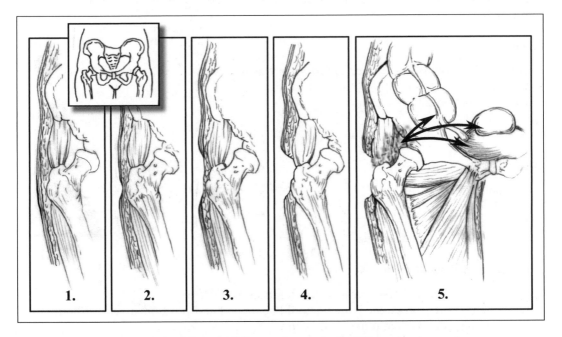

FIGURE 7–36. Levels of ulceration graded according to depth of tissue involvement

📖 MECHANISM OF DEVELOPING A PRESSURE ULCER

Local soft tissue ischemia results due to prolonged pressure over bony prominences, that exceed supra capillary pressure (70mm Hg)

1. Ischemia: lack of blood supply to the tissue
 – Frequently associated with hyperemia in the surrounding tissue
 – Increased local O2 consumption occurs

2. Pressure
 – Prolonged pressure over bony prominences, exceeding supracapillary pressure (70 mm Hg pressure continuously for 2 hours) results in occlusion of the microvessels of the dermis
 – Occlusion of the microvessels occurs when the force exerted on the vessel wall is greater than the intraarterial pressure
 – This results in immediate epidermal ischemia
 Ischemia causes hyperemia of the surrounding tissue

📖 **Tissues vary with regard to their sensitivity to pressure**
  Muscle is more sensitive to pressure, skin is more resistant to pressure

Important Facts
📖 **Note: 70 mm Hg pressure continuously × 2 hour: results in tissue damage**

Muscle is more susceptible to pressure ischemia than skin

3 📖 Friction (shearing force):
 – Removes corpus striatum (stratum corneum) of the skin
 – Friction mechanically separates the epidermis immediately above the basal cells
 – Friction is a factor in the pathogenesis since it applies mechanical forces to the epidermis

Common Locations of Pressure Ulcers (Figure 7–37)

During the *acute* period after SCI the most common locations of ulcers are due to the patient lying supine:
#1 Sacrum
#2 Heels

In *chronic* SCI patients the locations of ulcers are as follows:
Ischial decubitus (30 %)
Greater trochanter (20%)
Sacrum (15%)
Heels (10%)

Risk Factors

• Immobility
• Incontinence
• Lack of sensation
• Altered level on consciousness

Prevention of Pressure Ulcers

• Minimize extrinsic factors—pressure, maceration, and friction
• Decrease pressure forces, the patient should be turned and positioned every 2 hours
• Pressure relief every 30 minutes when sitting
• Proper cushioning and wheelchair seating (see wheelchairs)
• WC pushups

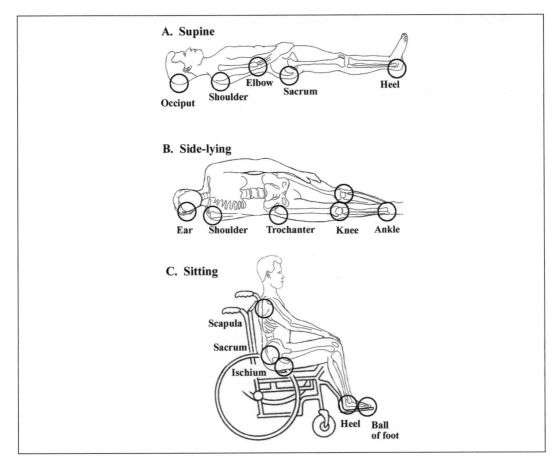

FIGURE 7–37. Common locations of pressure ulcers

Treatment

- Prevention of pressure ulcers should always be the first line of defense
- Once a lesion has developed, however, rational treatment should be prescribed to reduce the progression of the ulcer; the extrinsic factors that contributed to the formation of the ulcer should be identified and treated
- In general, healing will be promoted if the wound remains clean, moist, and debrided—a noninfected wound will also promote healing.

TABLE 7-6. Treatment: According to Shea Classification

Grade	I	II	III	IV
Depth of Ulcer	**Superficial epidermis** and dermal layers	**Extends to adipose** tissue	**Full thickness defect** to and including muscle	**Destruction down** to bone and/or joint structures
Treatment	Alteration of mattress Wet to dry dressing	Sharp/enzymatic debridement of ulcer	Sharp/enzymatic debridement of ulcer	Surgery/surgical consultation
Alternative Treatment		Possible surgical consultation	Surgical consultation	

📖 POST OP MANAGEMENT OF SACRAL DECUBITUS GRAFTING

- Positioning—Patient should be prone for 2–4 weeks
  If this is not tolerated, pressure relief bed should be prescribed to prevent iatrogenic pressure.
- Control the patient's spasticity.
- Antibiotic treatment—Used to address issues of infection
- Bowel and bladder management—To avoid contamination of the wound

Pressure Ulcer Complications

- Osteomyelitis
- Dehydration

REFERENCES

American Spinal Injury Association. *International Standards for Neurological and Functional Classification of Spinal Cord Injury.* ASIA/IMSOP: 1996.

Bohlmann HH. Acute fractures and dislocations of the cervical spine: An analysis of three hundred hospitalized patients and review of literature. *J Bone Joint Surg Am.* 1979; 61(8): 1119–1142.

Bors E., Comarr AE. Neurologic Disturbance of Sexual Dysfunction with Special Reference to 529 Patients with Spinal Cord Injury. *Urol Surv* 1960;10:191-222.

Braddom RL, Rocco JF. Autonomic dysreflexia: A survey of current treatment. *Am J Phys Med Rehabil* 1991; 70: 234–241.

Claus-Walker J, Spencer WA, Carter RE, Halstead LS, Meier RH 3rd, Campos RJ. Bone metabolism in quadriplegia: Dissociation between calciuria and hydroxprolimiria. *Arch Phys Med Rehabil* 1975; 56:327–332.

Corbett JL, Frankel HL, Harris PJ. Cardiovascular reflex responses to cutaneous and visceral stimuli in spinal man. *J Physiol* 1971 June; 215(2):395–401.

Ditunno JF Jr, Stover SL, Freed MM, Ann JH. *Motor recovery of the upper extremities in traumatic quadriplegia: a multicenter study.* Arch Phys Med Rehabil 1992;May 73 (5): 431–436.

Duckworth WC, Jallepalli P, Solomon SS. Glucose intolerance in spinal cord injury. *Arch Phys Med Rehabil* 1983; 64:107–110.

Dworkin GE, Stass WE Jr. Post-traumatic syringomyelia. *Arch Phys Med Rehabil* 1985; 66:329–331.

Fishburn MJ, Marino RJ, Ditunno JF Jr. Atelectasis and pneumonia in acute spinal cord injury. *Arch Phys Med Rehabil* 1990; 71:197–200.

Fluter GG. Pulmonary embolism presenting as supraventricular tachycardia in paraplegia: A case report. *Arch Phys Med Rehabil* 1993; 74:1208–1210.

Goldhaber SZ. Pulmonary embolism. *N Engl J Med.* 1998; 339:93–104.

Hoppenfeld S. *Orthopaedic Neurology: A Diagnostic Approach to Neurologic Levels.* J.B. Lippincott Co. Philadelphia, 1977.

Jackson AB, et al. Incidence of respiratory complications following spinal cord injury. *Arch Phys Med Rehabil* 1994 Mar; 75 (3): 270–275.

Kirshblum S, O'Connor K. Predicting neurologic recovery in traumatic cervical spinal cord injury. *Arch Phys Med Rehabil* 79; 11: Nov. 1998

Langis Respiratory system in spinal cord injury. *Phys Med Rehab Clin* 1992: NA. 725–40.

Lee MY. Rehabilitation of quadriplegic patients with phrenic nerve pacers. *Arch Phys Med Rehabil* 1989; July; 70 (7); 549–552.

Lindan R, Joiner E, Freehafer AD, Hazel C. Incidence and clinical features of autonomic dysreflexia in patients with spinal cord injury. *Paraplegia* 1980;18:292.

Linsenmeyer TA, Perkash I. Infertility in men with spinal cord injury. *Arch Phys Med Rehabil* 1991 Sept; 72: 747–754.

Maynard FM Jr., Bracken MB, et al. International standards for neurological and functional classification of spinal cord injury patients (revised). *Spinal Cord* 1997; 35: 266–274.

Merli GJ, Herbison GJ. Deep vein thrombosis; prophylaxis in acute spinal cord injury patients. *Arch Phys Med Rehab* 1988; Sept 69 (9): 661–664.

Merli GJ et al. Immobilization hypercalcemia acute spinal cord injury treated with etidronate. *Arch Intern Med* 1984; June 144(6):1286–1288.

Roth EJ, Fenton LL, Gaebler-Spira DJ, Frost FS, Yarkony GM. Superior mesenteric artery syndrome in acute traumatic quadriplegia: Case reports and literature review. *Arch Phys Med Rehabil* 1991; May 72 (6): 417–420.

Roth EJ, Lawler MH, Yarkony GM. Traumatic central cord syndromes: clinical features and functional outcomes. *Arch Phys Med Rehabil* 1990; 71:18–23.

Umbach J, Halpern A. Review article: Postspinal cord injury syringomyelia. *Paraplegia* 1991; 29: 219–221.

Waters RL, Adkins RH, Yakura JS. Definition of complete spinal cord injury. *Paraplegia* 1991; 29:573–581.

Williams B. Post-traumatic syringomyelia. In: Frankel HL (ed). *Handbook of Clinical Neurology* 17 (61) Amsterdam: Elsevier Science Publishers, 1992; 375–398.

RECOMMENDED READING

Bohlmann HH, Ducker TB. Spine and spinal cord injuries. In Rothman RH (ed.). The Spine 3rd ed. Philadelphia: W.B. Saunders Co.; 1992; 973–1011.

Braddom RL. *Physical Medicine and Rehabilitation.* Philadelphia: W.B. Saunders Co.; 1996.

Burke DC, Murray DD. *Handbook of Spinal Cord Medicine.* New York: Raven Press; 1975.

Garrison SJ. *Handbook of Physical Medicine and Rehabilitation Basics.* New York: Lippincott-Raven; 1995.

Hoppenfeld S. *Physical Examination of the Spine and Extremities.* Appleton-Century-Crofts,1976.

International Standards for Neurological and Functional Classification of Spinal Cord Injury. 1996; American Spinal Injury Association. ASIA/IMSOP.

Kotke, FJ, Lehmann JF, eds. *Krusens Handbook of Physical Medicine and Rehabilitation* 4th ed. Philadelphia: W.B. Saunders; 1990.

Mange KC, et al. Course of motor recovery in the zone of partial preservation in spinal cord injury. *Arch Phys Med Rehabil* 1992; May 73 (5): 437–441.

Nesathurai S, ed. *The Rehabilitation of People with Spinal Cord Injury: A house Officer's Guide.* Boston: Arbuckle Academic Publishers; 1999.

O'Young B, Young MA, Stiens SA. *PM&R Secrets.* Philadelphia: Hanley and Belfus Inc.; Mosby, New York: Mosby; 1997.

8

PHYSICAL MODALITIES, THERAPEUTIC EXERCISE, EXTENDED BEDREST, AND AGING EFFECTS

Thomas E. Strax, M.D., Priscila Gonzalez, M.D., and Sara Cuccurullo, M.D.,

■

PHYSICAL MODALITIES

Modalities that use physical energy for their therapeutic effect.
Includes:
- Pressure
- Thermotherapy—Heat and cold
- Hydrotherapy
- Light therapy—ultraviolet radiation, laser
- Electrotherapy
- Manipulation, mobilization, traction, massage, acupuncture

These are used as adjuncts to a therapy program including exercise and patient education

THERMOTHERAPY

- The amount of energy a tissue gains or loses depends on several factors:
  - Nature of the tissue
  - Agent used
  - Duration of exposure
- Temperature has an effect on:
  - **Viscosity**
  - **Nerve conduction**—heat increases nerve conduction velocity; cold decreases it
  - **Blood flow**—heat increases arterial and capillary blood flow; cold decreases blood flow
  - **Collagen extensibility**—heat increases tendon extensibility, collagenase activity is increased; cold decreases enzyme activity
- Temperatures > 45–50°C (113–122 °F) or < 0°C (32 °F) can injure tissue

A. Heat

Therapeutic uses for heat are based on:
- Hyperemia
- Analgesia
- Hyperthermia
- Decreased muscle tone
- Increase in collagen elasticity

Applications for heat therapy

Generally used for chronic process

- Decrease muscle spasms
- Decrease pain (myofascial, low back, neck, post herpetic neuralgia)
- Reduction in joint stiffness, contractures
- Arthritis, collagen vascular diseases
- Chronic inflammation
- Superficial thrombophlebitis

Contraindications for heat therapy

- Ischemia—e.g., arterial insufficiency
- Metabolic requirement of the limbs is increased with the use of heat. (Note: for every 10° increase in skin temperature, there is a 100% increase in metabolic demand.)
- Bleeding disorders (e.g., hemophilia), Hemorrhage—there is an increased arterial and capillary blood flow with heat
- Impaired sensation—e.g., spinal cord injury (SCI) may predispose to burns
- Inability to communicate or respond to pain—e.g., dementia
- Malignancy—May increase tumor growth
- Acute trauma or inflammation—Diffusion across membranes is increased
- 📖 Scar tissue—Elevation of temperature increases the metabolic demand of the tissue. Scar tissue has inadequate vascular supply, and is not able to provide an adequate vascular response when heated, which can lead to ischemic necrosis.
- Edema—Diffusion across membranes is increased
- Atrophic skin
- Poor thermal regulation

📖 The temperature of an object can be altered by

📖 *Convection*

Contact between two surfaces at different temperatures with resultant flow of one past the other. Conveyance of heat in liquids or gases by the movement of heated particles. The flow increases the temperature gradient between the surfaces maximizing heating and cooling. More intense than conduction.

Examples:
Fluidotherapy
Hydrotherapy (whirlpool)
Contrast baths

Conduction

Transfer of heat between two bodies at different temperatures. Movement of heat without movement of conducting body.

Examples:
Hot water
Paraffin
Hot packs (hydrocollator packs)

📖 *Conversive heating*

Nonthermal energy converts to heat in the tissues.

Examples:
Radiant heat (heat lamps)
Shortwave diathermy

Ultrasound
Microwave

Therapeutic Heat Can Be Superficial or Deep

1. Superficial Heat
Maximum tissue temperature is achieved in skin and subcutaneous fat. Used to heat joints with little soft tissue covering (hand, foot), or cause a deeper effect through reflex mechanisms (for relief of muscle spasms)

Convective Agents
- Fluidotherapy
  - Hot air is blown through a container holding fine cellulose particles (bed of beads or corn husks), which produces a warm air-fluid mixture with properties similar to liquid
  - Advantages: massage action of the turbulent solid-gas mixture; freedom to perform ROM activities
  - Good for hands and feet
  - Agitation level and temperature can be controlled. The typical temperature range is 46.1–48.9° C/115–120° F
  - Study performed by Borell and Parker measured temperature in different body areas following 20 minutes of fluidotherapy at 47.8° C/118° F (Borell and Parker 1980)
  - *Results:*
    Peak temperature of hands and joint capsule is 42° C/107.6° F
    Peak temperature of foot and joint capsule is 39.5° C/103.1° F
  - Fluidotherapy should be avoided in infected wounds, and burn precautions should be maintained

- Hydrotherapy
  - External use of water to treat a physical condition. Water can be used to produce convective heating or cooling, massage, and gentle debridement
  - Unit size, water temperature, agitation intensity, and solvent properties can be adjusted to meet treatment goals:
    Whirlpool baths—for partial body immersion
    Hubbard tanks—used for total body immersion
  - The water temperature can be selected depending on the amount of body submerged, patient's health and goals of treatment:
    Whirlpool temperature for   Upper limbs is 37.8–40.6° C (100–105° F)
    Lower limbs is 37.8–38.9° C (100–102° F)
    Hubbard tanks—The temperature should be less than 39° C (102.2° F) to avoid systemic problems (can change core body temperature)
    Mild heating: 36.7–37.2° C (98–98.9° F).
    Vigorous heating: 37.8–38.3° F (100–100.9° F)
    Give treatment for approximately 10 to 20 minutes, depending on the patient's cardiopulmonary tolerance.
  - In general, temperatures from 33–36° C are considered neutral for wounds and burns and are well tolerated
    Contraindications for Hubbard tanks:
    - Patients incontinent of bowel and bladder
    - Skin infections
    - Unstable blood pressure
    - Uncontrolled epilepsy
    - Acute febrile episodes

- Upper respiratory infections
- Tuberculosis
- Multiple sclerosis

> **Be cautious with patients with vital capacity < 1 liter**

– Contrast baths: Distal limbs receive alternating heat and cold in a whirlpool tank to produce reflex hyperemia. Temperatures range from hot 38–44° C or 100.4 to 111° F, and cold 10–18° C or 50–64.4° F

Technique: begin with warm soaks to the extremity, then follow with four cycles of alternating 1–4 minute cold soaks and 4–6 minutes warm soaks

Uses: Rheumatoid arthritis, reflex sympathetic dystrophy, to toughen residual limbs; muscular strains and joint sprains.

Contraindications: small vessel disease caused by diabetes, arteriosclerotic endarteritis or Burger's disease.

Conductive agents

- Hot packs
  - Hydrocollator: canvas bags filled with silicon dioxide immersed in tanks of heated water (74.5° C/166° F)
  - Applied over several layers of insulating towels
  - Heat treatment lasts 30 minutes
  - Lehman (1966): Hot pack to posterior thigh increased temperature to 3.3° C at 1 cm depth, 1.3° C at 2 cm depth
  - Advantages: low cost, minimal maintenance, long life patient acceptance, ease of use
  - Disadvantages: Prolonged superficial heat can produce temporary or permanent skin mottling—erythema abigne. This condition is characterized by reticular pigmentation and telangiectasia.

- Kenny packs—Wool cloths soaked in 60° C water, then spun dried. These cool rapidly, and require repeated applications.

- Heating pads
  - Available as electric pads and pads with circulating heated fluid such as water.
  - Peak temperature is 52° C (125° F)
  - The temperature is maintained at a constant level, no spontaneous cooling
  - If used with moist towels there is a potential risk for electrical shock
  - If the patient lies on the pad there is a potential for burns. This is common in patients with decreased adipose tissue
  - Generally used for periods of 20 minutes

- Paraffin bath
  - Paraffin wax and mineral oil in a 7:1 or 6:1 ratio heated to 52.2–54.4° C (126–130° F)
  - Commonly used in irregular surfaces such as distal extremities
  - Three methods are available for use:
    a. Dipping: most common method. Involves placing the body part to be treated in a paraffin bath, followed by removing it and allowing the paraffin to cool and harden. Approximately 7 to 12 dips are done, followed by wrapping in wax paper or plastic, which is covered by towels or insulated mitts. Application time is 20 to 30 minutes. A decrease in temperature is noted after 15 to 20 minutes post dip

      b. Immersion: serial dips are done forming a thin glove, which is followed by immersion in the paraffin bath for approximately 30 minutes. Provides more vigorous heating than dipping

      c. Brushing: A brush is used to apply paraffin to larger body parts or parts that are difficult to manage with the bath (e.g., ankle)

- Abramson, 1967: Noted a 5.5° C temperature increase in forearm subcutaneous tissue, 2.4° C in Brachioradialis muscle with paraffin use
- Patients have good compliance, and home units are available
- Uses: contractures Rheumatoid arthritis (RA), Scleroderma

Conversive Agents

- 📖 Radiant heat (Infrared lamps)

Energy is absorbed through the skin and converted to superficial heat.

      Distance from the lamp to skin is usually 45–60 cm (18–24 inches), and is applied for 20–0 minutes. Most lamps act as point sources and their heating effectiveness decreases with the square of their distance from the body ($1/r^2$ law).

      Used in patients who cannot tolerate the weight of hot packs

      Precautions: general heat precautions, light sensitivity (dermal photo-aging) and skin drying, photosensitizing medications

2. Deep heat (Diathermy)

Tissue temperature can be increased to a depth of 3–5 cm or more without overheating subcutaneous tissue or skin. Produced by conversion of energy into heat, and may penetrate to deep structures such as ligaments, bones, muscles, and joint capsules.

Includes ultrasound, shortwave diathermy, and microwave diathermy

Ultrasound (US)

- Acoustic vibration with frequencies above the audible range (>20,000 Hz) can produce thermal (heating) and nonthermal (cavitation, acoustic streaming, and standing waves) effects

Thermal effects

- Ultrasound interacts with skin, fat, and muscle during treatment. Heating occurs at all of these tissue as a result of beam attenuation and absorption. Its effect is more pronounced at tissue interfaces where sound transmission discontinuities occur.
- Ultrasound is absorbed and attenuated more in bone, followed by tendon, followed by skin, muscle, and fat.
- Lehman (1967) found that US produces the highest temperature in cancellous bone (spongy bone).
- 📖 Absorption (heating) is greatest at the bone–muscle soft-tissue interface.
- Thermal effects include increased distensibility of collagen fibers.

Nonthermal effects

- Cavitation—produces gas bubbles in a sound field due to turbulence, which, by their forced oscillation and bursting, are capable of disrupting tissue

- Acoustic streaming—unidirectional movement of compressible material or medium due to pressure asymmetries caused by US waves

- Acoustic streaming and cavitation are associated with wound contraction and protein synthesis

- Standing waves—In a stationary US field standing waves produce fixed areas of elevated pressure and rarefaction. They have not been found to have physiological benefits

Ultrasound indications
- Bursitis
- Tendinitis (calcific tendinitis)
- Musculoskeletal pain
- 📖 Degenerative arthritis and contracture (adhesive capsulitis, shoulder periarthritis and hip contracture). Helps to maintain a prolonged stretch and increases ROM
- Subacute trauma
  Less established:
  - Scar tissue (keloids)
  - Postherpetic neuralgic pain
  - Plantar warts

Ultrasound Contraindications
- General heat contraindications
- Near brain, cervical ganglia, spine, laminectomy sites (can cause spinal-cord heating)
- Near the heart, reproductive organs
- 📖 Near pacemakers—may cause thermal or mechanical injury to the pacemaker
- 📖 Near tumors
- Gravid or menstruating uterus
- At infection sites
- On contact lenses, eyes (fluid filled cavity with risk of cavitation and heat damage).
- Skeletal immaturity—open epiphysis can be affected with decreased growth due to thermal injury
- 📖 Total hip arthroplasties with methylmethacrylate or high density polyethylene. These have a high coefficient of absorption, more than soft tissue, and the prosthesis may loosen due to unstable cavitation in the cement. (Lehmann, 1990)
- Arthroplasties—the effect on bony ingrowth arthroplasties is not well defined, for this reason the most prudent course is avoiding US over these areas

Ultrasound precautions
- Avoid intensities over 3 W/cm^2
- Use multiple ports over large joints
- Ultrasound can be used under water but only if water is degassed. This can be achieved by putting it into a container and allowing it to sit overnight.
- Use stroking technique

Ultrasound prescription
- Frequency—📖 Most common 0.8–1.1 MHz
- Intensity—0.5–2.0 W/cm^2. Spatial average intensity is described as the total power output divided by the effective radiating area. World Health Organization (WHO) suggested maximal intensity is 3.0W/cm2.
- 📖 For tendonitis/bursitis the intensity used is 1.2–1.8W/cm^2, or in the 0.5 to 2.0 W/cm^2 range
  - 📖 Generates temperatures up to 46° C/114.8° F in deep tissues. Ultrasound deep heating is superior to microwave and short wave diathermy. In general, 45° C temperature increases will be seen at 8 cm depth. Increased temperature will remain for 2 minutes following US application.
- Duration—5–10 minutes per site – depends on W/cm^2
- Delivery methods—continuous and pulsed
  Continuous—thermal effects (heat production)
  Pulsed—Mainly nonthermal effects, cavitation, media motion, standing waves

- Techniques—direct and indirect
  DIRECT—most common. The applicator is moved slowly over an area of 4 square inches in a circular or longitudinal pattern. Uses a coupling media (gel) to accommodate for impedance inconsistencies.
  INDIRECT—for uneven surfaces (hands and feet). Applicator and body part are immersed in a container of degassed water.
  SPECIALIZED—
  Phonophoresis—A technique that utilizes US to drive medications through the skin, by increasing cell permeability.
  - Frequency—1–2 MHz, delivery method is continuous, or pulsed
  - Intensity—1–3 W/cm^2 for 5 to 7 minutes
  - Medications: Corticosteroids (1% or 10% Hydrocortisone and Dexamethasone) Anesthetics—1% Lidocaine (Xylocaine®)
  - Uses: Tendinitis—Achilles, patellar, bicipital; Tenosynovitis; Epicondylitis (tennis elbow)

Shortwave diathermy (SWD)
  - 📖 Produces deep heating through the conversion of electromagnetic energy (radio waves) to thermal energy
  - Federal Communications Commission (FCC) limits use to 13.56 MHz (22m wavelength), 27.12 MHz (11M), and 40.68 MHz (7.5m)
  - 📖 The most commonly used frequency is 27.12 MHz
  - 📖 Provides deep heat to 4–5 cm depth, therefore is good for deep muscle.
  - The heating pattern produced depends on the type of shortwave unit and water content and electrical properties of the tissue

Shortwave units can be inductive or capacitive

1. *Induction method*—produces high temperatures in water-rich tissues (muscles, skin) via a coiled magnetic field. Applicators in the form of cables or drum. The body acts as a receiver, and eddy currents are induced in the tissues in its field.
  Increases tissue temperature 4–6°C above normal.
- 📖 Indicated when heat to more superficial muscles or joints is desired. Muscle tends to become warmer than fatty tissue

2. *Conduction method* (capacitive applicators)—produce high temperatures in water-poor tissues (fat, bone) with low conductivity, via rapid oscillation of an electrical field. The portion of the body to be treated is placed between two plates to which the shortwave output is applied.
  The body acts as an insulator in a series circuit.
- Indicated for subcutaneous adipose tissue and bone
- Most effective for deeper joints (i.e., hip joint)
- Treatment time is 20–30 minutes
  - 📖 Precise dosing for shortwave diathermy is difficult, and pain perception is used to monitor intensity. The best way to monitor frequency depends on the patient's response to warmth
  - Subcutaneous fat temperature rises to 15° C, 4–6° C increase in muscle at 4–5 cm depth (Lehman, 1968)
  - Terry cloths are used for spacing and to absorb sweat, which is highly conductive and may cause severe local heating

Shortwave indications
- Chronic prostatitis
- Refractory pelvic inflammatory disease
- Myalgia
- Back spasms

Shortwave contraindications
- General heat precautions
- Metal (jewelry, pacemakers, metallic intrauterine devices, surgical implants) are excellent electrical conductors and can potentially cause burns. Water is highly conductive and can have the same effect with resultant severe local heating
- Contact lenses
- Gravid or menstruating uterus
- Skeletal immaturity

Microwave diathermy
- Conversion of electromagnetic energy (microwaves) to thermal energy.
- FCC approved frequencies: 915MHz (33 cm wavelength) and 2456 MHz (12 cm)
- Microwaves do not penetrate tissues as deeply as US or SWD

Microwave indications
- Used to heat superficial muscles and joints, to speed the resolution of hematomas, and for local hyperthermia in cancer patients
- The lower frequency has a higher depth of penetration, and is better for muscle heating

Microwave contraindications
- General heat precautions
- Skeletal immaturity
- Microwave diathermy selectively heats fluid-filled cavities:
  Its use should be avoided in edematous tissue, moist skin, eyes, blisters, and fluid-filled cavities
- Eye protection should be worn by patient and therapist due to risk of cataract formation

Delateur, 1970 noted:
Average temperatures with microwaves at a depth of 1–3 cm. are 41° C/105.8° F.
At frequencies of 915MHz, subcutaneous fat temperatures may increase by 10°–12° C, and muscles at a depth of 3–4 cm. will be heated only 3°–4° C.

Summary of Diathery
Diathermy—Deeper local elevation of temperature within the tissues, produced without overheating subcutaneous tissue or skin. Classified as:

1. **Ultrasound**
2. **Shortwave**
3. **Microwave**

All are forms of heating by conversion

ULTRASOUND	SHORTWAVE	MICROWAVE
– Sound waves	– Radio waves	– Microwaves
– Frequency: 0.8–1.1 MHz	– Frequency: 27.12 MHz	– Frequency: 915–2456 MHz
– Heats at 8 cm depth	– Heats at 4–5 cm depth	– Superficial heat: 1–4 cm depth

(Deepest penetration)

Indications

ULTRASOUND	SHORTWAVE	MICROWAVE
– Chronic inflammation	– Chronic prostatitis	– Superficial heat for muscles and joints
– Musculoskeletal pain	– Refractory pelvic inflammatory disease	– Speed the resolution of hematomas
– Contractures	– Myalgia	– Provide local hyperthermia in cancer patients
– Subacute trauma	– Back spasms	

Contraindications

ULTRASOUND	SHORTWAVE	MICROWAVE
– General heat contraindications	– General heat precautions.	– General heat precautions
– Near heart, reproductive organs	– Metal	– Skeletal immaturity
– Near tumors	– Contact lenses	– Avoid in fluid-filled cavities (eyes, blisters, moist skin, edematous tissue)
– Near brain, spinal cord, laminectomy sites	– Gravid or menstruating uterus	
– Near pacemakers	– Skeletal immaturity	
– Gravid or menstruating uterus		
– Infection sites		
– Skeletal immaturity		
– Total hip arthroplasties with methylmethacrylate		
– Near pacemakers		

B. Cold

Therapeutic effects of cold are based on the following
- Immediate local vasoconstriction
- Local metabolism decrease
- Decreased acute inflammatory response
- Slows nerve conduction velocity—decreased motor and sensory nerve conduction.
- Decreased muscle spindle activity—decreased firing rates of Ia and II afferent fibers
- Decreased pain/muscle spasm—increases nerve pain threshold
- 📖 Decreased spasticity
- Increased tissue viscosity with decreased tissue elasticity
- Transient increase in systolic and diastolic blood pressure
- Release of vasoactive agents (histamine)

Indications for cold therapy
Generally used for acute process
- Acute traumatic conditions—reduction of inflammation and edema in the 24–48 hour period.
- Musculoskeletal conditions—arthritis, bursitis
- Acute and chronic pain

- Spasticity management
- Immediate treatment of minor burns

General precautions and contraindications for cold therapy
- Cold intolerance, hypersensitivity to cold (Raynaud's disease/phenomenon)
- Arterial insufficiency—areas with circulatory compromise such as ischemic areas in patients with peripheral vascular disease affecting the arterial system
- Impaired sensation—insensate skin is at risk for burns
- Cognitive and communication deficits that preclude the patient from reporting pain
- Cardiac, respiratory involvement—if severe HTN present, the patient's BP must be monitored closely
- Cryotherapy induced neuropraxia/axonotmesis, regenerating peripheral nerves
- Cryopathies: Cryoglobulinemia, Paroxysmal cold hemoglobinuria
- Open wounds after 48 hours
- Note: Reflex vasodilation with hyperemia can occur after removal of ice

Mechanisms of cold transfer
- Conduction: Cold packs, ice massage
- Convection: Cold baths (whirlpool)
- Evaporation: Vapo-coolant spray

The treatment modality depends on the size of the area to be treated and how accessible it is for cold application.

Conduction

1. Cold packs
- Include ice packs, wraps and sluices, endothermic chemical gel packs and hydrocollator packs
- The pack is wrapped in moist towels and treatment time is generally 20–30 minutes
- Surface skin temperature can decrease by 15° C after 10 minutes, subcutaneous temperatures decrease by 3°–5° C
- A study by Knuttson and Mattsson in 1969 showed muscle cooling by 5° C at a depth of 2 cm after 20-minute application of a hydrocollator pack

2. Ice massage
- For cooling of small areas (muscle belly, tendon, trigger point) before applying deep pressure massage. Combines the therapeutic effect of ice with the mechanical effects of massage
- Direct application of ice to a painful area using gentle stroking motion
- Study by Lowdon and Moore in 1975 showed a reduction of intramuscular temperature by 4.1° C at 2 cm. depth in the posterior thigh region, and up to 15.9° C reduction in biceps brachii after the 5-minute application time
- Treatment of analgesia can be obtained in 7–10 minutes

Convection

1. Cold baths
- An example of hydrotherapy; uses water-filled containers for distal limb immersion
- Best suited for circumferential cooling of the limbs
- Water temperature: 4°–10° C
- Can be uncomfortable and poorly tolerated
- Effective for treatment of localized burns due to rapid skin temperature reduction

2. Evaporation
  Vapo-coolant sprays
- Volatile liquids such as Fluori-methane spray are commonly used

- Used for spray-and-stretch techniques to treat myofascial pain ; also used for local anesthesia
- Produce an abrupt temperature change over a small surface area
- Precautions: risk for skin site irritation and local cutaneous freezing

3. *Other techniques*
   Cryotherapy Compression units
- Combines the benefits of cold with the advantages of pneumatic compression
- Uses sleeves with circulating cold water, attached to an intermittent pump unit. Edematous extremities are placed inside the sleeves
- Used primarily to treat acute musculoskeletal injury with soft tissue swelling. Also used after some surgical procedures
- Temperatures used are 45°F (7.2° C) and pressures up to 60 mmHg

LIGHT THERAPY

Ultraviolet Radiation

- Wavelength of 2000–4000 Å. Bactericidal wavelength is 2537 Å
- It can be produced by a small, hand-held mercury or "cold quartz" lamp
- Produces a nonthermal photochemical reaction with resultant alteration of DNA and cell proteins

- **Physiologic effects**
  - Bactericidal on motile bacteria
  - 📖 Increased vascularization of wound margins
  - Hyperplasia and exfoliation
  - Increased Vitamin D production
  - Excitation of calcium metabolism
  - Tanning

- **Indications**
  - For treatment of aseptic and septic wounds
  - 📖 Psoriasis treatment—utilizes Goeckerman's technique, where a coal-tar ointment is applied to the skin prior to UV treatment.
  - Acne treatment
  - Treatment of folliculitis

- **Precautions**
  - Fair skin
  - 📖 Scars, atrophic skin
  - Acute renal and hepatic failure
  - Severe diabetes
  - Hyperthyroidism
  - Generalized dermatitis
  - Advanced arteriosclerosis
  - Active, progressive pulmonary tuberculosis
  - Protect eyes from conjunctivitis, photokeratitis—shield from UV rays using goggles

- **Contraindications**
  - Pellagra
  - Porphyria
  - Sarcoidosis
  - Acute psoriasis
  - Lupus

- Eczema
- Herpes simplex
- Xeroderma pigmentosum

- Dosage is prescribed as the minimal exposure time required to cause erythema on the volar surface of the forearm (MED—Minimal Erythema Dosage). The MED subsides in 24 hours. Usual initial prescription is in the dose of 1–2 MEDs; and kept to less than 5
- 2.5 MED—exposure produces a second-degree erythema in 4–6 hours with pain and subsides in 2–4 days followed by desquamation
- 5 MED—third degree erythema in 2–4 hours with local edema, pain, and followed by local desquamation
- 10 MED—fourth degree erythema with superficial blister
- The treatment can be given 2–3 times a week

ELECTROTHERAPY

- Refers to the use of electricity to transcutaneously stimulate nerve or muscle, using electrodes

- **Physiologic effects**
  - Increases joint ROM
  - Muscle group contraction
  - Retards muscle atrophy
  - Increases muscle strength
  - Increases circulation
  - Decreases muscle spasm
  - Releases polypeptides and neurotransmitters (b-endorphins, Dopamine, enkephalins, Vasoactive Intestinal Peptide, Serotonin)
  - Decreases spasticity
  - Promotes wound healing
  - Induces osteogenesis—tissue regeneration, remodeling
  - Inhibits pain fibers—stimulates large myelinated Type A nerve fibers (gate control theory, please refer to next section on TENS)
  - Drives medicated ions across the skin

- **Indications**
  - Pain management—acute and chronic musculoskeletal pain; chronic neurogenic pain; general systemic pain
  - Joint effusion, interstitial edema (acute and chronic)
  - Muscle disuse atrophy
  - Dermal ulcers, wounds
  - Circulatory disorders—neurovascular disorders, venous insufficiency
  - Postherpetic neuralgia
  - Arthritis—osteoarthritis, rheumatoid arthritis
  - ROM and stretching exercises

- **Contraindications:**
  - Circulatory impairment—arterial or venous thrombosis, thrombophlebitis
  - Stimulation over the carotid sinus
  - Stimulation across the heart—especially if patient has pacemaker
  - Pregnancy
  - Seizure disorder
  - Fresh fracture
  - Active hemorrhage
  - Malignancy
  - Decreased sensation—direct current can cause burns (electrochemical)
  - Atrophic skin
  - Patients inability to report stimulation-induced pain
  - Known allergies to gel or pads

Transcutaneous Nerve Stimulation (TENS)

  - Stimulates nerve fibers for the symptomatic relief of pain
  - Uses a pocket-size programmable device to apply an electrical signal through lead wires and electrodes attached to the patient's skin.
  - Electrode placement is subjective:
      Typically placed over peripheral nerve distribution
      Locations can be distal or proximal to pain site

Proposed mechanism of pain control

1.-📖 Placebo effect is 30–35%
2. 📖 Based on the Gate Control Theory by Melzack and Wall (1965) (Figure 8-1)
   Pain signals can be blocked at the spinal cord before they are transmitted to the brain.
   📖 TENS stimulates large Ia myelinated afferent nerve fibers that stimulate the substantia gelatinosa in the spinal cord, closing the gate on pain transmission to the thalamus.
3. Release of endogenous opioids via TENS

Cheng and Pomerantz (1979)—demonstrated that pain relief produced at 4 Hz stimulation (low frequency) was blocked by naloxone; pain relief induced at 200 Hz was not blocked by naloxone

Gate-Control Theory

- Attempts to account for mechanisms by which other cutaneous stimuli and emotional states alter the level of pain.

Types of Stimulators (Table 8–1)

- *Conventional*
  - 📖 High-frequency, low-intensity stimulation—most effective type of stimulation
  - Amplitude is adjusted to produce minimal sensory discomfort
  - Pain relief begins in 10–15 minutes and stops shortly after removing stimulation
  - Useful for neuropathic pain
  - Duration of treatment is 30 minutes to hours

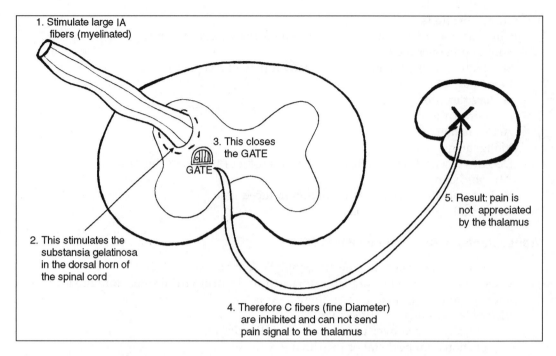

FIGURE 8–1. Simplistic Visualization of the Gate Control theory as described by Melzack and Wall. Pain signals can be blocked at the level of the spinal cord before they are transmitted to the thalamus. (Follow steps 1-5 in above figure.)

- *Acupuncture*
  - Low frequency, high intensity stimulation
  - Amplitude high enough to produce muscle contraction
  - Onset of pain relief can be delayed several hours
  - Pain relief persists hours after removing stimulation
  - Useful for acute musculoskeletal conditions
  - Treatment sessions last 30–60 minutes
  - Hyperstimulation
  - High frequency, high intensity stimulation
  - It is considered that this mode stimulates C-fibers causing counter-irritation
  - Rarely tolerated more than 15–30 minutes

- *Pulse or burst mode*
  - High frequency stimulation bursts at low frequency intervals
  - Delayed onset of pain relief
  - Treatment can range 30–60 minutes

- *Modulated*
  - Impulses vary in intensity and frequency
  - Attempts to avoid neuro-habituation

TABLE 8-1. Types of Stimulators

Type	Frequency	Width (msec)	Amplitude
Conventional	50–100	<200	Low
Acupuncture	1–10	200–300	High
Hyperstimulation	50–150	100–200	High
Burst	50–100* 1–10†	75–100	High
Modulated	Variable	<200	Variable

* Carrier frequency
† Burst frequency
From Weber D, Brown AW. Physical Agent Modalities. In Braddom RL. *Physical Medicine and Rehabilitation.* Philadelphia: W.B. Saunders; 1996, p. 485 table 23-5, with permission.

Treatment time with TENS is normally 30 minutes to 1 hour per session with a maximum of 2 hours per session, for a total of 8 hours per day. The treatments are continued for 3 weeks and gradually reduced over 8–12 weeks.

📖 Patients may report discomfort or skin irritation if the intensity is too high. Skin irritation can be resolved if the electrode positions are shifted or if a different conducting gel is used. Electrode shifting can increase current intensities to uncomfortable levels.

Neuromuscular Electrical Stimulation

Consists of transcutaneous electrical stimulation for muscles with or without intact PNS, or central control. It is more powerful than a regular TENS unit.

When the electrical stimulation is used to provide functional use of paretic muscles, it is called FES (functional electrical stimulation) or FNS (functional neuromuscular stimulation). Multiple muscles can be activated in a coordinated fashion through the use of electrical stimulation to attain certain functional goals (ambulation, transfers).

Uses
- Maintains muscle mass after immobilization. 📖 FES in patients with SCI increases muscle bulk
- 📖 FES prevents complications from immobility such as deep vein thrombosis (DVT), and osteoporosis
- 📖 FES slows the rate of bone loss in patients with SCI, where osteoporosis is common below the level of injury and may lead to fractures
- Strengthens muscles—effects have been noted even without voluntary muscle action. Changes of type II muscle fibers into type I fibers are temporarily noted with the treatments
- Increases ROM or maintains it
- 📖 Provides feedback to enhance voluntary muscle control (muscle reeducation). Feedback is used to adjust neuromuscular stimulation and is provided by the patient

- **Open-loop system**—Manual feedback. Most units are open-loop type
  The user observes the results of the stimulation and based on this adjusts the stimulation intensity. Each cycle of activity starts with the use of manually activating switches that send signals to control the unit.

- **Closed-loop system**—Control unit depends on movement sensors that send signals from the patient's body as results are obtained. Stimulation is adjusted to improve the programmed result. Lack of effective sensors may pose a problem. Advantages include correction of unexpected problems such as muscle spasms and fatigue.

- FES inhibits spasticity and muscle spasm
- FES can be used for orthotic training and functional movement

MASSAGE

Pressure and stretching are provided in a rhythmic fashion to the soft tissues

- 📖 **Physiologic effects include: reflexive, mechanical, and psychological**

Reflexive effects
- 📖 Reflex vasodilation with improvement in circulation
- Decrease in pain by means of the gate control or release of endogenous opiates or
- neurotransmitters
- General relaxation
- Increased perspiration

Mechanical effects
- 📖 Assists in venous blood return from the periphery to the CNS
- Increase lymphatic drainage
- Decrease muscle tightness
- Prevents or breaks adhesions in muscles, tendons, and ligaments
- Softens scars
- Loosening of secretions—example COPD

Psychological effect
"Laying of hands" promotes a sense of general well-being
There is no effect on the metabolism. Massage will not affect muscle strength, mass, or rate of atrophy of denervated muscle

Contraindications

- Do not use over malignancies
- Avoid open wounds, infected tissues, burns
- Nerve entrapments. Severe pressure over trigger points has produced hematoma formation with subsequent nerve entrapment, in severe cases.
- Acute inflammatory conditions: gout, rheumatoid arthritis, cellulitis, thrombophlebitis.
- DVT
- Severe varicose veins
- Severe clotting disorders or patients on anticoagulation
- Treatments can be provided to the extremities—5–15 minutes, or given to the trunk (neck, back, abdomen) which ranges from 15–30 minutes

Common techniques of therapeutic massage

Classical massage
- Effleurage—Gliding movement of the skin without deep muscle movement; used for muscle relaxation
- Pétrissage—Kneading, to increase circulation and reduce edema
- Tapotement—Percussion. Helps with desensitization, allows clearing of secretions, and improves circulation. Used for chest therapy in conjunction with postural drainage
- Friction massage—Prevents adhesions in acute muscle injuries and breaks adhesions in subacute and chronic injuries. Also reduces local muscle spasm, and decreases edema. Can be applied transverse or perpendicular to the muscle, tendon, or ligament fibers

– Soft tissue mobilization—Forceful massage of the fascia-muscle system. Massage is done with the fascia-muscle in a stretched position, rather than relaxed or shortened. Used for reduction of contractures
– Myofascial release—Prolonged light pressure is applied in specific directions of the fascia system to stretch focal areas of muscle or fascial tightness
– Accupressure—Finger pressure is applied over trigger points or acupuncture points to decrease pain

TRACTION

Spinal traction provides a pulling force to the cervical or lumbar spine.

Physiologic effects

– Vertebral joint distraction—Elongation of the cervical spine of 2–20 mm, can be achieved with 25 pounds or more of tractive force
– Reduction of compression and nerve root and disc irritation
– Reduction of pain, muscle spasm, and inflammation
– Loosening of adhesions in the dural sleeves

Contraindications

General
– Malignancy in the region of the spine
– Osteopenia
– Infectious process
– Congenital spinal deformity

Cervical spine traction contraindications
– Cervical ligamentous instability—RA, Down's Syndrome, Marfan Syndrome, Achondroplastic dwarfism
– Infectious process of the spine
– Atlantoaxial subluxation with spinal cord compromise
– Vertebrobasilar insufficiency

Lumbar spine traction contraindications
– Pregnancy
– Cauda equina compression
– Aortic aneurysms
– Restrictive lung disease
– Active peptic ulcer disease
– Hiatal hernia

• Traction can be achieved using manual technique or with the use of a pulley system or an electrical motorized device

Prescription parameters

Positioning

For cervical traction sitting or supine position is ordered. Depends on patient's comfort in different positions. ☐ To relieve symptoms of nerve root compression, 20°–30° of flexion optimally opens the intervertebral foramina.

For lumbar traction the supine position with 90° of hip and knee flexion is the most common position used. Reduces lumbar lordosis and the spine is relatively flexed, opening the intervertebral foramina.

Intermittent vs. continuous

Intermittent forces provide a greater pull. These are used for distraction, when neural foramina opening or retraction of herniated disc material is desired.
Continuous traction is used for prolonged muscle stretch, such as in muscle relaxation.

Amount of pull

Cervical spine—Distraction requires >25 pounds; amounts greater than 50 pounds do not provide additional advantage. ☐ For cervical radiculopathy may use 25 pounds with neck flexion described earlier.

Lumbar spine—For posterior vertebral separation requires forces > 50 pounds; for anterior separation forces > 100 pounds are needed.
☐ The effect of friction between the treatment table and the body should be counter-balanced before true traction in the spine is accomplished.

In a study by Judovich, it was reported that a pull equal to about one-half of the weight of the body part treated is needed to overcome friction. For the lower body this is approximately 26% of the total body weight. Another option may be the use of a split table, which eliminates the lower body segment friction. (Judovich, 1955)

Regardless of the effect of friction, another 25% or more of body weight is needed to cause vertebral separation.

Duration—Usually specified as 20 minutes.

■

THERAPEUTIC EXERCISE

Therapeutic exercises are prescribed to improve flexibility, increase endurance, aerobic capacity, and strengthening, among other purposes.

STRENGTHENING EXERCISES

Are designed to increase the maximal force that a muscle or muscle group can generate. Strength is affected by several factors, such as: the type of muscle contraction, speed of contraction, cross-sectional size of the muscle, length–tension relationship, and the recruitment of motor units.

☐ Physiology of muscle contraction (Figure 8-2)

- Transient muscle fiber shortening takes place whenever an action potential is generated and travels through the sarcolemma (muscle fiber cell membrane)

- Skeletal muscle fibers contain hundreds to thousands of myofibrils, each subdivided into functional units of contraction, called sarcomeres.
- The sarcomere contains contractile proteins, actin and myosin, that lie parallel to the axis of the fiber. Muscle shortening is produced by coordinated movement of the thin (actin) and thick (myosin) filaments within the myofibrils.
- The actin filaments attach to the outer margins of the sarcomere, (**Z line**), and the myosin filaments are located centrally.
- The sarcomere is measured from Z line to Z line.
- During muscle rest, the filaments overlap.

   The *A band* runs the length of the thick (myosin) filament. It has continuous overlap except at its center (*H zone*).

   The *I band* is composed of thin (actin) filaments that remain bare through the outermost portion of the sarcomere.
- Thick and thin filaments are linked to one another via cross bridges that arise from the myosin molecule. During muscle contraction, increasing amount of myosin overlap is observed, and muscle shortening occurs. Contraction results in the Z lines approaching each other, shrinking of the H zone and I band.

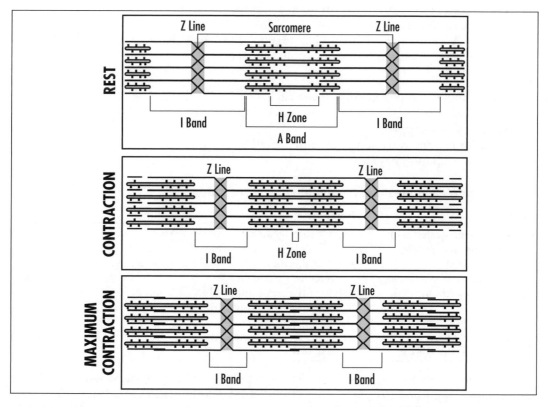

FIGURE 8–2. Sarcomere represented schematically under different conditions: Rest, Contraction and Maximum Contraction. During contraction Z lines approach each other and H zone and I band shrink.

Muscle Fiber Types
- Based on the speed of contraction two main categories can be established: fast units and slow units.

Fast units
Peak tension and relaxation achieved rapidly
Large muscle fiber diameter
Innervation provided by large, fast conducting motor neurons
Large number of muscle fibers
Can be divided into: fast fatigable (fatigue easily) and fatigue-resistant (slow to fatigue, can be compared to slow units)

Slow units
Slower peak tension and relaxation

Fibers innervated by fast motor units—type II fibers—fast twitch
- High activity of myofibrillar adenosine-triphaphatase (ATPase)—high energy release for contraction
- High levels of glycogen and phosphorylase—high breakdown of glycogen for anaerobic activities.
- Used for high-intensity, short-duration activities
- Subdivided into: type IIA and IIB
  Type II A—fatigue resistant, fast oxidative-glycolytic. These have a higher level of oxidative enzymes and capillary supply is better.
  Type II B—fast fatigable

Slow units innervate type I fibers—slow twitch
- Slow oxidative
- Rich capillary supply
- Used for low-intensity, long-duration activities.
- High in oxidative enzymes

Strengthening exercises can be divided into three categories

Isotonic	Isometric	Isokinetic
Muscle force generated with:	Muscle force generated with:	Muscle force generated with:
– Visible joint movement	– No visible joint movement	– Visible joint movement
– Variable speed	– Internal force doesn't	– Constant speed
– Constant external resistance	overcome external force.	– Variable external resistance
(constant weight through	– Exertion against immovable	Example: Cybex, Nautilus
ROM)	objects, or by holding an	
Example: weight lifting	object in a static position	
📖 Delorme's Progressive	Example: isometric contractions	
Resistive Exercises (PREs)	done in bed	

📖 Delorme exercises—progressive resistive technique—The greatest weight that can be lifted, pulled, or pushed 10 times through full ROM is determined. The patient performs one set of repetitions at 50% of the 10 RM (repetition maximum), a second set of 75% of the 10 RM, and a final set of 10 repetitions of full 10 RM. Each session consists of the three sets with breaks between sets. The 10 RM is determined each week with progressive advancement as strength increases.

Eccentric and concentric contractions are muscle contractions that may be isokinetic or isotonic.

A. ECCENTRIC CONTRACTIONS	B. CONCENTRIC CONTRACTIONS
• Muscle lengthening—resists a stretching force • 📖 Fast eccentric contractions—generate greatest force • 📖 Cause more tissue destruction • Muscle soreness increases up to 48 hours after initial muscle contraction. It can be minimized by beginning with low-intensity exercise and encouraging the patient to continue to exercise on a regular basis • Muscle soreness decreases with muscle conditioning. It is best relieved by mild exercise of the affected muscle groups rather than rest • Low metabolic cost: less VO_2 required, therefore, more energy efficient	• Muscle shortening. Tension develops to overcome resistance. • High metabolic cost • Generates little force

Improvement of muscle performance including strength can be increased by the following:
1. Increasing the amount of weight lifted
2. Increasing the amount of repetitions or sets
3. Increasing contraction velocity

The following graph shows the relationship between force generation and velocity during eccentric, concentric, and isometric contractions: (Figure 8-3)

Conditioning, Total Body Endurance Exercises, or Cardiopulmonary Endurance Exercises

These exercises use large muscle groups, and are continuous and rhythmic, providing low intensity and high repetition, to improve overall cardiopulmonary fitness. They can be divided into aerobic and anaerobic endurance exercises.

Cardiovascular effects of conditioning exercises

• Decreased resting heart rate and submaximal effort
• Increased peak BP during maximal exercise, decreased BP at rest and submaximal effort.
• Increase in stroke volume during maximal exercise
• Reduced myocardial oxygen consumption at rest and submaximal activities

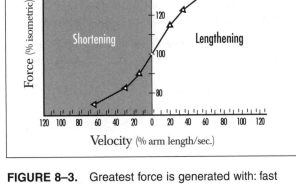

FIGURE 8–3. Greatest force is generated with: fast eccentric contractions > slow eccentric contractions > isometric contractions > slow concentric contractions. Fast concentric contractions generate the least force.

Exercise and the effect on cardiopulmonary function (Table 8-2)

TABLE 8–2

Exercise	HR	VO₂ max	SBP	DBP	Max vital capacity
Aerobic	↑	↑	↑	↑	↑
📖 Isometric	No change	No change	↑	↑	No change
Isotonic	↑	No change	↑	No change or ↓	No change
Effects after aerobic training	↓	↑	↓	No change or ↓	No change

Aerobic endurance exercises

- Combination of cardiopulmonary endurance exercise with strengthening
- Should consist of a warm-up period, a training period and a cool-down period:
  Warm-up 5 to 10 minutes
  Training period—20 to 30 minutes at 40%–60% (low intensity), 60%–70% (moderate intensity), or 70%–85% (heavy intensity) of their VO₂ max
  Cool-down period 5 to 10 minutes

Guidelines for the quantity and quality of aerobic exercise programs for healthy adults as proposed by the American College of Sports Medicine

- Mode—any exercise that uses large muscle groups, continuous and rhythmic in nature. Examples: running, swimming, walking, stair climbing.
- Frequency—3–5 days/week
- Duration—20–60 minutes
- Intensity—60%–90% HR max
  50%–85% of VO₂ max or 50%–85% of HR reserve max

Anaerobic exercises

High-resistance, short-duration exercises at 80% of maximum exertion capacity.
Deplete the glycolytic system, which functions during the first two minutes of exercise.

Mobility exercises: exercises to improve flexibility

- Flexibility is defined as the ability to move body joints through their entire range of motion (ROM)
- Each joint of the body has a specific ROM
- Flexibility exercises maintain mobility within the available ROM
- Flexibility exercises should be done at least three times a week, should consist of three to five repetitions once or twice a day

AVERAGE RANGE OF JOINT MOTION (IN DEGREES) (Table 8-3)

TABLE 8-3

SHOULDER	° Of Joint Motion	THUMB	° Of Joint Motion
Flexion	158	Abduction	58
Extension	53	IP flexion	81
Abduction	170	MP flexion	53
Adduction	50	MC flexion	15
Horizontal flexion	135	IP extension	17
Arm at side		MP extension	8
Internal rotation	68	MC extension	20
External rotation	68	**FINGERS**	
Arm in 90° abduction		DIP flexion	80
Internal rotation	70	PIP flexion	100
External rotation	90	MCP flexion	90
ELBOW		DIP extension	0
Flexion	70	PIP extension	0
Hyperextension	90	MCP extension	45
FOREARM		**HINDFOOT**	
Pronation	71	Inversion	5
Supination	84	Eversion	5
HIP		**FOREFOOT**	
Flexion	113	Inversion	33
Extension	28	Eversion	18
Abduction	48	**GREAT TOE**	
Adduction	31	IP flexion	60
Horizontal flexion	60	IP extension	0
Hip in flexion		MTP flexion	37
Internal rotation	45	MTP extension	63
External rotation	45	**2ND TO 5TH TOES**	
Hip in extension		DIP flexion	55
Internal rotation	35	PIP flexion	38
External rotation	48	MTP flexion	35
KNEE		Extension	40
Flexion	134	**CERVICAL SPINE**	
Hyperextension	10	Flexion	38
ANKLE		Extension	38
Plantar flexion	48	Lateral bending	43
Dorsiflexion	18	Rotation	45
WRIST		**THORACIC AND LUMBAR SPINE**	
Extension	71	Flexion	85
Flexion	73	Extension	30
Ulnar deviation	33	Lateral bending	28
Radial deviation	19	Rotation	38

Table reprinted with permission from American Academy of Orthopaedic Surgeons: Joint Motion: Method of Measuring and Recording. Chicago, AAOS, 1965.

TECHNIQUES TO IMPROVE FLEXIBILITY

- Can be done through anatomic planes of motion, combined planes of motion (similar to peripheral neuro-facilitation patterns), or through functional teaching activities

Stretching Exercises

- Increase ROM by lengthening tendon and muscle beyond the available range

- Include static stretching, static stretching with contraction of the antagonist muscle (reciprocal inhibition), static stretching with contraction of the agonist muscle, and ballistic stretching

- Ballistic stretching—utilizes repetitive bouncing movements with a rapid stretch. More tension is developed, and more energy is absorbed into the muscle and tendon, which can lead to bone avulsion or muscle–tendon tears. High risk of injury

- Static stretch—The joint is moved to the end of the ROM where the position is slowly held for 5 to 60 seconds. Can be done actively or passively. Safe technique

- Reciprocal inhibition—The joint is also moved to the end of ROM, and this is followed by a symmetric contraction of the antagonist muscle group for 5 to 30 seconds

- Static stretching with contraction of the agonist—The joint is moved to the end of ROM and followed by an isometric contraction of the agonist muscle for 5 to 30 seconds

■

EFFECTS OF EXTENDED BEDREST—IMMOBILIZATION AND INACTIVITY

MUSCLE

- 📖 Strength—immobilization decreases strength by 1.0%–1.5% per day. Strength can decrease as much as 20%–30 % during only a week to nine days of bedrest. Five weeks of total inactivity costs 50% of the previous muscle strength. A plateau is reached 25%–40% of original strength. One contraction a day at 50% of maximal strength is enough to prevent this decrease
- Strength is lost especially in the quadriceps and extensors
- A decrease in fiber diameter is found affecting type I fibers (slow twitch) during early immobilization. A decrease of percentage of type I fibers is noted. A decrease in oxidative enzymes is also noted. All these changes also lead to a reduction in muscular endurance. 📖 Percentage of muscle mass lost per week is estimated at 5%–10%
- Muscle torque can be affected: In a study by Gogia (1988) the effect of bedrest on extremity muscle torque in healthy men was evaluated after they were strapped down for 5 weeks and allowed to sit only for bowel movements. A 26% decrease in gastrocnemius and 24% decrease in soleus muscle torque was found
- Restricted activities affect muscle strength and recruitment patterns of muscles distant from specific sites of injury. In studies by Beckman (1995), and Nicholas (1976), effects of hip musculature strength and recruitment pattern were affected for several months after ankle sprain

BONE AND JOINTS

- Lack of gravitational force and muscle pull on bone cause osteopenia. As a result of osteopenia, hypercalcemia develops. 📖 Calcium is excreted in the urine and feces starting at 2–3 days after immobilization, and peaking at 3–7 weeks. After activity is resumed, calcium levels remain high for 3 weeks, reaching normal values at 5–6 weeks
- 📖 When comparing calcium to nitrogen and protein changes in the urine, it is noted that calcium improves last. Nitrogen loss is 2g N/day. Loss begins at 5–6 days after immobilization, peaks in the second week. After activity is resumed, loss continues for 1 week, normalizes during the second week, below normal values are obtained at 4 weeks, and returns to normal values in 6 weeks
- Calcium excretion in addition to phosphorus loss causes atrophy and a reduction in fracture threshold of bone
- Joints show a decrease in periarticular connective tissue extensibility after inactivity. Articular cartilage begins to deteriorate due to lack of nutritional support. The hyaline cartilage in synovial joints is not supplied by vascular blood flow. It depends on nutrition from the synovial fluid through loading and unloading of pressure
- Ligaments undergo biochemical changes noted as early as two weeks after immobilization. In the case of surgically repaired ligaments, improvement in strength is affected by immobilization. Immobilization causes ligament strength to decrease, compliance to increase, and collagen degradation to increase.

GASTROINTESTINAL (GI)—Decreased GI motility leads to constipation and loss of appetite.

GENITOURINARY—Urinary stasis, leading to an increased risk of urolithiasis and urinary tract infections.

PULMONARY—Diminished diaphragmatic movement and chest expansion, due to loss of strength of diaphragm and intercostal muscles, leading to impaired secretion clearance.

- Reduced cough and bronchial ciliary activity. Patients can develop hypostatic pneumonia.
- Reduction in pulmonary function with decreased tidal and minute volumes, decreased vital capacity.
- A-V shunting and regional changes in ventilation-perfusion occur.

📖 CARDIAC

- Reduction in blood and plasma volumes.
- Redistribution of body fluids leads to postural hypotension. Venous blood pooling occurs in the legs. In addition, β-adrenergic sympathetic activity is increased.
- 📖 Cardiovascular efficiency is decreased, increased HR, decreased stroke volume. Heart rate increases approximately 0.5 beats/minutes/day, leading to immobilization tachycardia and abnormal HR with minimal or submaximal workloads. Stroke volume decrease may reach 15% in 2 weeks of bed rest, as a result of blood volume changes and venous pooling in the lower extremities. There is also a decrease in maximal oxygen extraction (VO_2 max) that can occur as early as 3–5 days.
- Thromboembolism secondary to a decrease in blood volume and increased coagulability.

INTEGUMENTARY—skin atrophy and pressure sores develop.

■

EVALUATION OF FUNCTIONAL INDEPENDENCE

- Difference between impairment, disability, and handicap:
  - Impairment—physical or psychological abnormality, usually the manifestation of a disease or injury. Example Cerebral Vascular Accident (CVA)
  - Disability—loss of ability to perform a particular activity or function, such as walking
  - Handicap—inability to fulfill a usual role or life activity as a result of the impairment and disability. Example: inability to perform a certain job due to inability to ambulate

Term	Definition	Example
Disease	Sickness	Radial nerve palsy
Impairment	Physical, anatomic, or psychological abnormality	Wrist Drop
Disability	Loss of function	Inability to write
Handicap	Loss of role in society	Loss of job as an artist

- The evaluation of functional independence is important in the process of assessing a safe return home after a patient has been hospitalized
- 📖 One of the measurement scales used for this assessment is the FIM score (Functional Independence Measure) (Figure 8-4). It documents the severity of disability as well as the outcomes of rehabilitation treatment as part of a uniform data system.
  - Consists of 18 items organized under 6 categories:
    - Self care (eating, grooming, bathing, upper body dressing, lower body dressing, and toileting)
    - Sphincter control—(bowel and bladder function)
    - Mobility (bed, chair, wheelchair, tub or shower, and toilet transfers)
    - Locomotion (ambulation, wheelchair mobility, and stair management)
    - Communication (comprehension and expression)
    - Social cognition (interaction, problem solving, memory)
  - Patients obtain points on each category on a scale of 1 (total assistance required) to 7 (complete independence)

FIM™ instrument

LEVELS	7 Complete Independence (Timely, Safely) 6 Modified Independence (Device)	NO HELPER
	Modified Dependence 5 Supervision (Subject = 100%+) 4 Minimal Assist (Subject = 75%+) 3 Moderate Assist (Subject = 50%+) **Complete Dependence** 2 Maximal Assist (Subject =25%+) 1 Total Assist (Subject = less than 25%)	HELPER

	ADMISSION	DISCHARGE	FOLLOW-UP
Self-Care A. Eating B. Grooming C. Bathing D. Dressing - Upper Body E. Dressing - Lower Body F. Toileting			
Sphincter Control G. Bladder Management H. Bowel Management			
Transfers I. Bed, Chair, Wheelchair J. Toilet K. Tub, Shower			
Locomotion L. Walk/Wheelchair M. Stairs	W Walk C Wheelchair B Both	W Walk C Wheelchair B Both	W Walk C Wheelchair B Both
Motor Subtotal Score			
Communication N. Comprehension O. Expression	A Auditory V Visual B Both V Vocal N Nonvocal B Both	A Auditory V Visual B Both V Vocal N Nonvocal B Both	A Auditory V Visual B Both V Vocal N Nonvocal B Both
Social Cognition P. Social Interaction Q. Problem Solving R. Memory			
Cognitive Subtotal Score			
TOTAL FIM Score			

NOTE: Leave no blanks. Enter 1 if patient not testable due to risk

FIGURE 8–4. FIM Score documents the severity of disability as well as the outcomes of rehabilitation treatment.

▪

PHYSIOLOGIC EFFECTS OF AGING

📖 CARDIAC

- Progressive decline in maximal heart rate, possibly related to decreased chronotropic response to adrenergic stimuli. Max HR = 220 – age
- Increased left ventricle end systolic volume and decreased ejection fraction with exercise. When this is added to a decreased HR response, cardiac output during exercise is more dependent on an increased stroke volume by using the Frank-Starling mechanism (higher end-diastolic volumes). Cardiac output decreases with aging
- Rate of diastolic early filling is decreased; more dependent on late filling through atrial contraction. Patients are more susceptible to atrial fibrillation or atrial tachycardia, and CHF
- Maximal oxygen consumption (VO_2 max) decreases regardless of the level of activity, but more physically active patients have smaller decreases compared to sedentary patients
- Progressive, gradual increases in systolic and diastolic BP, mostly due to decreased arterial elasticity than to circulating catecholamines
- Decreased baroreceptor sensitivity. Associated with orthostatic hypotension—diminished reflex tachycardia with position change, in association to blunted plasma renin activity and reduced vasopressin and angiotensin II levels. Decreased baroreceptor sensitivity is also associated to cough and micturition syncope syndromes
- 📖 Patient's medications should be monitored during the evaluation of causes of orthostatic hypotension: antihypertensives, Levodopa, Phenothiazines, TCA. Evaluate for fluid loss, and aldosterone/cortisol level dysfunction

📖 PULMONARY

- Decreased vital capacity
- Decreased PO_2—Linear decline associated to a mild degree of impaired gas exchange. No changes in PCO_2 or pH, and oxygen saturation remains normal or slightly reduced
- Decreased forced expiratory ventilation-FEV_1. This decreases consistently at 33 cc/yr
- Decreased maximum minute ventilation. These declines reflect changes in related organ systems, which are stressed by voluntary ventilation required during these tests Examples: stiffening of the rib cage, weakening of the intercostal muscles, small airway narrowing due to decreased elastic recoil
- Increase in residual volume and functional residual capacity—Related to loss of elastic recoil
- No change in total lung capacity
- High incidence of pneumonia—Immunologic decline, impaired mucociliary action, ↓ chest wall compliance with decreased ability to clear secretions; reduced level of consciousness; dysphagia, esophageal disorders

INTEGUMENTARY—Decreased elasticity of connective tissue leads to increased risk for pressure ulcers and skin breakdown. Decreased moisture, decreased skin sensation.

MUSCULOSKELETAL—Overall muscle mass decreases, including number of myofibrils, and concentration of mitochondrial enzymes

- Decreased number of motor units
- Increased fat—15% increase at age 30, 30% increase at age 80. Patients retain more fat-soluble medications and have increased side effects
- Muscle endurance increases or remains stable due to muscle fiber type regrouping, increasing type II fibers with age
- High prevalence of osteoporosis and Degenerative Joint Disease (DJD)—decreased water content of cartilage and ratio of chondroitin-4-sulfate to chondroitin -6-sulfate . Chemical alteration of cartilage with decreased ability to bear weight without causing ulceration of cartilage and eventual exposure of bone
- Decreased peak bone mineral density at mid-30's. Base of stance is increased due to valgus deformity at the hips

THERMOREGULATORY

- Impaired temperature regulation with decreased autonomic vasomotor control and impaired sensitivity to changes in temperature
- Patients are vulnerable to hypothermia and hyperthermia. Hypothermia is affected by impaired sweating and aggravated by medical conditions, such as malnutrition, hypoglycemia, and hypothyroidism; or medications such as narcotics, ethanol, and benzodiazepines

NEUROLOGIC

- Decreased short-term memory and incidental learning
- Slowing in the rate of central information processing tasks requiring new information processing tend to decline progressively after 20 years of age
- Increase in choice reaction time is noted. The more complex the task, the greater the age effect
- Older adults are capable of learning but at a slower rate
- Decrease in proprioception and gait, leading to problems with coordination and balance. There is associated decrease in nigrostriatal neurons with age
- Loss of speed of motor activities

GENITOURINARY

- Reduction in bladder capacity
- Decreased urethral and bladder compliance
- Reduced urinary flow rate
- Decreased ability to postpone voiding
- Incontinence does not result from normal aging; it is the result of underlying disease. Confusional states, Urinary tract infection (UTIs) , atrophic urethritis, drugs (sedatives, anticholinergics, calcium channel blockers), limited mobility, and constipation can contribute. Approximately 70% of the elderly patients with urinary incontinence have detrusor instability
- Sexuality—decreased sexual function with aging. Older men have decreased ability to have psychogenic erections, and require more intense stimulation. Erections may be partial; the force of ejaculation is decreased, with a less intense sensation of orgasm. Many medications can contribute to impotence

– Women undergo postmenopausal changes such as increased vaginal wall fragility and decreased vaginal lubrication. Other reasons for decreased sexual function may include partner's impotence, decreased libido, and decreased opportunities for sexual encounters.
– Benign prostatic hyperplasia develops under hormonal influence and is almost universal in men over 40 years of age.

RENAL

– Atrophy of the glomeruli and decrease in renal tubular cell mass, leading to decreased glomerular filtration rate and decreased tubular function
– These factors result in an increase in the half life of renally excreted drugs, such as penicillin (PCN), aminoglycosides, digoxin, cimetidine, lithium, procainamide, chlorpropamide
– 📖 Digitalis toxicity in the elderly is commonly secondary to impaired renal function. Toxicity manifests with anorexia, nausea, vomiting, abdominal pain, fatigue, depression, drowsiness, lethargy, headache, and confusion. There are also ocular disturbances and cardiac dysrhythmias
– 📖 NSAIDs are also related to injury, with the most common finding as prerenal azotemia. In settings where the renal blood flow is dependent on the activity of vasodilating prostaglandins, the use of NSAIDs can precipitate acute renal failure. In states of prostaglandin inhibition, the patients develop hyporeninemic hypoaldosteronism

GASTROINTESTINAL

– Impaired esophageal function—decreased amplitude of peristaltic contractions
– Delayed esophageal emptying, and incomplete sphincter relaxation are associated with disease
– Colon—decreased force of muscle contraction with impaired rectal perception of feces. It is important to explore contributing factors for development of constipation: decreased dietary fiber and fluid intake, diseases associated with decreased bowel function (Parkinson's, CVA); medications (calcium, iron, antacids, NSAIDs, opiates, antihypertensives [calcium channel blockers], anticholinergics [TCAs], sympathomimetics [isoproterenol, terbutaline, pseudoephedrine])
– Fecal incontinence is secondary to fecal impaction in most cases. Other causes such as decreased cognitive function, diarrhea, and decreased sphincter tone need to be evaluated. Diarrhea is commonly seen in association with fecal impaction, infection, and drugs, such as laxatives, antibiotics, and digoxin toxicity

EFFECTS OF ACUTE HOSPITALIZATION AND DECONDITIONING IN THE ELDERLY

• Multiple chronic illnesses have a cumulative effects on the organ reserves, to which the elderly patient may try to adapt in order to be functional under the circumstances. Sometimes the patient's reserve capacity is limited and with minor acute complications or disease processes may develop functional decompensation
• Adverse effects of hospitalization in the elderly include:
– Disorientation
– Insomnia—usually treated with hypnotics, which may cause side effects or may adversely affect the patient's health. 📖 Sleep related disorders in the elderly are frequently related to depression
– Increased incidence of iatrogenic complications—adverse drug interactions are usually the result of polypharmacy
– Emotional sequelae—Anxiety and confusion are common in relation to illness, prognosis, and hospitalization. Patients tend to develop depression. Many times patients are dependent for functional activities

– Social support system and discharge disposition—patient's functional abilities may be impaired. This can be added to a decrease in patient's motivation, which can lead to a more difficult return to a prior living situation

– Deconditioning effects, as previously discussed, tend to appear earlier, are more severe, and take longer to reverse in the elderly. This is due to a greater degree with age and a diminished reserve

- Deconditioning effects include:
  – Decreased VO_2 max
  – Shortened time to fatigue during submaximal work
  – Decreased muscle strength
  – Decreased reaction time/balance/flexibility

- Multiple factors associated with falls are secondary to deconditioning. Falls in the community are associated with decreased static balance, leg strength, and hip/ankle flexibility. In nursing homes, falls are related to decreased muscle strength at the knee and ankles

SUMMARY OF ADAPTATIONS TO EXERCISE IN THE ELDERLY

Aerobic Conditioning

– Decreased minute ventilation during submaximal exercise—decrease of 9% to 15%

– Heart rate decreases with submaximal exercise—decrease of 9–20 beats/minutes, and stroke volume increases 8%

– Minute ventilation increases with maximal exercise—decrease 20%–30%

– With maximal exercise *stroke volume* and *cardiac output* increase. SV 6%–8%; CO up to 34%

– Total hemoglobin and blood volume increase. Hg 7%; blood volume 8%

– Systemic vascular resistance during submaximal exercise decreases 5%–18%

– Muscle enzymes increase oxidative enzymes, 0–45%, glycogen stores, 10%–28%

Strength Training

– Increase in muscle cross-sectional area, type I and II fibers, capillary density per fiber, and oxidative enzymes

– Age-related decrease in sarcoplasmic reticulum Ca^{2+} – ATPase is prevented

– Strength and torque velocity increase

MANAGEMENT OF COMPLICATIONS IN THE ELDERLY

- **Depression**—presents as sleep disturbance, loss of appetite, constipation, impaired concentration, poor memory, and psychomotor retardation. Rates of major depression vary from 16%–30% in geriatric populations. Prevalence rates in community-dwelling elderly ranges from 2%–5%. This risk is increased threefold if the patient has a disability

  – For prolonged depression, trazodone and selective serotonin reuptake inhibitors (low anticholinergic effect) are good, or the use of Tricyclic Antidepressants (TCAs) with the lowest anticholinergic effect

  – ☐ Of the common TCAs, Nortriptyline (Pamelor®), is preferred over others such as Amitriptyline. Nortriptyline is less anticholinergic, has decreased sedation effect, and causes less orthostatic hypotension (which is a result of α-1 blockade)

- ☐ Agitation—If medications are required, the TCA called Elavil® (amitriptyline) is recommended over other medications such as Valium®. Due to the fact that fat-soluble drugs tend to accumulate more in the elderly as a result of changes in metabolism and body composition, benzodiazepines accumulate with the adverse side effects such as drowsiness

REFERENCES

Abramson DI, Tuck S Jr, Lee SW, Richardson G, Levin M, Buso E. Comparison of wet and dry heat in raising temperature of tissues. *Arch Phys Med Rehabil* 1967 Dec:48(12):654–661

Beckman SM, Buchanan TS. Ankle inversion injury and hypermobility: effect on hip and ankle muscle electromyography onset latency. *Arch Phys Med Rehabil* 1995 Dec:76(12):1138–1143.

Borell RM, Parker R, Henley EJ, Masley D, Repinecz M. Comparison of in vivo temperatures produced by hydrotherapy, paraffin wax treatment, and Fluidotherapy. *Phys Ther* 1980 Oct:60(10):1273–1276

Cheng RS, Pomeranz B. Electroacupuncture analgesia could be mediated by at least two pain-relieving mechanisms; endorphin and non-endorphin systems. *Life Sci* 1979 Dec 3:25(23):1957–1962.

DeLateur BJ, Lehmann JF, Stonebrid JB, Warren CG, Guy AW. Muscle heating in human subjects with 915 MHz. Microwave contact applicator. *Arch Phys Med Rehabil* 1970:51(3):147–151

Downey JA, Myers SJ, Gonzalez EG, Lieberman JS. *The Physiological Basis of Rehabilitation Medicine* 2nd ed. Newton, MA: Butterworth-Heineman: 1994:134.

Gogia P, Schneider VS, LeBlanc AD, Krebs J, Kasson C, Pientok C. Bed rest effect on extremity muscle torque in healthy men. *Arch Phys Med Rehabil* 1988:69(12):1030–1032.

Judovich BD. Lumbar traction therapy—elimination of physical factors that prevent lumbar stretch. *JAMA*; 159: 549–550.

Knutsson E, Mattsson E. Effects of local cooling on monosynaptic reflexes in man. *Scand J Rehabil Med* 1969:1(3):126–132

Lehmann JF, Delateur BJ, Stonebridge JB, Warren CG.Therapeutic temperature distribution produced by ultrasound as modified by dosage and volume of tissue exposed. *Arch Phys Med Rehabil* 1967:48(12):662–666

Lehmann JF, DeLateur BJ. Diathermy and Superficial Heat, Laser, Cold Therapy. In: Kotke FJ, Lehmann JF. Krusens's *Handbook of Physical Medicine and Rehabilitation* 4th ed. Philadelphia: W.B. Saunders, 1990.

Lehmann JF, Guy AW, DeLateur BJ, Stonebridge JB, Warren CG. Heating patterns produced by short-wave diathermy using helical induction coil applicators. *Arch Phys Med Rehabil* 1968:49(4):193–198.

Lehmann JF, Silverman DR, Baum BA, Kirk NL, Johnston VC. Temperature distributions in the human thigh, produced by infrared, hot pack and microwave applications. *Arch Phys Med Rehabil* 1966:47(5):291–199

Lowdon BJ, Moore RJ. Determinants and nature of intramuscular temperature changes during cold therapy. *Am J Phys Med*. 1975:54(5):223–233.

Melzack R, Wall PD. Pain Mechanisms: a new theory. *Science* 1965:50: 971–979.

Nicholas JA, Strizak AM, Veras G. A study of thigh muscle weakness in different pathological states of the lower extremity. *Am J Sports Me* 1976:4(6):241–248.

Shepard RJ. *Physiology and Biochemistry of Exercise*. New York: Praeger Publishers, 1982:140–142.

RECOMMENDED READING

Basford JR. Physical Agents. In: DeLisa JA, Gans BM. *Rehabilitation Medicine: Principles and Practice*, 2nd ed. Philadelphia: J.B. Lippincott, 1993.

DeLateur B. Therapeutic Exercise to Develop Strength and Endurance. In: Kotke FJ, Lehmann JF. *Krusen's Handbook of Physical Medicine and Rehabilitation* 4th ed. Philadelphia: W.B. Saunders, 1990.

Lehmann JF, DeLateur BJ. Diathermy and Superficial Heat, Laser, Cold Therapy. In: Kotke FJ, Lehmann JF. *Krusen's Handbook of Physical Medicine and Rehabilitation* 4th ed. Philadelphia: W.B. Saunders, 1990.

Tan JC. *Practical Manual of Physical Medicine and Rehabilitation*. St. Louis: Mosby-Year Book, Inc., 1998.

Weber D, Brown AW. Physical Agent Modalities. In: Braddom RL. *Physical Medicine and Rehabilitation*. Philadelphia: W.B. Saunders, 1996.

9

PULMONARY/CARDIAC/ CANCER REHABILITATION

PULMONARY—Priscila Gonzalez, M.D. and Sara Cuccurullo, M.D.
CARDIAC—Iqbal Jafri, M.D.
CANCER—Priscila Gonzalez, M.D. and Lisa Luciano, D.O.

■

PULMONARY REHABILITATION

GOALS OF PULMONARY REHABILITATION

- Improvement in cardiopulmonary function
- Prevention and treatment of complications
- Increased understanding of the disease
- Increased patient responsibility for self-care and compliance with medical treatment
- Improvement in level of activity and quality of life, return to work

📖 BENEFITS OF PULMONARY REHABILITATION

- Improvement in exercise tolerance, symptom-limited oxygen consumption, work output, mechanical efficiency, and vital capacity
- 📖 Exercise increases arterial venous oxygen (AVO_2) difference, increasing oxygen extraction from arterial circulation
- Reduction in dyspnea and respiratory rate
- Improvement in general quality of life; decreased anxiety and depression, improvement in Activities of Daily Living (ADLs)
- Improvement in ambulation capacity
- Decreased hospitalization rates
- Focus on conditioning peripheral musculature in order to improve their efficiency and reduce stress on the heart and lungs (Alba 1996)

CANDIDATES FOR PULMONARY REHABILITATION

Motivated nonsmokers or patients who have quit smoking and whose activities are limited because of dyspnea are good candidates for a pulmonary rehabilitation program.

- Functional evaluation to assess pulmonary disability is recommended prior to starting the program:

📖 Classification of functional pulmonary disability—Moser Classification

1. Normal at rest—dyspnea on strenuous exertion
2. Normal ADL performance—dyspnea on stairs/inclines

3. Dyspnea with certain ADLs, able to walk one block at slow pace
4. Dependent with some ADLs; dyspnea with minimal exertion
   Note: 1—4 have no dyspnea at rest
5. Housebound—📖 dyspnea at rest, assistance with most ADLs
- 📖 Patients who benefit the most from a pulmonary rehabilitation program have at least one of the following:
  - Respiratory limitation of exercise at 75% of predicted maximum O_2 consumption
  - Irreversible airway obstruction with a Forced Expiratory Volume in one second (FEV_1) < 2000 ml or an FEV_1/FVC ratio of less than 60% (See Lung Volume Definitions below)
  - Restrictive lung disease or pulmonary vascular disease with carbon monoxide diffusion capacity <80% of predicted value (Bach, 1993)

QUICK REVIEW OF PULMONARY PHYSIOLOGY

Central control of respiratory function

Voluntary control of respiration originates in the cortex and descends through the spinal cord to the respiratory muscles

The medullary respiratory center—serves to integrate different chemoreceptors

Central chemoreceptors (stimulated by hypercarbia)
Peripheral chemoreceptors (stimulated by hypoxia) located in the carotid and aortic bodies

Muscles of respiration

Inspiratory muscles
- Accessory muscles of respiration—sternocleidomastoid, trapezius, pectoralis major
- 📖 Diaphragm—innervated by the phrenic nerve. Works at rest. Primary muscle of respiration
- External intercostals—act during exercise

Expiratory
- Abdominal muscles—primary expiratory muscles
- Internal intercostals

Muscles of the upper airway
- Keep the upper airway open
- Include muscles of the mouth, tongue, uvula, palate, and larynx

Acute ventilatory failure may result from

- Severe respiratory infections
- Pulmonary edema
- Diffuse parenchymal injury
- ARDS (Acute Respiratory Distress Syndrome)
- Acute pulmonary circulatory failure (i.e., acute pulmonary embolism)
- Head trauma or medications that can cause dysfunction of respiratory drive
- Patients with SCI with lesions above C3 present with diaphragmatic failure
  Note: Chronic respiratory failure—considered when ventilatory failure exceeds 30 days

Pulmonary function evaluation

- The magnitude of functional impairment can be assessed through the use of pulmonary function tests
- Respiratory excursions during normal breathing and during maximal inspiration and expiration are observed

– Evaluation of lung volume changes can be used to classify respiratory dysfunction into obstructive and restrictive pulmonary disease

Lung Volume Definitions (Figure 9–1)

Vital capacity (VC): the greatest volume of air that can be exhaled from the lungs after maximum inspiration

Forced vital capacity (FVC): vital capacity measured with the subject exhaling as rapidly as possible

Total lung capacity (TLC): amount of gas within the lungs at the end of maximal inspiration

Tidal volume (TV): amount of gas moved in normal inspiratory effort

Functional residual capacity (FRC): amount of gas in the lungs at the end of normal expiration

Residual volume (RV): amount of gas in the lungs at the end of maximal expiration

Forced expiratory volume in one second (FEV$_1$): amount of air expelled in the first second of FVC

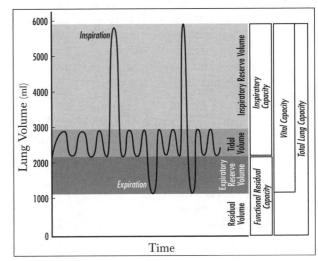

FIGURE 9–1. Illustration of respiratory excursions during: Normal breathing; Maximal inspiration; Maximal expiration

Maximal mid expiratory flow rate (MMEF): average flow rate, between 25% to 50% of FVC

Maximal voluntary ventilation (MVV): the maximum volume of air exhaled in a 12-second period in liters per second

Maximal static inspiratory pressure (PI max): static pressure measured near RV after maximal expiration

Maximal static expiratory pressure (PE max): static pressure measured near TLC after maximal inspiration

Minute volume: tidal volume × rate of breathing per minute

Other important definitions

📖 **Maximal Oxygen consumption**

Expired gases during maximal exercise are collected and analyzed for oxygen content.

VO$_2$ max-volume of consumed O$_2$. Can be calculated using the Fick equation:

VO$_2$ max = (HR × SV) × AVO$_2$ difference (Note: SV=Stroke Volume; HR=Heart Rate)

- Individual VO$_2$ max is dependent on body weight, age (peak is reached at approximately 20 years of age), sex (values for females are approximately 70% those of males), and natural endowment (the most important)
- Training or the presence of pathological conditions can affect this potential
- Endurance exercise training increases VO$_2$ maximum, cardiac output, and physical work capacity of untrained healthy individuals

📖 CLASSIFICATION OF RESPIRATORY DYSFUNCTION

Obstructive Pulmonary Disease (OPD)—Intrinsic Lung Disease

- 📖 Characterized by increased airway resistance due to bronchospasm resulting in air trapping, low maximum midexpiratory flow rate, and normal to increased compliance
- 📖 Impaired blood oxygenation secondary to perfusion-ventilation mismatching. Gas exchange surface of the lung is decreased as a result of air trapping. With decreased diffusion, hypoxia is present with normal or increased ventilation
- Usually eucapnic or hypocapnic, despite severe hypoxia. Hypercapnia occurs in acute respiratory failure or end-stage disease
- 📖 Flattening of the diaphragm, with increased airway resistance, expiratory effort, respiratory muscle fatigue

Incidence: 10% to 40% of all Americans

Fifth leading cause of death in the United States

Fifty percent have limitations in activity level and 25% are limited to bed activities.

Caused by a combination of factors
- Genetic predisposition
- Respiratory infections
- Chemical inflammation (cigarette smoke, asbestos)
  Cigarette smoke is the most common cause of chronic bronchitis and emphysema.
  Causes chronic inflammation and decreased mucociliary clearance
  Smokers are more likely to die from COPD than nonsmokers (3.5 to 25 times more likely)
  Smoking cessation is linked to improvement in the following:
  - Improvement in symptoms
  - Improvement in pulmonary function
  - Decreased risk of respiratory tract infection
  - Decreased reduction in rate of loss of FEV_1, (long term)
- Allergic processes (asthma)
- Metabolic deficiencies (Alpha 1-antitrypsin deficiency)

📖 Causes of Chronic Obstructive Pulmonary Disease (COPD)
- Chronic bronchitis
- Emphysema
- Cystic fibrosis
- Asthma

> REMEMBER ALL FORMS OF COPD INVOLVE AIR TRAPPING

Chronic Bronchitis
- Chronic mucous hypersecretion and respiratory infections as a result of tracheobronchial mucous gland enlargement.
- Production of >100 ml of sputum/day for >3 mo., for at least two consecutive years.

📖 *Emphysema (Figure 9–2)*
- Distention of air spaces distal to the terminal nonrespiratory bronchioles with destruction of alveolar walls. This is secondary to the unimpeded action of neutrophil derived elastase
- Loss of lung recoil, excessive airway collapse on exhalation, and chronic airflow obstruction
- Decreased gas exchange surface of the lung, arterial PO_2 decrease
- Increase in pulmonary vascular resistance in the presence of pulmonary tissue hypoxia, leading to severe pulmonary artery hypertension and right ventricular failure

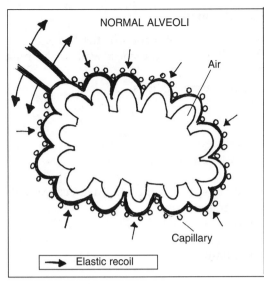

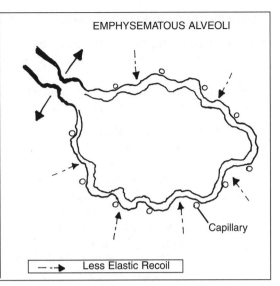

Note:
1. Abundance of capillaries
2. Good elastic recoil
3. Maximum alveolar surface area
4. Standard alveolar gas volume for normal function

Note:
1. Fewer capillaries
2. Decreased elastic recoil
3. Decreased alveolar surface area
4. Increased alveolar gas volume

FIGURE 9–2 Normal Single Alveoli as Compared to Emphysematous Single Alveoli.

📖 *Cystic Fibrosis (CF)*
- Generalized disease of the exocrine glands. Respiratory involvement is caused by failure to adequately remove secretions from the bronchioles, resulting in widespread bronchiolar obstruction and subsequent bronchiectasis, overinflation, and infection
- 📖 Aerobic exercise for cystic fibrosis patients helps to increased sputum expectoration. Patients have increased ciliary beat with improved mucous transport
- Aerobic exercise also improves exercise capacity, respiratory muscle endurance, and reduces airway resistance

Asthma
- Hypertrophy of bronchial muscle, mucosal edema, and infiltration with eosinophils and mononuclear cells, which cause changes in the basement membrane. Chronic bronchitis can result from asthma
- Episodic widespread narrowing of airways, and paroxysmal expiratory dyspnea at night

The magnitude of functional impairment in COPD patients can be assessed using Pulmonary Function Tests (PFTs)
- When the predicted FEV_1 is close to 4 liters, the patient should not have a history of significant exercise impairment
- Impairment develops when FEV_1 falls below 3 liters per second
- Between 2 to 3 liters the patient may experience mild exercise limitation (able to walk significant distances, but not at high speed)
- FEV_1 between 1 to 2 liters, the patient may experience moderate degree of exercise impairment (intermittent rest periods are required to walk significant distances or to climb stairs)
- $FEV_1 < 1$ liter, severe exercise impairment (very short distance ambulation)

Restrictive Pulmonary Disease—Mechanical Dysfunction

- ▢ Impaired lung ventilation as a result of mechanical dysfunction of the lungs or the chest wall, with respiratory muscle dysfunction. Stiffness of the chest wall or the lung tissue itself
- Hypercapnia precedes hypoxia, causing oxygenation abnormalities
- Almost all lung volumes are decreased

▢ **Causes of Restrictive Pulmonary Disease**
- Chest Wall Disease (increased stiffness of chest wall)
  - Neuromuscular disease (e.g., Duchenne's muscular dystrophy)
  - Thoracic deformities (e.g., kyphoscoliosis)
  - If scoliotic angle is >90 degrees, patients have dyspnea; with >120 degrees patients present with hypoventilation and may have cor pulmonale
  - Ankylosing spondylitis (limited expansion of the chest wall)
  - Cervical spinal cord injury
- Intrinsic Lung Disease (increased stiffness of lung tissue)
  - Interstitial lung disease
  - Pleural disease
  - Surgical removal of lung tissue
    Note: Intrinsic lung disease can lead to pulmonary HTN, Right Ventricular Hypertrophy, and cor pulmonale

Examples of Chest Wall Disease

Neuromuscular Disease
- Weakness of respiratory muscles impairs the bellows activity of the chest wall, limiting ventilatory capacity and causing hypoventilation
- Respiratory muscle weakness causes impaired cough
- Examples: Duchenne's Muscular Dystrophy (DMD), Amyotrophic Lateral Sclerosis (ALS), Guillain-Barré Syndrome (GBS), Myasthenia Gravis (MG)

Duchenne's Muscular Dystrophy—sex-linked recessive
- ▢ Patients present with several respiratory complications including:
  - Atelectasis
  - Pneumonia
  - Chronic alveolar hypoventilation (CAH) with hypoxemia
  - Ventilatory failure
- About 73% of the patients die from severe carbon dioxide retention due to CAH
- DMD patients develop progressive scoliosis, which limits expansion of the chest wall and interferes with respiration

Amyotrophic Lateral Sclerosis
- Most common form of motor neuron disease that causes respiratory failure. Respiratory failure usually develops late in the disease and is the most common cause of death
- Respiratory muscle weakness causes ventilatory limitation and impaired cough
- If symptoms begin with limb weakness the disorder may progress to respiratory failure in 2–5 years

Thoracic Deformities (i.e., Kyphoscoliosis)
- Severe Kyphoscoliosis limits expansion of chest wall, reduces lung volumes, and compromises respiratory muscle efficiency
- If scoliotic angle is > 90 degrees, patients suffer dyspnea
- If scoliotic angle is > 120 degrees, patients suffer hypoventilation and cor pulmonale

Ankylosing Spondylitis
- There is limited expansion of chest wall secondary to the ankylosing process.

Cervical Cord Injury
- Diaphragm is innervated by the phrenic nerve (at C3–C5)
- Spinal cord trauma sparing phrenic nerve innervation leaves diaphragm function intact and adequate ventilation can be sustained
- Although lower cervical and high thoracic cord lesions leave diaphragm function intact, they eliminate intercostal and abdominal muscle function, severely impairing cough mechanism
  – These patients have difficulty clearing secretions and ventilatory failure ensues
- Lesions above C3 eliminate all but accessory muscles of breath
- RV increases in C-spine injury

PULMONARY FUNCTION EVALUATION

Normal lung volumes	Restrictive lung disease	Obstructive disease (COPD)
INSPR RESERVE VOL / TV / EXP. RESERVE VOL / RESIDUAL VOL — VC — TLC	INSPR RESERVE VOL / TV / EXP. RESERVE VOL / RESIDUAL VOL — VC — TLC	INSPR RESERVE VOL / TV / EXP. RESERVE VOL / RESIDUAL VOL — VC — TLC
📖 **Normal changes noted with aging**	**Key point:** **All volumes are decreased**	📖 **Key point:** **Air trapping occurs**
• Decreases in VC MVV FEV_1 PO_2 • **FEV_1 decreased at a rate of 30cc/yr** • **No changes in** TLC PCO_2 • **Increases in** RV FRC	**Increased stiffness of chest wall** Ankylosing spondylitis Cervical SCI Neuromuscular disease including: DMD, ALS, MG, GBS Kyphoscoliosis **Increased stiffness of lung** Pulmonary edema Interstitial lung disease • **Decreases in** 📖 VC 📖 TLC 📖 RV FRC FVC MVV (decreases in severity) All volumes are decreased, this is distinctive for restrictive lung disease • 📖 FEV_1 is normal Note: RV increases in C-spine injury	**Limitation in expiration before air is fully expired** Emphysema Cystic fibrosis Asthma Chronic bronchitis **Flattening of the diaphragm** Increased: Airway resistance Expiratory effort Respiratory muscle fatigue Impaired gas exchange as a result of air trapping leads to resp. muscle fatigue. • **Decreases in:** VC FEV_1 MVV FVC • **FEV_1 decreases 45 to 75 cc/yr. in COPD patients** • **Increases in:** 📖 RV FRC 📖 TLC

Key: Refer to lung volume definitions for abbreviations.
Note: MVV decreases in most pathological states and aging.

LUNG VOLUME CHANGES PRESENT IN DIFFERENT CONDITIONS

Tobacco use with normal aging

- 📖 The rate of decrease in FEV_1 is approximately 30cc/year
- In smokers this can increase to 2–3 times this value. Smokers with an age < 35 years can increase lung function if they quit smoking. If patient is > 35 years of age and quits smoking, the rate of decline of lung function slows to the normal rate associated with aging

Cervical spinal cord injury

Cervical spinal cord injured patients have restrictive lung disease.
- 📖 Pulmonary changes seen in C5 quadriplegics
- Diaphragm remains intact and the expiratory muscles are paralyzed
- Patients retain approximately 60% of their inspiratory capacity and ventilate well, but have weak cough and difficulty clearing secretions during respiratory infections
- All volumes are greatly reduced because of limited expansion of the chest wall
- Decreased TLC and VC
- Increased RV
- 📖 In patients with spinal cord injury, the abdominal contents may sag due to the greater strength of the diaphragm relative to the weakness of the abdominal wall muscles. This decreases diaphragmatic excursion and the vital capacity in the sitting position.
- 📖 The reduction in vital capacity is most severe in quadriplegics with cervical cord injury and during the acute injury period. Severity of reduction increases with higher level of injury. A study by Maloney reported that in the sitting position the use of an abdominal binder improved vital capacity. (Figure 9–3) (Maloney, 1979)
- The goal of pulmonary rehabilitation of the SCI patient is to:
  - Increase vital capacity
  - Maintain good pulmonary hygiene
  - Subjectively improve dyspnea as it relates to patient functional mobility and self-care
  - Reduce average number of hospital stays

Duchenne's muscular dystrophy

- Vital capacity plateaus between 1,100 and 2,800 ml between 10 and 15 years of age
- Independent of chest deformity, the vital capacity is then lost at a rate of 200 to 250 ml/year. The rate of loss tapers below 400 ml
- 📖 No clear guidelines have been established for determining the point at which ventilatory support should be instituted in patients with Duchenne's muscular dystrophy, but various studies suggest the following:

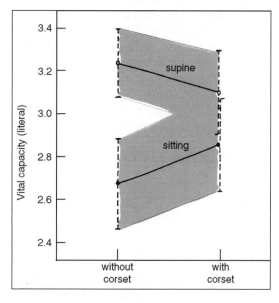

FIGURE 9–3. Comparison chart of actual vital capacities with and without wearing a corset in supine and sitting position. The chart shows the interaction of the position and the use of the corset. Note the significant difference in vital capacity in the patient without the corset in the supine vs. the seated position. The vital capacity is improved in the seated position with corset.

- Dyspnea at rest
- Vital capacity, 45% predicted
- Maximal inspiratory pressure < 30% predicted
- Hypercapnia

Amyotrophic lateral sclerosis (ALS)

- Routine pulmonary function tests, including functional vital capacity, should be monitored closely in ALS
- The earliest changes noted are decreases in maximum inspiratory and expiratory muscle pressures, followed by reduced vital capacity and maximum breathing capacity
- When VC falls to 25 ml/kg of body weight, the ability to cough is impaired, increasing the risk of aspiration pneumonia
- ☐ Functional vital capacity is the best prognostic indicator for noninvasive ventilation in patients with ALS. Patients may lose VC at a rate 1,000 ml or more per year.
- Blood gases remain normal until the patient is near respiratory arrest (Bach 1996)

REHABILITATION OF THE PATIENT WITH COPD

1. Evaluate Nutritional State

- Respiratory muscle weakness is associated with metabolic deficits
- Decreased magnesium, calcium, potassium, and hypophosphatemia are associated with respiratory muscle weakness which is reversible after replacement
- Serum albumin level correlates better with hypoxia than spirometric values. Indicates visceral protein depletion and is a good predictor of rehabilitation potential
- Impaired nutritional status is associated with increased morbidity and mortality
  - More frequent infections: Impaired cell-mediated immunity
  - Decreased macrophage action in the pulmonary alveolar region
  - Increased bacterial adherence and colonization in upper and lower airways
  - Pseudomonas species commonly colonize in patients with poor nutrition
- Poor nutritional state affects lung repair mechanisms, including surfactant synthesis
  Can lead to generalized weakness, affecting respiratory function, and finally, hypercapnic respiratory failure, and problems with weaning from mechanical ventilation

2. Optimize Pharmacologic Treatments Prior to Starting the Rehabilitation Program

- ☐ For reversible bronchospasm
  - methylxanthines
  - Beta-2 agonists
  - Anticholinergics—e.g., Atrovent® or Ipratropium®, can be used alone or added to a regimen, including beta-2 agonists. Block smooth muscle muscarinic receptors
- Theophylline—has a bronchodilator effect, decreases diaphragm fatigue; increases cardiac output, and improves mucociliary clearance in COPD
- ☐ Young patients with moderate asthma, who have tried B-2 agonists during exercise, may benefit from theophylline use
- Systemic steroid inhalers. Important to instruct inhaler use with the patients—>60% of COPD patients use them incorrectly
- Expectorants and mucolytics may be used for secretion management
- Increase fluid intake
- Low flow nasal supplemental O_2 can be used during therapy to reduce dyspnea and improve exercise performance, especially in patients with documented Coronary Artery Disease (CAD)

- ▢ O_2 is recommended for patients who desaturate during exercise. The most accepted guideline for O_2 use during exercise is if the patient exhibits an exercise induced SaO_2 below 90%
- Inspiratory phase or pulsed oxygen therapy, especially if provided transtracheally, decreases mucosal drying and discomfort. O_2 delivery is of 0.25 to 0.4 L/ min. compared to 2–4 L/min. via face mask or nasal cannula
- Supplemental O_2 use is also recommended for patients with a continuous PO_2 of 55 to 60 mm Hg
  ▢ Benefits of home oxygen use include:
  1. Reduction in polycythemia
  2. Improvement in pulmonary hypertension
  3. Reduction of the perceived effort during exercise
  4. Prolongation of life expectancy
  5. Improvement in cognitive function
  6. Reduction in hospital needs
- Cessation of smoking should be emphasized

3. Train in Controlled Breathing Techniques

- COPD patients exhibit an altered pattern of respiratory muscle use. The rib cage inspiratory muscles generate more pressure than the diaphragm. Expiratory muscles are also involved
- ▢ Controlled breathing techniques are used to reduce dyspnea, reduce the work of breathing, improve respiratory muscle function and pulmonary function parameters. Different types may be used in patients with obstructive pulmonary disease and restrictive disease

Techniques to Improve Pulmonary Function Parameters
Diaphragmatic breathing
- Used to reverse altered pattern of respiratory muscle recruitment in COPD patients.
- Patient uses the diaphragm, relaxes abdominal muscles during inspiration:
  Lying down, or at 15% to 25% head-down position, the patient places one hand over the thorax below the clavicle to stabilize the chest wall, and the other over the abdomen. The patient takes a deep breath, and expands the abdomen using the diaphragm.
  Feedback of abdominal and rib cage movement is obtained through hand placement as described previously
  ▢ *Benefits:* increased tidal volume, decreased functional residual capacity, and increase in maximum oxygen uptake.

Segmental breathing
- Obstructions, such as tumors and mucous plugs, should be cleared prior to practicing this technique
- The patient is asked to inspire while the clinician applies pressure to the thoracic cage to resist respiratory excursion in a segment of the lung. As the clinician feels the local expansion, the hand resistance is decreased to allow inhalation. This facilitates the expansion of adjacent regions of the thoracic cavity that may have decreased ventilation

Techniques to Reduce Dyspnea and the Work of Breathing
Pursed-lip breathing
Patient inhales through the nose for a few seconds with the mouth closed, then exhales slowly for 4–6 seconds through pursed lips. By forming a wide, thin slit with the lips, the patient creates an obstruction to exhalation, slowing the velocity of exhalation and increasing mouth pressure. Expiration lasts 2–3 times as long as inspiration.

☐ **Benefits:** Prevents air trapping due to small airway collapse during exhalation and promotes greater gas exchange in the alveoli. Increases tidal volume, reduces dyspnea and work of breathing in COPD patients. When added to diaphragmatic breathing, reduces the respiratory rate and can improve blood ABGs. (Bach, 1996)

4. Maintain an Adequate Airway Secretion Management Program

Airway clearance techniques (Controlled cough, Huffing)
Controlled cough
The patient assumes an upright sitting position, inhales deeply, holds the breath for several seconds, contracts the abdominal muscles ("bears down" increasing intrathoracic pressure), then opens the glottis and rapidly and forcefully exhales while contracting the abdominal muscles and leaning slightly forward.
This is repeated two or three times and followed by normal breaths for several minutes before attempting controlled cough.
Coughing generates high expulsive forces promoting secretion retention and may exacerbate air trapping; also leads to fatigue if the cough is weak.

Huffing
An alternative is huffing—following a deep inhalation, the patient attempts short, frequent exhalations by contracting the abdominal muscles and saying "ha, ha, ha".
The glottis remains open during huffing, and does not increase intrathoracic pressure, therefore, in COPD patients where airways can collapse. This is a more efficient means of secretion removal.

Secretion Mobilization Techniques (Postural Drainage, Percussion, Vibration)
Indications: Sputum production >30 ml/day
             Aspiration
             Atelectasis
             Moderate sputum production in debilitated patients that are unable to raise their own secretions

Postural Drainage
Use gravity-assisted positioning to improve the flow of mucous secretions out of the airways.
The affected lung segment is placed uppermost to increase oxygenation and drainage.
Best done after awakening in the morning (secretions accumulate at night) and one to two hours after meals to avoid gastroesophageal reflux.

☐ *Positions for postural drainage (Figure 9–4)*
A common position is the Trendelenburg or head-down posture, which can be done with the patient supine or prone, and different postural variations such as side lying or trunk bending.

To drain the upper lobes:
Patient is positioned sitting up
Exceptions:
- Right anterior segment—Patient supine
- Lingular—Patient in lateral decubital Trendelenburg
- Both posterior segments—Prone

To drain the right middle lobe and lower lobes:
Patient is positioned in the lateral decubital Trendelenburg

Exceptions:
- Superior segment of the lower lobe—Patient prone with buttocks elevated
- Posterior lower segment—Patient in prone Trendelenburg position with buttocks elevated
- Anterior segment—supine Trendelenburg

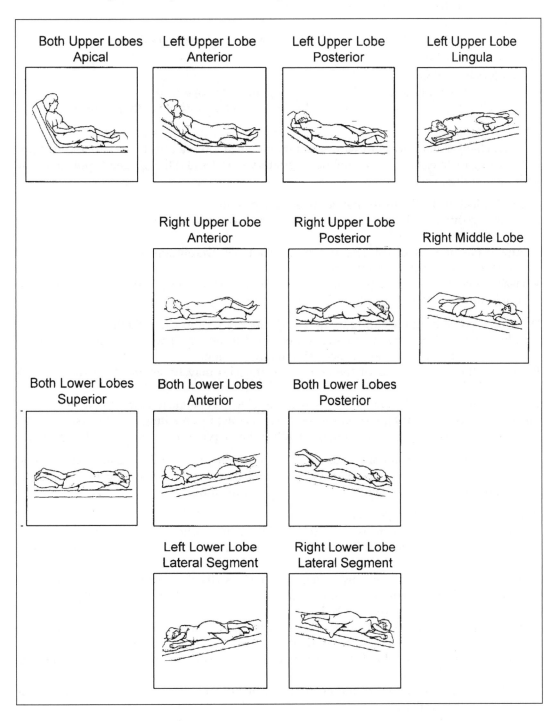

FIGURE 9–4. Postural Drainage Positions.

Precautions for postural drainage:

Head-down—Trendelenburg

Head-down tilt can range from 10° to 45°. COPD patients can tolerate up to 25° tilt.

Avoid in: Pulmonary edema

        CHF

        HTN

        Dyspnea

        Abdominal problems—hiatal hernia, obesity, recent food ingestion, abdominal distention.

Side-lying position

        Contraindications: Axillofemoral bypass graft

                                  Musculoskeletal pain—e.g., rib fractures

📖 *Postural Changes*

Postural changes not only help with secretion mobilization but affect the work of breathing by changing the mechanical load on the respiratory muscles and the oxygen supply and consumption in these areas

1. Mechanical load—Pressure changes related to position

• Upright position—Abdominal contents remain in low position due to gravity; diaphragm can compress them easily

• Supine position—Redistributes abdominal contents. Diaphragm is in a slightly longer resting position further up into the thorax

• Head-down Trendelenburg—Diaphragm at its longer resting position, displaced by the weight of the abdominal contents into the thorax

With progression from the sitting to the Trendelenburg position, the diaphragmatic work of breathing is increased (the abdominal content load increases). The diaphragm will accommodate to the increase in load by increasing its contraction.

In obesity, the external load of the abdominal muscles may be greater than the muscle's capacity of contraction.

In neuromuscular disease, the muscles may not be able to generate tension against the abdominal content load, requiring changes in posture to assist in breathing. This is also valid for COPD patients where postural changes can affect the diaphragmatic mechanical response.

📖 The weight of the pulmonary tissue also contributes to overall pressure on the most dependent alveoli. The dependent alveoli expand in size when changing from sitting to supine position, increasing ventilation at the base of the lung.

2. Blood flow—gravity dependent

Maximum flow is greatest at the most gravity dependent portions of the lung.

• Upright sitting—Ventilation/Perfusion (V/Q) mismatch, most effective at the middle lung fields

Blood flow is more at the lower fields, while gas distribution is initially distributed through the apices. With inspiration, the fall in pressure will draw the greatest gas volume to the more dependent areas of the lung.

• In some patients changing from supine to prone positioning displaces the weight of the abdominal contents, reversing blood flow distribution to the anterior segments

  – 📖 The difference in blood flow distribution is based on the pressure affecting the capillaries: (Figure 9-5)

  – The pressure of the surrounding tissues can influence the resistance to blood flow through the capillaries

  – Blood flow depends on pulmonary artery pressure, alveolar pressure, and pulmonary venous pressure

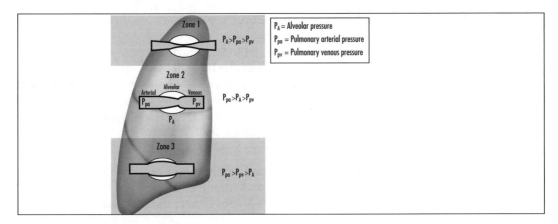

FIGURE 9–5. 3 Zone Model of the Lung: The difference in blood flow distribution is based on the pressure affecting the capillaries.

Zone 1: Alveolar Pressure (PA) exceeds Pulmonary Artery Pressure (Ppa), and no flow occurs because the vessels are collapsed.

Zone 2: Arterial Pressure (Ppa) exceeds alveolar pressure but Alveolar Pressure (PA) exceeds Pulmonary Venous Pressure (Ppv). The arterial-alveolar pressure difference (Ppa–PA) determines the flow in Zone 2. This steadily increases down the zone.

Zone 3: Pulmonary Venous Pressure (Ppv) exceeds alveolar pressure and flow is determined by the Arterial Venous Pressure (Ppa) difference (Ppa–Ppv) which is constant down this pulmonary zone. Note the pressure across the vessel walls increases down the zone so their caliber increases. As the caliber of the vessel wall increases, so does the flow.

- The perfusion of the lung is dependent on posture.
- The perfusion of the 3-zone model of the lung in the upright position is described below. (Figure 9–6A)
  Zone 1: Ventilation occurs in excess of perfusion
  Zone 2: Perfusion and ventilation are fairly equal
  Zone 3: Is the most gravity dependent region of the lung where

Pulmonary Artery Pressure > Pulmonary Venous Pressure, which is > Alveolar Pressure

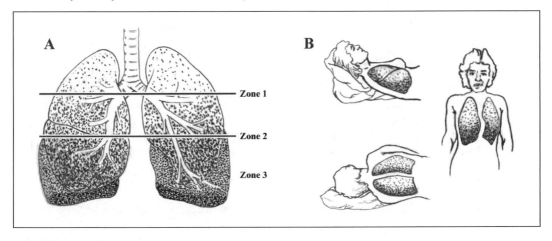

FIGURE 9–6. A: Perfusion of the lung is dependent on posture. This diagram shows the perfusion of the lung in the upright position. **B:** Perfusion of the lung is effected on positioning of the patient. The gravity-dependent segments have the greatest amount of perfusion.

- 📖 When changing from a sitting to supine position, venous pressure increases in relation to the arterial pressure in dependent areas of the lung
- Blood flow is governed by the pulmonary arterial to venous difference
- When supine, the apical blood flow increases, but the bases remain virtually unchanged. There is an almost uniform blood flow throughout the lung. However, posterior segment flow will exceed anterior segment perfusion in this position.
- The normal ratio of ventilation/perfusion is 0.8. Areas of low ratios (perfusion > ventilation) act as a shunt. Areas of high ratios act as dead space.

Percussion
Mechanical percussor or a cupped hand can be used to rhythmically strike the thoracic cage during the entire respiratory cycle to loosen mucus within the lungs.
Delivered at a frequency of 5 Hz for 1 to 5 minutes or longer over the chest area desired to be drained.
Used on patients who are unable to mobilize and expectorate excess secretions, or to help expand areas of atelectasis.

Precautions:
Coagulation disorders
Anticoagulation therapy
Platelet count below 50,000
Fractured ribs
Flail chest
Severe osteoporosis

Contraindications:
Cardiovascular instability or failure
Aortic aneurysm
Increased intracranial pressure
Increased intraocular pressure
Cannot do percussion over a tumor

Vibration
Rapid shaking back and forth, (not downward) on the thorax over a segment of the lung, causing mucus to move toward the trachea. Applied to the thorax or airway to facilitate secretion elimination.
Can be applied manually or through the use of a mechanical vibrator.

Mechanically:
Vibrator can be used at frequencies ranging from 10–15 Hz up to 170 Hz
Most animal studies favor the 10–15 Hz frequency range

- Uses very little or no pressure on the thorax, and constitutes an alternative in cases where percussion is contraindicated
- The effects of mechanical chest percussion and vibration are frequency dependent
- Side effects of percussion and vibration can include increased obstruction to airflow in COPD patients

Preoperative and Postoperative Chest Therapy Program
Airway clearance and secretion mobilization techniques can be applied prior to surgery, and after the procedure
📖 A preoperative and postoperative chest therapy program has the following advantages:
- Decreases the incidence of pneumonia

- Reduces the probability of developing postoperative atelectasis following thoracic and abdominal surgery

Pre-operative Program: The patient is taught standard postoperative treatment.

Deep breathing—Taught with the patient in the semi-Fowler position, in which the abdominal muscles are on slack. This allows greater diaphragmatic excursion. Most important modality of postoperative pulmonary hygiene.

Rolling—Allows patient mobility and minimizes trunk movement

Coughing—Decreased cough effectiveness can be a result of anesthesia
Two-stage cough, preceded by a deep diaphragmatic breath. First cough raises the secretions, second cough facilitates expectoration. May use splinting techniques for coughing, splinting the surgical incision with the use of a pillow or hands.

Huffing
Incentive spirometry—Provides the patient with visual feedback of the air volume inspired during a deep breath. Patients practice deep inspiration every hour in addition to their chest physical therapy sessions.

Post-operative Treatment
Most therapy programs start one day postoperatively. Diaphragmatic and segmental breathing are used to assist the ventilator.
Breathing exercises are provided.
Secretion management techniques include postural drainage, vibration and percussion.
If the patient underwent abdominal surgery, one hand is placed between the incision site and the area to be percussed to decrease discomfort during the treatment. A pillow over the incision may also be used.
Vibration is preferred post operatively because it is less traumatic.
These treatments are contraindicated in patients with cardiac or hemodynamic instability or in cases of pneumothorax.

5. Provide Therapeutic Exercises

Used to improve respiratory muscle endurance, strength, and efficiency

Inspiratory resistive loading
- Uses an inspiratory muscle trainer. The patient inhales through its inspiratory orifices, which progressively decrease in size. Exhalation is performed without resistance
- Treatment is provided 1 to 2 times per day for approximately 15 to 30 minutes, with a rate of 10 to 20 breaths per minute. If the patient is able to tolerate 30-minute sessions, the intensity is increased by varying the orifice size. To increase endurance and orifice size that allows a longer exercise duration is chosen

Threshold inspiratory muscle training
A threshold loading device allows inspiration only after a predetermined mouth pressure is reached. Produces inspiratory resistance without relying on inspiratory flow rates. Benefits include increased ventilatory strength and endurance.
- Inspiratory muscle training has been proven beneficial in patients with cystic fibrosis, where FVC, TLC, and inspiratory muscle strength have been improved
- Inspiratory muscle training has appeared to prevent the weakness associated with steroid use in patients with this type of medication, as documented in one controlled study

 – In patients with asthma, a reduction in asthma symptoms has been noted in addition to the documented improvement in the inspiratory muscle strength and endurance. A reduction in hospitalizations and emergency room visits, increase in school and work attendance, and reduction in medication use has also been found.

6. Instruct In Reconditioning Exercises

This type of exercise allows the patient to increase the ability to perform ADLs. The patient is engaged in a progressive program for which he or she is made responsible.

 – Activities may include: aerobic conditioning (bicycle, pool exercise program, walking, stair climbing, calisthenics), ROM exercises (coordinated with diaphragmatic breathing) and upper extremity strengthening exercises
 – A daily 12-minute walk with a record of time spent and distance achieved; and 15 minutes a day of inspiratory training is also advised. The 12-minute walk can be used to estimate exercise tolerance
 – Pulse parameters include: increase of at least 20% to 30% during the activity with a return to baseline within 5 to 10 minutes after exercise
 – The program is reevaluated weekly for 10 to 12 weeks, and modifications are made along with patient education
 – Upper extremity exercise reduces the metabolic demand and increased ventilation associated with arm elevation, and dyspnea
 – Unsupported upper extremity activities produced the most benefits, including decreased O_2 consumption. These type of activities include self-care, lifting, reaching, carrying, and athletic activities
 – All exercises should be performed to tolerance (symptom limited, subjective dyspnea)
 – Should hold exercise for a HR >120 beats/minute
 – Hold exercise if the patient has premature beats > 6/minute
 – Hold exercise for oxygen saturation less than 92%. If the patient desaturates during exercise (<90%) may use supplemental O_2 to enhance exercise performance and protect patients with CAD from dysrhythmia
   📖 Aerobic exercise in patients with cystic fibrosis may include:
   – Exercises involving the trunk muscles such as sit-ups
   – Swimming
   – Jogging
 – 📖 Patients with CF that participate in a structured running program show significant improvements in exercise capacity, respiratory muscle endurance, and a reduction in airway resistance. In addition, studies in children with CF have found increased sputum expectoration and an improvement in lung function after several weeks of strenuous regular aerobic exercise.

7. Muscle Rest Periods Should Be Added to the Exercise Program

Monitor hypercapnia as an indicator for the need of a rest period.
Ventilatory assistance provides relief to tired respiratory muscles decreasing their energy expenditure. Diaphragm rest can be achieved by assisting ventilation noninvasively with the use of body ventilators, mouthpiece, or nasal intermittent positive pressure ventilation (IPPV) or tracheostomy IPPV.
Although assisting ventilation can exacerbate air trapping in COPD patients, the benefits of resting respiratory muscles and decreasing oxygen consumption may outweigh this in importance

Two groups of COPD patients may benefit from ventilatory assistance

1. Medically and psychologically stable patients who require assistance around the clock, usually by tracheostomy route
2. Patients with need of nocturnal assistance only
   The nocturnal use of ventilators supports weak respiratory muscles
   Potential benefits include:
   - increased vital capacity, respiratory muscle strength and endurance, and decreased need for hospitalizations

Ventilatory assistance for COPD patients includes Positive Pressure Airway Ventilators and Negative Pressure Body Ventilators

Positive Pressure Airway Ventilation can be intermittent (IPPV), continuous (CPAP), or bilevel (BiPAP).

- Intermittent Positive Pressure Ventilation (IPPV) is the most common method of noninvasive support
  For mouthpiece IPPV, a mouthpiece is set up near the mouth, where the patient can easily grab it up to 6 to 8 times a minute for full ventilatory support. It is an ideal inspiratory muscle aid for day time use.
  For nocturnal use, nasal IPPV with CPAP mask (adequate seal is a problem) or mouthpiece IPPV with lip seal retention (seal is adequate, but patient cannot talk).
- ▣ Continuous Positive Airway Pressure ventilation (CPAP) may be used to help maintain patent airways in patients with sleep disordered breathing (obstructive sleep apnea). It produces splinting of the pharyngeal airway with positive pressure delivered through a nose mask. This method prevents desaturation.
- Bilevel positive airway pressure (BiPAP) permits independent adjustment of inspiratory (IPAP) and expiratory positive airway pressure (EPAP)

Negative Pressure Body Ventilators (NPBV) used during the day or night have provided the following benefits:
   - Improved respiratory endurance with decrease in dyspnea
   - Improved in quality of life, 12-minute walking distance
   - Improved transdiaphragmatic pressure, and maximum inspiratory and expiratory pressures

NPBV ventilators assist respiratory muscles by creating atmospheric pressure around the thorax and abdomen

NPBV are also an alternative to intubation and tracheostomy for patients with acute respiratory failure (Bach 1998)

REHABILITATION OF THE PATIENT WITH RESTRICTIVE LUNG DISEASE

Respiratory complications are the most common causes of death in advanced restrictive lung disease. The major cause of acute respiratory failure for these patients is impaired secretion clearance. Rehabilitation of the patient with restrictive lung disease is based on prevention of complications and assistance with secretion management.

1. Patient Education

- Prevents development of pneumonia, respiratory failure, and subsequent intubation and mechanical ventilation
- Importance of vaccinations should be stressed:
  Influenza, pneumococcal, and the possible use of antiviral agents
- Avoid crowded areas or exposure to respiratory tract pathogens
- Avoid sedatives at night and the risk of possible aspiration

- Avoid oxygen therapy. Central ventilatory drive can be suppressed, exacerbation of carbon dioxide can occur, and the risk of respiratory failure can be increased
  Studies indicate that O_2 therapy can prolong hypopneas and apneas by 33% during rapid eye movement (REM) and by 19% otherwise, even in patients with mild neuromuscular disease
- Avoid obesity and heavy meals
- Develop goals and start planning for the future

2. Keep A Good Nutritional State

- Respiratory muscle insufficiency can be exacerbated by hypokalemia
- Patients with Duchenne muscular dystrophy have decreased total body potassium, and commonly develop hypokalemia during acute illnesses

3. Instruct In Controlled Breathing Techniques

Glossopharyngeal breathing

- This is a noninvasive method to support ventilation, and it can be used in the event of ventilator equipment failure
- The patient takes a deep breath, and uses the pistoning action of the tongue and pharyngeal muscles to project air boluses into the lungs. Rhythmic opening and closing of the vocal cords occurs with each air bolus
- Each breath usually consists of 6 to 9 air boluses (or up to 65), with each bolus consisting of 30 to 150 ml of air (usually 60 to 200 ml.)
- Requires intact oropharyngeal muscle strength, and the patient should not be tracheostomized

📖 Other uses of glossopharyngeal breathing

- Enables the patient to breathe without mechanical ventilation (up to 4 or more hours if the lungs are normal; if lungs are affected may only tolerate minutes). This time off the ventilator can be used to transfer to different types of aids
- Improves the volume of the voice and the rhythm of speech, allowing the patient to shout
- Helps prevent micro-atelectasis
- Allows the patient to take deeper breaths for more effective cough
- Improves or maintains pulmonary compliance

Use deep breathing and insufflations

- A program of air stacking hyperinflations 2 to 4 times a day with progressively increasing volumes helps prevent atelectasis and can benefit VC
- Regular maximal insufflations can be provided with manual resuscitators, portable ventilators, and mechanical insufflators-exsufflators. A mouthpiece may be used, or a nosepiece may be provided for larger volumes and when patients have weak oral muscles

4. Use Adequate Secretion-Management Techniques

Manually assisted cough

- The clinician's or the assisting person's heel of the hand or arm is placed at various sites along the anterior chest or abdomen to provide pressure, and is coordinated with the patient's coughing or expiratory effort
- Location of the areas of pressure:
  - Heimlich-type or abdominal thrust assist—Patient in the side-lying position, pressure is applied at the navel while pushing up the diaphragm
  - Costophrenic assist—Patient in any position, pressure applied to the costophrenic angles
  - Anterior chest compression assist—Patient lying on the side or the three-quarter supine position, pressure applied to the upper and lower anterior chest

– Counter rotation assist—Pressure is applied to the pelvis or shoulder during inspiration followed by reversing the pressure direction to compress the thorax in all planes to facilitate expulsion

Suctioning
– Should be done in conjunction with other secretion clearing techniques, or when other techniques fail to remove secretions appropriately
– May lead to complications such as: airway membrane irritation, airway edema and wheezing, hypoxemia, bradycardia or tachycardia, hyper- and hypotension, increased intracranial pressure
– ONLY suction as you withdraw the catheter
Chest percussion, postural drainage may also be used.

Mechanical insufflator-exsufflator
– Most effective method of mechanical assistance for secretion clearance in paralyzed patients
– A deep inspiration (positive-pressure insufflation) is provided via a mask or through the tracheal tube, followed by rapid controlled suction (negative pressure exsufflation)
– Insufflation and exsufflation can be independently adjusted
– A desired decrease in pressure from insufflation to exsufflation is approximately 80 cm H_2O. This may be sustained for 2 to 3 seconds. The duration of exsufflation is longer than with other methods of assistance
– The decrease in pressure creates flows of approximately 7 to 11 L/second, helping to bring secretions to the upper airways where those can be suctioned
– It can be used in patients with scoliosis, dysphagia , impaired glottis function, and severe upper respiratory tract infections
– Allows continued ventilatory support without tracheostomy, and improves pulmonary volumes and SaO_2

5. Use Noninvasive Ventilation

Mechanically assisted ventilation provides respiratory muscle rest, decreasing the energy expenditure of the respiratory muscles.
Body ventilation—includes positive, negative/positive, and negative pressure ventilation

Positive pressure body ventilators
Provide positive pressure on the abdomen to assist diaphragmatic cephalad movement, promoting expiration. Passive inspiration occurs after removing the abdominal pressure.

- ▢ **Intermittent abdominal pressure ventilator (IAPV)**
  Examples: Pneumobelt, Exsufflation belt.
  – Abdominal corset containing a battery operated rubber air sac. It helps to create forced expiration by moving the diaphragm cephalad. When deflated, the diaphragm and the abdominal contents fall to resting position, resulting in passive inspiration
  – Worn from the xiphoid to above the pelvic arch. Cycles are 40% inspiration and 60% expiration. Approximately 250 to 1,200 ml of tidal volume can be provided
  – Depends on gravity to assist inspiration, and is only effective when the patient is in the sitting position. A trunk angle of 75° from the horizontal is optimal but may be used with 45° in some cases
  – This is the most useful mode of ventilation for wheelchair-bound patients with less than 1 hour of ventilator-free time during the day. Benefits also include liberating the mouth and hands for other activities
  – Contraindicated in severe scoliosis and severe obesity. The patient should have a mobile abdomen

- Not useful in patients with decreased pulmonary compliance or increased airway resistance
- Most beneficial when used during the day in addition to nocturnal noninvasive IPPV. Inspiration may be supplemented by the use of available inspiratory muscles and or glossopharyngeal breathing

Negative and positive pressure body ventilator

📖 *Rocking bed*

Rocks the patient along a vertical axis (15 to 30 degrees from the horizontal) utilizing the force of gravity to assist ventilation.
- When the head of the bed is up, inspiration is assisted by using gravity to pull the diaphragm down. This creates a negative pressure
- With the head down, exhalation assist is obtained. Cephalad movement of the abdominal contents pushes the diaphragm up with production of positive pressure
- It is used in patients with diaphragm paralysis with some accessory muscle function
- Benefits: prevents venous stasis, improves clearance of bronchial secretions, weight shifting prevents development of pressure ulcers, benefits bowel motility. It is easy to apply
- Disadvantages: heavy (not portable); not effective in patients with poor lung or chest wall compliance or in those with increased airway resistance

External oscillation ventilator (Hayek oscillator)
- Flexible chest enclosure (cuirass) with external oscillating ventilator
- Pressure change is developed between the cuirass and the chest wall. Negative pressure helps chest wall expansion and inspiration. Positive pressure causes chest compression and aides expiration
- Inspiratory pressure is always negative, but the expiratory pressure can be adjusted to positive, zero or subatmospheric, and negative
- By increasing the number of oscillations per minute it may be used for secretion clearance
- Patients with decreased lung compliance may use this type of assistance

Negative pressure ventilators

- Create intermittent extrathoracic pressure over the chest wall and abdomen, helping inspiration
- Main use is at night
- Provides rest to fatigued respiratory muscles
- Cor pulmonale may be prevented
- The patient may be able to function during the day without respiratory assistance
- Contraindicated in upper airway obstruction cases, where it may increase the frequency and severity of airway collapse and obstruction during the night. This may lead to obstructive apnea and desaturation
- Not useful in children < 3 years old due to recurrent pneumonias and atelectasis
- Not useful in patients with excessive airway secretions

Tank Ventilators (Emerson iron lung, LifeCare Porta-lung)
- Patient's entire body is enclosed in a chamber that produces intermittent subatmospheric pressure (Iron lung) or has a separate negative pressure generator (Porta-lung).
- Uses: Management of acute respiratory failure patients
     Ventilatory support in patients with decreased pulmonary compliance, significant scoliosis, and severe infections

Wrap Ventilators (Poncho, Pneumosuit)
- Plastic grid that covers abdomen and thorax. The wrap is sealed around the patient's wrists, neck and abdomen, or legs. A negative pressure ventilator creates subatmospheric pressure under the grid and wrap

– Provides greater volumes
– Only used with nocturnal assisted ventilation

Uses: In patients with scoliosis or with sensory deficits

Disadvantages: Difficult to don, decreased access to the body by the medical personnel; difficult to turn the patient

Cuirass or Chest Shell Ventilators
– Firm shell that covers the chest and abdomen attached to a negative pressure ventilator that generates a sub-atmospheric pressure under the shell
– It is the only Negative Pressure Body Ventilator (NPBV) that can be used during the day for ventilatory support in the seated position

Advantages: The patient can get on and off without assistance

Disadvantages: In insensate patients can cause pressure ulcers around the area anterior to the axilla

Not effective in: Patients with complete respiratory paralysis
Impairment of pulmonary compliance
Patients with apnea
Patients with intrinsic lung disease
Severe back deformity
Morbid obesity

MANAGEMENT OF SLEEP DISORDERED BREATHING

• Weight reduction can improve obstructive sleep apnea for obese patients
• Use of independently varying inspiratory positive airway pressure and expiratory positive airway pressure ventilators is very effective in patients with hypercapnia. The greater the difference between Inspiratory Positive Airway Pressure (IPAP) and Expiratory Positive Airway Pressure (EPAP), the greater the inspiratory muscle assistance
• To allow for an adequate fit, custom molded nasal interfaces may be provided
• Portable volume ventilators may be used in morbidly obese patients or patients who require high peak ventilators pressures
• An orthodontic splint that brings the mandible and tongue forward is helpful to maintain the hypopharynx open, as a long-term resource

INVASIVE VENTILATORY SUPPORT

Invasive ventilation is used when noninvasive methods fail or are inadequate
Tracheal intubation or tracheostomy is indicated when the ABGs show PaO_2 < 55 mm Hg, or PCO_2 > 50 mm Hg.

COPD and restrictive lung disease patients may need intubation for other reasons:
– Noninvasive mechanical ventilator does not deliver O_2 adequately due to poor access to oral or nasal routes, i.e., orthopedic conditions (osteogenesis imperfecta, inadequate bite or mouthpiece entry), presence of NGT, or upper airway obstruction
– Severe intrinsic pulmonary disease requiring high Frequency of Inspired Oxygen (FiO_2)
– Inadequate oropharyngeal muscle strength
– Uncontrolled seizures or substance abuse
– Assisted peak cough flow < 160 L/minute
– When mechanical exsufflator is not available or contraindicated
– Unreliable access to assisted coughing
– Depressed cognitive status

Tracheal intubation with tracheostomy tube

The choice of tracheostomy tube depends upon the patient and the duration of use

Types of tracheostomy tubes

Metal (e.g. Jackson, Holinger)
- Cuffless, reusable tubes made of stainless steel or silver
- Cause less local irritation, and tissue reaction as compared to plastic
- May be left in place longer
- Help to keep the tracheostomy stoma open until the tracheostomy is not needed, in patients who breathe spontaneously

Plastic (e.g., Bivona, Shiley, Portex)
- Disposable, made of PVC, nylon, silicone, and Teflon
- Available single or double cannulated, with/without cuff

Cuff inflated versus uncuffed

Cuff-inflated Tracheostomy Tubes
- Provide a good air seal, protects lower airways from aspiration, and prevents air leaking through the upper airway. Creates the least positive pressure against the tracheal wall.
- Patients cannot speak with cuff-inflated tracheostomy tube.
- Two types: High pressure/low volume
  - Low pressure/high volume-conform more to the shape of the trachea and inflate more uniformly

Uncuffed Tracheal Tubes
- Some patients may be able to talk while on mechanical ventilation
- Should not be used in patients at risk for aspiration because it provides a loose fit
- Used after tracheostomy, when a looser fit of the tube on the stoma is needed, or to prevent subcutaneous emphysema
- Used in patients with increased secretions
- Should not be used in patients known to aspirate

Fenestrated versus nonfenestrated tubes

Fenestrated
📖 This tracheostomy tube is good for patients who are able speak and require only intermittent ventilatory assistance.
- A continuous inner cannula can be used with an outer fenestrated cannula. The fenestrations should lie within the lumen of the trachea, and should not touch the tracheal wall (may develop granulation tissue around the holes and become clogged with secretions)
- The inner cannula can be attached to a positive pressure ventilator
- When the inner cannula is out and the tube is plugged, the patient can breath through the fenestrations and is able to phonate. This is possible because the air is directed though the upper respiratory tract

Nonfenestrated
- Used in patients who require continuous mechanical ventilation, or are unable to protect the airway during swallowing
- 📖 If the patient wants to talk, a one-way talking valve may be used on the tracheostomy tube. These devices open on inhalation and close during exhalation to produce phonation

📖 **Talking tubes (TT) versus speaking valves**

Speaking Tracheostomy Tubes (e.g., Portex "Talk" tube, Bivona Fome-cuff with side-port airway connector, Communi-trach)
- Used in alert and motivated patients, who require an inflated cuff for ventilation and who have intact vocal cords and the ability to mouth words
- Airflow is through the glottis, supporting vocalization with airflow over the vocal cords while maintaining a closed system for ventilation
- Talking trachs supply pressurized gas mixtures through a cannula that travels through the wall of the talking tube, then enters the trachea through small holes above the inflated tube cuff so the patient can use the larynx to speak while the cuff is inflated (thus leaving mechanical ventilation undisturbed)
- The quality of speech is altered (e.g., lower pitch, coarser). Patients need to speak short sentences (because constant flow through the vocal cords can cause the voice to fade away)
- The patient requires some manual dexterity and minimal strength to occlude the external port

One-way speaking valves (e.g., Passy-Muir speaking valve, Olympic Trach-Talk)
- Passy-Muir valve is the only valve that has a biased, closed position; opens only on inspiration
- All the other valves are open at all times until they are actively closed during expiration (when enough force is placed)
- The air is directed into the trachea and up through the vocal cords, creating speech as air passes through the oral and nasal chambers
- Requires less work—opening and closing the valve is not needed
- Do not use the speaking valves with COPD patients because the lung has lost elasticity and the patient cannot force air out due to lack of lung compliance

TABLE 9-1. Characteristics Of One-Way Speaking Valves

Valve*	Type	Attachment To Trachs	Valve Characteristics
Passy-Muir speaking valve Passy-Muir, Inc.	One-way valves, #005 for tracheostomy use, #007 for ventilator use (only valve for ventilator)	Fits on 15 mm hub or can be placed in line with ventilator tubing	One-way silastic membrane with biased closed position—opens on inspiration. Creates positive closure feature.
Montgomery Boston Medical Products, Inc.	One-way valve	Fits standard 15 mm hub or Boston cannula system	Silicone membrane is hinged; maintains open position but opens more fully upon inspiration, closing upon expiration. Special cough release feature.
Trachoe ® distributed by BostonMedica Products, Inc.	Two types of fenestrated inner cannulas, which contain hinged valves	Tracheostomy tube with attachment that occludes inner cannula of tube. Two designs.	Tracheostomy tube is modified by the placement of an inner cannula that contains a one-way valve
Kistner One Way valve Philling-Weck	One-way valve	Fits Jackson metal tubes or Kistner plastic* tubes (made by Philling)	Hinged valve maintains open position, opening more fully upon inspiration, closing during expiration
Olympic "Talk Trach" Olympic Medical	T-shaped device that that fits on tracheostomy tube and can be attached to T-piece	Fits standard 15mm hub	Spring loaded valve mechanism maintains open position. Closes upon expiration to direct air into the upper airway.
Hood Hood Laboratories	One-way valve	Fits standard 15 mm hub	Valve contains a ball that moves, opening upon inspiration and closing upon exhalation

* All valves must be used with deflated tracheostomy tube cuffs.
(Table reprinted from Dikeman KJ, Kanandjan MS. Communication and Swallowing Management of Tracheostomized and Ventilator-dependent Adults. San Diego: Singular Publishing Group, Inc., 1995: 168, Table 5-8, with permission)

Guidelines for Decannulation

- Patients are ready for decannulation when they no longer need mechanical ventilation and can adequately clear airway secretions
- Patient should be evaluated for aspiration risk
- Should be able to cough secretions out of the tracheal tube
- Gradual cuff deflation allows weaning from cuffed to uncuffed TT. The cuffless TT is down sized to a smaller size and the patient evaluated for ability to cough secretions
- When the patient does not need excessive suctioning and the outer diameter of the TT is 8 mm., you may discontinue the TT or place a tracheal button temporarily

Tracheal buttons—extend only to the inner surface of the anterior tracheal wall without causing tracheal lumen obstruction. They are used when there is doubt about the success of the tracheostomy weaning. When plugged, the patient may breathe through the upper airway without resistance from the tracheostomy tube.

📖 Another means of invasive ventilatory support is electrophrenic respiration with the use of a diaphragmatic pacer, used in patients with intact phrenic nerves and diaphragm. This is discussed in detail in the spinal cord injury chapter.

■

CARDIAC REHABILITATION

DEFINITION

Cardiac rehabilitation is the process by which persons with cardiovascular disease (including but not limited to patients with coronary heart disease) are restored to and maintained at their optimal physiological, psychological, social, vocational, and emotional status. (American Association of Cardiovascular and Pulmonary Rehabilitation–AACPR)

GOALS

The goal is to improve or maintain a good level of cardiovascular fitness, thereby returning the individual to a normal and productive life.
- For those able to return to work:
  1. Return to productive employment as soon as possible
  2. Improve and maintain as good cardiovascular fitness
- For those not able to return to work:
  1. Maintain as active a life as possible
  2. Establish new areas of interest to improve quality of life
- Patient Education and Reduction of Coronary Risk Factors

Risk Factors for Coronary Artery Disease (CAD)	
Irreversible	**Reversible**
Age Male gender Family history of CAD Past history of CAD, PVD, CVA	Hypertension Cigarette Smoking Hypercholesterolemia Hypertriglyceridemia Diabetes Mellitus Obesity Sedentary lifestyle Type A personality

EPIDEMIOLOGY

- Cardiovascular disease is the leading cause of morbidity and mortality in the United States, accounting for almost 50% of all deaths
- Coronary Heart Disease (CHD) with its clinical manifestations of stable angina pectoris, unstable angina, acute myocardial infarction (MI), and sudden death affects about 13.5 million Americans. Nearly 1.5 million Americans sustain myocardial infarction each year, of which almost 500,000 episodes are fatal
- 50% of MI occurs in people under age 65
- Annually, 1 million survivors of MI and more than 7 million patients with stable angina pectoris are candidates for cardiac rehabilitation, as are patients following coronary artery bypass graft (CABG) (309,000 patients in 1993), and a similar number will require angioplasty
- Although several million patients with CHD are candidates for cardiac rehabilitation services, only 11% to 20% have participated in cardiac rehab programs
- The mortality rate for CAD has fallen 47% since 1963; 30% of that decrease occurring from 1979–1989
- The Framingham study credits three factors as playing possible roles in this marked decrease in those with CAD. (Wilson et al., 1987)
  1. The modification of risk factors in those with CAD:
     - Lower cholesterol
     - Lower blood pressure
     - Better hypertension management
     - Reduced cigarette smoking
  2. Improved treatment methods
  3. Improved prevention

PHASES OF CARDIAC REHAB

Phase I	During acute inpatient hospitalization
Phase II	Supervised ambulatory outpatient lasting 3 to 6 months
Phase III	Maintenance phase in which physical fitness and risk factor reduction are accomplished in a minimally supervised or unsupervised setting

Phase I (Inpatient Period)

This stage of rehabilitation can last from as short as one day to as long as 14 days for cardiovascular patients undergoing invasive procedures or suffering from acute events

Phase II (Immediate Outpatient Period)

This period is the convalescent stage following a hospital discharge. The length is partly determined by risk satisfaction and monitoring need. By definition this period is the most closely monitored phase of rehabilitation.

Phase III and Phase IV (Intermediate and Maintenance Periods)

The third stage of recovery is an extended outpatient period that may be divided into two components, intermediate and maintenance. The intermediate stage follows immediate outpatient cardiac rehabilitation, that is, when the patient is not intensely monitored and/or supervised but is still involved in regular endurance exercise training and lifestyle change. The transition to Phase IV varies according to the individual outcomes and medical needs.

📖 EXERCISE PHYSIOLOGY

- Total Oxygen Consumption (VO_2) represents the oxygen consumption of the whole body, therefore it mainly represents the work of the peripheral skeletal muscles rather than myocardial muscles.
- Aerobic capacity (VO_2 max) is a term used to measure the work capacity of an individual. As the individual increases the workload (exercise) the VO_2 increases in a linear fashion until it levels off and reaches a plateau, despite further increases in the workload. This is the aerobic capacity of the individual. It is usually expressed in the millimeters of O_2 consumed per kilogram of body weight per minute.
- Myocardial Oxygen Consumption (MVO_2) is the actual oxygen consumption of the heart. It can be measured directly with cardiac catheterization. In a clinical setting, however, the rate pressure product (RPP) can be used since the heart rate and systolic blood pressure correlates well with the MVO_2.
- Double Product, also called Rate Pressure Product (RPP) refers to the work required of the heart, which closely parallels the systolic blood pressure (SBP) × heart rate (HR).
- Rate Pressure Product (RPP) = SBP × HR
- Cardiac Output (CO) = HR × stroke volume
- Metabolic equivalent (met): Resting metabolic unit—1 met = 3.5 ml O_2 consumed per kilogram of body weight per minute (Pashkow, 1993)

📖 OUTCOMES OF CARDIAC REHABILITATION SERVICES

The results of cardiac rehabilitation services, based on reports in the scientific literature. The most substantial benefits:

Improvement in Exercise Tolerance

Cardiac rehabilitation exercise training improves objective measures of exercise tolerance in both men and women, including elderly patients with CHD and heart failure.

Improvement in Symptoms

Cardiac rehabilitation exercise training decreases symptoms of angina pectoris in patients with CHD and decreases symptoms of heart failure in patients with left ventricular systolic dysfunction. Improvement in clinical measures of myocardial ischemia, as identified by ECG and nuclear cardiology techniques, following exercise rehabilitation.

Improvement in Blood Lipid Levels

Multifactorial cardiac rehabilitation in patients with CHD, including exercise training and education, results in improved lipid and lipoprotein levels. Exercise training as a sole intervention has not effected consistent improvement in lipid profiles. Optimal lipid management requires specifically directed dietary and, when medically indicated, pharmacological management as a component of multifactorial cardiac rehabilitation.

Reduction of Cigarette Smoking

Education, counseling, and behavioral intervention are beneficial for smoking cessation.

Improvement in Psychosocial Well-being and Stress Reduction

Improvement in psychological status and functioning, including measures of emotional stress and reduction of the Type A behavior pattern

Reduction in Mortality

Multifactorial cardiac rehabilitation service can reduce cardiovascular mortality in patients following myocardial infarction.

Safety

The safety of exercise is established by the very low rate of occurrence of myocardial infarction and cardiovascular complications during exercise training.

TABLE 9-2. Absolute Contraindications for Entry into Inpatient and Outpatient Exercise Training

- Unstable angina
- Resting systolic blood pressure > 200 mm Hg or resting diastolic blood pressure > 110 mm Hg
- Significant drop (20 mm Hg) in resting systolic blood pressure from the patient's average level that cannot be explained by medication
- Moderate to severe aortic stenosis
- Acute systemic illness or fever
- Uncontrolled atrial or ventricular arrhythmias
- Uncontrolled tachycardia (> 100 bpm)
- Symptomatic congestive heart failure
- Third-degree heart block without pacemaker
- Active pericarditis or myocarditis
- Recent embolism
- Thrombophlebitis
- Resting ST displacement (> 3 mm) (as seen on ECG)
- Uncontrolled diabetes
- Orthopaedic problems that would prohibit exercise

Candidates for Inpatient Cardiac Rehabilitation

- Patients who have had myocardial infarction
- Coronary artery bypass surgery (CABG) or angioplasty patients
- Coronary patients with or without residual ischemia
- Heart failure and arrhythmias
- Patients with dilated cardiomyopathy
- A variety of patients with nonischemic heart disease
- Patients with concomitant pulmonary disease
- Patients who have received a pacemaker or an automatic implanted cardioverter-defibrillator
- Patients who have had heart-valve repair or replacement
- Aneurysm, aneurysm resection, organ transplantation

Modified from "Exercise Prescription for Cardiac Patients" In ACSM Guidelines for Exercise Testing and Prescription (5th ed) p.179, Philadelphia; Lea & Febiger, 1995, with permission.

INPATIENT VERSUS OUTPATIENT REHABILITATION

1. Inpatient program: Strictly supervised inpatient hospitalization lasting 1–2 weeks (phase I)
2. Structured outpatient program: Supervised ambulatory out-patient program lasting 3–6 months (phase II)
3. Maintenance program: Minimally supervised or unsupervised setting (phase III/IV)

Inpatient Program 7–14 Days

Acute Period—CCU (Coronary Care Unit):
- Activities of very low intensity (1–2 mets)
    Passive ROM (1.5 mets)
    Upper extremity ROM (1.7 mets)

Lower extremity ROM (2.0 mets)
Avoid: isometrics (increases heart rate), valsalva (promotes arrhythmia), raising the legs above the heart (can increase preload)
- Use protective chair posture—can reduce the cardiac output by 10%
- Bedside commode (3.6 mets) versus bedpan (4.7 mets)

The goal of an inpatient rehabilitation program is to provide a coordinated, multifaceted program designed to assist and direct patients and their families early in the recovery process following an acute cardiovascular event. The focus is on the medical care, physical activity, education, and psychological issues.

Subacute Period—Physical program can vary among institutions. Transfer from the CCU to either a telemetry unit or to the medical ward.
- Activities or exercises of intensity (3–4 mets)
  Calisthenics of known energy cost
  ROM exercise: intensity can be gradually increased by increasing the speed and/or duration; may add mild resistance or low (1–2 lbs.) weight
  Early ambulation: starting in the room and then corridors of the ward, treadmill walking at 0% grade starting at 1 mph and gradually increasing to 1.5 mph, 2 mph, 2.5 mph as tolerated
- Energy cost of low grade ambulation:
  1 mph (slow stroll) = 1.5–2 mets
  2 mph (regular slow walk) = 2–3 mets
  Propelling wheelchair = 2–3 mets
- Serial progression of the self-care activities should parallel to the intensity of the monitored program, particularly with earlier hospital discharge

Bypass Surgery—Rehabilitation regime is differentiated into Aggressive vs. Slow to Recover Fig. 9–7).

EXERCISE TESTING

📖 Graded Exercise Testing

Graded exercise stress tests (GXTs) assess the patient's ability to tolerate increased physical stress. The GXT may be used for diagnostic, prognostic, and therapeutic application, with or without addition of radionuclide or echocardiography assessment.
- 📖 The cardiac rehabilitation health professionals usually use GXTs as a functional rather than diagnostic tool
- 📖 GXTs also provide useful information when applied to risk stratification models. GXTs also allow the establishment of appropriate limits and guidelines for exercise therapy and the assessment of functional change over time
- Submaximal GXT is recommended for inpatients and prior to outpatient cardiac rehabilation programs
- GXTs may be submaximal or maximal relative to patient effort in addition to common indications for stopping the exercise test (see Contraindications to Exercise Testing). Endpoint criteria for submaximal testing may include heart rate limits, perceived exertion, and predetermined met levels
- 📖 Most of the activities of daily living in the home environment require less than 4 mets (*Guidelines for Cardiac Rehabilitation* 2nd ed. 1995)
- The American Heart Association suggests a heart rate limit of 140 and 130 beats per minute for patients not on beta-blocking agents, or Borg rating of perceived exertion (RPE) of 13–15 (Table 9–7), as additional end point criteria for low-level testing

- The low-level test provided sufficient data to permit most activities of daily living and serve as a baseline for ambulatory exercise therapy.
- The frequency of the test should be relative to the patients clinical course rather than a fixed schedule.

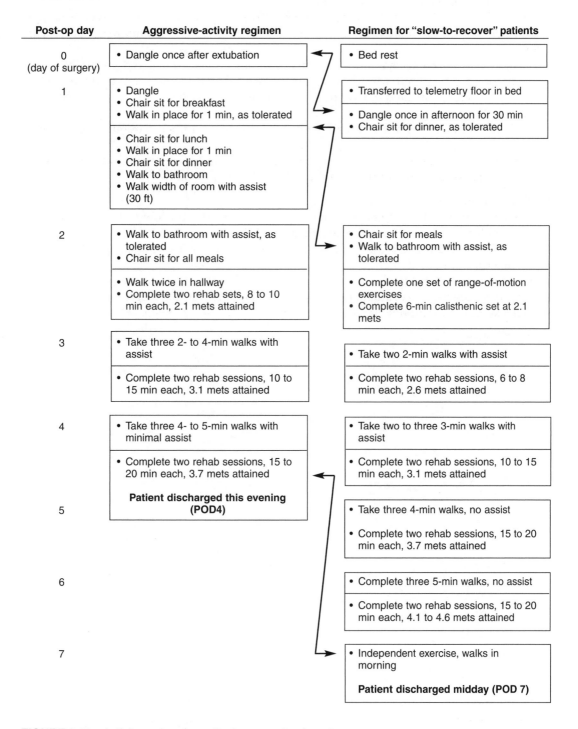

Post-op day	Aggressive-activity regimen	Regimen for "slow-to-recover" patients
0 (day of surgery)	• Dangle once after extubation	• Bed rest
1	• Dangle • Chair sit for breakfast • Walk in place for 1 min, as tolerated	• Transferred to telemetry floor in bed
	• Chair sit for lunch • Walk in place for 1 min • Chair sit for dinner • Walk to bathroom • Walk width of room with assist (30 ft)	• Dangle once in afternoon for 30 min • Chair sit for dinner, as tolerated
2	• Walk to bathroom with assist, as tolerated • Chair sit for all meals	• Chair sit for meals • Walk to bathroom with assist, as tolerated
	• Walk twice in hallway • Complete two rehab sets, 8 to 10 min each, 2.1 mets attained	• Complete one set of range-of-motion exercises • Complete 6-min calisthenic set at 2.1 mets
3	• Take three 2- to 4-min walks with assist	• Take two 2-min walks with assist
	• Complete two rehab sessions, 10 to 15 min each, 3.1 mets attained	• Complete two rehab sessions, 6 to 8 min each, 2.6 mets attained
4	• Take three 4- to 5-min walks with minimal assist	• Take two to three 3-min walks with assist
	• Complete two rehab sessions, 15 to 20 min each, 3.7 mets attained	• Complete two rehab sessions, 10 to 15 min each, 3.1 mets attained
5	**Patient discharged this evening (POD4)**	• Take three 4-min walks, no assist • Complete two rehab sessions, 15 to 20 min each, 3.7 mets attained
6		• Complete three 5-min walks, no assist • Complete two rehab sessions, 15 to 20 min each, 4.1 to 4.6 mets attained
7		• Independent exercise, walks in morning **Patient discharged midday (POD 7)**

FIGURE 9–7. Activity regime for patients recovering from bypass surgery.

📖 Exercise Testing Protocols

A variety of exercise testing protocols are available, whether the test is conducted using treadmill, cycle, or arm ergometer.

- 📖 Amputee patients use arm ergometer
- 📖 Treadmill testing provides a more common form of physiologic stress, (i.e., walking), in which subjects are more likely to attain a slightly higher VO_2 maximum and peak heart rate
- 📖 The cycle ergometer has the advantage of requiring less space and generally is less costly than the treadmill. Minimized movements of the arm and thorax facilitates better quality EKG recording and blood pressure monitoring. (*Guidelines for Cardiac Rehabilitation* 2nd ed. 1995)
- 📖 To perform a stress test in an above-knee amputee, an upper extremity ergometer is used
- Balke-Ware protocols that increase metabolic demands by 1 met per stage are appropriate for high-risk patients with functional capacity of less than 7 mets

📖 Bruce Protocol

Metabolic demands of > 2 mets per stage may be appropriate for low to intermediate risk patients with functional capacity greater than 7 mets

📖 The widely used Bruce Protocol of 2–3 mets per stage is useful with stable patients with functional capacities of 10 mets.

Pharmacological testing in debilitated patients for whom exercise testing cannot be performed, has been used to evaluate ischemia. The data from pharmacologic testing cannot be used in exercise presumption. (Froehlicher, 1987)

TABLE 9-3. Approximate met Costs for Sample Exercise Testing Protocols

FUNCTIONAL CLASS	CLINICAL STATUS	O₂ COST ml/kg/min	METS	BICYCLE ERGOMETER (1 WATT = 6 KPDS) FOR 70 KG BODY WEIGHT KPDS	BRUCE 3 MIN STAGES MPH / %GR	KATTUS MPH / %GR	BALKE-WARE % GRADE AT 3.3 MPH 1-MIN STAGES	ELLESTAD 3/2/3 MIN STAGES MPH / %GR	USAFSAM MPH / %GR	"SLOW" USAFSAM MPH / %GR	McHENRY MPH / %GR	STANFORD % GRADE AT 3 MPH	STANFORD % GRADE AT 2 MPH	METS
NORMAL AND I (HEALTHY, DEPENDENT ON AGE, ACTIVITY)							26							
		56.0	16		5.5 / 20		25	6 / 15						16
		52.5	15	1500	5.0 / 18		24	5 / 15						15
		49.0	14	1350			23		3.3 / 25					14
		45.5	13	1200	4.2 / 16	4 / 22	22	5 / 10			3.3 / 21			13
		42.0	12	1050		4 / 18	21		3.3 / 20		3.3 / 18	22.5		12
		38.5	11	900			20			2 / 25	3.3 / 15	20.0		11
		35.0	10	750	3.4 / 14	4 / 14	19		3.3 / 15	2 / 20		17.5		10
	SEDENTARY HEALTHY	31.5	9	600		4 / 10	18	4 / 10			3.3 / 12	15.0		9
		28.0	8	450			17	3 / 10	3.3 / 10	2 / 15	3.3 / 9	12.5		8
II	LIMITED	24.5	7	300	2.5 / 12	3 / 10	16		3.3 / 5	2 / 10	3.3 / 6	10.0	17.5	7
		21.0	6	150		2 / 10	15			2 / 5		7.5	14	6
III		17.5	5		1.7 / 10		14	1.7 / 10	3.3 / 0			5.0	10.5	5
		14.0	4		1.7 / 5		13					2.5	7	4
	SYMPTOMATIC	10.5	3		1.7 / 0		12		2.0 / 0	2 / 0	2.0 / 3	0.0	3.5	3
IV		7.0	2				11							2
		3.5	1				10							1

Reprinted from Froehlicher VF. Exercise and the Heart. Clinical Concepts p.15, Year Book Medical Publishers, Inc. Chicago 1987., with permission.

TABLE 9-4. Contraindications to Exercise Testing

Absolute Contraindications
1. A recent significant change in the resting ECG suggesting infarction or other acute cardiac events
2. Recent complicated myocardial infarction
3. Unstable angina
4. Uncontrolled ventricular dysrhythmia
5. Uncontrolled atrial dysrhythmia that compromises cardiac function
6. 3rd degree A-V block
7. Acute congestive heart failure
8. Severe aortic stenosis
9. Suspected or known dissecting aneurysm
10. Active or suspected myocarditis or pericarditis
11. Thrombophlebitis or intracardiac thrombi
12. Recent systemic or pulmonary embolus
13. Acute infection
14. Significant emotional distress (psychosis)
Relative Contraindications
1. Resting diastolic blood pressure > 120 mmHg or resting systolic blood pressure >200 mmHg
2. Moderate valvular heart disease
3. Known electrolyte abnormalities (hypokalemia, hypomagnesemia)
4. Fixed-rate pacemaker (rarely used)
5. Frequent or complex ventricular ectopy
6. Ventricular aneurysm
7. Cardiomyopathy, including hypertrophic cardiomyopathy
8. Uncontrolled metabolic disease (e.g. diabetes, thyrotoxicosis, or myxedema)
9. Chronic infectious disease (e.g. mononucleosis, hepatitis, AIDS)
10. Neuromuscular, musculoskeletal, or rheumatoid disorders that are exacerbated by exercise
11. Advanced or complicated pregnancy

Modified from "Guidelines for Exercise Test Administration" In ACSM Guidelines for Exercise Testing and Prescription (5th ed) p. 42, 1995, Philadelphia: Lea & Febiger, with permission.

TABLE 9-5. Indications for Stopping an Exercise Test

Symptom-limited maximal test
1. Progressive angina (stop at 3+ level or earlier on a scale of 1–4)
2. Ventricular tachycardia
3. Any significant drop (20 mm HG) of systolic blood pressure or a failure of the systolic blood pressure to rise with an increase in exercise load
4. Light-headedness, confusion, ataxia, pallor, cyanosis, nausea, or signs of severe peripheral circulatory insufficiency
5. 3mm horizontal or downsloping ST depression or elevation (in the absence of other indicators of ischemia)
6. Onset of second- or third-degree A-V block
7. Increasing ventricular ectopy, multiform PVCs, or R on T PVCs
8. Excessive rise in blood pressure: systolic > 250 mm Hg; diastolic pressure > 120 mmHg
9. Chronotropic impairment
10. Sustained supraventricular tachycardia
11. Exercise-induced left bundle branch block
12. Subject requests to stop
13. Failure of the monitoring system
Additional Criteria for Stopping Low-level/Hospital Discharge Exercise Test
1. Exercise heart rate > 130 bpm
2. Borg RPE (Rate perceived exertion) 15 (15 grade scale) (Table 9–7)

Continued

Suggested Endpoint Criteria for a Submaximal Exercise Progress Evaluation
1. Appearance of any criteria that indicate ending an exercise test
2. Exercise heart rate in excess of previous GTX peak heart rate
RPE = Rate Perceived Exertion > 16 (Borg 15 grade scale)
(Elaboration of Borg Scale—see below)

Modified from "Guidelines for Exercise Test Administration" ACSM Guidelines for Exercise Testing and Prescription (5th ed) p. 78 Philadelphia: Lea & Febiger, 1995, with permission and from Fletcher GF, Hartley, LH, Haskell WL, Pollock ML. "Exercise Standards, a Statement for Health Professionals from the American Heart Association" Circulation 1990; 82: 2297.

Structured Outpatient Program/Maintenance Program

Traditionally, outpatient cardiac rehabilitation has been divided into three phases:
Phase II (immediate)
Phase III (intermediate)
Phase IV (maintenance)

Phase II (immediate) will define the stage of cardiac rehabilitation that occurs immediately after discharge, in which higher levels of surveillance, monitoring of ECGs, and intensive risk factor modification occurs

Phase III (intermediate) is the period of rehabilitation when ECG monitoring occurs only if signs and symptoms warrant, although endurance training and risk factor modification continue

Phase IV (maintenance) is the stage in the program that is structured for patients who have plateaued in exercise endurance and achieved stable risk factor management

Physical Activity Program

Slow walk	2 mph	2–3 mets
Regular speed walk	3 mph	3–4 mets
Brisk walk	3–5 mph	4–5 mets
Very brisk walk	4 mph	5–6 mets
Sexual intercourse*		3–4 mets
Outdoor work—shovel snow, spade soil		7 mets
Jog, walk	5 mph	9 mets
Mop floor		2–4 mets
Push power lawn mower		4 mets

* Note: met level for sexual intercourse varies depending upon reference source. Tardif (1989) states that patients who reach 5–6 mets on stress-testing without ischemia or arrhythmias can, in all likelihood, resume their normal sexual activities without any risk.

The goal is the improvement of the cardiovascular capacity through physical exercise training whether in a minimally supervised or unsupervised setting.

Types of Physical Activities

- Begin with the last exercise program performed during the supervised cardiac exercise program
- Aerobically trained, clinically stable candidates may participate in resistive or circuit training. An overall lifestyle that includes proper diet, weight control, stress management, and smoking cessation should be maintained along with good physical fitness
- Active participation, within prescribed limits, in sport activity is encouraged

Sport Activity	Energy Cost in Mets
Golf	2–5
Bowling	4–5
Volleyball	3–4
Ping pong	3–6
Tennis	4–7
Roller-skating	5–6

CARDIAC FUNCTIONAL CLASSIFICATION

Class I
- NY Heart Association—Patient's cardiac disease does not limit physical activity. Ordinary physical activity does not cause undue fatigue, palpitation, dyspnea, or anginal pain.
- Specific Activity Scale
Patients can perform to completion any activity requiring > or = 7 mets:
Can carry 24 lbs. up 8 steps
Can carry objects that weigh 80 lbs.
Do outdoor work (shovel snow, spade soil)
Do recreational activities (skiing, basketball, squash, handball, jog at 5 mph)

Class II
- NY Heart Association—Patient's cardiac disease results in slight limitation on physical activity. They are comfortable at rest. Ordinary physical activity results in fatigue, palpitation, dyspnea, or anginal pain.
- Specific Activity Scale
Patient can perform to completion any activity requiring > or = 5 mets, but cannot and does not perform to completion of activities requiring > or = to 7 mets:
Sexual intercourse to completion without interruption
Garden, rake, weed
Roller-skate, walk at 4 mph on level ground

Class III
- NY Heart Association—Patient's cardiac disease results in marked limitation of physical activity. They are comfortable at rest. Less than ordinary physical activity causes fatigue, palpitation, dyspnea, or anginal pain.
- Specific Activity Scale
Patient can perform to completion any activity that requires > or = 2 mets and < 5 mets:
Shower without interruption
Strip and make bed
Clean windows
Walk 2.5 mph
Bowl, golf
Dress without stopping

Class IV
- NY Heart Association—Patient's cardiac disease results in inability to carry on any physical activity without discomfort. Symptoms of cardiac insufficiency or of the angina syndrome may be present even at rest. If any physical activity is undertaken, discomfort is increased.
- Specific Activity Scale
Patient cannot or does not perform to completion activities requiring > or = 2 mets. Cannot carry out activities in Class I – III.

TABLE 9-6. Criteria for Determination of the Specific Activity Scale Functional Class

	Any yes	No
1. Can you walk down a flight of steps without stopping (4.5-5.2 METs)?	Go to #2	Go to #4
2. Can you carry anything up a flight of eight steps without stopping (5-5.5 METs)? Or can you	Go to #3	Class III
(a) have sexual intercourse without stopping (3-4 METs);		
(b) garden, rake, weed (5.6 METs);		
(c) roller skate, fox-trot (5-6 METs); or		
(d) walk at a 4 mph rate on level ground (5-6 METs)?		
3. Can you carry at least 24 lb up eight steps (10 METs)? Or can you	Class I	Class III
(a) carry objects that are at least 80 lb (8 METs);		
(b) do outdoor work—shovel snow, spade soil (7 METs);		
(c) do recreational activities such as skiing, basketball, touch football, squash, handball (7-10 METs); or		
(d) jog/walk 5 mph (9 METs)?		
4. Can you shower without stopping (3.6-4.2 METs)? Or can you	Class III	Go to #5
(a) strip and make a bed (3.9-5 METs);		
(b) mop floors (4.2 METs);		
(c) hang washed clothes (4.4 METs);		
(d) clean windows (3.7 METs);		
(e) walk 2.5 mph (3-3.5 METs);		
(f) bowl (3-4.4 METs);		
(g) play golf (walk and carry clubs) (4.5 METs); or		
(h) push a power lawn mower (4 METs)?		
5. Can you dress without stopping because of symptoms (2-2.3 METs)?	Class III	Class IV

From Goldman L., Hashimoto B., Cook EF., Loscalzo A. Comparative reproducibility and validity of systems for assessing cardiovascular functional class: advantages of a new specific activity scale. *Circulation* 1981 Dec; 64(6): 1227–37 © American Heart Association, with permission.

Contraindications to Exercise Testing

Exercise Prescription
Exercise for the cardiac patient should specify the type of exercise, the intensity, duration and frequency

📖 Type of Exercise
Exercise for cardiovascular conditioning should be isotonic, rhythmic, and aerobic; should use large muscle masses and should not involve a large isometric component
- Sessions of exercise should incorporate aerobic activity such as walking/jogging, stationary cycling or water aerobics. Sessions should also incorporate warm-up and cooldown periods. In addition to aerobic activity, resistance exercise (using light weights) may be added on an individual basis
- 📖 Resistance exercises have been shown to be a safe and effective method for improving strength and cardiovascular endurance in low-risk patients. Surgical and myocardial infarction patients should wait three to six weeks before beginning resistance training. Patients diagnosed with the following conditions should be excluded from resistance training:

CHF
Uncontrolled arrhythmias
Severe vascular disease
Uncontrolled hypertension
Systolic blood pressure > 160 mm/Hg, or diastolic blood pressure > 100 mm/Hg
Aerobic capacity less than 5 mets

- Results in increase in aerobic capacity of all muscle fibers exercised: both type I and type II fibers. Type I fibers continue to show approximately five times the aerobic capacity of type II fibers, as before exercise. (Flores and Zohman, 1993)

Exercise Intensity

- Exercise intensity is usually prescribed as some percentage of the maximum capacity obtained on exercise testing, (i.e., O_2 consumption, heart rate workload and/or degree of exertion)

O_2 Consumption

Threshold	40–50% max VO_2	60% max HR
Optimum	55–65% max VO_2	70% max HR
Ceiling	80–90% max VO_2	90% max HR

For the deconditioned cardiac patient, exercise even at 40% to 50% of max VO_2 will result in improvement

Target Heart Rate (THR)
Exercise intensity is based on target heart rate
Note: Clearance Heart Rate (HR) is the clinical maximum HR attained on stress test.
Target HR is the following range:
Clearance HR × .7 = beginning range
Clearance HR × .85 = end range
  1. For the cardiac patient, 70% of the maximum HR attained on the exercise stress test
  2. For the healthy patient, 70% to 85% of the predicted age-adjusted maximum HR:
     Average maximum = 220 – age
  3. Karvonen formula—useful for those on chronic beta blockade or with abnormally high resting heart rate
- The age-predicted formula of (220 – age = HR maximum) has the potential for over- and underestimating the actual exercise intensity and, therefore, places patients with heart disease at risk for exercise-induced cardiovascular complications
- The percent HR maximum reserve method of establishing a target HR uses the subject's potential heart-rate increase and assumes that the resting heart rate represents zero intensity. Thus, this method corrects for the nonzero value of resting heart rate associated with the percent HR maximum method
Karvonen Method:
THR range = 0.7 to 0.85 (HR maximum - resting HR) + resting HR
  Example: Patient is a 60 year old with a HR maximum of 160 and a resting HR of 60.
  $(160 - 60) \times 0.7 + 60 = 130$ for lower limit
  $(160 - 60) \times 0.85 + 60 = 145$ for upper limit
  Therefore, the target HR (THR) range = 130–145
Age Predicted Method:
THR range = 0.7 (220 – age) to 0.85 (220 – age)
  Example: same as previous patient
  $(220 - 60) \times 0.7$ to $(220 - 60) \times 0.85$
  THR range = 112–136

Perceived Exertion Method
1. Borg RPE scale (Table 9–7): A linear scale of rating from 6–20. This scale is a valid indication of physical exertion and correlates linearly with HR, ventricular O_2 consumption, and lactate levels. The new exerciser can proceed with exercise to level 13, (somewhat hard) provided he has been given clearance to do so from his exercise stress test.
2. Conversational exercise level: Patient should be able to talk while exercising (Talk Test) The conversational level is of adequate intensity to induce a training effect but allows the exerciser to talk without becoming excessively out of breath while exercising at the same time

The American Heart Association suggest a heart rate limit of 130–140 beats per minute (b/min) for patients not on beta-blocking agents, or Borg rating of perceived exertion (RPE) of 13–15 as an additional point criteria for low-level testing

Duration and Frequency of Exercise
- The duration depends on the level of fitness of the individual and the intensity of the exercise
- The usual duration when exercise is at 70% of maximum heart rate is 20–30 minutes at conditioning level
- In the poorly conditioned individual, daily exercise as low as 3–5 minutes can bring about improvement. For the conditioned individual who prefers to exercise at higher intensities, duration of exercise may be reduced to 10–15 minutes

Format of an Exercise Session
- There should be a warm-up phase before and a cool-down phase after the period of training
- The warm-up period is usually at the lower intensity levels of exercise to be performed, gradually increasing to the prescribed intensity
- At the cool-down period, there is gradual reduction in exercise intensity to allow the gradual redistribution of blood from the extremities to other tissue and to prevent sudden reduction in venous return, thereby reducing the possibility of postexercise hypotension or even syncope. (*Guidelines for Cardiac Rehibilitation* 2nd ed. 1995)

Predicted Age-Adjusted Maximum Heart Rate

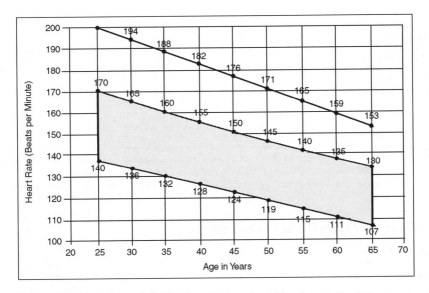

FIGURE 9–8. Exercise intensity based on the predicted age-adjusted rate. Shaded area is 70–80% of Age Adjusted Maximum Attainable Heart Rate. Top solid line is Age Adjusted Maximum Attainable Heart Rate.

TABLE 9–7.   Borg Scale of Rate Perceived Exertion

Borg Scale: 15-Grade Rating of Perceived Exertion
6 No exertion at all
7
8
9 Very light
10
11 Light
12
13 Somewhat hard
14
15 Hard (heavy)
16
17 Very hard
18
19 Extremely hard
20 Maximal exertion

From Borg, G. An Introduction to Borg's RPE Scale. Ithaca, NY: Mouvement Publications; 1985, with permission. Copyright 1985 by Gunnar Borg.

TABLE 9–8   Patient Rating Scales: Angina, Dyspnea, Intermittent Claudication

Angina Scale
0 – No angina
1 – Light, barely noticeable
2 – Moderate, bothersome
3 – Severe, very uncomfortable
4 – Most pain ever experienced

Dyspnea Scale
0 – No dyspnea
1 – Mild, noticeable
2 – Mild, some difficulty
3 – Moderate difficulty, but can continue
4 – Severe difficulty, cannot continue

Intermittent Claudication
0 – No claudication pain
2 – Initial, minimal pain
2 – Moderate, bothersome pain
3 – Intense pain
4 – Maximal pain, cannot continue

Reprinted with permission from American Association of Cardiovascular & Pulmonary Rehabilitation, 1999, *Guidelines for Cardiac Rehabilitation and Secondary Prevention Programs.* 3rd ed. (Champaign, IL: Human Kinetics), 64 and "Guidelines for Exercise Test Administration" In *ACSM Guidelines for Exercise Testing and Prescription.* 5th ed. (Philadelphia: Lea & Febiger).

CARDIAC REHABILITATION OF SPECIAL GROUPS

Heart Transplantation

Pathophysiology
The heart is denervated (loss of vagal inhibition to the SA node), therefore, physiologic response is somewhat different then the one seen in a post-CABG patient.
1. High resting heart rate
2. Lower peak exercise heart rate

3. Postexercise recovery rate—slow return to resting level
   - At maximum effort—the work capacity, cardiac output, systolic BP, and the total O_2 consumption (VO_2) are lower
   - Pretransplantation, rehabilitative strength training may enhance pre-operative and operative recovery
   - Five- and ten-year survival is about 82% to 74% respectively
   - Accelerated arthrosclerosis occurs following transplantation

Exercise Prescription

1. Heart-rate guidelines are not used
2. Intensity of exercise is based on the following:
   - Borg RPE scale 11 to 14 (Table 9–7)
   - Percentage of maximum oxygen consumption or maximum workload performed on stress test
   - Anaerobic threshold
   - Duration frequency and types of exercise follow the same principles as those with other types of cardiac problems
   - During exercise testing, ischemia is not presented as angina, therefore, ECG changes and other symptoms should be followed

Outcome

Generally favorable, typically reporting increased work output and improved exercise tolerance.

Most Common Major Physical Disabilities That Often Exist with Coronary Artery Disease

1. Amputation
2. Stroke

1. Amputee
   - The atherosclerotic vascular disease that affects the cardiovascular system also predisposes these patients to limb loss (dysvascular lower extremity amputation)
   - Diabetes, in addition to causing accelerated atherosclerotic vascular disease, is a major risk factor for amputation. It has been estimated that 50% to 70% of all amputations are the result of complications of diabetes
   - **Energy Cost of Ambulation for the Amputee** is based on percentage increase above the cost of normal ambulation at 3 mets (Table 9–9)

TABLE 9-9   Energy Cost of Ambulation for the Amputee

AMPUTATION	% INCREASE IN ENERGY	METS
No prosthesis with crutches	50%	4.5
Unilateral BK with prosthesis	9–28%	3.3–3.8
Unilateral AK with prosthesis	40–65%	4.2–5.0
Bilateral BK with prosthesis	41–100%	4.2–6.0
BK plus AK with prostheses	75%	5.3
Bilateral AK with prostheses	280%	11.4
Unilateral hip disarticulation with prosthesis	82%	5.5
Hemipelvectomy with prosthesis	125%	6.75

(Flores and Zohman, 1998)

Amputee Exercise Test
- Pharmacological stress testing using dipyridamole—for patients that are unable to perform any exercise stress test
- Upper extremity cycle ergometer stress test—first determine the safety and ability of mobility
- Telemetry monitoring of ambulation training:
  1. Preprosthetic period
  2. Prosthetic period
  3. Postprosthetic period

2. Stroke
- Acute MI and acute stroke
- CABG and acute stroke
- According to the studies, as much as 77% of stroke patients have some form of co-existing cardiac disease
- Roth et al., showed the overall incidence of cardiac complications of 27% to 34% during inpatient rehabilitation. The incidence was higher in patients with known CAD
- Complications include:
  Hypertension
  Angina
  Myocardial infarction
  CHF
  Rhythm disturbances

Stroke Exercise Testing Modality
- Treadmill ambulation, if tolerated
- Stationary bicycle/ergometer modified for involved leg (ace wrap)
- Portable leg ergometers that allow for seating in a wheelchair or arm chair
- Arm ergometer modified for involved hand or using one-handed arm ergometer
- Telemetry monitoring of level surface ambulation or general conditioning classes

Hemiplegic Ambulation Compared to Normal Ambulation
- Speed—40% to 45% slower
- Energy cost—50% to 65% higher

Cardiovascular Conditioning of the Physically Impaired

Choice of Modalities Used for Assessment Depends on Number of Variables
- Upper extremity cycle ergometer—impaired lower extremity with normal upper extremity
- Air dyne arm—leg cycle ergometer for lower extremity weakness
- Hemiparetic—strap the affected extremity to foot pedal and/or handle bar
- Wheelchair bound—extra wide treadmills that can accommodate a wheelchair

EVALUATION FOR RETURN TO EMPLOYMENT
- Evaluation of the patient
- Evaluation of the job
- Matching the patient and the job
- Other conditions

Evaluation of the Patient
- Clinical Evaluation – Functional Cardiac Classification
  Class I—can perform 7 mets or greater
  Class II—can perform 5 mets or greater but not 7 mets
  Class III—can perform 2 mets or greater but not 5 mets
  Class IV—cannot perform 2 mets or greater

- Functional Exercise Stress Test
  Recommendations are made based on the maximum work load performance.
  > 7 mets—can return to work to most jobs in the USA
  > 5, but < 7 mets—can return to sedentary job and household chores
  3–4 mets—not suitable to return to employment (Flores and Zohman, 1998)

Evaluation of the Job

- Physical Task Performed
  Regular work or steady activity not to exceed endurance limits
  Peak activity – not to exceed prescribed maximum intensity
  Duration of each task
- Environmental Conditions at Areas of Work
  Temperature and humidity
    Hot and humid environment can increase the energy cost of work two to three times
  Air pollution
  High altitude
  Motivation and emotional attitude of patients
  Transportation to and from work
  Household chores after work

Matching the Patient and the Job

- Matching the cardiac functional class and/or result of stress test to the requirement of the job
- Simulated job monitoring
- Monitoring the actual tasks at the job site

Other Conditions

- Emotional Disorders
- Alcoholism
- Financial compensation (security gain)
- Retirement age
- Legal aspect
- Strenuous job requirements
- Patient motivation

AMERICAN HEART ASSOCIATION DIET

Step 1 Diet

On this diet you should eat:
  8% to 10% of the day's total calories form saturated fat
  30% or less of the day's total calories from fat
  Less than 300 mg of dietary cholesterol a day
  Just enough calories to achieve and maintain a healthy weight

Step 2 Diet

  If you do not lower your cholesterol enough on Step 1 diet or if you are at a high risk for heart disease or already have heart disease:
  Less than 7% of the day's total calories from saturated fat
  30% or less of the day's total calories from fat
  Less than 200 mg of dietary cholesterol a day
  Just enough calories to achieve and maintain a healthy weight

BENEFITS DERIVED FROM LONG-TERM OUTPATIENT CARDIAC REHABILITATION

- Increased oxygen extraction and wider AVO_2 difference. Skeletal muscles take up more oxygen from entering blood supply so that the venous return carries less back to the heart. The heart is thus doing less work to bring adequate oxygen to the tissue
- Improved utilization of oxygen by active muscles resulting from increased oxidative enzymes and number of mitochondria in the muscles
- Increased maximal oxygen consumption (VO_2 max) or aerobic capacity and physical work capacity
- The conditioned patient generally has a slower pulse and low blood pressure and lower rate pressure product; $RPP = HR \times SBP$. Because RPP is a good indicator for the myocardial oxygen demand (MVO_2), the trained cardiac patients function at a lower myocardial oxygen demand. Thus, an angina patient may be below the angina threshold in daily life and is able to perform certain activities without angina or silent ischemia
  - Decreased MVO_2 at rest and any submaximal workload
  - Increased cardiac output at maximal exercise; cardiac output remains the same at rest and at submaximal exercise
  - Cardiac output = Heart rate × stroke volume
  - Fick equation $VO_{2\ max}$ = (HR × stroke volume) × AVO_2 difference
  - Fick equation measures cardiac output × AVO_2 difference
  - Increased stroke volume at rest, submaximal and maximum work. This increase is due mostly to a combination of increased blood volume and prolonged diastolic filling time. (Flores and Zohman, 1993; Garden and Gillis, 1996)
  - Exercise training, combined with intensive dietary intervention, with and without lipid-lowering drugs results in regression or limitation of progression of angiographically documented coronary atherosclerosis
  - Cardiac rehabilitation exercise training decreases myocardial ischemia as measured by exercise, ECG, and radionuclide perfusion imaging
  - Cardiac rehabilitation exercise has no apparent effect on development of a coronary collateral circulation and produces no consistent changes in cardiac hemodynamic measurement at cardiac catheterization
  - Exercise training in patients with heart failure and decreased ventricular systolic function resulted in documented improvement in functional capacity. Data reinforces that the favorable training effects in these patients are due predominantly to adaptation in the peripheral circulation and skeletal muscles rather than adaptation in the cardiac musculature. (Cardiac Rehabilitation: Clinical Practice Guidelines Number 17; 1995)

■

CANCER REHABILITATION

GOALS OF REHABILITATION:

The general rehabilitation goals of patients with cancer are similar to the general goals of patients with disabilities caused by other diseases.

Rehabilitation of the patient with cancer should begin when disability is anticipated, rather than after it has occurred. The number of individuals surviving five years or more with a history of cancer continues to grow. Survivors may face significant physical and psychosocial problems that affect their quality of life. Rehabilitation goals can be appropriately assessed according to the different stages of the disease manifestation.

In **preventative rehabilitation therapy** the goal is to achieve maximal function in patients considered to be cured or in remission.

Supportive rehabilitation therapy is geared for those patients whose cancer is progressing; the goals of supportive rehabilitation therapy include providing adaptive self-care equipment in an attempt to offset what can be a steady decline in a patient's functional skills. Range of motion and bed mobility can be taught to patients hospitalized or confined to bedrest to prevent the adverse effects of immobility.

In **palliative rehabilitation therapy** the goals are to improve or maintain comfort and function during the terminal stage of the disease

Through retrospective analysis and observation, over 1/2 of all cancer patients had some form of difficulty addressable by physical medicine and rehabilitation. Physical medicine problems occur for patients with all tumor types. In patients with Central Nervous System (CNS), breast, lung, head and neck tumors, physical medicine problems may occur in over 70%. Often, there is a gap in rehabilitative patient care which is changed dramatically by introducing a physiatrist to the oncologic management team.

There is little literature studying the effectiveness of cancer rehabilitation. In a study published by Marciniak (Garden, 1994), comprehensive inpatient rehabilitation resulted in significant functional gains in patients who suffered from cancer or its treatment, regardless of metastases or cancer type. Other studies report improvement in functional independence and productivity in patients suffering from brain injury after post acute outpatient rehabilitation. (Marciniak, 1996)

EPIDEMIOLOGY

- Approximately 1,268,000 new cases were expected to be diagnosed in 2001
- Since 1990 approximately 15 million new cancer cases have been diagnosed
- The National Cancer Institute estimates that approximately 8.4 million Americans alive today have a history of cancer
- The five-year relative survival rate for these cancers is approximately 60% (American Cancer Society, 2002)
- The most common rehabilitation problems for the patient with cancer were described in a study by Lehman including a sample of 805 patients: general weakness 35%, ADL deficits 30%, pain 30%, difficulty with ambulation 25%. Other problems include: speech, swallowing, respiratory, neurologic impairments, skin problems, nutritional deficiencies, lymphedema, skeletal disease, and psychological disorders. (Lehman, 1978)

CAUSES AND MANAGEMENT OF DISABILITY ASSOCIATED WITH CANCER

Immobility and Related Problems

These complications are pertinent in the cancer patient secondary to longer time periods of illness, treatment, and recovery

Immobility may predispose patients to
- Muscle Atrophy
- Decreased Endurance
- Joint Contractures
- Orthostatic Intolerance
- Protein Loss
- Deep Venous Thrombosis (DVT)

- Pulmonary Embolism (PE)
- Impaired Glucose Tolerance
- Pressure Ulcers
- Difficulty Voiding
- Constipation
- Compression Neuropathies
- Sleep Disturbance
- Depression
- Dysphagia

Traditional rehabilitation intervention may allow patients to maintain independence and AVOID complications associated with bedrest or immobility associated with prolonged hospitalization and medical treatment. Traditional rehabilitation intervention is geared toward countering the effects of bedrest and maximizing ADLs and functional mobility. The following apply:

- Patients may perform strengthening exercises using an elastic band or mild resistive exercises against gravity while in bed
- Bed mobility and frequent repositioning with cushions or pillows is employed to avoid skin breakdown and joint contractures
- Evaluation for an air mattress for those patients at high risk for the presence of skin breakdown
- AROM exercises are performed in the upper and lower extremity and are initiated whenever possible
- The tilt table may be used to facilitate weight bearing and gradual upright positioning in those patients with orthostatic hypotension
- OT and PT evaluations are necessary for equipment assessment, transfers, balance, ROM, bed mobility, and to maximize independence in ADLs and ambulation, as well as for patient and family education
- 📖 A high index of suspicion for swallowing disorders should be maintained. Swallowing disorders may result from a variety of reasons in patients with cancer. Swallowing difficulty can be associated with cognitive impairment, central nervous system involvement, radiation treatment, and in patients with generalized deconditioning secondary to bedrest. When aspiration is suspected, a dysphagia evaluation is performed. A follow-up barium swallow may be required. If silent aspiration is suspected a barium swallow is necessary. Calorie counts should also be performed to ensure adequate nutrition. A gastrostomy may be required for long-term nutritional management in some patients
- 📖 A high index of suspicion should be maintained for metastatic involvement of the extremities and spine. Complaints of bony pain or discomfort warrant further investigation prior to initiating a skilled rehabilitation program. Extremities with possible tumor involvement should be positioned for non-weight bearing and ROM withheld until a workup is completed
- Patient-specific cardiac and pulmonary precautions should be ordered along with any skilled rehabilitation program (Lehman, 1978)

CENTRAL NERVOUS SYSTEM INVOLVEMENT IN CANCER

Brain Tumors

Primary tumors in adults—gliomas comprise approximately 60% of all primary CNS tumors Cerebellar astrocytoma is the most common primary CNS solid tumors in young adults

Primary brain tumors in children
Brain tumors (17%) are only second to leukemia (25%) as the most prevalent malignancy in childhood.

– Cerebellar astrocytoma is the most common posterior fossa tumor in childhood and has the best prognosis
– ▢ Medulloblastoma is the next most common posterior fossa tumor in childhood and is the most prevalent brain tumor in children less than 7 years of age
– Brain stem gliomas are the third most frequent posterior fossa tumor in children

Brain metastasis

– Brain metastasis occurs in approximately 25% of patients with cancer
   Lungs, gastrointestinal, and urinary tract tumors account for most brain metastasis in men
   Breast, lung, gastrointestinal, and melanoma account for most brain metastasis in women
   Rehabilitation of patients with primary brain tumors or metastatic lesions is based on the location of the lesion and resultant neurological deficits. (Takakura et al., 1982)

Some of the presenting signs and symptoms of brain involvement are headaches, weakness, seizures, and cognitive impairment.
- ▢ Headaches are the most common symptom
- ▢ Weakness is the most common focal sign
- ▢ Seizures are frequently the first presenting sign of CNS involvement
- ▢ Contrast CT or MRI is the best diagnostic test
- Cognitive impairment, aphasia, dysarthria, and dysphagia require intervention through speech therapy, communicative evaluations, and dysphagia management. Deficits usually reflect the specific location of the lesion
- Chemotherapy and radiation may produce neurologic deficits including impaired visual perceptual skills, memory, and judgment. (Table 9-10)
- Rehabilitation efforts are also geared towards the prevention of skin pressure breakdown through effective bed mobility, progressive ambulation and mobilization, maximizing ADLs, safety and equipment assessment, and family training to improve the patient's quality of life

Spinal Cord Involvement

Tumors
Tumors of the spinal cord are rare. The majority of tumors are extradural (95%) and arise from the vertebral body. Approximately 70% of metastatic tumors are in the thoracic cord.

Radiation effects
Radiation therapy may also damage the spinal cord.

▢ *Induced Transient Myelopathy*
The most common form of radiation damage is referred to as **induced transient myelopathy**. The syndrome develops after 1–30 months, with a peak onset at 4–6 months. There is transient demyelination of sensory neurons in the posterior column and lateral spinothalamic tract. Patients may report symmetrical paresthesias that radiate to the extremities. CT scans are normal and induced transient myelopathy usually resolves over a period of 1–9 months.

▢ *Delayed Radiation Myelopathy*
Delayed radiation myelopathy is irreversible. The symptoms begin at 9–18 mo. after radiation treatment. Most cases occur within 30 mo. Symptoms begin with lower extremity paresthesias followed by bowel dysfunction and weakness. Midback pain may also be associated with radiation myelopathy. Resultant deficits depend on the level of neurological involvement. (Takakura et al., 1982)

Involvement of the Peripheral Nerve

- Peripheral neuropathy can occur due to tumor or from chemotherapeutic agents
- Peripheral polyneuropathy has been associated with lung cancer, multiple myeloma, and breast and colon cancer
    Polyneuropathy is associated with inflammation and degeneration of the dorsal root ganglia
    Symptoms include gait dysfunction, paresthesias, sensory loss, with sparing of the face, bowel, and bladder
- EMG reveals fibrillation potentials, and polyphasic motor unit potential
- Subacute motor neuropathy usually occurs with lymphoma. Anterior horn cells degenerate, resulting in weakness; however, stabilization occurs with gradual improvement

Treatment

Treatment for involvement of the peripheral nervous system usually focuses on treatment of the underlying malignancy, treatment of pain or paresthesias, and supportive rehabilitation, intervention including orthotics, assistive and adaptive equipment, endurance, energy conservation, ROM, skin protection, and maintenance of strength.

Chemotherapy (Table 9–10)

- ▣ Chemotherapy can cause a peripheral or plexus neuropathy that is generally distal and symmetrical and is commonly associated with vincristine. Vincristine may also cause distal axonal degeneration, severe neuropathic pain, and in rare cases motor involvement may lead to quadriparesis
- Cisplatin and vincristine may also cause autonomic neuropathies resulting in fluctuating blood pressure or heart rate

Radiation

- ▣ Radiation may cause peripheral nerve damage due to effects on the nerve itself, or by involvement of the surrounding connective tissue and vascular supply. Symptoms include muscle atrophy, hyperesthesia, paresthesias, decreased strength and decreased range of motion
- ▣ Brachial Plexopathy is uncommon; however, it can occur as a result of radiation treatment or through direct tumor extension
    - ▣ Direct extension must be excluded especially in the presence of severe pain. In 90% of patients with direct tumor extension, pain is the initial symptom
    - ▣ In postradiation plexopathy, numbness and paresthesias are the usual initial symptom. The upper trunk is predominately involved with radiation plexitis and the lower trunk is predominately involved in 75% of patients with invasive tumor
    - ▣ One example of tumor extension is seen in Pancoast's syndrome, which is caused by a lesion in the superior pulmonary sulcus. It produces pain in the C8, T1, T2 nerves as well as Horner's syndrome. Patients report pain beginning in the shoulder and vertebral border of the scapula. Radiation and surgery are the usual treatment. (O'Young et al., 1997)
    - ▣ Myokymia on EMG is pathognomonic of radiation plexitis
    - ▣ An MRI may be used to reveal invasive lesions but is not 100% sensitive in tumors resulting in a plexopathy. A CT reveals focal lesions in over 90% of the cases

TABLE 9-10. Chemotherapeutic Agents and Side Effects

Cytoxan	Hemorrhagic cystitis, bladder fibrosis, bladder carcinoma, cardiac necrosis (massive doses), stomatitis
Nitrogen Mustard	Skin necrosis if extravasated, dermatitis, neurologic toxicity (rare)
Nitrosoureas	Stomatitis, lung fibrosis, ataxia, organic brain syndrome, optic neuritis
Platinum complexes	Nephrotoxicity, ototoxicity, peripheral neuropathy, loss of taste, seizures
Azacitidine	Hepatic dysfunction, rhabdomyolysis, lethargy, weakness, confusion, fever, skin rashes, stomatitis, phlebitis, hypotension
Cytarabine	Arachnoiditis with intrathecal administration, stomatitis, esophagitis, hepatic dysfunction (mild, reversible), thrombophlebitis
Fluorouracil	Diarrhea, stomatitis, esophagitis, intestinal bleeding, dermatitis, photosensitivity, loss of nails or dark band on nails, "black hairy tongue," lacrimation, lacrimal duct stenosis, cerebellar ataxia, myocardial ischemia
Mercaptopurine	Cholestasis, stomatitis, diarrhea, dermatitis, fever, hematuria, Budd–Chiari-like syndrome
Methotrexate	Stomatitis, diarrhea (intestinal hemorrhagic, ulceration, perforation), renal tubular necrosis, liver cirrhosis, osteoporosis (in children), dermatitis, furunculosis, fever, headache, pneumonitis Intrathecal: arachnoiditis with radicular syndrome, myelitis, seizures Previously irradiated areas: skin erythema, pulmonary fibrosis, transverse myelitis, cerebritis
Thioguanine	Cholestasis
Actinomycin D	Stomatitis, cheilitis, glossitis, proctitis, diarrhea, skin erythema, desquamation, hyperpigmentation, necrosis with SQ injection
Bleomycin	Shaking chills, fever, anaphylaxis-like reaction with hypotension, fever, delirium, bronchospasm in lymphoma patients, severe pneumonitis, pulmonary fibrosis, skin hyperpigmentation, hardening/loss of fingernails, erythroderma, desquamation
Doxorubicin (Adriamycin), Daunorubicin, Adriamycin	Cardiomyopathy, stomatitis Extravasation: severe ulceration and necrosis Erythema, desquamation in previously irradiated skin areas, diarrhea
Mitomycin C	Necrosis with SQ injection, stomatitis, rash, pulmonary fibrosis, hepatic and renal dysfunction
Vinblastine	Local vesication if injected SQ, stomatitis, glossitis, neurologic toxicities similar to vincristine
Vincristine	📖 Peripheral neuropathy with severe paresthesias, paralytic ileus, abdominal pain, local vesicant if injected SQ
Vindesine	Neurotoxicity as per vincristine, but less severe
VP-16-213 (etoposide, VP-16)	Orthostatic hypotension with rapid infusion
L-Asparaginase	Allergic reactions, hepatitis (< 50%), pancreatitis (5%), coagulation deficits, CNS depression, glucose intolerance
Dacarbazine (DTIC)	Local irritant if injected SQ, flulike syndrome, hepatotoxicity, diarrhea, cerebral dysfunction
Hexamethyl-melamine (HMM)	Rash, neurotoxicity
Hydroxyurea	Stomatitis, rash, headaches, increased blood urea nitrogen
Mitotane	Diarrhea, depression, lethargy, dermatitis, permanent cerebral dysfunction (rare)
Procarbazine	Lethargy, depression, muscle cramps, arthralgia, sensitization of tissue to radiation, peripheral neuropathy, vertigo, headache, seizures, dermatitis (hyperpigmentation), stomatitis, dysphagia, diarrhea
Streptozocin	Nephrotoxicity, renal tubular acidosis, renal failure, hepatotoxicity, diarrhea
Adrenocortico-steroids	Peptic ulcer disease, Na^+ retention, hypertension, K^+ wasting, glucose intolerance, weight gain, proximal myopathy, Psychologic effects: euphoria, depression, psychosis Osteoporosis, avascular hip necrosis, skin fragility, susceptibility to infection
Androgens Estrogens Progestins Taxol® Suramin	Virilization, fluid retention, hepatotoxicity Fluid retention, feminization, uterine bleeding, hypercalcemic flare (breast cancer) Mild fluid retention Hypersensitivity reactions, peripheral polyneuropathy, myalgia, arthralgias, bradycardia Peripheral polyneuropathy, coagulopathy, adrenal insufficiency, renal toxicity

(Cascioto, 1988)

RADIATION THERAPY SIDE EFFECTS

- 📖 Cognitive effects of radiation are probably dose related. Young children are at higher risk than adults as myelin is developing rapidly and, therefore, is susceptible to CNS insult. It usually presents slowly, in delayed fashion, and can be difficult to distinguish from tumor recurrence.

    It is estimated in approximately 34% after radiation therapy, especially if combined with chemotherapy.
- Fibrosis and contractures—maintain patient on a prophylactic stretching program, and continue therapeutic stretching after surgery.
- Postradiation osteonecrosis—uncommon; may lead to pathologic fractures

MYOPATHY: PARANEOPLASTIC POLYMYOSITIS AND DERMATOMYOSITIS

- These are well-recognized syndromes that can be associated with malignancies of the breast and lung
- Rehabilitation treatment includes traditional rehabilitation, intervention, stretching, isometric exercises, assistive devices, energy conservation, bracing, as well as social and vocational counseling. Specific attention must be paid to avoid exercise to fatigue
    - 📖 Carcinomatous Myopathy—A syndrome seen in metastatic disease that is consistent with muscle necrosis and presents with proximal muscle weakness
    - 📖 Carcinomatous neuropathy affects peripheral nerves as well as muscle. Signs and symptoms include distal motor and sensory loss, proximal muscle weakness, decreased reflexes and sensation. It most often occurs with lung cancer. Type II muscle atrophy is present as well as a distal peripheral polyneuropathy. Rehabilitative measures focus on supportive intervention including adaptive equipment, orthosis and functional mobility
    - Chemotherapy-related myopathies, such as steroid myopathy, result from atrophy of type II muscle fibers in the proximal musculature
    - Isometrics may be used to improve muscle metabolism and enhance strength and recovery

BREAST CANCER REHABILITATION

Lymphedema

Lymphedema is a frequent complication of breast cancer management and is manifested by upper extremity swelling associated with a sense of arm fullness. It usually develops over an extended period of time, postmastectomy or lumpectomy in up to one-third of women.

📖 Lymphedema is a result of damage or blockage of the lymphatic system in which an accumulation of protein occurs in the interstitium. This changes the colloidal pressure and detracts fluid into the interstitial space.

Lymphedema is described in three grades:

Grade 1   Pitting edema that is reversed by elevation

Grade 2:   Nonpitting edema. The skin may now become hardened secondary to the development of fibrotic tissue as a result of chronic excess protein in the interstitial spaces and deposition of adipose tissue. Appears as brawny edema unresponsive to elevation.

Grade 3:   Swelling of the involved extremity described as lymphostatic elephantiasis. Cartilage-like.

Without intervention the limb enlargement progresses and continues, which may result in significant social, physical, and psychological disability.

Intervention focuses on prevention by not interfering with lymph outflow by constricting the arm, protecting the arm from infection, excess scarring, and avoidance of vasodilation from extreme heat exposure.

Treatment

Treatment involves elevation, retrograde massage or manual lymph drainage, isometric external compression garment.

- 📖 Compression therapy by sequential graded pumps has been shown to be effective in reabsorption of water form the interstitium into the venous capillaries. The downfall to this is that large protein molecules remain interstitial, continuing to change the colloidal pressure. If a pneumatic or graded pump is used, it must be used daily (2–6 hours) followed by placement of a compression garment to prevent re-accumulation of fluid. This must be done daily for the remainder of the patient's life

- Precautions should be taken when using a compression pump and its use should proceed after manual lymph drainage has been performed.

When initiating the compression pump, patients with cardiovascular compromise should be monitored closely for shortness of breath, increasing heart rate, fluctuation of blood pressure, or complaints of increasing pain

Caution should be taken in the presence of residual tumors

Pumping should be discontinued if edema increases above the pump's sleeve

Pumps should not be used in the presence of infection

Pumps are contraindicated in bilateral mastectomy patients because truncal edema may result

- 📖 When more than one lymphedematous area is involved there is no place for fluid resolution and other areas may become edematous
- 📖 Following mastectomy, immediate postoperative therapies can safely consist of hand pumping, hand and elbow ROM exercises, positioning techniques, postural exercises, and shoulder ROM exercises to 40 degrees of flexion and abduction. Active assistive exercises can be initiated when the surgical drains have been removed.
- Additional management includes antibiotic treatment as needed for cellulitis or dermatolymphangitis.

METASTATIC BONE INVOLVEMENT

In Patients with Metastatic Bone Disease
- 75% have breast, lung or prostate cancer

  25% have renal, thyroid, or other cancer

  60% of all bone metastasis in males are secondary to prostate cancer, and approximately > 90% of patients with advanced prostate cancer will develop bone metastases

  50% to 85% of bone metastasis in females are secondary to breast cancer
- More than 50% of all patients with breast, lung, or prostate cancer will eventually develop bone metastasis. Skeletal metastasis arise through hematogenous spread. Bone is the third most common site for metastasis
- 📖 The most consistent symptom is pain, which is most severe at night or upon weight-bearing. In patients with spinal involvement, pain may be worse lying down and improves with sitting
- Metastatic Bone Disease causes pain, pathological fractures, neurologic injury, and functional disability. Pathological fractures occur in 10% to 30% of patients with bone lesions
- 📖 Skeletal metastases are rarely solitary. The metastasis usually involves the axial skeleton, proximal femur, and humerus. 70% of spinal metastases occur in the thoracic spine. 95% are extradural in origin and involve the vertebral body anterior to the spinal canal

Evaluation of Metastatic Bone Disease

- Bone scan is done usually at the time of diagnosis with correlation of involved areas on bone scan with X-rays. Most patients with high risk for conus medullaris involvement are

followed serially with bone scans to detect bony involvement before physical manifestation is present.
- Complaints of pain warrant X-rays and a bone scan at any time during the disease
- If the clinician suspects metastatic involvement, the patient is placed non-weight bearing on the involved extremity until a full evaluation and work-up is completed.
- 📖 Bone scans usually pick up metastatic disease early. Up to one-third of patients with positive bone scans have no X-ray changes on plain films. If a patient complains of persistent back pain and radiographs are normal, an MRI is indicated. Not all lesions are painful. Bone scans are highly sensitive but not highly specific for tumor involvement. False negatives occur in the setting of bone destruction without ongoing repair or bone metabolism.

Involvement of the Upper Extremity
📖 More than 90% of upper extremity metastases involve the humerus.
- In the upper extremity the majority of symptomatic lesions are from:
  1. Breast Cancer (Ca)
  2. Multiple Myeloma
  3. Renal Ca

Involvement of the Lower Extremity
📖 Most metastases of the lower extremity involve the hip and femur.
- In the lower extremity the majority of symptomatic lesions are from:

HIP	FEMUR
Prostate Ca	Breast Ca
Breast Ca	Renal Ca
Lung Ca	Multiple Myeloma
Lymphoma	Prostate Ca

📖 Note: It is possible to have a negative bone scan with positive X-rays (Any complaint of pain warrants a bone scan and plain film)

Treatment Once Bony Involvement is Identified

- Once metastatic bone disease is identified, treatment may consist of radiation, chemotherapy, immobilization, splinting, bracing, and/or surgical intervention. If an unstable lesion is identified or suspected a surgical opinion should be sought

Immobilization—Relieves pain and assists with prevention of pathological fractures. Different types of immobilization consist of:
- Slings, splinting and/or concommitant weight-bearing precautions with appropriate assistive devices
- Spinal orthosis: halo bracing, cervical bracing, Philadelphia collars, sternal-occipital-mandibular immobilizers (SOMI brace)
- Body jackets such as the plastic molded body jackets (TLSO—thoracolumbar sacral orthosis) can be used for lesions involving the cervical and thoracic regions. A thoracic extension can connect a SOMI or Philadelphia collar to a custom molded body jacket

General Indications for Surgical Treatment of Metastatic Bone Disease
1. Intractable pain
2. Impending pathological fracture
3. Fracture has occurred

Surgical Intervention Is Indicated When:

	Size of Lesion	Amount Cortex Involved
• Upper Extremity	> 3 cm	> 50%
• Lower Extremity (Fig. 9–9)	> 2.5 cm	> 30% to 50%
–Femoral Neck	> 1.3 cm	> 1.3 cm in axial length
– Surgical intervention is indicated if greater than 50% to 60% of medullary cross-sectional diameter is involved – This determination is enhanced by CT sections		

(Gerber and Vargo, 1998)

- 📖 Lytic lesions are generally considered to be more prone to fracture than blastic lesions Lytic lesions typically occur in tumors of the:
  - Breast
  - Lung
  - Kidney

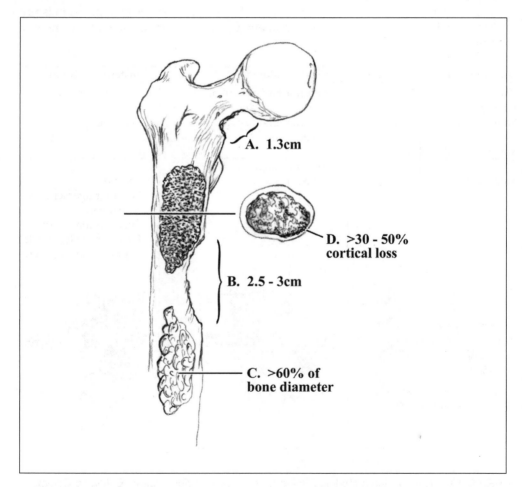

FIGURE 9–9. Lytic lesions of the femur that meet criteria for instability. **A.** Cortical destruction exceeds 1.3 cm in the femoral neck. **B.** Cortical destruction exceeds 2.5-3 cm elsewhere in the femur. **C.** Lytic lesion exceeds 60% of the total bone width (diameter). **D.** Lytic lesion exceeds >30–50% involvement of the cortex.

- Thyroid
- Gastrointestinal tumors
- Neuroblastoma
- Lymphoma
- Melanoma
- Blastic lesions typically occur in prostate cancer

Involvement of the Axial Skeleton

- Requires evaluation of the extent of metastatic involvement of the vertebral column. An MRI will clearly delineate epidural vertebral involvement even if radiographs are normal
- Denis (1984) described stability of thoracic and lumbar injuries by utilizing the three-column model described as (Figure 9–10):
  - The spine is considered stable when only one column is involved except if it is the middle column
  - The spine is considered unstable when two or more columns are involved or the middle column is severely involved
  - The spine is also considered unstable if greater than 20 degrees of angulation is present
  - These basic principles can be applied in evaluating metastatic bony involvement of the spine.

Anterior Column	Middle Column	Posterior Column
Anterior longitudinal ligament	Posterior half of vertebral body	Spinous process
Anterior half of vertebral body	Posterior annulus/ posterior disc	Laminae
Anterior annulus fibrosis		Facets
Anterior disc	Posterior longitudinal ligament	Pedicles
		Posterior ligamentous structures:
		Ligamentum flavum
		Intraspinous ligaments
		Supraspinous ligaments

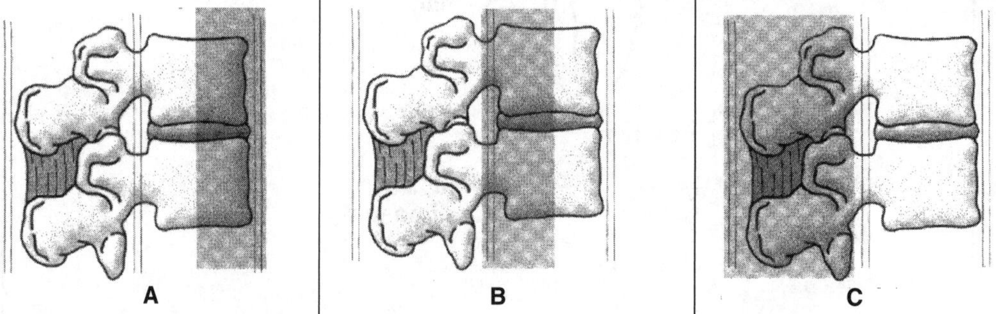

FIGURE 9–10. Three Column Model of Spine Stability. **A.** Anterior Column. **B.** Middle Column. **C.** Posterior Column.

PRIMARY BONE TUMORS

- Metastatic cancer to the skeletal system is more common.
- Primary bone tumors consist of 0.5% of all cancers in the United States each year

Osteosarcomas

📖 Most common primary malignant tumor of bone in children. (Garden and Gillis, 1996)
  - Occur in adolescence and commonly involve the knee and proximal humerus
  - Five-year survival has increased to nearly 80%
  - **Tx.** Involves surgical intervention through amputation or limb salvage. Amputee and prosthetic management—see Prostheties and Orthotics

Multiple Myeloma

  - Represents 10% to 25% of patients with pathologic fractures
  - Characterized by presence of cells resembling plasma cells originating in the bone marrow. This abnormal protein leads to termination of cells
  - Occurs most commonly in patients 50 to 70 year old males > female
  - Usually progresses with gradual development of pain
  - Frequently involves the lumbar spine, pelvis/sacrum, chest, skull, and ribs
  - Often, there may be no early findings and pathologic fracture may be the presenting manifestation of the disease
  - Course of disease is insidious and eventually leads to extensive marrow replacement, anemia, thrombocytopenia, and hemorrhages

Complications:
  - Renal failure occurs as a result of tubular blockage by protein cast deposition
  - Bone involvement on roentgenograph reveals diffuse osteoporosis and multiple lytic lesions
  - Early films are often negative
  - Bone scans may be normal. However, a skeletal survey may reveal diffuse "punched out" lytic lesions with black sclerotic borders
  - Amyloid deposits may also infiltrate peripheral nerves causing a peripheral neuropathy

Treatment:
  - Radiotherapy
  - Chemotherapy
  - Intramedullary fixation – may be difficult or impossible because of the remaining abnormal bone
  - Rehabilitation concerns are similar to those for patients with metastatic involvement or other primary malignancies. A high index of suspicion is necessary to identify patients at risk for pathologic fractures

REHABILITATION OF PATIENTS WITH ONCOLOGIC BONE DISEASE

- Goals are to protect the affected bone and promote strength and mobility
- Intervention includes:
  - Crutches, walkers, wheelchairs, and required assistive devices and equipment to provide safety, joint protection, and function
  - Orthosis for patients with spinal instability—Corsets may be beneficial for pain relief and support when spinal stability is not a concern
  - Exercise programs should avoid high impact, torsion, and manual resistive exercises Isometric and nonresistive isotonic exercises: swimming, walking, or stationary biking are recommended within reason of each patient's current limitation. Exercises should improve endurance and strength

- Fall prevention and proper body mechanics are also components of the rehabilitation program
- Physical modalities used to relieve pain—soft tissue massage, electrical stimulation (TENS)
- Heat modalities, such as ultrasound, diathermy, microwave therapy—considered contraindicated in the presence of malignancy

CANCER PAIN

Cancer pain may result from direct tumor invasion, chemotherapy, peripheral neuropathy, plexopathy, postsurgical pain or procedure related pain or can be unrelated to any of these factors. The World Health Organization (WHO) estimates that 25% of all cancer patients die with unrelieved pain. (World Health Organization 1990)

Pain can be effectively treated in 85% to 95% of patients with an integrated program of systemic, pharmacologic, and anticancer therapy.

Treatment:

The WHO has devised a 3-step analgesic ladder to outline the use of nonopioid analgesics, and adjuvant therapy for the treatment of progressively more severe pain. (Figure 9-11)

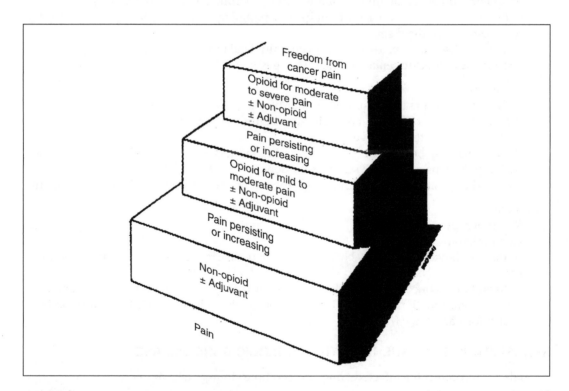

FIGURE 9–11. The Three-Step Analgesic Ladder.

Nonopioid Analgesics
Nonopioid analgesics are limited by maximum dosages
This group is made up of anti-inflammatory agents (aspirin and NSAIDs) and acetaminophen

Opioid Analgesics

Opioid analgesics have no ceiling, and dosing is guided by pain relief and is limited by side effects

Breakthrough pain is treated with "rescue doses." Dosing should be titrated to a level in which pain is either controlled or side effects limit increasing the dosage of the medication. Oral administration is the first choice; however, there are options for transdermal, rectal, IV, and spinal (epidural and intrathecal) routes. These routes may be indicated in those patients in which oral administration is not possible. An example of opiate analgesic agents and their conversion follows. (Table 9–11)

TABLE 9–11.

	Parenteral (mg)	Oral (mg)	Conversion Factor (IV to po)	Duration (parenteral, oral) (hr)
Narcotic Agonists				
Morphine	10	30	3.0	3–4
Controlled-released morphine MS Contin® Roxanol SR®	– –	30 30	– –	12 8
Methadone (Dolophine®)	10	20	2.0	4–8
Hydromorphone (Dilaudid®)	1.5	7.5	5.0	2–3
Fentanyl	100µg	–	–	1
Meperidine (Demerol®)	75	300	4.0	2–3
Levorphanol (Levo-Dromoran®)	2	4	2.0	3–6
Codeine	130	200	1.5	3–4
Oxycodone (Roxicodone®, component of Percodan®, Tylox®)	–	30	–	3–5
Hydrocodone (Lortab®, component of Vicodin®)	–	200	–	3–5
Propoxyphene (Darvon®, component of Darvocet®)	–	200	–	3–6
Mixed Agonist-Antagonists				
Pentazocine (Talwin®)	60	180	3.0	2–4
Nalbuphine (Nubain®)	10	–	–	4–6
Butorphanol (Stadol®)	2	–	–	4–6

(Garden and Gillis, 1996)

Adjuvant Drugs

Adjuvant drugs include antidepressants, anticonvulsants, Benzodiazepines, neuroleptics, antihistamines, corticosteroids, calcitonin, psychostimulants, and alpha-blockers. These supplement analgesics or treat side effects.

Patients who do not respond to oral medications or have difficulty with limiting side effects may benefit from nerve blocks, TENS, or surgical intervention such as cordotomy, dorsal column stimulation implantation, or centra-spinal opioid injections.

Measuring and Assessing Pain

Appropriate analgesic therapy is based on the pain level of the patient and the dosage of current medications. Pain can be measured on a scale of 0–10. Pain ratings of 1–4 are considered mild pain. Pain levels of 5–6 are consistent with moderate pain, 7–10 is consistent with severe pain. (Wall, 1999)

Using the 3-Step Analgesic Ladder (WHO)
The 3-step analgesic ladder (WHO) should be used to determine the appropriate initiation of analgesic therapy.

Step 1
Patients not on any analgesic therapy with mild/moderate pain are treated with Step 1 nonopiate analgesics. Adjuvant pain medication may be added to facilitate better control or treat side effects or specific pain-related symptomatology. For example, Elavil® has been shown to help with neuropathic pain and insomnia.

Step 2
If a patient has mild to moderate pain despite taking a nonopioid analgesic, dose the nonopioid analgesic should be maximized and a Step-2 opioid analgesic should be added.

Step 3
Patients who have moderate to severe pain despite therapy with Step-2 opioids require an increase in the dose of opioid, or a change to Step-3 opioid when pain is severe. Patients who have mild-moderate pain while taking a Step-3 opioid should have the dose increased to an effective level. (Levy, 1996)

Oral and Parenteral Dose Equivalents of Opioid Analgesic Drugs
Step-2 and Step-3 Opioid Analgesics

TABLE 9-12

Drug	Dose	
	Oral	*Parenteral*
Recommended for routine use		
Step 2 opioids		
Codeine	100 mg every 4 hr	50 mg every 4 hr
Dihydrocodeine	50–75 mg every 4 hr	N/A
Hydrocodone	15 mg every 4 hr	N/A
Oxycodone	7.5–10 mg every 4 hr	N/A
Step 3 opioids		
Morphine	15 mg every 4 hr	5 mg every 4 hr
Oxycodone	7.5–10 mg every 4 hr	N/A
Hydromorphone	4 mg every 4 hr	0.75–1.5 mg every 4 hr
Fentanyl	N/A	50 µg/hr every 72 hr
Not recommended for routine use		
Propoxyphene		N/A
Meperidine		50 mg every 2 hr
Methadone		5 mg every 6 hr
Levorphanol		1 mg every 6–8 hr
Oral opiates begin relief at 30 minutes and last approximately 4 hours		
IV opioids begin relief at 5 minutes an last 1–2 hours		

Treatment of Chronic Pain

- In order to treat chronic cancer pain, the physician should titrate around the clock medications with supplemental rescue doses for breakthrough pain. Rescue doses are based on one-sixth of the 24-hour total daily dose. Sustained-release medication should not be given PRN.

  Example: A patient taking 90 mg of controlled-release morphine every 12 hours would receive 30 mg of immediate-release morphine every 4 hours. The patient who is given Q 12 hour controlled-release morphine or oxycodone appreciates analgesic effect in 1 hour, peaks in 2–3 hours, and lasts for 12 hours when the next schedules dosing is due.

- Patients should be monitored closely, even daily, when beginning or changing an analgesic regimen. The optimal therapeutic regimen should be titrated based on unrelieved pain and side effects. It is important not to abruptly withdraw opioids. If pain has subsided, the dosage may be decreased 25 to 50% each day. If a patient has severe side effects from opioid use, 1 or 2 doses can be withheld and overall doses reduced by 50% to 75%. Avoidance of abrupt discontinuation is essential to prevent physical withdrawal syndrome.

Adequate pain relief, appropriate rehabilitative programs and goals, as well as supportive psychosocial intervention continue to play an important role in improving the quality of life in patients with cancer.

MANAGEMENT OF GASTROINTESTINAL COMPLICATIONS

Nutrition

- The nutritional status of the cancer patient can become compromised as a result of radiation and chemotherapy. Radiation therapy causes alteration in the saliva production and in taste. It may also cause nausea, cramps, and diarrhea
- Chemotherapy may lead to folic acid and vitamin K deficiency
- Patients who receive radiation therapy may benefit from a lactose-free, low-residue oral diet
- It is advisable to start parenteral nutrition when > 20% of body weight has been lost.

Emesis

- 📖 Effective anti-emetic management of the cancer patient includes the use of serotonin antagonists. One agent commonly used is ondansetron hydrochloride (Zofran®), which blocks 5-HT receptors. Advantages of specific serotonin antagonists over conventional anti-emetics include lack of extrapyramidal side effects, akathisia, and other CNS effects. Mild headache is, however, more common with these agents.

REFERENCES

Alba AS. Concepts in Pulmonary, Rehabilitation. In: Braddom RL. *Physical Medicine and Rehabilitation.* Philadelphia: W. B. Saunders; 1996:671–686.

American Cancer Society, Inc. Cancer Facts and Figures 2001. Available at http://www.cancer.org. Accessed August 28, 2002.

American College of Sports Medicine. *Guidelines for Exercise Testing and Prescription* 5th ed. Philadelphia: Lea & Febiger; 1995.

Bach JR. Rehabilitation of the Patient with Respiratory Dysfunction. In: DeLisa JA. *Rehabilitation: Principles and Practice* 2nd ed. Philadelphia: Lippincott Williams & Wilkins; 1993:952–972.

Bach JR. *Pulmonary Rehabilitation: The Obstructive and Paralytic Conditions.* Philadelphia: Hanley & Belfus; 1996.

Borg G. *An Introduction to Borg's RPE Scale.* Ithaca, NY: Mouvement Publications; 1985.

Cardiac Rehabilitation: Clinical Practice Guidelines, number 17. U.S. Department of Health and Human Services, Public Health Service, Agency for Health Care Policy and Research, National Heart, Lung, and Blood Institute. Rockville, MD; 1995.

Casciato DA, Lowitz BB. *Manual of Clinical Oncology* 2nd ed. Boston: Little Brown; 1988.

Denis F. Spinal Instability as defined by the three-column concept in acute spinal trauma. *Clin Orthop* 1984 (189): 65–76.

Dikeman KJ, Kanandjian MS. *Communication and Swallowing Management of Tracheostomized and Ventilator-dependent Adults.* San Diego: Singular Publishing Group, Inc.;1995.

Fletcher GF, Hartley LH, Haskell L, Pollock ML. Exercise standards, a statement for health professionals from the American Heart Association. *Circulation* 1982, 82: 2297.

Flores AM, Zohman LR. Rehabilitation of the cardiac patient. In: DeLisa JA. *Rehabilitation Medicine Principles and Practice* 2nd ed. Philadelphia: Lippincott Williams & Wilkins: 1993; 934–951.

Flores AM, Zohman LR. Rehabilitation of the cardiac patient. In: DeLisa JA, Gans BM eds. *Rehabilitation Medicine: Principles and Practice* 3rd ed. Philadelphia: Lippincott-Raven; 1998: 1337–1357.

Froehlicher VF. *Exercise and the Heart: Clinical Concepts.* Chicago: YearBook Medical Publishers, 1987.

Gerber LH, Vargo M. Rehabilitation for Patients with Cancer Diagnoses. In: DeLisa JA, Gans BM eds. *Rehabilitation Medicine: Principles and Practice* 3rd ed. Philadelphia: Lippincott-Raven; 1998: 1293–1317.

Garden F, Grabois M. Cancer Rehabilitation, *Physical Medicine and Rehabilitation State of the Art Reviews.* Philadelphia: Hanley and Belfus; 1994.

Garden FH, Gillis TA. Principles of Cancer Rehabilitation. In Braddom RL. *Physical Medicine and Rehabilitation.* Philadelphia: W. B. Saunders, 1996:1199–1214.

Goldman L, Hashimoto B, Cooke F, Loscalzo A. Comparative reproducibility and validity of systems for assessing cardiovascular functional class: advantages of a new specific activity scale. *Circulation.* 1981: Dec; 64(6): 1227–34.

Guidelines for Cardiac Rehabilitation Programs 2nd ed. American Association of Cardiovascular and Pulmonary Rehabilitation: Human Kinetics, Champaign, IL; 1991, 1995.

Lehman, JF, DeLisa JA, Warren CG. Cancer rehabilitation: assessment of need, development and evaluation of a model of care. *Arch Phys Med Rehabil* 1978; 59:410–419.

Levy, MH, Drug Therapy: Pharmacologic Treatment of Cancer Pain: *NEJM* 1996, 1124–1132.

Maloney FP. Pulmonary function in quadriplegia: effects of a corset. *Arch Phys Med Rehabil* 1979; 60(6): 261–265.

Marciniak CM, Sliwa JA, Spill G, Heinemann AW, Semik PE. Functional outcome following rehabilitation of the cancer patient. *Arch Phys Med Rehabil* 1996, 77(1): 54–57.

Takakura K, Sono K, Holo S, et al. *Metastatic Tumors of the Central Nervous System.* Tokyo: Igaku-shoin; 1982.

O'Young B, Young MA, Stiens SA. *PM&R Secrets.* Philadelphia: Hanley and Belfus; 1997.

Pashkow FJ. Issues in Contemporary Cardiac Rehabilitatio: A historical perspective. *J Am Coll Cardiol.* 1993; 21(3): 822–834.

Tardif GS. Sexual activity after a myocardial infarction. *Arch Phys Med Rehabil* 1989; 70(10): 763–766.

Wall PD, Melzack R. *Textbook of Pain* 4th ed. New York: Churchill Livingstone; 1999.

Wilson PW, Castelli, Kannel WB. Coronary risk prediction in adults (The Framingham Heart Study). *Am J Cardiol* 1987; 59(14): 91G–94G.

World Health Organization. *Cancer Pain Relief and Palliative Care.* WHO Expert Committee Technical Report Series, No. 804, 1990.

10

PEDIATRIC REHABILITATION

Roger Rossi, D.O., Michael Alexander, M.D.,
and Sara Cuccurullo, M.D.

This chapter is designed to review various pediatric topics within the field of rehabilitation medicine that may be helpful when studying for the physical medicine and rehabilitation boards. The chapter is broken down into different sections to encompass childhood development and growth, and the major childhood disabilities within the field of rehabilitation medicine. The ten subsections presented include:

Genetics and Chromosomal Abnormalities
Development and Growth
Limb Deficiencies
Diseases of the Bones and Joints
Connective Tissue and Joint Disease
Burns
Cancers
Traumatic Brain Injury
Cerebral Palsy
Spina Bifida
Neuromuscular Disease

■

GENETICS AND CHROMOSOMAL ABNORMALITIES

- Normal humans have 46 chromosomes (23 maternal and 23 paternal) in every cell except gonads, which have 23 chromosomes. Errors during cell division will result in chromosome abnormalities
- Chromosome abnormalities can be found in approximately 0.5% of all newborns
- The numerical chromosome abnormalities are most frequently trisomy or monosomy
- Chromosome abnormality should be suspected in children with any of the following:
  - Dysmorphic features
  - Congenital malformations
  - Developmental delay
  - Mental retardation
  - Prenatal and/or postnatal growth retardation
  - Abnormal sexual characteristics
- Fragile X syndrome, XXY and XYY often are associated with excessive growth

PHENOTYPIC FEATURES OF SELECTED CHROMOSOMAL SYNDROMES (Table 10–1)

TABLE 10–1. Signs of Selected Chromosomal Syndromes

Syndromes	Signs
📖 Trisomy 21 Down Syndrome	Mongoloid slant of eyes, Brushfield spots of iris, protruding tongue, 3rd fontanelle, low set auricles, excess nuchal skin, Simian lines, single flexion crease and incurving (clinodactyly) of 5th fingers, increased distance between 1st and 2nd toes, mottling of skin, hypotonia, congenital heart disease (CHD), (endocardial cushion defect, Ventricular Septal Defect [VSD], other)
Trisomy 13 (Edwards)	Intrauterine Growth Retardation (IUGR) in all 3 parameters, coloboma of iris (pupil of keyhole shape), capillary hemangioma, skin defect of skull, hyperconvex nails, polydactyly, rocker bottom feet, arrhinencephaly, cleft lip and palate, CHD, urinary tract abnormalities
Trisomy 18	IUGR, antimongoloid slant of eyes, short palpebral fissure, small mouth, micrognathia, low set, abnormal auricles, prominent occiput, short sternum, abnormal position of fingers (2nd overlapping 3rd and 5th overlapping 4th), hypoplastic finger nails, rocker bottom feet, CHD, spasticity, feeding problems
📖 Turner Syndrome 45X	Triangular face, antimongoloid slant of eyes, abnormal shape of ears, webbed or wide neck, broad "shield" chest, wide set nipples, edema of hands and feet, shortened 4th and 5th metacarpals and metatarsals, cubitus valgus, short stature, primary amenorrhea, CHD especially coarctation of aorta, mostly normal IQ, infertility
📖 Klinefelter Syndrome 47XXY 47XYY	Tall stature, postpubertaly small testicles, gynecomastia, eunuchoid build, increased risk for mild mental retardation (MR), learning and behavior problems, infertility No characteristic physical findings, except for tall stature, increased risk for behavior problem, mild MR

From Merenstein GB, Kaplan DW, Rosenberg AA. Handbook of Pediatrics 18th ed. Stamford, CT: Appleton & Lang; 1997: p. 776, with permission

- Prenatal diagnosis includes amniocentesis at 14–16 weeks of pregnancy or chorionic villi sampling at 9–10 weeks of gestation
- The exposure of a genetically susceptible fetus to a potential teratogen increases the chance of malformations. Although many environmental agents are potentially teratogenic, very few are proven teratogens. These include:
  - 📖 Infectious agents (rubella virus, cytomegalic virus, toxoplasma, herpes virus, varicella virus)
  - Drugs and medications (including alcohol, cocaine, anticonvulsants, vitamin A derivatives)
  - Maternal diseases (such as diabetes mellitus and phenylketonuria)
  - Uterine conditions (malformed uterus, twinning)

INDICATION FOR REFERRAL FOR GENETIC COUNSELING

1. Child with birth defects and/or developmental delay/mental retardation
2. Dysmorphic child
3. Parent or child affected with known or suspected genetic disorder
4. Positive family history of birth deficits or retardation in aunts, uncles, grandparents or other relatives, especially if multiple members are affected
5. Possible teratogenic exposure or other abnormalities of pregnancy
6. Advanced maternal age (> 35 years) or other indications for prenatal diagnosis

▪

DEVELOPMENT AND GROWTH

Development includes maturation of organs and systems, acquisition of physical, intellectual, and interpersonal skills, ability to adapt more readily to stress and assumption of personal responsibility, and capacities for creative expression. Growth signifies increase in size.

HEIGHT

- Birth length doubles by approximately age 4 years and triples by age 13 years
- The average child grows approximately 10 inches (25 cm) in the first year of life, 5 inches (12.5 cm) in the second and 3–4 inches (7.5–10 cm) in the third and approximately 2–3 inches (5–7.5 cm) per year thereafter until growth spurt of puberty

WEIGHT

- The average infant weighs approximately 7 pounds 5 ounces (3.33 kg at birth)
- Within the first few days of life the newborn loses up to 10% of the birth weight
- Birth weight doubles between 4 and 5 months of age, triples by the end of the first year, and quadruples by the end of the child's second year. Between ages 2 and 9 years the annual increment in weight averages about 5 pounds (2.25 kg) per year

HEAD AND SKULL

- At birth the head is approximately two-thirds to three-fourths of its total mature size, whereas the rest of the body is only one-quarter of its adult size
- Six fontanels (anterior, posterior, two sphenoid and two mastoid) are usually present at birth
- The anterior fontanel normally closes between 10 and 14 months of age but may close by 3 months or remain open until 18 months
- The posterior fontanel usually closes by 4 months but in some children may not be palpable at birth
- Cranial sutures do not ossify completely until later childhood

OSSIFICATION CENTERS

- At birth the average full-term infant has five ossification centers: distal end of the femur, proximal end of the tibia, calcaneus, talus, and cuboid
- The clavicle is the first bone to calcify in utero, calcification beginning during the fifth fetal week

INFANTILE REFLEX DEVELOPMENT

- In neonates and infants, motor behavior is influenced by primitive reflexes as a result of the immature central nervous system (CNS)
- During the first six to eight months of life as CNS maturation progresses, these reflexes become gradually suppressed
- Concurrently, more sophisticated postural responses emerge between 2 to 14 months that are used and incorporated into volitional motor behavior (Table 10–2)
- 📖 Obligatory or persistent primitive reflexes are the earliest markers of abnormal neurological maturation. (See Table 10–28)

PHYSIOLOGIC POSTURAL REFLEX RESPONSES

TABLE 10–2. Postural Reflex Responses

Postural Reflex	Stimulus	Response	Age of Emergence	Clinical Significance
Head righting	Visual and vestibular	Align face/head vertical, mouth horizontal	Prone—2 months Supine—3–4 months	Delays or absent in CNS immaturity or damage
Head and body righting	Tactile, vestibular proprioceptive	Align body parts in anatomic position relative to each other and gravity	4–6 months	Same as above
Protective extension tone or parachute reactions	Displacement of center of gravity outside supporting base in sitting, standing	Extension/abduction of lateral extremity toward displacement to prevent falling	Sitting anterior-5–7 months Lateral—6–8 months Posterior—7–8 months Standing—12–14 months	Same as above
Equilibrium or tilting reactions	Displacement of center of gravity	Adjustment of tone and posture of trunk to maintain balance	Sitting—6–8 months Standing—12–14 months	Same as above

From Molnar GE, Alexander MA. Pediatric Rehabilitation 3rd ed. Philadelphia: Hanley & Belfus; 1999: page 21, table 2-4 with permission.

MILESTONES IN CHILD DEVELOPMENT

Developmental milestones can be grouped in 4 distinct areas of function:

1. Gross motor behavior
2. Fine motor, adaptive behavior
3. Language behavior
4. Personal-social behavior

TABLE 10–3. Milestones in Child Development

Age	Gross Motor	Fine Motor Adaptive	Personal/Social	Speech and Language	Cognitive	Emotional
NEWBORN	Flexor tone predominates In prone, turns head to side Automatic reflex walking Rounded spine when held sitting	Hands fisted Grasp reflex State-dependent ability to fix and follow bright object	Habituation and some control of state	Cry State dependent quieting and head turning to rattle or voice	Sensorimotor 0–24 months Reflex stage	Basic trust vs. basic mistrust (first year) Normal symbiotic phase – does not differentiate self and mother
4 MONTHS	Head midline Head held when pulled to sit In prone, lifts head to 90° and lifts chest slightly Turns to supine	Hands mostly open Mid-line hand play Crude palmar grasp	Recognizes bottle	Turns to voice and bell consistently Laughs, squeals Responsive vocalization Blows bubbles, raspberries	Circular reaction, the interesting result of an action motivates its repetition	Lap baby, developing a sense of basic trust
7 MONTHS	Maintains sitting, may lean on arms Rolls to prone Bears all weight, bounces when held erect Cervical lordosis	Intermediate grasp Transfers cube from hand to hand Bangs objects	Differentiates between familiar person and stranger Holds bottle Looks for dropped object Talks to mirror image	Uses single-word and double-consonant vowel combinations		At 5 months begins to differentiate mother and self—individualization Sense of belonging to a central person

(continued)

TABLE 10-3. Milestones in Child Development (*Continued*)

Age	Gross Motor	Fine Motor Adaptive	Personal/Social	Speech and Language	Cognitive	Emotional
10 MONTHS	Creeps on all fours Pivots in sitting Stands momentarily, cruises Slight bow leg Increased lumbar lordosis, acute lumbosacral angulation	Pincer grasp, mature thumb to index grasp Bangs two cubes held in hands	Plays peek-a-boo Finger feeds Chews with rotary movement	Shouts for attention Imitates speech sounds Waves bye-bye Uses *mama* and *dada* with meaning Inhibits behavior to "no"	Can retrieve an object hidden from view	Practicing phase of separation—individuation, practices imitating separations
14 MONTHS	Walks alone, arms in high guard or midguard Wide base, excessive knee and hip flexion Foot contact on entire side Slight valgus of knees and feet Pelvic tilt and rotation	Piles two cubes Scribbles spontaneously Holds crayon full length in palm Casts objects	Uses spoon with over pronation and spilling Removes a garment	Uses single words Understands simple commands	Differentiates available behavior patterns for new ends, e.g., pulls rug on which is a toy	Rapprochement phase—individuation; ambivalence behavior to mother Stage of autonomy vs. shame and doubt Pleasures in control of muscle and sphincter
18 MONTHS	Arms at low guard Mature supporting base and heel strike Seats self in chair Walks backward	Emerging hand dominance Crude release Holds crayon butt end in palm Dumps raisin from bottle spontaneously	Imitates housework Carries, hugs doll Drinks from cup neatly	Points to named body part Identifies one picture Says "no" Jargons	Capable of insight; problem solving by mental combinations, not physical groping	

	Gross Motor	Fine Motor/Adaptive	Personal-Social	Language	Cognitive	
2 YEARS	Begins running Walks up and down stairs alone Jumps on both feet in place	Hand dominance is usual Builds 8-cube tower Aligns cubes horizontally Imitates vertical line Places pencil shaft between thumb and fingers Draws with arm and wrist action	Pulls on garment Uses spoon well Opens door turning knob Feeds doll with bottle or spoon Toilet training usually begun	2-word phrases are common Uses verbs Refers to self by name Uses *me, mine* Follows simple directions	Preoperational period- 2–7 years Able to evoke an object or event not present Object performance established Comprehends symbols	
3 YEARS	Runs well Pedals tricycle Broad jumps Walks up stairs alternating feet	Imitates 3-cube bridge Copies circle Uses overhand throw with anteroposterior arm and motion Catches with extended arms hugging against body	Most children toilet trained day and night Pours from pitcher Unbutton; washes and dries hands and face Parallel play Can take turns Can be reasoned with	3-word sentences are usual Uses future tense Asks who, what, where Follows prepositional commands Gives full name May stutter; eager Identifies sex of self Recognizes 3 colors	Preoperational period continues: Child is capable of deferred limitation symbolic play, drawing of graphic images, mental images, verbal evocation of event	Stage of initiative vs. guilt 3–5 years Deals with issue of genital sexuality
4 YEARS	Walks down stairs alternating feet Hops on one foot Plantar arches developing Sits up from supine position without rotating	Handles a pencil by finger and wrist action, like adults Copies a cross Draws a froglike person with head and extremities Throws underhand Cuts with scissors	Cooperative play- sharing and interacting Imaginative make-believe play Dresses and undresses w/ supervision distinguishing front and back of clothing and buttoning Does simple errands outside of home	Gives connected account of experience Asks why, when, how Uses past tense, adjectives, adverbs Knows opposite analogies Repeats four digits		

(continued)

TABLE 10-3. Milestones in Child Development (*Continued*)

Age	Gross Motor	Fine Motor Adaptive	Personal/ Social	Speech and Language	Cognitive	Emotional
5 YEARS	Skips, tiptoes Balances 10 seconds on each foot	Hand dominance expected Draws man with head, body, extremities Throws with diagonal arm and body rotation Catches with hand	Creative play Competitive team play Uses fork for stabbing food Brushes teeth Is self-sufficient in toileting Dresses w/o supervision except tying shoelaces	Fluent speech Misarticulation of some sounds may persist Gives name, age, address Defines concrete nouns—composition, classification, use Follows 3-part commands Number concept to 10		Stage of industry vs. inferiority 5 years–adolescence Adjusts himself to the inorganic laws of the tool world
6 YEARS	Rides bicycle Roller skates	Prints alphabet; letter reversals still acceptable Mature catch and throw of ball	Teacher is important authority Uses fork appropriately Uses knife for spreading Plays table games	Shows mastery of grammar Uses proper articulation		Stage of industry vs. inferiority continues
7 YEARS	Continuing refinement of skills		Eats with fork and knife Combs hair Is responsible for grooming		Period of concrete operational thought 7 years–adolescence Child is capable of logical thinking	

From Molnar GE, Alexander MA. Pediatric Rehabilitation 3rd ed. Philadelphia: Hanley & Belfus; 1999: page 23, table 2-5 with permission.

■

PEDIATRIC LIMB DEFICIENCIES

CONGENITAL LIMB DEFICIENCY (Table 10–4)

The genesis of limb deficiency occurs primarily in the first trimester, with mesodermal formation of the limb occurring at day 26 of gestation and continuing with differentiation until 8 weeks gestation. Maternal diabetes is a risk factor for limb deficiency as is the drug thalidomide.

Original (Classic) Classification

When describing limb deficiency, classic terms include the following:
- Amelia—absence of a limb
- Meromelia—partial absence of a limb
- Hemimelia—absence of half a limb
- Phocomelia—flipper-like appendage attached to the trunk
- Acheiria—missing hand or foot
- Adactyly—absent metacarpal or metatarsal
- Aphalangia—absent finger or toe

Frantz Classification

Another classification system is the Frantz system, which describes deficiencies as either terminal, representing the complete loss of the distal extremity, or intercalary, denoting the absence of intermediate parts with preserved proximal and distal parts of the limb.
Those classifications are then divided into horizontal and longitudinal deficits.

ISPO Classification System (International Society for Prosthetics and Orthotics)

Divides all deformities into transverse or longitudinal.
Transverse deficiency has no distal remaining portions, whereas the longitudinal deficiency has distal portions.
Transverse level is named after the segment beyond which there is no skeletal portion.
Longitudinal deficiencies name the bones that are affected.
Any bone not named is present and of normal form.
📖 The ISPO Classification is the preferred classification system.

TABLE 10–4. Examples of Common Deficiencies Named by 3 Classification Systems

Original (Classic)	Frantz	ISPO
Upper Extremity Amelia	Terminal transverse	Transverse upper arm, total
Fibula Hemimelia	Intercalary/normal foot Longitudinal/absent rays Fibular deficiency	Longitudinal fibular deficiency, total or partial
Upper Extremity Phocomelia	Complete upper extremity phocomelia Distal/absent radius ulna Proximal/absent humerus	Longitudinal total, humerus, ulna, radius Carpal, metacarpal, phalangeal (total or partial)

From Molnar GE, Alexander MA. Pediatric Rehabilitation 3rd ed. Philadelphia: Hanley & Belfus; 1999: page 333, table 16-1, with permission.

CONGENITAL UPPER EXTREMITY DEFICIENCY

- Incidence 4.1 per 10,000 live births
- Most cases of congenital upper extremity deficiency have no hereditary implications.
- Exceptions to the above statement include:
  Deficiencies that involve hands and feet
  Central ray deficiencies
  Adactyly involving the first 4 digits with the fifth intact.
- Craniofacial anomalies are associated with limb deficiencies (Table 10–5).
- There are 5 associated syndromes seen with some limb deficiencies

TABLE 10–5. Associated Syndromes Seen with Limb Deficiencies

Upper Extremity Syndromes	Associated Problem
TAR Syndrome (thrombocytopenia with absence of radius)	Thrombocytopenia
Fanconi's Syndrome Anemia and leukopenia developing at 5–6 years of age	Anemia, Leukopenia
Holt-Oram Syndrome Congenital heart disease, especially atrial septal defects and tetralogy of Fallot	Congenital heart disease
Baller-Gerold Syndrome Craniosynostosis	Craniosynostosis
VACTERL (or VATER) Multi-organ symptom involvement	Vertebral defects Anal atresia Cardiac defects Tracheo Esophageal fistula Renal dysplasia Limb deficiency

Adapted from Molnar GE, Alexander MA. Pediatric Rehabilitation 3rd ed. Philadelphia: Hanley & Belfus; 1999: page 334, table 16-3, with permission.

Transradial Deficiency

- 📖 The most common congenital limb deficiency is a left terminal transradial deficiency
- 📖 Prosthetic fitting should follow the attainment of normal developmental milestones with the first fitting for a unilateral deficiency occurring when the child achieves sitting balance at around 6–7 months. The initial prosthesis has a passive mitt in which the infant can practice placing objects

- 📖 A more sophisticated prosthesis and terminal device is provided around 11–13 months when the child begins to walk, performs simple grasp and release activities, and has attention span greater than 5 minutes
- The initial transradial prosthesis is usually self-suspending using a supracondylar design and a hand, which is preferred by parents
- By age 4–5 years, the child can operate all types of prosthetic components and controls

Transhumeral Deficiency

- For the transhumeral deficiency, the initial prosthesis may be suspended either by a harness or by silicone suction suspension
- Prosthetic fitting should follow the attainment of the normal developmental milestones. By comparison to the transradial level it is advisable to delay progression slightly to achieve optimal results. A transhumeral design can be more of an encumbrance than the transradial design and may impede the infant, i.e., difficulty in rolling over
- Terminal device should be activated shortly after the child begins to walk. Terminal devices are the same as for the transradial
- Body-powered hooks are used successfully at 2–3 years once the child is strong enough and has the cognitive ability to operate them
- At age 4–5 years, a body-powered elbow may be used

Revision Amputation is required in 10% of upper extremity congenital limb deficiencies
Examples:
    The radial club hand
    The ulnar club hand
These represent longitudinal deficiencies of the forearm.
Treatment is directed at centralization of the hand and reconstructing the thumb.

📖 **Krukenberg Procedure:** Reconstructs the forearm and creates a sensate prehensile surface for children with absent hands by separating the ulna and the radius in the forearm. Because of cosmetic appearance, the procedure is used rarely with unilateral conditions.
Indications: absent hands, visual impairment

Vilkke Procedure: attaches a toe to the residual limb.
In general the higher the limb absence, the less the child accepts the prosthesis, i.e., transradial patients wear their prostheses more than transhumeral.

CONGENITAL LOWER EXTREMITY (LE) DEFICIENCY

Fibula

- 📖 Fibular longitudinal deficiency or fibula hemimelia is the most common congenital lower limb deformity (bilateral fibular longitudinal deficiency occurs 25% of the time). Unilateral fibular deficiency creates a problem with limb length discrepancy. (If leg length inequality is severe, a Syme's amputation may be performed with fitting of a Syme's prosthesis.)

Tibia

- Transtibial deficiency (or transverse deficiency of tibia) is more common than transfemoral (or transverse deficiency of the thigh)
- Longitudinal deficiency of the tibia occurs in 1 per 1,000,000 births. Clinical picture includes a varus foot; a short leg; and an unstable knee, ankle or both. Treatment of choice is a knee disarticulation
- Partial tibial deficiency: 30% of partial tibial deficiency occurs as an autosomal dominant inherited pattern. Segment length of the tibia is important. If the tibial segment is long enough, the surgeon creates a synostosis with the intact fibula and amputation of the foot. This provides a stable walking surface for the child without a prosthesis

Femur

- 📖 Longitudinal deficiency of the femur or partial proximal femoral focal deficiency (PFFD) occurs in 1 per 50,000 births 10%–15% bilateral. PFFD is the absence of development of the proximal femur, including stunting or shortening of the entire femur. The femur is typically short and held in flexion, abduction, and external rotation.

Treatment

Severe forms of PFFD usually require fusion of the shortened femur to the tibia. Removal of the foot (via Syme's amputation), leaves a stump that will accept an appropriate above-the-knee prosthesis.

Options

- Van Ness Rotation: (controversial) allows simulation of below knee function by rotating the foot by 180 degrees so ankle motion can control the prosthesis
- Nonstandard prosthesis or shoe lifts with no surgical conversion

Fitting Timetable of LE Amputee

- The lower limb deficient child is fit with a prosthesis when ready to pull up to standing position at 9–10 months. It is advisable to fit a jointless above-the-knee prosthesis to the toddler
- The normal child does not establish heel-to-toe gait until around 2 years
- Prosthetic heel-strike to toe-off gait is not attained until 5 years or when the child can demonstrate sustained one-legged standing
- A knee joint is usually added between 3–5 years old

Components

- The most common foot prescribed for the child amputee has been the solid ankle cushion heel (SACH foot): although energy-storing feet for children are becoming more popular
- Some knees that can be used in children include:
  Single axis knees: (with or without lock) are durable and lightweight
  Polycentric knees: good in situations in which residual limb is long and the knee centers are difficult to match
  Fluid controlled knees: offers a smoother gait and the ability of the knee to adapt to different walking speeds. Fluid controlled knees are reserved until adolescence secondary to size and weight restraints
- Suspension system should be easily adjustable to allow for growth. Suspension sleeves and silicone suction suspensions provide good adjustability because they allow for growth and provide excellent suspension. A suction socket is not prescribed until a child can assist in donning a prosthesis, at about 5 years of age. The pelvic belt is an acceptable way to suspend an above-knee prosthesis
- Below-knee amputees may use a patellar tendon-bearing prosthesis with a supracondylar cuff. It should be noted that one-third of limb deficient children using this type of suspension develop a dislocated patellae
- Major causes of gait deviations are growth or worn prosthetic parts
- Prostheses need to be replaced every 15–18 months on the growing child. Some children may require a new prosthesis annually until age 5, then every 2 years between 5–12 years, and every 3–4 years until adulthood
- Children may assume gait deviations to relieve pressure if they have an ill-fitting prosthesis

ACQUIRED AMPUTATIONS

Causes

- The most common cause of pediatric acquired amputation is trauma, occurring two times more than disease-related amputation. Motor vehicle accident, motorcycle, as well as train accidents account for the majority of childhood acquired amputations. Single limb loss occurs in more than 90% with 60% involving the lower extremity. Boys are affected greater than girls with a ratio of 3:2
- Childhood tumors are the most frequent cause of disease-related amputation with the highest incidence of malignancy in the 12–21 age group. Osteogenic sarcoma and Ewing's sarcoma occur most commonly (please see pediatric cancer section)
- Home accidents (i.e. burns, fireworks)
- Vascular insufficiency—gangrene
- Neurologic disorders—i.e., neurofibromatosis with associated nonunion of fracture.
- Emboli from meningococcemia may cause auto-amputation of limbs or digits. This usually affects all four limbs

Complications

Terminal overgrowth at the transected end of a long bone is the most common complication after amputation in the immature child: occurring most frequently on the humerus, fibula, tibia, and femur, in that order. The appositional growth may be so vigorous that the bone pierces the skin causing ulcers. Treatment of choice is surgical revision.

Other complications include: bone spur formation, development of adventitious bursae and stump scarring requiring socket modifications.
- Fitting the child with an acquired amputation follows the same time table as a congenital amputee except for the fact that a child who undergoes an amputation will require a temporary or preparatory prosthesis while post-op swelling subsides
- Intra-operative prosthetic fitting for a lower extremity amputee:

Advantages
Allows amputee to begin walking soon after surgery
Decreased edema and calf pain
Good candidates include teenagers or young adults undergoing amputation for a tumor

Disadvantages
Weight-bearing restrictions and activity restrictions that may put the stump at risk
Poor candidates for this procedure include young children who do not understand the restriction, immunocompromised children, children with insensate limbs or infections

GENERAL FUNCTIONAL ISSUES

- The child with bilateral upper extremity deficiency, substitutes fine motor tasks with the feet
- Amputees preserve their energy expenditure by decreasing their walking speed.
- Motorized wheelchairs traditionally are used when the child is around 5–6 years old
- The child with isolated limb deficiency or amputation is capable of achieving age-level academic skills

PHANTOM PAIN

- Congenital limb-deficient children do not develop phantom sensation or pain, even after the surgical conversion of the limb

- Acquired amputees: these children retain some awareness of the amputated part. This sensation has been described as uncomfortable or painful. The older the child is at the time of the amputation, the greater the chance that he or she may experience phantom pain, especially if the amputation occurs after the age of 10

■

DISEASES OF THE BONES AND JOINTS

THE FEET AND TOES

Metatarsus varus (Fig 10–1)

- Characterized by adduction of the forefoot on the hindfoot, with the heel in normal position or slightly valgus
- Flexible deformities are secondary to intrauterine posture and usually resolve
- Rigid deformities may require splinting
- 85% correct by age 3–4 years

Club foot (talipes equinovarus) consists of three associated deformities

1. Equinus or plantar flexion of the foot at the ankle
2. Varus or inversion deformity of the heel
3. Forefoot varus
- Incidence is around 1 per 1,000. Club foot follows a hereditary pattern and may be part of a generalized syndrome or be associated with anomalies especially of the spine
- 50% of children eventually require surgical correction

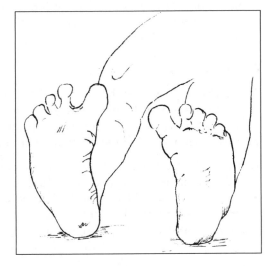

FIGURE 10–1. Metatarsus Varus.

Talipes calcaneovalgus

- Excessive dorsiflexion at the ankle and eversion of the foot
- Usually due to intrauterine position
- Treatment includes stretching and rarely splinting

Flat foot

Normal condition in infants

Cavus foot

- Usually high longitudinal arch
- May be hereditary or associated with neurologic conditions such as poliomyelitis, Charcot-Marie-Tooth disease (CMT) or Friedreich's ataxia
- Usually associated contracture of toe extensors (claw toes)

Claw toes

- Metatarsophalangeal joints are hyperextended and interphalangeal joints flexed
- Usually congenital and seen in disorders of motor weakness such as CMT or pes cavus foot deformity

THE LEG

Genu varum (bowleg)

- Infants generally have bowing of the legs as a normal finding
- By 12–18 months of age the legs have straightened and progressed to mild knock-knee
- They then gradually assume their ultimate configuration by 6–7 years of ag

📖 Blount's disease (tibia vara) (Figure 10–2)

- Due to abnormal function of the medial portion of the proximal tibial growth plate and results in bowing in the proximal tibia
- It is the most common morphologic cause of bowing in the young child and is found most commonly in obese children who walk at 9–10 months
- It is more common in African-Americans than other racial groups; and should be suspected in all children with persistent bowing after 2 years of age
- Treatment is usually osteotomy of the proximal tibia and fibula, which may have to be repeated one or more times.

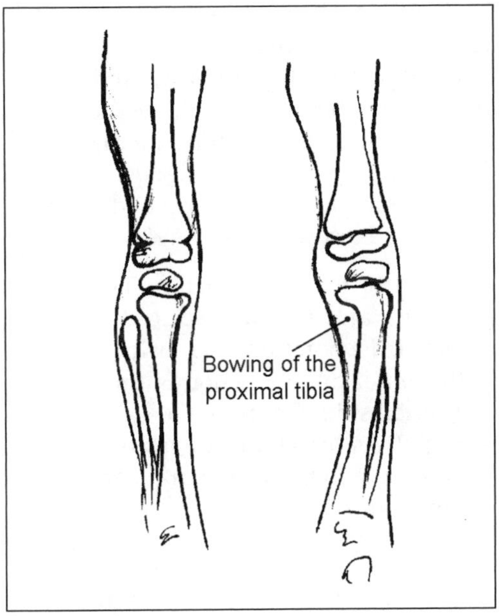

THE HIP

Developmental Dysplasia of the Hip (DDH)

FIGURE 10–2. Blount's Disease (Tibia Vara).

- Preferred term for previously known congenital dislocation of the hip. Includes hip subluxation, hip dislocation, and acetabular dysplasia; all of which imply instability of the hip
- Hip dislocation is usually diagnosed at birth, but acetabular dysplasia may present several months later
- Hip dislocation occurs in around 1 per 1,000 births; more commonly in breech babies and females more than males
- If the mother had a history of dislocated hip, the risk to the baby is increased to 1 per 25 nonbreech and 1 per 15 breech
- Children with coincident metatarsus adductus or torticollis at birth have increased incidence of hip dysplasia

Galeazzi (Allis) test: (Figure 10-3) Flex hip and knees bilaterally looking at the level of the knees. In the diagram, the level of the left knee is obviously lower, which usually indicates that hip dysplasia is present in this leg. Note: The same sign is seen in a congenital short femur, but this is a much less common finding.

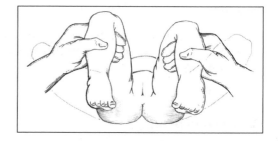

FIGURE 10–3. The Galeazzi or Allis Test.

Barlow Test and Ortolani Test

Barlow test and Ortolani test are the principal tests for instability of the hip

Barlow Test: (Figure 10–4) At rest, the hip is reduced and abduction is near normal or normal. With the leg in a flexed and adducted position, push laterally with the thumb. If the hip dislocates, as shown in the diagram, the Barlow test is positive. Reduction usually occurs immediately with hip abduction after a positive Barlow test is found.

Ortolani test: Used to determine if a dislocated hip can be readily reduced

• Step 1: Femoral head is dislocated at rest, therefore, hip abduction is limited on the affected side (Figure 10–5)

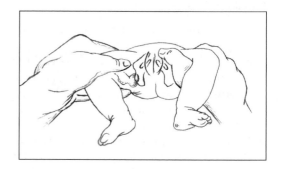

FIGURE 10–4. The Barlow Test.

• Step 2: As hip abduction is attempted, the long finger over the greater trochanter pushes anteriorly to lift the femoral head over the posterior lip of the acetabulum and reduce the hip (Figure 10–6)

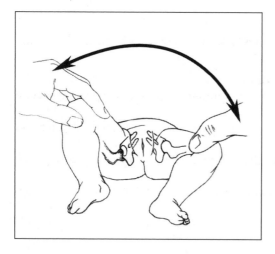

FIGURE 10–5. Ortolani Test—Step 1: Femoral head is dislocated at rest, therefore hip abduction is limited on the affected side.

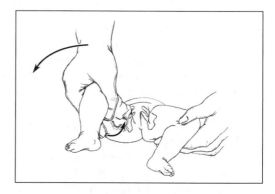

FIGURE 10–6. Ortolani Test—Step 2: As abduction of the hip is attempted reduction of the femoral head over the posterior lip of the acetabulum is attempted by applying anterior pressure over the greater trochanter.

- A positive Ortolani test is present when a palpable "clunk" is noted by the examiner as the hip reduces. A high-pitched "click" at full abduction is not a positive but is probably due to fascia lata slipping over the greater trochanter

Diagnosis/Treatment

- If diagnosis of hip instability is made in the first few months of life, generally closed reduction and use of a Pavlik harness or hip spica cast to maintain reduction with greater than 90° flexion and moderate abduction for three to four months usually produces good results
- If diagnosis is not made until walking age, surgery may be needed

THE NECK

Congenital Torticollis or "wry neck"

- Physical sign of an underlying problem usually due to muscular fibrosis, the presence of a hemivertebra, or atlantoaxial rotary subluxation. The head is tilted laterally toward one shoulder, with the chin rotated away from that shoulder
- 📖 The most common cause of congenital torticollis is fibrosis of the sternocleidomastoid muscle (SCM).
- Suggested causes of this fusiform muscular swelling and fibrosis include birth trauma and ischemia due to the intrauterine position of the head and neck. The SCM is enlarged on the side toward which the head is laterally tilted. Since there is a slightly higher incidence of developmental dysplasia of the hip in children with muscular torticollis, the hips need to be evaluated

X-ray Evaluation

- Xrays of the cervical spine in congenital muscular torticollis will reveal rotation of C1-C2 related to the torticollis position
- Early treatment includes stretching exercises. If normal range of motion is obtained by 1 year of age, facial asymmetry should resolve. Failure to regain full cervical range of motion will lead to persistent facial asymmetry
- In older children with persistent torticollis, surgical lengthening of the affected SCM is indicated
- A less common cause of torticollis in the infant is the presence of a cervical hemivertebra. If a hemivertebra is present, stretching exercises are of no benefit. Surgical fusion is used if the cervical scoliosis increases with growth

TRAUMATIC CONDITIONS

Subluxation of the radial head (nursemaid's elbow) (Figure 10–7)

- The radial head and neck is displaced distal to the annular ligament, usually in children less than 6 years old
- It results from longitudinal pull or sudden traction applied to the upper extremity; most commonly from children being lifted by the hand over a curb or object
- Sudden onset of pain results, the child refuses to move the arm, hand function is normal and elbow X-ray usually reads as normal
- Reduction usually is achieved by supination of the forearm

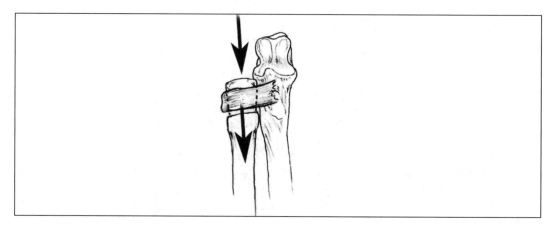

FIGURE 10–7. Subluxation of the radial head (Nursemaid's elbow).

Medial epicondylitis (Little Leaguer's elbow)

- Results from repetitive stress on the apophysis of the medial humeral epicondyle ossification center, usually from throwing a baseball; causing the elbow to assume a valgus position
- Treatment consists primarily of rest

Osgood-Schlatter's disease (Figure 10–8)

- This is a disease of the anterior tibial tubercle
- A common self-limited condition in active children 11–14 years old that presents with pain on the anterior aspect of the lower knee after sports activities
- Pain results secondary to repeated microfractures in the apophyseal cartilage between the proximal tibia and the secondary ossification center where the patella tendon attaches
- These microfractures occur as the cartilage is less able to resist the stress of repeated knee extensions
- Inflammation results followed by pain, tenderness, and calcification in the area of cartilage involved
- Physical exam reveals tenderness to palpation directly over the tibial tubercle. The anterior tubercle becomes prominent
- The lateral X-ray may be normal or reveal a pattern of fragmentation of the ossified portions of the tibial tubercle
- Treatment consists primarily of strenuous activity restriction, 4–8 weeks, especially activities requiring deep knee bending

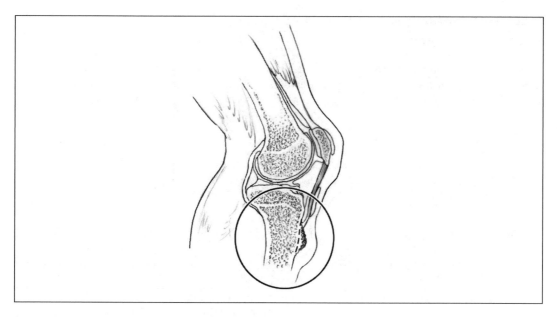

FIGURE 10–8. Osgood Schlatter's Disease.

📖 NONTRAUMATIC HIP PAIN OR LIMP (Table 10–6)

- 📖 Transient (Toxic) synovitis of the hip—the most common cause of limping and pain in the hip of children
- Avascular necrosis of the proximal femur (Legg-Calvé-Perthes disease)—due to rapid growth in relation to blood supply, the secondary ossification centers in the epiphysis are subject to avascular necrosis
- Epiphysiolysis (slipped capital femoral epiphysis) (Figure 10–9)—the most common hip disorder of preadolescent and adolescent children. Separation of the proximal femoral epiphysis through the growth plate (physis). More common in obese children

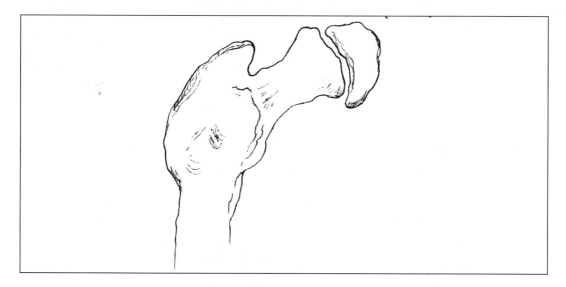

FIGURE 10–9. Slipped Capital Femoral Epiphysis.

TABLE 10–6. Causes of Non-Traumatic Hip Pain or Limp

	📖 Acute Transient/Toxic Synovitis (ATS)	📖 Legg-Calvé Perthes Disease	📖 Slipped Capital Femoral Epiphysis
Etiology	Unclear	Avascular necrosis ossification center femoral head	Separation of proximal femoral epiphysis through the growth plate; Obesity 80% children; delayed development of secondary sex characteristics
Incidence		1:750	
Age Onset	3–6 years; boys greater than girls	4–10 years; boys greater than girls (4:1)	9–15 years; boys greater than girls; blacks greater than whites
Symptoms	Pain/Limp ATS is the most common cause of acute hip pain in children	Pain/limp	Pain/limp; most common hip disorder in preadolescents–adolescents
Physical Exam	Limited internal rotation of hip	Pain in groin and radiates anterior/medial thigh toward knee Decreased internal rotation, extension and abduction	Decreased internal rotation, abduction, affected leg in external rotation
WBC	Normal or slight increase	Normal	Normal
ESR	Slight increase	Normal	Normal
X-ray	Normal	Smaller ossified femoral head, sclerotic femoral head, widening of hip joint space	Physis (growth plate) on involved side wider and irregular; narrowing epiphysis (femoral head)
Treatment	Rest, NSAIDs, usually resolves in 3–5 days Full activity should be avoided until hip is pain free.	*Conservative*: rest, abduction brace; the goal of treatment is to retain the normal spherical shape of the femoral head. Current therapy allows child to continue weight bearing, but with the femur in abducted position so that the head is well contained by the acetabulum. Surgical: varus osteotomy	Surgical pinning is preferred treatment preventing further epiphyseal displacement by stabilizing the epiphysis with screws or pins.
Prognosis	Good, less than 10% have second episode	Good prognosis in children detected earlier, ie., less than 6 years old and with less than 50% of femoral head involvement; poor prognosis in children detected later, with involvement of the lateral portion of the femoral head (especially > 40% of the structural part)	Variable

SCOLIOSIS

- Scoliosis can be considered either functional or structural (Table 10–8)

Functional Scoliosis

- Due to malpositioning or unilateral paraspinal muscle pull. This may be associated with back pain and muscle spasm
- In this type of curve, there is no significant vertebral body rotation, and scoliosis is reversible

Structural Scoliosis

- Not reversible
- May be idiopathic, congential, or acquired

Idiopathic Scoliosis (Table 10–7)

- Accounts for approximately 80% of patients with structural scoliosis
- Etiology is unclear
- It is a multifactorial condition with a genetic predisposition. There is an autosomal dominant component with incomplete penetrance
- It is subdivided according to the age of onset with three well-defined periods:
  1. Infantile: 0–3 years old
  2. Juvenile: 4 years old–puberty onset
  3. Adolescent: puberty to just prior to closure of epiphyseal plates

TABLE 10–7. Clinical Features of Idiopathic Scoliosis

	Infantile	Juvenile	Adolescent
Incidence	Least common		Most common
Onset/Diagnosis	Less than 3 years	4–10 years	Greater than 11 years
Ratio	Males greater than females	Males equal to females	Males equal to females, however, females worsen 8–10 times more frequently
Curve Pattern	Left thoracolumbar	Right thoracic or double curve	Right thoracic 1; Right thoracic/Left lumbar 2

Congenital Scoliosis

- Results from abnormal spinal formation during embryonic development
- The most common presentation is a hemivertebra in which one lateral half of the vertebra fails to form
- Congenital scoliosis is associated with a number of congenital anomalies
- About 30% of infants with congenital scoliosis have a congenitourinary abnormality; most commonly unilateral renal agenesis
- About one-third of children with congenital scoliosis also have a spinal cord abnormality
- In children with VATER syndrome (vertebral defects, imperforate anus, tracheoesophageal fistula, radial and renal dysplasia) congenital scoliosis is an additional finding

- All children with any congenital vertebral anomaly should have a renal ultrasound to assess possible anomalies of the genitourinary system

Acquired Scoliosis—secondary (disease related)

Neuromuscular Scoliosis

- Most commonly seen in CP, muscular dystrophy, spina bifida, and spinal muscular atrophy. Scoliosis is uncommon in children with neuromuscular disease who are able to walk
- In CP, scoliosis is primarily seen in the spastic quadriplegic who is unable to stand or walk
- In Duchenne's muscular dystrophy, scoliosis is unusual until the child becomes wheelchair bound
- Children with spina bifida who have no neurologic function below the thoracolumbar region have a high incidence of progressive scoliosis

Classifying Scoliosis (Table 10–8)

Functional	Structural

Muscle Spasm
  Paraspinal strain
  Herniated disc (unilateral)
Postural
	Congenital
	  Bar
	  Block
	  Hemivertebra or other body anomaly
	Idiopathic
	  Adolescent (spinal cord or brainstem disease?)
	  Juvenile
	  Associated with congenital heart disease
	Acquired
	  Degenerative
	    Posttraumatic (fracture)
	    Overuse (repetitive microtrauma)
	    Senile
	  Secondary (disease related)
	    "Paralytic" neuromuscular disease (spinal muscular atrophy, muscular dystrophy, myelomeningocele, etc.) connective tissue disease (Ehlers-Danlos, chondrodysplasia, Marfan's, etc.)

From O'Young, Young, Stiens. PM&R Secrets. Philadelphia: Hanley & Belfus; 1997, p. 313, with permission.

Evaluation of Scoliosis

The Adams test (forward bending test)

- The child bends forward with legs straight at the knees and hands together as if trying to touch the toes
- Because scoliosis is a three-dimensional deformity, there is a rotation of the involved vertebrae as well as a lateral curvature
- This vertebral rotation leads to a prominence on the posterior trunk that corresponds to the convex side of the curve

Cobb Method (Figure 10–10)

- A radiographic measurement on a PA view of the spine is used to quantify the angle of curvature
- One line is drawn along the superior endplate of the vertebra tilted the most at the top of the curve and a similar line is drawn along the inferior endplate of the vertebra tilted the most at the bottom of the curve. Large scoliosis will allow these two lines to intersect forming the angle *a*, otherwise, if the curve is not large enough, strike perpendiculars to form the angle *A*

Pulmonary Function Studies

- If a thoracic scoliosis exceeds 50°–60°, abnormalities in pulmonary function tests (PFTs) may appear
- The most common abnormality is a decreased vital capacity probably related to decrease in size of the hemithorax on the convex side of scoliosis

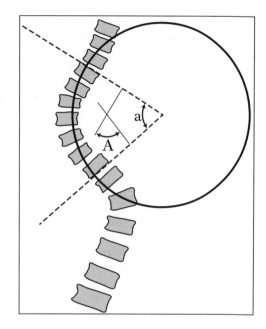

FIGURE 10–10. Cobb Method.

Treatment Of Scoliosis (Table 10–9)

Goal

Early diagnosis, keep curvature controlled during the growth spurt.

TABLE 10–9. Treatment of Scoliosis

Degree of Curvature	Idiopathic	Muscular Dystrophy	Cerebral Palsy
1°–20°	Observation	Observation	Observation
20°–40°	Brace	Surgery (sooner if rapidly progressive)	
>40°	Surgery		Surgery (may wait until 60° or more in some cases)

From O'Young, Young, Stiens. PM&R Secrets. Philadelphia: Hanley & Belfus; 1997, p. 403, with permission.

- During the period of rapid adolescent growth, progressive curves increase at the rate of approximately 1° per month
- Studies have shown that if thoracic curvatures can be kept less than 50° and lumbar curvature is less than 40° by the completion of growth, the likelihood of the curve increasing during adult life is small.

SCHEUERMANN'S DISEASE

- Scheuermann's disease or kyphosis occurs in 0.5%–8% of the population with an increased prevalence in males
- Radiographically, Scheuermann's disease is demonstrated when greater than or equal to three consecutive vertebrae are wedged greater than 5°. Radiographic picture includes irregular vertebral endplates, and protrusion of disc material into the spongiosum of the vertebral bodies, i.e., *Schmorl's nodes*. Other radiographic findings include narrowed disc spaces and anterior wedging of the vertebral bodies

- The cause is unknown, but thought to result from repetitive microtrauma and fatigue failure of the immature thoracic vertebral bodies
- When Scheuermann's disease is associated with pain in the presence of one or more irregular vertebral bodies, physical exercises are prohibited
- Sometimes a thoracolumbosacral orthosis may be required for pain control along with conservative measures of rest, ice, gentle stretching, and NSAIDs

SPONDYLOLISTHESIS

- Spondylolisthesis is a forward slip of one vertebral body relative to the vertebral body below it
- Difficulty with forward bending is often the presenting symptom
- Pain may present in the back with radiation to the buttocks or posterior thigh
- Radiographs are usually the only studies used to diagnose and manage spondylolisthesis in children and adolescents
- ▭ In adults, degenerative spondylolisthesis is most common, however, in children, dysplastic and isthmic types are most frequent and occur most frequently at L5-S1 and then L4-L5
- The isthmic type is the result of a slip at the site of a previous spondylolysis, or bony defect in the pars interarticularis (Figure 10–12.)
- The dysplastic type has lengthening of the lamina but no spondylolysis initially; Spondylolysis may occur later as the slip increases (Figure 10–11)
- Spondylolisthesis is two to four times more common in males but progression is more common in females
- Pars defect is at L5 in 67% of people, at L4 in 15%–30%, and L3 in 2%
- The frequency of pars defect in children is about 4.5% (in adolescents 6%, but increases to 12% in gymnasts)
- Generally, all children with over 50% of slippage require surgical fusion
- If the slippage is less than 50%, treatment depends on the severity of symptoms
- A body jacket, rest, and transient restriction of activities may relieve symptoms
- Surgery is rarely needed with less than 25% slippage

Dysplastic Spondylolisthesis

(Figure 10–11)
Attenuation or lengthening of the lamina. More likely to cause compression of the cauda equina as the L5 vertebra moves forward on the sacrum.

Isthmic Spondylolisthesis

(Figure 10–12)
Follows a stress fracture at the pars interarticularis.

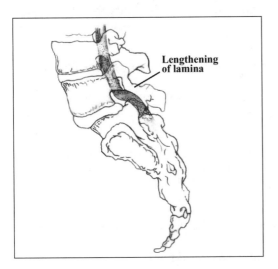

FIGURE 10–11. Dysplastic Spondylolisthesis.

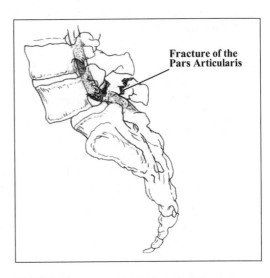

FIGURE 10–12. Isthmic Spondylolisthesis.

■

CONNECTIVE TISSUE AND JOINT DISEASE

JUVENILE RHEUMATOID ARTHRITIS (JRA) (Table 10–10, see also Rheumatology Chapter)

- 📖 The most common connective tissue disease in children
- It is the presence of arthritis lasting ≥ 6 weeks with an onset less than 16 years of age
- Childhood onset accounts for 5% of rheumatoid arthritis cases
- The incidence is 13.9 per 100,000 per year with prevalence of 113.4 per 100,000
- The cause remains unknown; genetic predisposition, immunologic abnormalities, infection, and trauma are possible contributing factors

Clinical Presentation

There are five types of onset in juvenile rheumatoid arthritis.
1. Polyarticular RF negative
2. Polyarticular RF positive
3. Pauciarticular Type 1 (Early Onset)
4. Pauciarticular Type 2 (Late Onset)
5. Systemic Onset

Polyarticular Disease

- Onset accounts for 35% of children with JRA; with girls more affected than boys, and greater than or equal to five joints involved in the first six months

Polyarticular RF Negative
- Comprises 25% of all patients with JRA
- Children may complain of stiffness but many do not complain of pain with inflamed joints
- Hip involvement occurs in 50% of children and is a cause of late disability from the erosion of the femoral head

Polyarticular RF Positive
- Onset occurs in 10% of children with JRA; and is characterized by onset greater than 11 years of age with female predominance
- Findings include symmetric joint involvement, subcutaneous nodules and erosive disease

Pauciarticular Disease

- The pauciarticular group accounts for the largest percentage of children with JRA (45%)
- Involvement is limited to less than or equal to four joints
- There are two subgroups: early onset and late onset

Pauciarticular Type I Early Onset
- The early onset group are usually preschool-aged girls who present less than 4 years of age
- This accounts for 30% of all children with JRA
- 📖 There is a high risk of iridocyclitis which may be asymptomatic
- These children require routine eye examinations

Pauciarticular Type II Late Onset
- The late onset group occurs in 15% of JRA, and in 9–10-year-old boys
- These children are at risk for acute iridocyclitis
- There is an association with HLA-B27 in 90%; with 50% later developing ankylosing spondylitis or other seronegative spondyloarthropathies

Systemic Onset JRA

- Systemic-onset JRA (20%) is characterized by acute onset of spiking fevers, rash, hepatosplenomegaly, lymphadenopathy, arthritis, fatigue, myalgia, irritability, and pericarditis
- Systemic symptoms may precede arthritis by several months
- Small joints are most often involved
- Still's Disease; a form of JRA characterized by high fevers, systemic illness, and skin lesions which are small erythematous macules and papules

TABLE 10–10. Five Types of Onset of Juvenile Rheumatoid Arthritis

	Polyarticular Rheumatoid Factor NEGATIVE	Polyarticular Rheumatoid Factor POSITIVE	Pauciarticular Type I Early onset	Pauciarticular Type II Late onset	Systemic onset
% of JRA pts. Sex	25% Predominantly females	10% Predominantly females	30% Predominantly females	15% Predominantly males	20% Females/Males
Age at Onset	Throughout childhood	Late childhood	Early childhood	Late childhood	Throughout childhood
Joints	≥ 5 joints including small joints of the hand and especially hip	≥ 5 joints including small joints of the hand	≤ 4 joints including large joints; knee, ankle, elbow	≤ 4 joints including large joints; hip girdle sacroiliac	Any
Sacroiliitis	No	No (rare if any)	No	Common	No
Iridocyclitis	No (rare if any)	No	📖 50% chronic	📖 10%–20% acute	No
Rheumatoid Factor	Negative	100% positive	Negative	Negative	Negative
Antinuclear Antibodies	Positive (25%)	Positive (75%)	Positive (60%)	Negative	Negative
HLA Studies	Inconclusive	HLA DR4	HLA DR5 DR8	📖 HLA B27	Inconclusive
Ultimate Morbidity	Severe Arthritis 10–15%	📖 Severe Arthritis >50%	Ocular damage—10%; Chronic Orotos—risk of vision loss Arthritis—good outcome	May progress to spondylo-arthropathy	Severe Arthritis 25%

Adult Rheumatoid Arthritis (RA) vs. Juvenile Rheumatoid Arthrits (JRA)

- Systemic features are more common in children
- Adults have joint destruction earlier, whereas children have synovitis with erosive disease later
- Children have large joints involved more frequently than adults with RA
- Wrist and hand deviations differ from adults with RA; Children have ulnar deviation at the wrist with loss of extension. Radial deviation of the fingers occurs at the metacarpal-phalangeal (MCP) joints with finger flexion
- Tenosynovitis is more common in children than bursitis
- Rheumatoid nodules occur less frequently than in adults
- The cervical spine is more commonly involved in children than adults
- Arthritis in children tends to be ANA-positive, RF-negative; whereas adult RA is generally RF-positive
- In children, periarticular bone demineralization is seen radiographically once 50% demineralization occurs

Management of Juvenile Rheumatoid Arthritis

The goals of management of JRA are to minimize deformity while maintaining as close to a normal lifestyle as possible. (Figure 10–13, Table 10–11)

TABLE 10–11

Rehabilitation of the Child With Juvenile Rheumatoid Arthritis
Rest
Splinting
Passive ROM
Active exercises for strengthening
Adaptive equipment
Functional training for ADLs and ambulation
Postsurgical rehabilitation
Nutrition
Counseling: family and child

From Molnar GE, Alexander MA. Pediatric Rehabilitation 3rd ed. Philadelphia: Hanley & Belfus; 1999: page 370, Table 10–12, with permission.

Medications (Table 10–12)

• Aspirin and NSAIDs

Aspirin is used less frequently because of the occurrence of Reye's syndrome with influenza and varicella infections. Of the NSAIDs, naproxen, Tolmetin, and ibuprofen are approved for use in children. More than 50% of children improve with NSAID therapy. Treatment is continued for one to two years after suppression of disease activity.

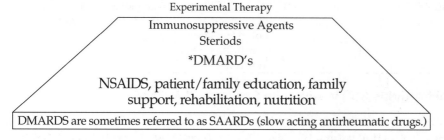

Experimental Therapy
Immunosuppressive Agents
Steriods
*DMARD's
NSAIDS, patient/family education, family support, rehabilitation, nutrition

DMARDS are sometimes referred to as SAARDs (slow acting antirheumatic drugs.)

FIGURE 10–13. Pyramid Approach to management of the child with JRA.

• DMARDs

The second line of drug therapy is termed the **D**isease **M**odifying **A**nti**R**heumatic **D**rugs (DMARDs). These include gold salts, antimalarials, D-penicillamine, and sulfasalazine. Studies have not demonstrated that disease progression is modified with (DMARDs). Of children receiving gold salts, 60%–70% show improvement. Side effects include skin rash, proteinuria, and bone marrow suppression. Oral gold (auranofin) has been found to be safe for use in children but with less efficacy than IM administration

Hydroxychloroquine is the most commonly used antimalarial drug. Oral D-penicillamine induces remission in 60%–70% of cases.

• Cyclosporine

Cyclosporine blocks production of interleukin-2 and the proliferation of synovial T cells. Cyclosporine may have disease modifying as well as anti-inflammatory effects.

• Azathioprine

Azathioprine is an effective treatment for children with refractory disease and can reduce the use of steroids. It was not found to alter the cause of iridocyclitis.

TABLE 10–12. Drug Therapy in Juvenile Rheumatoid Arthritis

Drug	Side Effects
Aspirin	Drowsiness, tinnitus, hyperventilation, concern of Reye's syndrome if used during varicella or influenza, reduced platelet function, gastrointestinal irritation
Naproxen	Gastrointestinal irritation, cutaneous pseudoporphyria, cutanea tarda
Ibuprofen	Gastrointestinal irritation, rash, aseptic meningitis
Tolmetin	Gastrointestinal irritation
Indomethacin*	Headache, epigastric pain, difficulty paying attention
Diclofenac*	Mild gastrointestinal effects
Piroxicam*	Side effects not established in pediatric population
Gold Salts	Mucosal ulcers, rash, proteinuria, nephropathy, leukopenia, thrombocytopenia, anemia
Auranofin*	Gastrointestinal irritation, rash
Hydroxychloroquine	Macular degeneration
D-Penicillamine	Bone marrow suppression, renal, rash, autoimmune, proteinuria
Sulfasalazine*	Gastrointestinal irritation, rash, hypersensitivity, renal toxicity, headache
Methotrexate*	Avoid use with NSAID because it may potentiate bone marrow suppression, gastrointestinal, side effects hepatotoxicity
Azathioprine*	Gastrointestinal irritation, side effects liver, side effects dose-related leukopenia
Cyclophosphamide*	Alopecia, nausea, vomiting, bladder side effects, pulmonary fibrosis, leukopenia, thrombocytopenia
Cyclosporine	Immunosuppression, hypertension, renal insufficiency
Corticosteroids	Growth failure, adrenal suppression, osteopenia, cushingoid appearance, avascular necrosis, weight gain, cataracts, psychosis, myopathy
Prednisone	Same side effects as for corticosteroids
Pulse steroid methylprednisolone	Same side effects as for corticosteroids

* Not approved for use in children From Molnar GE, Alexander MA. Pediatric Rehabilitation 3rd ed. Philadelphia: Hanley & Belfus; 1999, page 369, table 18.2, with permission.

- Corticosteroids
Systemic corticosteroids reduce symptoms but do not cause remission. Intra-articular steroids can suppress synovitis.

Additional Aspects of Managing JRA

- Joint pain is caused by stretching of the capsule. Pain can be assessed using the child visual analogue scale (VAS) or the Varni/Thompson Pediatric Pain Questionnaire, which takes into account the child's cognitive level of development
- Heat can reduce stiffness, increase tissue elasticity, and decrease pain and muscle spasm. Water temperature should be 90°–100°F. There remains concern that heat can increase inflammation and accelerate the disease process that leads to articular destruction. Moist heat can be provided to a tissue depth of 1 cm with a hot pack. Ultrasound can provide deep heat but there is concern regarding the effect on the growth plate in children. Cold can provide pain relief, increase pain threshold, and decrease muscle spasm and swelling by vasoconstriction
- Splinting: The upper extremity is splinted in a functional position with the wrist in 15°–20° extension, the fingers in some flexion, 25% at the MCP joint and a few degrees at the proximal interphalangeal joint (PIP) joints; ulnar deviation controlled, and the thumb in opposition

Specific Joints of Involvement in JRA

- Cervical Spine—Involved more in children than adults. Subluxation of the atlantoaxial joint can occur when its involvement leads to erosion of the transverse ligament
- Temporomandibular joint (TMJ)—involved in up to 50% of children with JRA. Micrognathia results from reduced mandibular growth
- Shoulder—Uncommon, occurring in only 8%. Children lose abduction and internal rotation in contrast to adults who lose external rotation
- Elbow—≥ 90% of flexion range is needed at the elbow for ADLs
- Wrist—Common in children. Early loss of extension with progression of flexion contracture at the wrist develops. (Note: In children, the wrist deviates in ulnar direction)
- Hand—Swan-neck deformity: hyperextension at the PIP joint is more common in adults. Boutonnierè deformity: flexion at PIP joint with hyperextension at DIP. (Note: Radial deviation of the fingers occurs at the MCP joint)
- Hip—occurs in 50% of children with polyarticular arthritis. Hips develop flexion contractures with internal rotation and adduction compared to adults with external rotation and abduction
- Knee—The knee is held in flexion at 30 degrees as this position minimizes intra-articular pressure
- Ankle/Foot—Involvement at the metatarsophalangeal joint causes decreased push off resulting in flat foot gait

Outcome (Table 10–13)

TABLE 10-13. American College of Rheumatology Revised Criteria for Classification of Functional Status in Rheumatoid Arthritis

CLASS I	Completely able to perform usual activities of daily living (self-care, vocational, avocational)
CLASS II	Able to perform usual self-care and vocational activities but limited in avocational
CLASS III	Able to perform usual self-care activities but limited in vocational and avocational
CLASS IV	Limited in ability to perform usual self-care, vocational, and avocational activities

(Hochberg MC, Chang RW, Dwosh I, Lindsey S, Pincus T, Wolfe F. The American College of Rheumatology 1991 revised criteria for the classification of global functional status in rheumatoid arthritis. Arthritis Rheum 1992;35:498–502. Reprinted by permission of John Wiley & Sons, Inc.)

- 31% of children have severe limitations in Class III or IV. Remission occurs in up to two-thirds of children whereas adults usually progress
- Poor outcome is related to:
  - Delay in treatment
  - Later age at disease onset
  - Longer duration of disease as remission is unlikely after greater than seven years
  - RF-positive status
  - Unremitting course
  - Multiple small joint involvement
  - Early appearance of erosion
  - Hip involvement
- Death occurs in 2%–4% of children

JUVENILE ONSET SERONEGATIVE SPONDYLOARTHROPATHY

HLA-B27 associated syndromes in children less than 16 years old with findings related to arthritis, enthesitis, and tenosynovitis involving joints in the lower extremity, spine and sacroiliac joint. RF and ANA are negative, usually more common in boys than girls. These include the following four entities: Ankylosing Spondylitis (AS), Reiter's Syndrome, arthritis with irritable bowel disease, and psoriatic arthritis.

Ankylosing Spondylitis

- Incidence: 2 per 100,000 in the United States and occurs more often in boys greater than eight years old. 90% of white patients with ankylosing spondylitis are HLA-B27 positive
- Cause: Unknown. There is a strong genetic susceptibility. Axial symptoms (spine and SI joint) and radiographic sacroiliitis develop
- Children often have peripheral joint involvement (82%) with lower extremity and hip most often involved
- Enthesitis, pain at the insertion of tendon to bone, occurs more commonly in children than adults
- Up to 27% have associated uveitis
- Radiographic findings of bilateral SI joint involvement are necessary for the definitive diagnosis
- Hip disease is an indicator for poor outcome

Reiter's Syndrome

- Characterized by conjunctivitis, urethritis, and symmetric arthritis
- More frequent in boys greater than eight years old
- Postinfectious or reactive cause secondary to infection with Chlamydia trachomatis, Chlamydia pneumoniae, Salmonella, Shigella flexneri, and Yersinia enterocolitica
- Uncommon in children
- Oligoarthritis of the knee or ankle most common

Arthritis associated with irritable bowel disease

- Occurs in 10%–20% of children with ulcerative colitis and Crohn's disease
- No sex predilection

Psoriatic arthritis

- Inflammatory arthritis in children less than 16 years old associated with psoriasis, either preceding onset or within 15 years
- Girls are slightly more affected than boys. 50% present with nonarticular arthritis; but most progress to involve greater than five joints in asymmetric pattern
- Psoriasis occurs with nail pitting, hyperkeratosis, and anterior uveitis
- A positive ANA may be associated with poor functional outcome

SYSTEMIC LUPUS ERYTHEMATOSUS (SLE)

- Multisystem autoimmune disease with episodic inflammation and vasculitis associated with positive ANA
- Cause is unclear
- Incidence 0.5–0.6 per 100,000 with 20% of cases beginning in childhood
- Females are predominately affected 4.5:1 in all age groups; a closer ratio exists in prepubertal patients
- 11 Diagnostic criteria for SLE (Table 10–14)

TABLE 10–14. 📖 11 Diagnostic Criteria For Systemic Lupus Erythematosus*

Malar rash
Discoid lupus rash
Photosensitivity
Oral or nasal mucocutaneous ulceration
Nonerosive arthritis
Nephritis
Encephalopathy
Pleuritis or pericarditis
Cytopenia
Positive immunoserology: LE cells, antinative DNA antibodies, anti-Sm antibodies, false-+ test for syphilis
Positive antinuclear antibody

*Four or more criteria required for clinical diagnosis. From Molnar GE, Alexander MA. Pediatric Rehabilitation 3rd ed. Philadelphia: Hanley & Belfus; 1999: page 381, table 18-5, with permission.

- The presence of four criteria has 90% sensitivity and 98% specificity
- One-third of children have an erythematous rash in a butterfly distribution over the bridge of the nose and cheeks (malar rash)
- Nephritis is present in 75% and is the main factor in determining outcome in children
- Ten-year survival is greater than 80%
- Hematuria, proteinuria, persistent hypertension, pulmonary hypertension, chronic active disease and biopsy-proven diffuse proliferative glomerulonephritis are associated with a poor outcome

JUVENILE DERMATOMYOSITIS

- Multisystem inflammatory disease of unknown cause, involving primarily the muscle, skin, and subcutaneous tissues.
- Clinical features: histologic presence of vasculitis, the onset of calcinosis and lack of association with malignancy in childhood
- It occurs more commonly in girls between 5–14 years old
- A vascular process leading to arteritis and phlebitis and may involve any organ
- Diagnostic features of juvenile dermatomyositis include:
  - Proximal muscle weakness
  - Elevated muscle enzymes
  - A characteristic heliotropic discoloration of eyelids or other skin rash
  - Electromyogram evidence of inflammatory myopathy
  - Evidence of vasculitis or chronic inflammation on muscle biopsy

- Other symptoms may include fever, muscle tenderness and pain, malaise and weight loss, arthralgia and arthritis, dyspnea, dysphagia, myocarditis with abnormal EKG, and +ANA
- The clinical course of this disease is variable

Treatment Options

- Steroid therapy is indicated in acute or active disease
- Prednisone therapy with a slow taper over two years once muscle enzyme elevations have normalized is standard. Immunosuppressive agents may be used in refractory cases
- Physical therapy is important to treat or prevent contractures and is instituted once the muscles are less inflamed
- The prognosis is good with less than 7% mortality
- Those with chronic form of disease have calcinosis and functional disability in adulthood

SCLERODERMA

- A collagen disease that chiefly affects the skin, but may involve any organ
- Although uncommon in children, it affects girls > boys with fibrosis of involved tissue
- The cause is unclear
- Average age of onset is between 8–10 years old with duration of 7–9 years

Types of Scleroderma

Morphea
Local or general, small lesions occur with minimal sclerosis (guttate morphea), self-limiting over two to three years

Linear sclerosis
Atrophic erythematosus, which later becomes fibrotic with binding of the skin to underlying tissue. En coupe de sabre is unilateral linear involvement of the face and scalp.

Systemic sclerosis
Characterized by Raynaud's phenomenon, symmetric cutaneous involvement, involvement of lungs, gastrointestinal (GI) tract, kidneys, loss of joint function, pulmonary and renal complications are causes of death in these children.

Mixed connective tissue disease
Combines features of SLE, RA, dermatomyositis, and scleroderma

CREST syndrome
Calcinosis, Raynaud's, esophageal dysfunction, sclerodactyly, telangiectasia

INFECTIOUS ARTHRITIS

Lyme disease

- Cause: the spirochete Borrelia burgdorferi, transmitted by the deer tick, Ixodes dammini
- Incidence: 5.2 per 100,000
- Initial phase is characterized by fever, fatigue, headache, arthralgias, myalgia, and stiff neck
- Erythema migrans is the characteristic round, red skin lesion with central clearing
- Late phase: is characterized by arthritis, cardiac disease, and neurologic disease
- Cardiac manifestations of heart block occur in 5%–10% of children and chronic neurologic manifestations in 15%
- Bell's palsy is seen more frequently in children than adults
- In 85% of children the arthritis resolves before the end of the initial treatment, but a chronic inflammatory phase develops in 10%
- Treatment: Antibiotic therapy: Doxycycline, Amoxicillin, Erythromycin (late disease IV—ceftriaxone)

Rheumatic fever (RF)

- RF occurs in children greater than four years old with boys and girls affected equally
- Arthritis presents with pain, swelling, warmth, and decreased joint range of motion in large joints more commonly knees, elbows, ankles, and wrists
- Associated findings are carditis, fever, rash, chorea, and nodules
- There often is a history of a prior streptococcal infection. Diagnosis is clinical by the Jones criteria

📖 **Jones Criteria For The Diagnosis Of Rheumatic Fever** (Table 10–15)

TABLE 10–15. Jones Criteria

Major	Minor	Preceding Group A Streptococcal Infection
Carditis	Fever	Throat culture
Polyarthritis	Arthralgia	Rapid streptococcal antigen
Chorea	Elevated Erythocyte Sedimentation Rate (ESR) or C-Reactive Protein (CRP)	Elevated streptococcal antibody
Erythema marginatum	Prolonged PR interval	
Subcutaneous nodules		

Two of the major criteria or one major and two minor are required for diagnosis with evidence of preceding streptococcal infection.
From Molnar GE, Alexander MA. Pediatric Rehabilitation 3rd ed. Philadelphia: Hanley & Belfus; 1999: page 385, table 18-10, with permission.

Treatment

Management including anti-inflammatory meds (salicylates, corticosteroids), physical therapy

Prognosis: Arthritis does not result in long-term morbidity, but prognosis is related to the extent of cardiac involvement

Septic arthritis (Table 10–16)

- Occurs most often in children less than two years old with boys > girls and joint involvement by hematogenous spread
- Transient synovitis occurs mainly in boys three to ten years old with pain in the hip or referred pain in the thigh or knee
- Bacterial septic arthritis accounts for 6.5% of arthritis in children. Monoarticular involvement is most common
- Common pathogens are Haemophilus influenzae and Staphylococcus aureus

TABLE 10–16. Causes of Septic Arthritis in Children

Age	Most Common Bacteria
Newborn	Staphylococcus aureus—(less commonly, gram negative enteric bacteria)
2 months–2 years	Hemophilias influenzae
> 2 yrs	Staph aureus
Sexually active adolescents	Gonococcal disease

HEMOPHILIAS

- The hemophilias are the most common and serious of the congenital coagulation disorders. They are associated with genetically determined deficiencies of factor VIII, IX, or XI. (gene is carried on the X chromosome)
- Classification:
  - Classic Hemophilia; hemophilia A; is a deficiency of factor VIII
  - Christmas Hemophilia; hemophilia B; is a deficiency of factor IX
  - Hemophilia C
- 📖 The hallmark of hemophilia is HEMARTHROSIS
  Hemarthrosis: hemorrhaging into the joints causing pain, swelling, and limited movement of the joint.
  This may be induced by minor trauma, but can also occur spontaneously.
  Repeated hemorrhages may produce degenerative changes with osteoporosis, muscle atrophy, and ultimately a fixed nonfunctional joint
- Treatment:
  - Prevention of trauma (avoid contact sports)
  - Avoid aspirin and other platelet-affecting drugs because they may provoke severe hemorrhage
  - Bleeding episodes:
    - Factor VIII replacement therapy is essential to prevent pain, disability, or life-threatening hemorrhage
    - Aim of factor VIII replacement is to increase the level of factor VIII in the plasma to a level of securing hemostasis (i.e., IV infusion)
  - When hemophiliac child has significant bleeding:
    - Factor VIII should be given as soon as possible
    - Local measures should include application of cold and pressure
    - Initially immobilize
    - Within 48 hours, passive exercises should begin to prevent joint stiffness and fibrosis
    - Aspiration of joint is controversial
    - There is compelling evidence that early treatment with Factor VIII concentrates will reduce disability and deformity. Parents or older patients can be trained to give IV concentrates at home
- Severe disease presents with < 1 % factor activity
- Moderate disease presents with > 1 % factor activity
- Mild disease presents with > 5 % factor activity
  - Complications of treatment with factor VIII replacement:
    - Abnormalities of hepatic enzyme activities are found in 50% of patients
    - 30% of hemophiliacs are currently infected with HIV
- Hepatitis B and C are transmissible by factor concentrate

KAWASAKI DISEASE

- A systemic vasculitis that affects young children with annual incidence of 6–7.6 per 100,000
- 80% of affected children are less than four years old. It is more common in boys
- The cause is unknown

Diagnostic Criteria in Kawasaki Disease (Molnar, 1999)

- Fever lasting > 5 days
- Mucocutaneous changes of the oral cavity strawberry tongue, red peeling lips, pharyngeal erythema
- Conjunctival injection
- Peripheral extremity; Edema of the hands or feet, erythema of the palms or soles, desquamation
- Rash
- Cervical lymphadenopathy

▪

PEDIATRIC BURNS

EPIDEMIOLOGY

- Burns are the number one cause of non-motor vehicle deaths in children ages 1 through 4 and the second most common cause of death in children ages 4 through 14
- Scald injuries represent 40–50% of all burns with the highest incidence in toddlers
- Increased burn size raises the risk of mortality in children
- Children < 4 years of age have a higher risk of death independent of burn size. In children < 4, male to female ratio is 2:1 and increases to 4:1 in adolescence
- Inhalation injury is an important predictor of burn mortality

Scald burns are the single most common cause of pediatric burn injury. Immersion scald burns have been associated with child abuse or neglect.
- 16% of all burn injuries are non-accidental and 50% of these are a result of abuse
- Flame burns resulting from playing with matches, gasoline, firecrackers, flammable aerosols continue to occur in the 6 to 14 year old group. Education programs are geared toward this age group
- Wall-outlet caused electrical injuries represent < 15% of all pediatric electrical injuries

BURN CLASSIFICATION

Calculation of burn size is relative to total body surface area and varies depending on age. The modified Lund and Browder chart is most often used in estimating extent of burn size in children. (Table 10–17)

TABLE 10–17. Child Burn Size Estimation Chart (% Body Surface Area)

Burn Area	Age in years				
	1	1–4	5–9	10–14	15
Head	19	17	13	11	9
Neck	2	2	2	2	2
Anterior Trunk	13	13	13	13	13
Posterior Trunk	18	18	18	18	18
Genitalia	1	1	1	1	1
Upper Extremity (each)	9	9	9	9	9
Lower Extremity (each)	14.5	15.5	17.5	18.5	19.5

From Molnar GE, Alexander MA. Pediatric Rehabilitation 3rd ed. Philadelphia: Hanley & Belfus; 1999: page 353, table 17-2, with permission.

📖 Rule of 9s: (Figure 10–14)

- The rule of 9s is another frequently used method of estimating burn size. It is modified for use with children
- 9% is taken from the legs and added to the head of a child < 1-year-old. For each subsequent year, 1% is returned to the legs until 9 years old at which time the head is in proportion to the adult

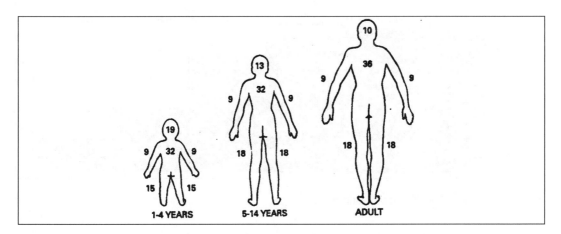

FIGURE 10–14. The Rule of 9's.

Classification by Severity (Figure 10–15)

• The depth of thermal injury through epidermis and dermis determines classification

Superficial burns (formerly first degree)
Typified by sunburn are dry, warm, painful, and hypersensitive. They heal without treatment.

Partial thickness (formerly second degree)
Burns affect epidermis and variable but not complete elements of the dermis. Partial thickness burns can be superficial, resulting in burns that are red, painful, and potentially blistered; or deep, resulting in dry, white, and hyposensitive burns. Treatment depends on depth of damage.

Full thickness (formerly third-degree burns)
Affects all epidermal and dermal elements, and are anesthetic, white, avascular, dry, and leathery appearing. Skin grafting helps ameliorate the uneven and hard fibrotic scar formation as healing proceeds.

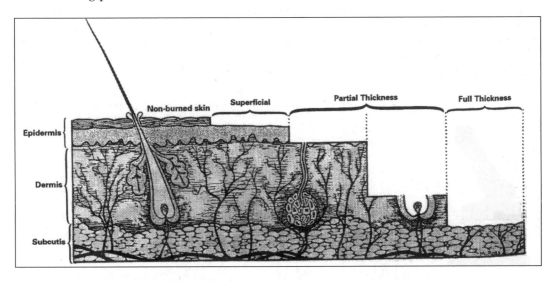

FIGURE 10–15. Classification of Burns.

The American Burn Association established a guideline for hospitalization of a burn patient based on the 5-10-20 rule:

INDICATIONS FOR HOSPITALIZATION

• > 20% Total Body Surface Area (TBSA)
• > 10% Total Body Surface Area in children or elderly
• > 5% Full thickness injury
• Any burns to the eyes, ears, face, hands, feet, genitalia
• All inhalation injuries
• All electrical burns
• All burns complicated by other medical problems
• Any burns associated with concomitant trauma (Molnar, 1999)

POSITIONING IN THE PEDIATRIC BURN PATIENT (Table 10–18)

Proper Positioning

- Proper positioning of the burned child during the acute phase of care is essential in preventing contractures and deformity, and controlling edema. Typically, the position of comfort is one that promotes deformity and should be avoided
  Remember, in burn patients, COMFORT = CONTRACTURE

TABLE 10–18. Proper Positioning of a Pediatric Burn Patient

Area Involved	Contracture Predisposition	Contracture Preventing Position
Anterior neck	Flexion	Extension, no pillows
Anterior axilla	Shoulder adduction	90° abduction, neutral rotation
Posterior axilla	Shoulder extension	Shoulder flexion
Elbow/Forearm	Flexion/Pronation	Elbows extended, forearm supinated
Wrists	Flexion	15°–20° extension
Hands:		
MCPs	Hyperextension	70°–90° flexion
IPs	Flexion	full-extendsion
Palmar Burn	Finger Flexion, thumb opposition	All joints full extension, thumb radially abducted
Chest	Lateral/Anterior Flexion	Straight, no lateral or anterior flexion
Hips	Flexion, adduction, external rotation	Extension, 10° abduction, neutral rotation
Knees	Flexion	Extension
Ankles	Plantarflexion	90° dorsiflexion

From Molnar GE, Alexander MA. Pediatric Rehabilitation 3rd ed. Philadelphia: Hanley & Belfus; 1999: page 356, table 17–4, with permission.

REHAB PRINCIPLES

- **Splinting:**
  Positioning splints with goals of contracture prevention are useful adjuncts for the pediatric burn victim
  Splinting is generally initiated at the first indication of developing skin tightening
  In contrast to adult and adolescents, small children do not tend to lose strength or joint mobility when immobilized in splints for extended periods, provided that the splints are removed for regular exercise or activity session
- **Range of Motion ROM:**
  Once the child is medically stable, ROM should move from gentle, repetitive action to more aggressive stretching
  Active or active assisted ROM is preferable to passive however, it may be necessary to combine both
- **ADLs:**
  Children who have sustained burn injury should be encouraged to participate in ADLs as soon as they are medically stable

- **Exercise:**
  Children frequently experience loss of strength and motor function as a result of their initial burn injury
  Exercise programs should emphasize flexibility, strength, and endurance
  Ambulation should begin as soon as the child's physical condition allows, often by 48–72 hours after injury, when vital signs are stable and fluid resuscitation is complete
- **Physical Modalities:**
  Fluidotherapy and paraffin may be helpful additions to scar therapy. Heat tolerance must be assessed.
  Extreme caution should be taken if using ultrasound. Ultrasound (US) may be useful in softening connective tissue. Care should be given to avoid overexposure of the epiphyseal plates to US. This exposure can cause premature closure of the epiphyseal plates.

BURNS REQUIRING SPECIAL ATTENTION

Neck

Correct positioning is essential so as not to develop neck flexion contracture
In the acute phase, the child should be placed in hyperextension, this can be accomplished by placing a 2nd mattress overlying the first, with the end of the top one slightly above the shoulders. The head then rests on the bottom mattress – do not allow the jaw to drop open.
Watch occiput for pressure areas
📖 Occiput is the prime location for decubiti to occur acutely in children
No pillows
The appropriately fabricated thermoplastic neck conformers do not inhibit function. Soft collars and Philadelphia collars are also used.

Axilla

Burns of the axilla are often difficult to treat in the pediatric population
Of all the burn-related contractures, the axilla is most commonly involved
The most successfully used device in an active patient is the airplane splint

Hands and Feet

The size of the hand and feet in children combined with a tendency toward rapid contractures in partial and full thickness burns makes this area difficult to treat
In hand and foot burns, the development of considerable edema can quickly lead to deformities
During the acute phase, fingers and toes should be wrapped separately to maintain average spaces
Splinting is universally used to maintain ROM and preserve function

Splinting Hands and Feet (Table 10–19)

TABLE 10–19. Splinting of Hands and Feet

Body Part	Correct Splint Position
Dorsal hand	MCP flexion 70°–90°, IP extension, radial abduction of thumb
Volar hand	MCP/IP full extension, fingers abducted, palmar abduction of thumb
Dorsal foot	Ankle and toes plantar flexion
Sole of foot	Ankle dorsiflexion, toes neutral

From Molnar GE, Alexander MA. Pediatric Rehabilitation 3rd ed. Philadelphia: Hanley & Belfus; 1999: page 362, table 17-6, with permission.

■

PEDIATRIC CANCERS

Neoplastic disease is the second leading cause of death in the pediatric age group in the United States. Solid tumors represent 70% of cases and acute leukemia represents the remaining 30%. (Figure 10–16)

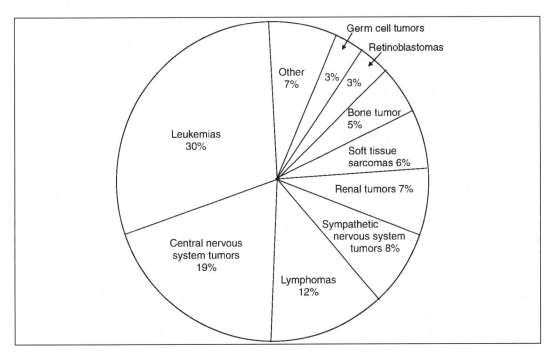

FIGURE 10–16. Major cancers in children less than 15 years old (approximate incidence).

SOLID TUMORS (70% OF ALL NEOPLASTIC DISEASE IN CHILDREN)

Brain Tumors

Brain tumors are the second most common type of childhood cancer, with leukemia being the most common. About 50% arise in the posterior fossa.
1. Cerebellar and fourth ventricle tumors often present with increased intracranial pressure along with cerebellar signs
2. Supratentorial tumors present with increased intracranial pressure along with seizures in 40%
3. Brain stem tumors often result in cranial nerve palsies along with hemiparesis and ataxia

Hodgkin's Disease

- Hodgkin's disease occurs two times more frequently in males than females, with peak incidence in the third decade, though reported in children as young as three years of age
- Painless cervical adenopathy is the most common presentation in children
- Etiology is not known

Non-Hodgkin's Lymphoma

Burkitt's tumor (African lymphoma) is a nonlymphoblastic lymphoma found principally in Africa. A viral cause has been proposed with the Epstein-Barr virus suggested.
The tumor is characterized by:
- Predilection for facial bones and mandible
- Primary involvement of abdominal nodes and viscera
- Massive proliferation of primitive lymphoid cells

Neuroblastoma

- This tumor arises from cells in the sympathetic ganglia and adrenal medulla
- It is the third most common pediatric neoplasm in children < 5 years of age with the highest incidence at 2 years of age
- Presentation in the abdominal area is commonly associated with distant metastasis and carries a poor prognosis

Wilm's Tumor (Nephroblastoma)

- In early childhood the most common abdominal masses encountered are hydronephrosis, neuroblastoma, and Wilm's tumor
- It develops within renal parenchyma and enlarges with distortion and invasion of adjacent renal tissue
- It occurs most often in children 2 to 5 years of age
- It occurs bilaterally in up to 5% and may be associated with congenital anomalies

Soft-Tissue Tumors

Rhabdomyosarcoma is the most common malignant soft-tissue tumor in children. It is associated with neurofibromatosis and most commonly occurs in the head and neck. Biopsy is necessary to distinguish this from other soft tissue sarcomas, lymphomas, and neuroblastomas.

Bone Tumors

- Metastasis of other tumors to bone commonly is seen in adults, however, it is uncommon in children
- Benign bone and cartilage tumors include osteochondroma, unicameral bone cyst, osteoid osteoma, eosinophilic granuloma, chondroblastoma, chondromyxoid fibroma, and fibrous dysplasia
- Malignant bone tumors—Osteosarcoma followed by Ewing's sarcoma are the most common types of malignant bone tumors in children and occur more often in children > 10 years of age than younger groups
  - Osteogenic sarcoma typically arises in the metaphysis of long bones. The distal femur is the most common site followed by the proximal tibia and proximal humerus
  - Ewing's sarcoma arises in long and flat bones including the pelvis and most typically in the diaphysis

- Figure 10–17 portrays each bone tumor and it's characteristic location in long bone

Retinoblastoma

- Retinoblastoma is a malignant ocular tumor that occurs at < 5 years of age in greater than 90% of cases
- The tumor may arise sporadically or be inherited
- Inherited retinoblastomas are often bilateral, whereas the non-inherited sporadic mutation form is unilateral

Germ Cell Tumors

- These tumors are derived from primordial germ cells and can be benign or malignant, gonadal or extragonadal
- Extragonadal midline sites are involved in about two-thirds of cases, including the sacrococcygeal area, mediastinum, retroperitoneum, and central nervous system

LEUKEMIAS (30% of all neoplastic disease in children)

- The majority (97.5%) of leukemias in childhood are acute
- Acute lymphoblastic leukemia (ALL) is the most common type accounting for 80% of cases
- The highest incidence of leukemia occurs between 2 and 5 years of age
- There is an increased risk of leukemia in patients with chromosomal abnormalities or immune deficiency states

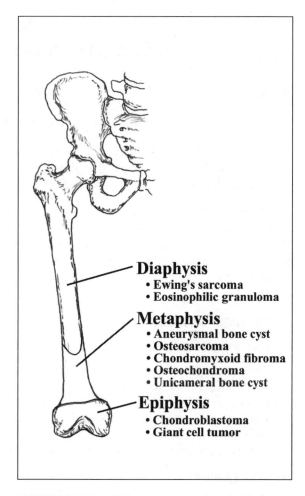

FIGURE 10–17. Bone tumor sites and their characteristic location in the long bone (not only in the femur, which is illustrated).

■

TRAUMATIC BRAIN INJURY (TBI)

EPIDEMIOLOGY

Traumatic brain injury is the leading cause of death in the United States in children > 1 year of age.

10 per 100,000 children die each year from brain injury, (which is five times the rate of death for leukemia, the next leading cause of death in children)

Annual incidence: 185 children per 100,000 per year

📖 Leading causes:

Transportation related (39%)
Falls (28%),
Sports and recreation (17%)
Assault (7%)
Other (9%)

MECHANISM OF INJURY

Primary Injuries

- Due to direct impact or to the initial deceleration or shearing forces applied to the brain
- 📖 The presence or absence of skull fractures is generally not indicative of the severity of brain injury
- Contrecoup is a cerebral contusion that occurs distant to the point of impact against an object. Shearing injuries also result in damage away from any point of impact and include diffuse axonal injury (DAI) and multiple punctate hemorrhages

Secondary Injury

- Occurs as a result of the sequelae of the initial injury and contributes to additional damage Causes: anything that interferes with cerebral perfusion or oxygenation: Hypotension, hypoxia, increased intracerebral pressure (ICP) secondary to cerebral edema, acute hydrocephalus, or mass lesion. Midline shift or herniation may lead to infarction because of pressure or traction on cerebral vessels
- In young children, incomplete myelination may result in a greater risk of shearing injury. Their relatively large heads may increase the likelihood of injury secondary to increased rotational forces
- Nonaccidental injuries are a result of acceleration-deceleration forces and are generally associated with retinal hemorrhages, fractures, and multiple injuries

Associated Injuries

- Because a large number of TBIs in children are due to Motor Vehicle Accidents (MVAs) or other high-speed accidents, almost one-half of all children who sustain a TBI sustain another injury as well
  The associated injuries can affect long-term outcome and complicate acute management. Other injuries sustained include:
  - Spinal Cord Injury (SCI) in 5%–10% of TBI children
  - Brachial plexus secondary to traction
  - Fractures because of impact
  - Perforated viscus
  - Liver and spleen lacerations

Congenital Brachial Plexus Injuries

📖 **Brachial Plexus injuries are also due to:**
General trauma
Obstetrical complications

📖 **Brachial Plexus Upper Root (Erb-Duchenne):**
Due to sudden traction to the arm causing injury to the upper trunk of the brachial plexus and/or C5–C6 cervical roots.

📖 **Brachial Plexus Lower Root (Klumpke's Paralysis):**
Due to violent upward pull of the shoulder causing damage to the lower trunk and/or C8–T1 cervical roots. Horner's Syndrome can be associated with injury of the C8 and T1 roots which results from injury to the superior cervical sympathetic ganglion. Klumpke's palsy is rare in the setting of traumatic birth palsy and results from a fall onto a hyperabducted shoulder, penetrating trauma or tumor.

Entire Brachial Plexus Injury: Secondary to injuries

SEVERITY OF INJURY

- The Glasgow Coma Scale (GCS) is usually determined within hours of injury. A score of ≤ 8 is considered to be coma and classified as severe injury
- A score of 9–11 as moderate injury and 12–15 as mild injury. (Table 10–20)

TABLE 10–20. 📖 Pediatric Coma Scale

Eyes Open	
Spontaneously	4
To speech	3
To pain	2
Not at all	1
Best Verbal Response	
Orientated	5
Words	4
Vocal sounds	3
Cries	2
None	1
Best Motor Response	
Obeys commands	5
Localizes pain	4
Flexion to pain	3
Extension to pain	2
None	1
Normal Aggregate Score	
Birth to 6 months	9
6–12 months	11
1–2 months	12
2–5 years	13
Over 5 years	14

From Menkes JH. Textbook of Child Neurology 5th ed. Baltimore: Williams & Wilkins; 1995, p. 564, table 8-5, with permission.

Adaptations of the Glasgow Coma Scale for verbal response have been developed for children. Table 10–21)

TABLE 10–21. Glasgow Coma Scale for Young Children: Modification of Scoring Verbal Responses

Verbal Score	Adult and Older Children	Young Child
5	Oriented	Smiles, oriented to sound, follows objects, interacts
4	Confused, disoriented	Cries but consolable, interacts inappropriately
3	Inappropriate words	Cries but is inconsistently consolable, moaning
2	Incomprehensible sounds	Inconsolable crying, irritable
1	No response	No response

From Molnar GE, Alexander MA. Pediatric Rehabilitation 3rd ed. Philadelphia: Hanley & Belfus; 1999: page 247, table 13-1, with permission.

Duration of consciousness is another measure of severity of injury. (Table 10–22)

TABLE 10–22. Rating of Severity of Brain Injury

	Mild	Moderate	Severe	Profound
Initial Glasgow Coma Scale	13–15 with no deterioration	9–12 with no deterioration	3–8	
Posttraumatic amnesia	< 1 hr.	1–24 hr.	>24	
Duration of unconsciousness	< 15–30 min.	15 min–24 hr.	1–90 days	>90 days

From Molnar GE, Alexander MA. Pediatric Rehabilitation 3rd ed. Philadelphia: Hanley & Belfus; 1999: page 248, table 13-2, with permission.

COMMON MOTOR DEFICITS

- Focal damage—hemiparesis
- Diffuse damage—deficit in balance, coordination, initiation. Overall 79% achieved independence in mobility
- Balance—impairment in cochlear and vestibular functions
- Tremor
- Dystonia—more common in children than adults status post TBI
- Spasticity/rigidity (38%), combined spasticity/ataxia (39%) results from upper motor neuron injury and manifested by hyperreflexia and velocity-dependent resistance to movement

COMMON SENSORY DEFICITS

- Anosmia—Impaired olfaction usually secondary to damage to olfactory bulbs and tracts, temporal lobes or subfrontal areas
- Hearing impairment—Secondary to central processing deficit, peripheral nerve damage, cochlear injury or disruption of the middle ear structures. Injuries to the VIII cranial nerve are frequently associated with basilar skull fracture
- Visual impairment—Secondary to injuries to cranial nerves, eyes, optic chiasm, tracts, radiations or cortical structures. Optic nerve injury occurs in 1.5% of cases

COGNITIVE DEFICITS

Cognitive and communication deficits are believed to be the largest cause of disability in traumatic brain injury.

- Impairment of arousal and attention—Experimental evidence exists that neurotransmitters decrease after brain injury. Trial of dopamine, norepinephrine, tricyclic antidepressants, and serotonin may be beneficial. Hyperactive children are more likely to sustain TBI. One study reveals 35% had a history of learning disability, attention deficit or emotional problems before the accident
- Agitation—Damage to frontal lobes and subcortical areas may result in agitation
- Memory impairment—Particularly affected in moderate to severe injuries. Academic performance is directly correlated to the severity of injury. Majority of improvement in IQ occurs in the first four months after TBI
- Communication impairment—Two-thirds present with difficulty in communication including naming, verbal fluency, and expression. One-third present with dysarthria. The age at injury may influence language outcome, as the young child has experienced less language development before injury
- Behavioral sequelae—Deficits in impulse control and disinhibition may relate to frontal lobe injury. Adolescents may exhibit hypersexuality
- Abnormal emotional expression—Initial lack of emotional expression may present as long term emotional lability
- Impairment in abstract reasoning—Also associated egocentricity
- Social isolation—Difficulty forming lasting social relationships

MEDICAL PROBLEMS ASSOCIATED WITH TBI

Neuroendocrine dysfunction

- Diabetes insipidus—Excessive water loss secondary to deficiency of antidiuretic hormone (ADH), which is produced in the hypothalamus
- Syndrome of inappropriate ADH (SIADH) characterized by decrease in urinary output, hyponatremia, and decreased serum osmolarity
- Cerebral salt wasting—direct neural effect on renal tubular function
- Precocious puberty—Initial signs may present 2–17 months after TBI. Girls more affected than boys (54.5% vs. 4.5%). Clinically show precocious secondary sexual development, accelerated linear growth, advanced bone ages > 2 years old, and shortened adult stature secondary to premature epiphyseal closure

Respiratory Dysfunction

- Acutely intubated as part of the initial management
- Pneumonia may be an early respiratory complication
- Late complications may be seen 2° to prolonged intubation, which may include stenosis of the trachea in the glottic area, tracheomalacia, and vocal-cord injury or paralysis

Gastrointestinal Concerns

- Nutritional concerns are that the TBI child is hypermetabolic
- Tube feedings are used because of decreased level of responsiveness
- Gastroesophageal reflux should be assessed before a gastrotomy tube is placed

Bowel Management

- It is important to establish routine bowel-management programs
- Early after injury, bowel motility decreases on the basis of the injury itself or because of narcotics

Bladder Management

- Acutely, short term bladder management to ensure that fluid intake and output are balanced
- Later, after injury, bladder management becomes a more cognitively based activity. If incontinence persists, the patient may have the presence of a neurogenic bladder. Clinical evaluation and treatment should then be performed

Central Autonomic Dysfunction (CAD)

- This is a clinical entity manifested by symptoms of unexplained hyperthermia, systemic hypertension, diaphoresis, generalized rigidity, decerebrate posturing, and rapid breathing
- It is found in 14% of children with severe acquired brain injury
- The mechanism is felt to involve hypothalamic or brain-stem dysfunction
- Presence of CAD after acquired brain injury is correlated with a more protracted period of unconsciousness and worse cognitive and motor outcomes > 1 year after injury

Heterotopic Ossification (HO)

- Ectopic bone formation occurring in 14%–23% of pediatric TBI patients
- More common in children > 11 years old, in those with more severe injury, and in those who had two or more extremity fractures
- It most commonly affects hips and knees, presents with pain, decreased range of motion, and sometimes swelling, and is associated with poor outcome
- HO is usually diagnosed a month or later after injury
- Deep venous thrombosis is unusual in children but may be seen in association with heterotopic ossification
- Treatment in children includes aggressive PROM, splinting and positioning, and NSAIDs. Do not use etidronate because it has been reported to result in a reversible rachitic syndrome in growing children.

Posttraumatic Epilepsy

- The incidence of seizures is increased both early and late (after one to two weeks), after TBI
- Patients with two or more seizures late after TBI are considered to have posttraumatic epilepsy (PTE). The risk of development of PTE is correlated with severity of TBI
- Late seizures occur in 1.6% of children with moderate and 7.4% with severe injury
- There has been no reported efficacy in prevention of PTE using phenytoin therapy
- Prophylactic anti-epileptic medication is not recommended

Cerebral Atrophy and Hydrocephalus

- Enlargement of the ventricular system is commonly seen after severe TBI in children
- This results from a decrease in brain volume (cerebral atrophy) or from obstruction of Cerebral Spinal Fluid (CSF) flow (hydrocephalus)
- Cerebral atrophy is more frequently seen after severe brain injury than true hydrocephalus

SURVIVAL

- More than two-thirds of deaths from brain injury occur at the scene or en route to the hospital

- For those children with significant injury, up to 47% of hospital costs are due to inpatient rehabilitation. Most children are discharged to home after TBI. Generally, all children who had even minimal responsiveness survive for years
- If it occurs, death in children with profound brain injuries is seen in those who remained in vegetative states greater than 90 days after anoxic or traumatic injury. In contrast to adults, in which 50% in vegetative states die within one year of injury, 50% of children still in vegetative states at one year after injury were still living seven to eight years later

LONG-TERM IMPAIRMENT

- By one year after injury, children who had minor brain injury rarely have impairment that can be attributed to the accident. Children with minor TBI are clinically indistinguishable from age-matched controls at one year postinjury
- In severe TBI, 87% of children unconscious more than six hours had a good recovery and were able to lead full independent lives with or without minimal neurological deficit. 73% became independent in ambulation and self-care within a year of injury.
- Children with profound brain injury, unconscious more than 90 days, have less favorable prognosis for recovery
- 75% of children with traumatic brain injury unconscious more than 90 days eventually regained consciousness, whereas only 25% of those with anoxic injury did so. In general, a traumatic cause of injury has a better prognosis than an anoxic etiology
- Survival and neurologic outcome are worse for abused children than after other causes of TBI
- Final outcome of children with diffuse TBI was worse in those youngest at age of injury

■

CEREBRAL PALSY (CP)

DEFINITION OF CP

- A disorder primarily of movement control and posture
- 📖 Resulting from a nonprogressive lesion to an immature brain
- Occurring in utero, near time of delivery, or within the first three years of life
- 📖 CP is the leading cause of childhood disability with an incidence of 2–3 per 1,000 births
- The brain injury resulting in CP is limited to prenatal, perinatal, or postnatal periods

RISK FACTORS OF CP: PRENATAL, PERINATAL, AND POSTNATAL (Table 10–23)

TABLE 10–22. Risk Factors of Cerebral Palsy

Prenatal Risk Factors	Perinatal Risk Factors	Postnatal Risk Factors

📖 The majority of CP cases (70%–80%) occur during the prenatal period Risk factors include the following:
 	
• **Prenatal Intracranial Hemorrhage**—outcome depends on degree of associated parenchymal injury
 	
• **Placental Complications**
 	
• **Gestational Toxins**—
  – Iodine deficiency can lead to Diplegia
  – Organic mercury intoxication can lead to quadriplegia
 	
• **Gestational Teratogenic Agents**
 	
• **Congenital malformations of the Brain and Cerebral vascular occlusions during fetal life**
 	
• **Acquired Congenital Infections**
  – Torch
  – Toxoplasmosis
  – Rubella
  – CMV
  – Herpes
 	
• **Maternal Causes**
  – Seizures
  – Hyperthyroidism
  – Mental retardation
 	
• **Socioeconomic Factors**
 	
• **Reproductive Inefficiency**
 	
• Prenatal Hypoxic-Ischemic injury as a result of:
  – Multiple pregnancies
  – Maternal bleeding
  – Maternal drug use
  – Idiopathic (most common)
 	
Note: Prenatal factors may lead to premature birth or intrauterine growth retardation of both term and preterm infants
	• 📖 **Complications of prematurity:**
	  Births at < 32 weeks gestation
	  Low birth weight < 2500 gms
	
	📖 Prematurity remains the most common antecedent of CP due to combination of:
	– Immaturity
	– Fragile brain vasculation
	– Physical stresses of immaturity, combine to predispose these children to compromise of cerebral blood flow
	
	Blood vessels are particularly vulnerable in the watershed zone next to the lateral ventricles in the capillaries of the germinal matrix
	
	• **Complications of full term infant**
	  – Placenta previa
	  – Abruptio placenta
	  – Meconium aspiration resulting in neonatal asphyxia
	
	• **Hyperbilirubinemia**
	  – Rh incompatibility
	  – G6PD
	  – ABO incompatibility
	
	Results in Kernicterus with disposition of bilirubin in the cranial nerve nuclei and basal ganglia with subsequent Athetoid CP
	
	• **Difficult Traumatic Delivery**
	  Mechanical trauma to the brain at birth can result in CP (i.e., spastic hemiplegia)
	
	• **Infection**
	  – Viral
	  – Bacterial
	
	• **Seizures**
	
	• **Bradycardia and Hypoxia**
	
	• **Perinatal Intracranial Hemorrhage**—Outcome depends on the degree of associated parenchymal injury
		• **Trauma**
		  – Fall
		  – Child abuse (i.e., shaken baby syndrome—look for retinal hemorrhage)
		  – MVA
		
		• **Toxins**
		  – Especially lead (heavy metals)
		  – organophosphates
		
		• **Stroke syndromes with hemiplegia which can result from**
		  – Sickle cell anemia
		  – AVM rupture
		  – Congenital heart disease (especially tetralogy of Fallot)
		
		• **Infection**
		  – Bacterial
		  – Viral
		  – Meningitis (especially in first 6 months)
		
		• **Neoplastic Disease**
		
		• **Anoxia**
		  i.e., near drowning can cause anoxic encephalopathy
		
		• **Intracranial hemorrhage**

CLASSIFICATION OF CP (see Tables 10–24 and 10–25)

- Current methods try to incorporate a functional basis for classification. CP may manifest itself differently as the child ages
- The modified neurologic classification system divides patients into the following categories:
  1. Spastic (pyramidal) cerebral palsy} 75%
  2. Dyskinetic (extrapyramidal) cerebral palsy
  3. Mixed types

📖 SPASTIC TYPE (75%)—manifest signs of upper motor neuron involvement

- Hyperreflexia
- Clonus
- Extensor Babinski response (abnormal at > 2 years).
- Persistent primitive reflexes.
- Overflow reflexes such as crossed adductor reflex

The spastic group can be further subdivided by the part of the body that is involved

Spastic monoplegia

- Rarely seen, however, has isolated upper or lower extremity involvement and usually a mild clinical presentation

Spastic diplegia

- Primarily lower extremity (LE) involvement with history of prematurity common
- Of premature infants that develop CP, 80% are spastic diplegics (most common lesion)
- History of intraventricular hemorrhage is typical especially at 28–32 weeks of gestation. MRI imaging in the spastic diplegic may show periventricular leukomalacia or post hemorrhagic porencephaly
- History of early hypotonia followed by spasticity is typical
- Developmental delays, commonly in the area of gross motor, result
- Lower extremity spasticity is caused by damage to pyramidal fibers within the internal capsule
- Mild incoordination problems result in the upper extremities (UE) with upper motor neuron findings in the lower extremities
- Diplegic gait pattern includes spastic adductors, gastrocnemius muscles, and hip flexors. Contractures result secondary to spasticity
- Ocular findings include strabismus in 50% and visual deficits in 63%
- Seizures occur in 20%–25% and cognitive impairment in 30%

Spastic triplegia

- Involves 3 extremities, classically both lower extremities and one upper extremity
- Spasticity results in the involved limbs with mild coordination deficits in the uninvolved limb
- Upper motor neuron signs result with characteristic scissoring and toe walking

Spastic quadriplegia

- All extremities are involved with quadriplegics, patterns of truncal hypotonia with appendicular hypertonia or total body hypertonia exist
- Often a history of difficult delivery with evidence of perinatal asphyxia
- Approximately 50% have a prenatal origin, 30% perinatal, and 20% postnatal
- MRI in the preterm child shows a periventricular leukomalacia

- Opisthotonic posturing may begin in infancy, often persisting in the severely involved. Oromotor dysfunction, pseudobulbar involvement and risk of aspiration with feeding difficulties occur and may require feeding tube placement
- Cognitive involvement results in a large percentage
- Seizures occur in 50% of affected children
- Spasticity and persistent primitive reflexes contribute to making these children the most severely involved of those with cerebral palsy

Spastic hemiplegia

- One side of the body is involved, usually the arm more than the leg
- The majority are congenital, 70%–90%
- 10%–30% are acquired secondary to vascular, inflammatory or traumatic causes
- MRI reveals evidence of unilateral lesions in 66% of cases
- In term infants, the cause is usually secondary to prenatal events
- In premature infants, asymmetric periventricular leukomalacia is a common cause. Hemiparesis is usually evident by 4–6 months of age with hypotonia usually being the first indicator; other indicators include preferential hand use
- There is a slightly higher incidence of right-sided involvement
- Cranial nerves may be involved, generally presenting as facial weakness
- Often growth retardation of the affected side with associated spasticity
- Sensory deficits on the ipsilateral side occur in 68%
- Visual deficits occur in 25% of hemiplegics, cognitive impairment in 28%, seizures in 33%
- Perceptual motor deficits are common, causing learning disabilities

⌨ DYSKINETIC TYPES

Dyskinesias are characterized by extrapyramidal movement patterns secondary to abnormal regulation of tone, defects in postural control and coordination deficits
- **Athetosis** or slow writhing involuntary movements, particularly in the distal extremities
- **Chorea**—Abrupt, irregular jerky movements, usually occurring in the head, neck, and extremities
- **Choreoathetoid**—Combination of athetosis and choreiform movements. Generally are large-amplitude involuntary movements. The dominating pattern is the athetoid movement
- **Dystonia**—A slow rhythmic movement with tone changes generally found in the trunk and extremities, associated with abnormal posturing
- **Ataxia**—Unsteadiness with uncoordinated movements, often associated with nystagmus, dysmetria, and a wide-based gait

Classic movement patterns emerge sometime between 1 and 3 years of age. Severely affected children have persistent hypotonia. Movement patterns typically increase with stress or purposeful activity. During sleep, muscle tone is normal and involuntary movement stops.

Pseudobulbar involvement presents with dysarthria, dysphasia, drooling, and oromotor dyskinesias. These children have normal intelligence 78% of the time.

⌨ There is a high incidence of sensorineural hearing loss which has been associated with hyperbilirubinemia and neonatal jaundice

MIXED TYPE

- This includes descriptions from both spastic and dyskinetic classifications. e.g., spastic athetoid (predominant dyskinetic movement pattern with underlying component of spasticity)

The modified neurologic classification system divides patients into the following categories:

TABLE 10–24. Classification of Cerebral Palsy (CP)

Type	Spastic (Pyramidal) CP	Dyskinetic (Extrapyramidal) CP	Mixed Types
% OF CP	75%	25% (both dyskinetic and mixed)	
CLINICAL SIGNS	Manifest signs of upper motor neuron involvement: Hyperreflexia Clonus Extensor Babinski response (abnormal at > 2yrs) Persistent primitive reflexes Overflow reflexes, such as crossed adductor reflexes 📖 Subgroups: **Spastic Monoplegia** **Spastic Diplegia** **Spastic Triplegia** **Spastic Quadriplegia** **Spastic Hemiplegia**	Dyskinesias are characterized by extrapyramidal movement patterns secondary to abnormal regulations of tone, defects in postural control, and coordination deficits: **Athetosis**—slow writhing, involuntary movements especially in the distal extremities **Chorea**—abrupt irregular jerky movements, usually occurring in the head, neck, and extremities **Choreoathetoid**—combination of athetosis and choreiform movements; generally are large-amplitude involuntary movements. The dominating pattern is the athetoid movement. **Dystonia**—a slow rhythmic movement with tone changes generally found in the trunk and extremities, associated with abnormal posturing **Ataxia**—unsteadiness with uncoordinated movements associated with nystagmus, dysmetria, and a wide based gait	This includes descriptions from both Spastic and Dyskinetic classifications e.g., spastic/athetoid—predominant dyskinetic movement pattern with underlying component of spasticity

TABLE 10–25. Major Categories of CP: Spastic, Dyskinetic, Mixed (and their subgroups)

SPASTIC: Subgroups combine to comprise approximately 75% of all cases of CP; Based on topographic distribution of spasticity			
Type	**Etiology**	**Will They Walk?**	**Associated Findings**
HEMIPLEGIC	– **Most cases congenital (some acquired 10%–30%)** – **Focal perinatal injury** – Highest incidence of CT/MRI abnormalities in distribution of MCA (middle cerebral artery) – **Infarction in a vascular distribution** (usually MCA) results in focal and multi-focal ischemic brain necrosis	Ambulation usually achieved by 2 years of age (unless severe retardation is associated)	– Most common presentation: Failure to use the involved hand (i.e. preferential hand used prior to 1 year of age) – Arm more involved than leg – Speech is preserved—children have the ability to switch dominance of hemisphere up until approximately age 6 – Asymmetric crawl seen – Refractory error, may have hemianopsia – Initial seizures may occur as late as 5 years of age – Mild mental retardation or no retardation – Cortical sensory deficit
DIPLEGIC (Little's Disease) 📖 Most common type of CP seen in premature infants	– **Ischemia**—due to hypoperfusion of the germinal matrix of the periventricular region of the premature fetus The periventricular white matter resides within the boarder zones between the penetrating branches of the major vessels and is exquisitely sensitive to decreases in cerebral perfusion. Result is periventricular leukomalacia (This region of white matter is transversed by the descending fibers of the motor cortex. In the corona radiata, descending fibers from the motor cortex are arranged with those subserving the LE medially and UE laterally.) – Therefore smaller lesions result in diplegic CP (i.e., involving mainly the LE) [Note: Larger lesions affect both the UE & LE]	Most diplegics ambulate—some require assistive devices	– Disproportionate involvement of the legs, although upper extremity motor perceptual dysfunction also seen – Developmental delay in gross motor skills – Ocular findings include strabismus in 50% of the cases (visual deficits in 63%) – Mild or no mental retardation – Seizures occur in 25% – Cognitive impairment in 30% (mild retardation) – UMN findings in the lower extremities – Initially there is a period of hypotonicity, later these patients manifest spasticity in the lower extremities

TABLE 10–25. *(Continued)*

SPASTIC: Subgroups combine to comprise approximately 75% of all cases of CP; Based on topographic distribution of spasticity			
Type	**Etiology**	**Will They Walk?**	**Associated Findings**
QUADRIPLEGIC 📖 This group has the highest incidence of significant disability 25% severely involved 50% moderately involved	**– Major hypoxic event** (perinatal asphyxia) usually a history of difficult delivery Result is a more severe degree of ischemia (more than diplegic CP) resulting in a more advanced form of periventricular leukomalacia. This larger lesion results in LE and UE involvement. Result is Quadriplegic CP. **– Parasagittal cerebral injury—injury to bilateral cortical zones.** Necrosis occurs within the border watershed zones. Injury to this region involves motor cortex that subserves proximal extremity function. UE more severely affected than LE. (Think of Homunculus.) **– Focal and multi-focal ischemic brain lesions.**	– One-quarter are independent in ambulation, modified ADL – One-half assisted ambulation, assisted ADL. – One-quarter are completely disabled	– Strabismus – Legs are usually more involved than arms— asymmetries not unusual – Mental retardation can be significant – Oromotor dysfunction, pseudobulbar involvement —risk of aspiration – Feeding difficulties—may need G-tube – UMN signs in all limbs – One-half have seizures. – Must be monitored for hip dislocation and scoliosis – These patients have an initial period of hypotonia which develops into extensor spasticity. The more persistent the tone, the poorer the prognosis. Opisthotonus and precocious head raising can be an early manifestation of extensor hypertonicity.
DYSKINETIC AND MIXED TYPES: Combine to comprise 25% of all cases of CP			
Type	**Etiology**	**Will They Walk?**	**Associated Findings**
DYSKINETIC: Dyskinetic disorders are characterized by extrapyramidal movement patterns. (Dyskinetic movements are defined previously in the modified neurological classification system.)	**– In the past, most cases were associated with Kernicterus due to Rh disease,** i.e., Bilirubin deposition in the basal ganglia. **– Diffuse anoxia resulting in hypoxia of the basal ganglia and thalamus.**	– One-half of children attain walking, most of them after 3 years of age UE function is adequate for ADLs – One-half of children are nonambulatory, dependent in ADLs.	– Athetosis—slow writhing, involuntary movements especially in the distal extremities – Seizures in 25%. – 📖 Sensorineural deafness (high incidence) – Paralysis of upward gaze. – These children are generally hypotonic at birth. – Classic movement patterns emerge some time between 1 and 3 years of age.

(continued)

TABLE 10–25. Major Categories of CP: Spastic, Dyskinetic, Mixed (and their subgroups) (*Continued*)

DYSKINETIC AND MIXED TYPES: Combine to comprise 25% of all cases of CP			
Type	Etiology	Will They Walk?	Associated Findings
DYSKINETIC (*continued*)			– The child develops involuntary movements first in the hands and fingers. Abnormal movements are usually evident in all extremities by 18 months– 3 years of age
			– Pseudobulbar signs are present with: Drooling Oromotor dyskinesias Dysarthria
			– During sleep, muscle tone is normal
			– DTR are normal to slightly increased
			– Tension athetosis when moving the limb increases tone
			– Children have normal intelligence 78% of the time
			– Nonambulatory patients are at risk for hip dysplasia and scoliosis
			– The UE are often more involved than the LE
MIXED TYPES: Include descriptions from both spastic and dyskinetic classifications, i.e. spastic-athetoid.	Mixed	Dependent on classification	– Ocular findings: – Kernicterus causes paralysis of upward gaze – Nystagmus is present in the ataxic type

GROSS MOTOR FUNCTION CLASSIFICATION SYSTEM

This is a functionally based system to standardize gross motor function in the CP child:

Level 1

Walks without restrictions: limitations in more advanced gross motor skills

Level 2

Walks without assistive devices: limitations walking outdoors and in the community

Level 3

Walks with assistive mobility devices: limitations walking outdoors and in the community

Level 4

Self-mobility with limitations: transported or use power mobility outdoors and in the community

Level 5

Self-mobility severely limited even with use of assistive devices

Typical Gait Abnormalities Include

Spastic diplegia
- Scissoring gait pattern
- Hips flexed and adducted
- Knees flexed with valgus
- Ankles in equinus

Spastic hemiplegia
- Weak hip flexion and ankle dorsiflexion
- Overactive posterior tibialis
- Hip hiking or hip circumduction
- Supinated foot in stance phase
- Upper extremity posturing

Crouch
- Tight hip flexors
- Tight hamstrings
- Weak quadriceps
- Excessive dorsiflexion in both diplegic and quadriplegics

Will My Child Walk?

This is usually the most frequent question asked by the parent of a newly diagnosed CP child. Several factors are relevant. The best indicator of how the child is going to do is how the child is doing.
- 📖 Sitting: Molnar has shown that if independent sitting occurs by age 2, prognosis for ambulation is good
- Crawl: Badell felt that ability to crawl on hands and knees by 1.5–2.5 years is a good prognostic sign
- Primitive Reflexes: Persistence of three or more primitive reflexes at 18–24 months is a poor prognostic sign (Table 10–28)
- Type of CP: See (Table 10–25)

ASSOCIATED DEFICITS (Table 10–26)

Mental Retardation

The incidence of associated disabilities in cerebral palsy varies. The overall incidence of mental retardation is approximately 50%. Microcephaly, seizures, and severe neuromuscular dysfunction are associated with increased risk of intellectual deficit. Spastic quadriparetics, rigid and atonic types have the highest rate of mental retardation, and spastic hemiparetics and diplegics the lowest.

📖 **Language development**, especially speaking in two–three word sentences by age three, is a good indication of intellectual potential.

Seizures

The overall incidence of seizure in children with CP is approximately 50%. Seizures are more common in spastic quadriparetics (50%) and less frequent in diplegics and dyskinetics (25%–33%). Grand mal with tonic clonic convulsions is a frequent type.

Visual Deficits

Deficits of extraocular movements and vision are also common in CP. Strabismus is the most frequent at 25%–60% of all cases with the highest rate in spastic diplegics and quadriparetics. Esotropia is more frequent than exotropia. Paralysis of conjugate upward gaze is a clinical manifestation of kernicterus. Nystagmus is present in the ataxic type. A homonymous hemianopsia occurs in hemiparetic CP in 25% of cases. Retinopathy of prematurity occurs in preterm infants.

📖 Hearing Impairment

The characteristic hearing loss in cerebral palsy is a sensory neural impairment, which occurs in 12% of CP children < age 15 with a fourfold increased prevalence in athetosis than in spasticity. Kernicterus is the most common cause of sensory neural hearing loss in athetosis. Other causes include intrauterine infections, especially rubella, cytomegalovirus, toxoplasmosis and syphilis, as well as perinatal hypoxia, meningitis, encephalitis, and ototoxic drugs.

Language Disorders

Developmental language disorders of verbal and written communication also occur. After one and one-half to two years of age, insults to the dominant hemisphere lead to aphasia. Although most children show significant recovery from aphasia acquired before 8–10 years, they rarely regain premorbid levels. Defective speech results from pseudobulbar palsy and supranuclear spastic paralysis or dyskinetic incoordination of the muscles innervated by the lower cranial nerves. Most athetoids and 50% of bilateral spastics have some dysarthria.

Respiratory Impairment

Respiratory impairment may also occur in CP children. Decreased vital capacity and aerobic working capacity is seen both in spastic and athetoid types. Restrictive pulmonary disease accompanies scoliosis.

Behavioral Disorders

Disorders of behavior may present with attention deficit, distractibility, disturbances of impulse control and overt hyperkinesis. Behavior disorders also include true emotional lability as part of an organic pseudobulbar palsy consisting of dysarthria, drooling and poor chewing. Poor peer acceptance leading to a negative self-image, school problems, depression, and anger may be exacerbated during normal periods of transition, i.e. preschool–kindergarten, early adolescence. The more mildly physically involved child may have more difficulty and need more psychosocial support.

Gastrointestinal Problems

Symptoms are frequent. Gastroesophageal reflux often requires medical management. Constipation is exaggerated by immobility and abnormal diet and fluid intake.

Bowel and Bladder Dysfunction

Management is usually related to dysfunction of central neuromotor control and cognitive development status of the child.

Oromotor Problems

May lead to difficulty swallowing, sucking, and chewing. The motor incoordination is manifested by poor lip closure, retraction or thrusting of the tongue, and decreased tongue movements. Feeding difficulties can contribute to malnutrition and aspiration. Dysphagia evaluation, modified barium swallow, fiber optic endoscopy evaluation may be needed. Gastric tube may be necessary in certain cases.

Dental Problems

Include malocclusion, enamel dysgenesis secondary to palatal distortions and abnormal oromotor reflexes. CP children are also at increased risk for cavities due to poor handling of secretions and food as well as chronic drooling. (Meds, i.e. Scopolamine patches can be used to address the problem of drooling).

TABLE 10–26. Associated Deficits in Cerebral Palsy

📖 **Mental retardation**	50% incidence, most common in rigid atonic, and severely spastic quadriplegia
Seizures	50% incidence, most frequent in hemiplegia and spastic quadriplegia
Oromotor	Difficulty sucking, swallowing, and chewing; poor lip closure, tongue thrust, drooling, dysarthria; most common in spastic quadriplegia, dyskinetic
Gastrointestinal	Reflux, constipation
Dental	Enamel dysgenesis, malocclusion, caries, gingival hyperplasia
Visual	Strabismus, refractory errors; hemianopsia in hemiplegia
Hearing impairment	Infection (TORCH), medications, bilirubin encephalopathy
Cortical sensory deficit	Hemiplegia
Pulmonary	Deficient ventilation, bronchopulmonary dysplasia in premature infants; microaspirations with oromotor dysfunction
Bowel and bladder	Dysfunction of central neuromotor control and cognitive developmental status of the child
Behavior	Attention deficit disorder, distractibility, impulse control, overt hyperkinesis, organic pseudobulbar palsy
Language disorders	Developmental, pseudobulbar supranuclear spastic paralysis, incoordination of muscles innervated by the lower cranial nerves

From Molnar GE, Alexander MA. Pediatric Rehabilitation 3rd ed. Philadelphia: Hanley & Belfus; 1999: page 204, table 11-12, with permission.

PROGNOSIS

- **Positive factors for independent living** include regular schooling, completion of secondary school, independent mobility and ability to travel beyond the house, good hand skills, living in a small community, and having spasticity as the motor dysfunction. (Mental retardation, seizures, and wheelchair dependency are factors that reduce the likelihood of independent living.)
- **Positive prognostic indicators for employment** include mild physical involvement, good family support, vocational training, and good employment contracts
- Immobility and severe or profound retardation reduce life expectancy. About 90% of children with CP survive to adulthood

THERAPEUTIC MANAGEMENT

Early intervention implies a system of programs that work with the infant and young child and the family to prevent or minimize adverse developmental outcomes. The **Individuals With Disabilities Educational Act** mandated early intervention for children 0–3 years of age who demonstrate developmental delay. There is no evidence that early intervention prevents disability or produces changes in brain organization. There is evidence that these strategies do minimize secondary complications and do support the families.

Therapeutic exercise methods:
- **Phelps**—Uses extensive bracing, withdrawing support as motion is performed with a minimum of tension, overflow and substitution
- **Deaver**—Uses extensive bracing, limiting all but two motions of an extremity
- **Doman and Delacato**—A series of set patterns repeated many times during the day, attempting to train cerebral dominance and normalization of function
- **Rood**—Emphasizes sensory and motor systems equally, activating muscles through sensory receptors
- **Bobath (most widely used)**—Neurodevelopmental treatment to normalize tone, inhibit abnormal primitive reflex patterns and facilitate automatic reactions and subsequent normal development
- **Vojta-European method**—Activates postural development and equilibrium reactions to guide normal development
- **Conductive education**—Based on theory that difficulties with motor dysfunction are problems of learning

Spasticity Management

- The mainstay of treatment is through the application of modalities, primarily therapeutic exercise, range of motion, hot and cold application, as well as casting and splinting

Nerve/Motor Point Blocks
Indicated for spasticity affecting specific muscle groups
They are commonly done to decrease scissoring due to adductor spasticity and equinovarus foot deformity during gait and hamstring tightness.
- Phenol and, less commonly, alcohol are neurolytic. They basically cause a chemical neurectomy that is effective for 3–6 months Distal regeneration from the site of injection results in loss of effect after 4–6 months (less for motor points)
- An electrical stimulator is usually used to identify the proper location for injection
- Potential benefits include prevention of deformity and improved function by facilitation of therapies, orthoses, etc.

– Disadvantages: temporary sensory dysesthesias (nerve block only), especially in the tibial and upper extremity nerves and permanent weakness leading to deformity (i.e., tibial block leading to calcaneo valgus foot)
– After this procedure an aggressive stretching and gait-training program is indicated

The Expected Effects of Specific Nerve Blocks – Lower Extremities
• Obturator nerve blocks (anterior and posterior branch)
  – Reduce adductor tone
  – Diminish scissored gait
  – Promote passive abduction as a means of protecting hip joint integrity
• Sciatic branch blocks to the medial hamstring (semimembranosus and semitendinosus)
  – Lessen crouch gait and internal rotation deformities
• Tibial blocks (and in recent past, tibial branch blocks to the heads of the gastrocnemius)
  – Diminish plantar flexion tone and allow better tolerance of AFOs
• Femoral nerve blocks
  – Diminish spastic recurvatum

Botulinum Toxin
• Botulinum toxin affects the neuromuscular junction (NMJ) with essentially the same results
  – It has been used extensively for blepharospasm ocular muscles and to treat torticollis
  – Botox acts by irreversibly blocking the NMJ presynaptictically preventing acetylcholine (ACh) release. Given as an IM injection, onset of effect occurs at 24–72 hrs. (due to a complex process of binding to presynaptic receptor sites, NMJ uptake by endocytosis and interruption of ACh mechanisms) which peaks at 2 weeks. Days after exposure, the axon fibrils begin to sprout and form junction plates on new areas of the muscle cell walls rendering weakness reversible over a period of 3 months
  – Advantages over nerve blocks include:
  Less technically demanding on clinicians
  Does not cause dysesthesia
  Decreased injection site pain and discomfort.

Surgical Procedures
• Note: surgery to improve ambulation remains problematic
• Surgery may be indicated to improve function and appearance and to prevent or correct deformities

Neurosurgical Procedures
Neurosurgical procedures have been employed for tone and management.

• Selective Posterior Rhizotomy (SPR)
  – SPR is a neurosurgical procedure designed to decrease the excitatory input to the motor neuron, thereby decreasing spasticity.
  – The procedure consists of a laminectomy and exposure of the cauda equina.
  – The dorsal roots are electrically stimulated and various criteria are used for determining which parts of the root contain more fibers involved with abnormal reflexes.
  – These rootlets are subsequently severed.
  – This technique allows for decreased tone without significant sensation loss.
  – Patient selection criteria include:
    ▪ Lack of dystonia and/or athetosis
    ▪ Preservation of functional strength independent of spasticity
    ▪ Presence of selective motor control

- Younger age (3-8 yrs.)
- Lack of significant joint contractures and few previous orthopaedic procedures
- Cognitive preservation, motivation and positive family supports are important.
- Poor Candidates for SPR Include children with poor head and trunk control and children who use spasticity for functional purposes, (i.e. extensor spasms to stand).

  - Negative effects of SPR include:
  - Hypotonia (usually transitory immediately post-op, but occasionally lasting 6 months)
  - Weakness (unmasked by reduction of tone)
  - Sensory changes and bladder dysfunction (both usually of brief duration)
  - Hip dislocation (thought to be exacerbated by sparing of L1 root leading to unbalanced hip flexor spasticity)
  - Spinal deformity (lordosis possibly secondary to sparing of L1)
  - After surgery, the children require an extensive physical and occupational therapy program to recover from post-op weakness to maximize functional gains.

Orthopaedic Procedure
- Orthopaedic intervention can be classified as either soft tissue or bony.
- Soft tissue procedures are done at the muscle or tendon level and consist of either releases, lengthenings or transfers.
- Bony procedures consist of either fusions (ankle or spine), (de)rotations (femur or tibia) or angulations (femur).

📖 Using both rhizotomy and orthopaedic surgery in combination is often required to gain the greatest improvement in gait. Gait lab analysis may help with determining the appropriate intervention

The Baclofen Pump
- The baclofen pump delivers baclofen directly to the spinal cord performing a chemically adjustable rhizotomy and minimizing side effects.
- Of course, implanted devices have their own problems and they need to be filled on a regular basis.

Ankle Foot Orthoses (AFO)
AFOs aid in gait by controlling the equinus or equino varus deformity.
- Tone Reducing AFOs (TRAFOs)
  TRAFOs have certain features designed to decrease abnormal reflexes, including a *foot plate* that extends past the toe to discourage toe flexion and a *metatarsal support* to discourage stimulation to a particularly reflexogenic area of the foot.
  They are most effective during gait, but use during rest helps prevent contractures.
- Knee Ankle Foot Orthoses (KAFO)
  KAFOs add direct control over knee flexion and extension as well as varus and valgus, but add bulk and weight.
- Hip Knee Ankle Foot Orthoses (HKAFO)
  HKAFOs add direct control over hip position. Neither of the two (KAFO or HKAFO) braces significantly improve gait but they do prevent deformity.

Medication
The management of spasticity in children with CP also includes an increasingly wide assortment of medication. The following table lists medications used for the management of spasticity (Table 10–27).

TABLE 10-27. Medications for Management of Spasticity

Medication	Site of Action	Mode of Action	Dose	Side Effects	Precautions	Comments
Baclofen	GABA receptors in spinal cord	↓ release of excitatory neurotransmitters from afferent terminals	Start with 2.5–5.0mg bid, increase by 2.5–5.0 mg q 3–5 d; max: 20 mg qid	Weakness, fatigue, confusion, constipation	May lower seizure threshold; abrupt withdrawal may precipitate seizures or hallucinations	Drug of choice for multiple sclerosis (MS) and spinal cord injury (SCI)
Baclofen: intrathecal	GABA receptors in spinal cord	↓ release of excitatory neurotransmitters from afferent terminals	Test dose 50 ug; pump dose 27–800 ug/d	Weakness, fatigue, confusion, constipation, cardiorespiratory depression	May lower seizure threshold; abrupt withdrawal may precipitate seizures or hallucinations, cardiorespiratory arrest	Approved for MS, SCI, cerebral palsy (CP), Traumatic Brain Injury (TBI)
Dantrolene	Intrafusal and extrafusal muscle fibers	↓ release of calcium from sarcoplasmic reticulum	Start with 0.5mg/kg bid; increase by 0.5 mg/kg q 5–7 d; max: 12 mg/kg/d to 400 mg	Weakness, fatigue, drowsiness, diarrhea	Hepatotoxicity 2%; frequent liver function tests	Drug of choice for spasticity of cerebral origin
Benzodiazepines	Receptors of brain stem, reticular formation, spinal cord	↑ GABA binding, potentiating presynaptic inhibition	Start with 1–2 mg bid; increase by 1–2 mg q 2-3; max: 20 mg qid	Drowsiness, fatigue, impaired memory, and recall	Tolerance and dependence, central nervous system (CNS) depression	Most helpful in incomplete SCI
Clonidine	Agonist in brain, brain stem, substantia gelatinosa of spinal cord	Inhibits short latency of motor neurons; augmentation of presynaptic inhibition	Start with 0.1mg patch for 7 d	Bradycardia, hypotension, depression	Blood pressure and pulse monitoring	Effective in reducing spasms and resistance to stretch MS, SCI, stroke

(continued)

TABLE 10–27. Medications for Management of Spasticity (*Continued*)

Medication	Site of Action	Mode of Action	Dose	Side Effects	Precautions	Comments
Tizanidine	Adrenergic receptors both spinally and supraspinally	Prevents release of excitatory amino acids from presynaptic terminal of spinal interneurons; may facilitate glycine, an inhibitory neurotransmitter	Start with 2–4 mg at bedtime; increase 2 mg q 2–4 d; max: 36 mg	Dry mouth, sedation, dizziness	Orthostatic hypotension, hallucination, elevated liver function tests	Dystonia, torticollis, blepharospasm, strabismus
Botulinum A toxin	Presynaptic acetylcholine (ACh) neuromuscular junction (NMJ)	Prevents release of acetylcholine by binding irreversibly to the presynaptic membranes of the ACh NMJ	1–12 units/kg depending on size of muscle; 50 units per site; no more frequent than every 3 months	Weakness, cramping, pain	Antibody formation, respiratory arrest (causes loss of effect) Targeted muscles No need for anesthesia	No sensory side effects No tolerance to repeat injections
Phenol	Peripheral nerve; motor end plate Denatures protein and disrupts myoneural junctions	4–6% aqueous solution; max: 20 ml	Pain, skin irritation, temporary sensory dysesthesias peripheral neuropathy, perm. weakness	Anesthesia, cardiac arrhythmia	Referred to as chemical neurolysis	

Modified from Stempien LM, Gaebler-Spira D. Rehabilitation of children and adults with cerebral palsy. In: Braddom RL (ed): Physical Medicine and Rehabilitation. Philadelphia, W.B. Saunders, 1996, with permission.

AGING WITH CEREBRAL PALSY

In general, health-related problems occur at about the same rate as in the regular population. One of the most common complaints is neck pain, occurring in 50% of spastic patients, and 75% in the dyskinetic group. Scoliosis has a much higher incidence in nonambulatory individuals. Data suggests that individuals with CP are capable of near normal reproduction. There is no correlation between degree of disability and level of sexual activity.

VOCATIONAL ASPECTS

Predictors of successful and unsuccessful employment include:

Competitive/able to work

- IQ > 80
- Ambulation with or without assistive device
- Speech hard to understand to normal
- Hand use normal to requiring assistance

Sheltered employment

- IQ between 50 and 79
- Ambulation with or without assistive devices
- Speech hard to understand to normal
- Hand use normal to requiring assistance

Unemployable/unable to work

- IQ < 50
- Nonambulatory and nonoral
- Requires assistance using hand

REFLEX DEVELOPMENT (Table 10–28)

TABLE 10–28. Reflex Development

Reflex	Stimulus	Response	Age of Suppression	Clinical Significance
Moro	Sudden neck extension	Shoulder abduction, shoulder, elbow, and finger extension followed by arm flexion adduction	4–6 months	Persists in CNS pathology, static encephalopathy
Startle	Sudden noise, clapping	Same as motor reflex	4–6 months	Persists in CNS pathology, static encephalopathy
Rooting	Stroking lips or around mouth	Moving mouth, head toward stimulus in search of nipple	4 months	Diminished in CNS pathology, may persist in CNS pathology
Positive supporting	Light pressure or weight bearing on plantar surface	Legs extend for partial support of body weight	3–5 months replaced by volitional weight bearing with support	Obligatory or hyperactive abnormal at any age, early sign of lower extremity spasticity, may be associated with scissoring
🕮 Asymmetric tonic neck	Head turning to side	Extremities extend on face side, flex on occiput side	6–7 months	Obligatory response abnormal at any age, persists in static encephalopathy
🕮 Symmetric tonic neck	Neck flexion	Arms flex, legs extend	6–7 months	Obligatory response abnormal at any age, persists in static encephalopathy
	Neck extension	Arms extend, legs flex		

(continued)

Reflex	Stimulus	Response	Age of Suppression	Clinical Significance
Palmar grasp	Touch or pressure on palm or stretching finger flexors	Flexion of all fingers, hand fisting	5–6 months	Diminished in CNS suppression, absent in lower motorneuron (LMN) paralysis; persists/hyperactive in spasticity
Plantar grasp	Pressure on sole distal to metatarsal heads	Flexion of all toes	12–14 months when walking is achieved	Diminished in CNS suppression, absent in LMN paralysis; persists/hyperactive in spasticity
Autonomic neonatal walking	On vertical support plantar contact and passive tilting of body forward side to side	Alternating automatic steps with support	3–4 months	Variable activity in normal infants, absent in LMN paralysis
Placement or placing	Tactile contact on dorsum of foot or hand	Extremity flexion to place hand or foot over an obstacle	Before end of first year	Absent in LMN paralysis or with lower extremity spasticity
Neck righting or body derotational	Neck rotation in supine	Sequential body rotation from shoulder to pelvis toward direction of face	4 months replaced by volitional rolling	Non-sequential leg rolling suggests increased tone
Tonic labyrinth	Head position in space, strongest at 45° from horizontal Supine Prone	Predominant extensor tone Predominant flexor tone	4–6 months	Hyperactive/obligatory abnormal at any age, persists in CNS damage/static encephalopathy

From Molnar GE, Alexander MA. Pediatric Rehabilitation 3rd ed. Philadelphia: Hanley & Belfus, 1999: page 20, table 2-3, with permission

■

SPINA BIFIDA

Spina bifida is the second most common childhood abnormality/disability disease, following cerebral palsy. It represents a group of neural tube deficits caused by congenital dysraphic malformations of the vertebral column and spinal cord (SC). It is the most frequent SC disorder in children.

EPIDEMIOLOGY

- Highest incidence occurs in the British Isles, Ireland, Wales and Scotland, and the lowest in Japan.
- In the U.S., the rate of neural tube deficits was about 0.6 per 1,000 births in 1989, with higher incidence in families of Irish, German, or Hispanic ancestry and lower among Asians and Pacific Islanders.

ETIOLOGY

- Both polycentric inheritance and environmental influences have been proposed. Increased familial incidence and recurrence rate and slightly greater number of affected females than males (1.2–1) points to a genetic etiology.
- Recurrence rate is 2.5 to 5% after the birth of one child with spina bifida and doubles after two affected children.
- Several environmental risk factors have been implicated:
  1. Low socioeconomic class
  2. Midspring conception
  3. Maternal obesity
  4. In utero exposure to anticonvulsant drugs (valproic acid, carbamazepine)
  5. Maternal febrile illness

📖 Studies have demonstrated that folic acid periconceptually and during early pregnancy significantly reduces the occurrence and recurrence of neural tube deficits (0.4 mg daily).

PRENATAL DIAGNOSIS

- Maternal serum measurement of alpha-fetoprotein (AFP) and acetylcholinesterase in the maternal serum and amniotic fluid and fetal ultrasound are methods of prenatal diagnosis. AFP is reliable in 80% of open neural tube deficits in weeks 13 through 15.
- Amniocentesis done by week 16 through 18 is nearly 100% accurate for detecting elevated amniotic fluid AFP. Amniocentesis does not detect closed neural tube defects without leakage of fetal cerebrospinal fluid (CSF).
- Fetal ultrasound between 16 to 24 weeks gestation is reported to have > 90% reliability.

PATHOGENESIS

- Theories about the pathogenesis of neural tube defects relate to embryonic development of the CNS.
- Neurulation of the anterior and posterior neuropores occurs during the third to fourth week after conception. The post neurulation phase takes place during the fourth through seventh post conceptional weeks. Defects occurring at this phase are skin covered lesions.
- Normal neural tube closure starts in the third week of gestation from the mid-cervical level and proceeds in both the cephalad and caudad directions.

- Defect of neural tube closure is thought to occur around day 26 and accounts for most lesions through mid-lumbar.
- The more distal caudal cell mass forms between days 26 and 30 eventually resulting in formation of the central canal in the embryonic tail.
- Caudal regression with rostral extension resulting in fusion with the neural tube results in formation of the spinal cord by day 53.
- Lesions of the lumbo-sacral levels occur before day 53.

CLINICAL TYPES (Table 10–29)

The two major types are spina bifida occulta and spina bifida cystica or aperta.

📖 Spina Bifida Occulta

In spina bifida occulta, dysraphism affects primarily the vertebrae. The neural and meningeal elements are not herniated to the surface. A frequent sign in 50% of children is the presence of a pigmented nevus, angioma, hirsute patch, dimple or dermal sinus on the overlying skin.

📖 Spina bifida occulta usually occurs in the lumbosacral or sacral segments. Unlike the cystic form, spina bifida occulta is not associated with Arnold-Chiari malformation.

📖 Spina Bifida Cystica

Spina bifida cystica collectively designates meningocele, myelomeningocele, and other cystic lesions. In spina bifida cystica, contents of the spinal canal herniate through the posterior vertebral opening.

CLINICAL SIGNS AND COURSE

Clinical signs can be discerned by careful examination in the newborn nursery.

- Motor and sensory deficits vary according to the level and extent of the spinal cord involvement. (Table 10–30)
- Motor paralysis is usually of the lower motor neuron type.
- Sensory deficit is present in the dermatomes that would be innervated by the defective spinal segments and nerve roots.

Table 10–29

FIGURE 10–18	SPINA BIFIDA OCCULTA	SPINA BIFIDA CYSTICA		
	SPINA BIFIDA OCCULTA	MENINGOCELE	MYELOMENINGOCELE	MYELOCELE
	Failure of fusion of the posterior elements of the vertebrae.	The protruding sac contains meninges and spinal fluid.	The protruding sac contains meninges, spinal cord and spinal fluid.	Cystic cavity is in front of the anterior wall of the spinal cord.
	SPINA BIFIDA OCCULTA	MENINGOCELE	MYELOMENINGOCELE	MYELOCELE
POSTERIOR ELEMENTS OF SPINE	Failure of Fusion	Failure of Fusion	Failure of Fusion	Failure of Fusion
MENINGES HERNIATE AND FORM A CYSTIC SAC	No Cystic Sac Formation	Cystic Sac Formation Present	Cystic Sac Formation Present	Cystic cavity is in front of the anterior wall of the spinal cord
CONTENTS OF CYSTIC SAC	No Cystic Sac Formation	Spinal Fluid Meninges	Spinal Fluid Meninges Spinal Cord	
ASSOCIATED FINDINGS	A frequent sign in 50% of the children is the presence of: A pigmented nevus Angioma Hirsute patch Dimple or dermal sinus overlying skin	With or without intact skin at site of sac Incomplete skin coverage leads to leakage of CSF	📖 Arnold Chiari malformation which is complicated by hydrocephalus in over 90% of the cases— with or without intact skin at site of sac	
CLINICAL SYMPTOMS	No neurologic deficit Rarely associated with sacral Lipoma and tethered cord, therefore these children must be followed	In the absence of other underlying malformation, neurologic signs are normal, but children must be followed Meningocele occurs in <10% of cases of spina bifida cystica	Motor paralysis Sensory deficits Neurogenic bowel and bladder	
📖 **SPINAL CORD LEVEL INVOLVED**	Lumbosacral or sacral Region (most common level is L5 and S1 levels)	75% of these lesions affect the lumbar and lumbosacral segments. (The remainder are located in the thoracic or sacral area but only rarely at the cervical level)	75% of these lesions affect the lumbar and lumbosacral segments. (The remainder are located in the thoracic or sacral area but only rarely at the cervical level)	75% of these lesions affect the lumbar and lumbosacral segments. (The remainder are located in the thoracic or sacral area but only rarely at the cervical level)
POPULATION AFFECTED	Normal variant in approx. 5-10% of the population	Meningocele occurs in <10% of cases of spina bifida cystica	Myelomeningocele affects an overwhelming majority of the group with spina bifida cystica	

SEGMENTAL INNERVATION

Musculoskeletal, sensory and sphincter dysfunction by segmental level (see Table 10–30)

TABLE 10–30

	T6–T12	L1	L2	L3	L4	L5	S1	S2	S3	S4
TRUNK	Abdominals Trunk flexion Lower trunk extensors									
HIP		Iliopsoas Hip flexion	Hip adductors		Gluteus maximus Hip abduction		Gluteus maximus Hip extension			
KNEE			Quadriceps Knee extension		Hamstring-hip extension Knee flexion					
ANKLE					Tibialis anterior Dorsiflexion, inversion	Peroneus Eversion	Triceps surae Plantar flexion	Tibialis posterior Plantar flexion, inversion		
FOOT					Toe extensors		Toe flexors	Foot intrinsics	Perineum sphincters	
% LEVEL OF INJURY	T6-T12 40%	L1-L2-L3 25%			L4-L5 25%		S1-S2		S3-S4 10%	
ASSOCIATED DEFICITS	– Complete leg paralysis (most often flaccid) – Kyphosis – Scoliosis Hip, knee flexion (frog leg position) contractures – Equinus foot – Bowel and bladder dysfunction	– Early hip dislocation – Hip flexion and adduction contractures – Scoliosis – Lordosis – Knee flexion contractures due to intrauterine positioning – Equinus foot – Bowel and bladder dysfunction			– Late hip dislocation – Scoliosis, lordosis – Calcaneovarus or calcaneus foot (ankles dorsiflexed) – Knee extension contractures – Hip, knee flexion contractures – Bowel and bladder dysfunction		– Bowel and bladder dysfunction – Pes Cavus foot and clawing of toes due to intrinsic muscle denervation		– Bowel and bladder dysfunction – Cavus foot and clawing of toes due to intrinsic muscle denervation	

From Molnar GE, Alexander MA. Pediatric Rehabilitation 3rd ed. Philadelphia: Hanley & Belfus; 1999: page 222, table 12-2, with permission.

Other Complications

- **Arnold Chiari Malformation Type II (ACMII)**
  Defined as downward displacement of the medulla and brainstem through the foramen magnum with associated kinking of the brainstem
  ACMII is present in almost all cases (80%–90%) of myelomeningocele and is complicated by hydrocephalus in over 90% of those cases

- **Hydrocephalus**
  Usually present at birth and becomes symptomatic during the 1st week.
  More than 80% of children require ventriculoperitoneal shunting with revision. Infection is the most frequent complication followed by obstruction
  Spontaneous arrest of hydrocephalus occurs in 50% by 15 yrs. although "prophylactic" shunt removal is contraindicated

- **Vasomotor changes over involved area**

- **Charcot joints**

- **Osteoporosis**

- **Malformations forebrain and hindbrain**

- **Tethered cord—abnormal attachment of spinal cord at distal end.**
  Retethering occurs in 10%–15%. Weakness is the number one symptom followed by sensory deficit and bladder dysfunction, spasticity

- **Benign lumbosacral tumors**
  Associated with neural tube deficits; include lipoma and fibrolipoma

- **Diastematomyelia or sagittal cleavage of the spinal cord**

- **Syringomyelia**
  A tubular cavitation in the spinal cord parenchyma lined with glial cells. Incidence 5%–40%; usually occurs in the cervical spine
  Presenting symptoms include deterioration of neurologic function, loss of sensory and motor function in the upper extremities, spasticity and pain

- **Scoliosis/kyphosis**
  Secondary to vertebral anomalies above the deficit

- **Central respiratory dysfunction**
  Most frequent single cause of death in myelodysplasia

- **Impaired fine hand coordination, ataxia**

- **Impaired visual function**
  (Strabismus, lateral rectus palsy and nystagmus)

- **Renal**
  Malformation of the urinary system, renal hypoplasia, horseshoe kidney, solitary kidney, ureteral or lower tract anomalies

Neurogenic bladder
📖 T10-T12 Sympathetic adrenergic innervation.
📖 S2-S4 Parasympathetic cholinergic innervation.
📖 S2-S5 Somatic innervation through pudendal plexus.
Disturbed bladder sensation interferes with perception of bladder filling.
Hypertonic bladder most common in thoracic lesions.
Hypotonic bladder most common in sacral lesions.
Urinary incontinence occurs in 95% with spina bifida.
Detrusor sphincter dyssynergia in 50%.
📖 Calcinosis is common with Proteus urinary tract infection.

Neurogenic bowel
There is autonomic innervation to the colon, rectum and internal anal sphincter. Voluntary somatic motor and sensory nerve supply to the external sphincter S2-S4 occurs via the pudendal plexus. Most children with spina bifida have fecal incontinence from poor rectal tone, absent cutaneous reflex response and perianal sensory deficit. In lesions above L2, intact spinal reflex arc can maintain sphincter tone despite absent rectal sensation.

Obesity
Secondary to reduced daily energy expenditure.

Precocious puberty
Secondary to premature activation of the hypothalamic pituitary gonadal axis from increased pressure on the hypothalamus. Occurs in 10%–20% of cases of myelomeningocele with hydrocephalus. Breast and testicular enlargement occurs < 8 to 9 years of age instead of the usual 11 to 11.6 years. There is an associated short stature.

Intellectual Function
- There is a 3x higher incidence of low IQ scores in children with spina bifida
- 📖 Intellectual function correlates inversely with the level of spinal cord dysfunction The higher the lesion, the lower the IQ score
- Hydrocephalus alone does not exclude normal cognitive function, however, its complications do, i.e. repeated CNS complications with meningitis can lead to significant cognitive deficits. Concentration and attention deficits are related to hydrocephalus. Higher scores are achieved on verbal tasks than visual and visual motor activities
- The term "cocktail party personality" represents children with good verbal ability that creates the impression of higher intellectual functioning than is found on formal testing.

TREATMENT

Neurosurgical Treatment (current philosophy)

Neurosurgical repair of cystic lesion is usually performed on the first day of life, with resultant lower mortality.
- 75%–85% require shunting for hydrocephalus. The average revision rate of shunting is 30%–50% for the first year and 50%–75% for the second year. Nearly all shunts are revised by five years of age

Urologic Treatment

- Neurogenic bladders are seen in all patients except very low sacral lesion and may be partial in low lumbar or high sacral lesions
- Renal ultrasound to define anatomy in infancy (2 weeks old)

- GU malformations associated with spina bifida, although rare, include hypoplastic kidneys, horseshoe kidneys, renal agenesis, ureteral duplications
- Intermittent catheterization should begin when the residual volume is ≥ to 20 cc
- ▣ Self-independent catheterization may be achieved at the age of 5 to 6 years with boys learning intermittent catheterization more easily than girls secondary to anatomic differences. 15%–20% reveal vesicoureteral reflux at birth
- IVP is recommended at about the age of 2 years
- Pharmacologic management includes anticholinergics which decrease detrusor contractions and enlarged bladder storage capacity and alpha adrenergic agents which increase outflow resistance
- Surgical measures may include bladder augmentation using the ileum or colon, suprapubic vesicostomy and artificial urinary sphincter
- Culture and sensitivities are done initially at 6 week intervals but can be lengthened to 6 month interval if symptom-free
- Long-term goal of bladder management is to prevent renal damage by preventing infections and reflux

Orthopaedic Management

Spine
Spinal deformities occur most commonly in thoracic lesions with 80–100% of patients affected by the age of 14 to 15 years.

Kyphosis may be structural or paralytic.

Structural Scoliosis may include vertebral anomalies such as wedge or hemi-vertebrae, block-vertebral, etc. and can occur alone or in combination. Paralytic Scoliosis occurs 2° to loss of truncal support and is seen in 70% above L2 and 40% below L4.

Treatment of spinal deformities:
- Mild scoliosis—Thoraco Lumbar Sacral Orthosis (TLSO) with regular follow-up
- Rapidly progressing scoliosis—check for tethered cord which can cause rapid scoliosis; requires surgical correction.
- Gibbous deformity—Kyphectomy

Hips
Hip dislocation and pelvic obliquity are common in paralytic scoliosis

At hips, *bilateral dislocation* without restriction of joint mobility is best left alone.

Unilateral dislocation or asymmetric contractures may be treated as these can lead to pelvic obliquity difficulty sitting and decubiti.

Knees
Flexion, or extension contractures of the knees are most common in thoraco-lumbar lesions. Serial casts can be tried early.

At the knees, soft tissue releases of flexion or extension contractures may increase mobility and allow sitting and/or bracing.

Osteotomies may be necessary late if shortening of the neurovascular bundle has occurred. Tibial osteotomy for severe tibial torsion may be helpful.

Foot
Rigid club foot is associated with thoracic or upper lumbar lesions.

Posterior transfer of tibialis anterior is performed at > 5 years of age for calcaneus foot deformity.

Equinus deformity is often treated with Achilles tendon lengthening.

Flexor tenodesis or transfer and plantar fascia fasciotomy is used to correct severe claw toe deformity and pes cavus.

Bowel Management

- Training in timed bowel program may be initiated by 2–3 years of developmental age
- Peristalsis and gastrocolic reflexes are usually intact making post-mealtime evacuation most successful
- Additional useful measures include bulk additives such as Metamucil®, Senokot®, suppositories PRN and enemas

Latex Allergy

- Latex sensitivity occurs in 59% with spina bifida and 55% in children who face multiple surgeries for other diagnoses
- Predisposing factors are atopic disposition with known allergies, multiple surgical procedures and previous frequent exposure to latex-containing gloves, nonsurgical equipment or toys
- Diagnostic tests include serum IgE antigen specific for rubber, skin pinprick test, and radioallergosorbent testing (RAST)
- Children should be carefully screened for any type of allergic reaction to latex, anaphylaxis

Motor Development

- During the first six months motor development is close to normal with children attaining head control and hand play. From six to twelve months, delays become obvious, requiring adaptive equipment

Rolling
Children with thoracic lesions usually roll by 18 months with compensatory strategies. Many with mid lumbar deficits and all with L5 or sacral lesions get up on hands and knees to crawl.

Sitting
T12 lesions allow trunk control. Children with mid lumbar lesions can usually sit with some delay and increased lordosis. If L4-5 is spared, the child can sit normally.

▢ Ambulation

Thoracic Lesions
Children with thoracic lesions require assistive devices for passive standing usually started at 12 to 18 months. These may include a parapodium which allows sitting and standing, a swivel walker, HKAFOs with spinal extensions and either a walker or Lofstrand crutches. Gait pattern established from as low as drag to as high as swing through.

Lower Thoracic and Lumbar Lesions
Lower thoracic and lumbar lesions often require devices such as a reciprocal gait orthosis used after the age of 3. Tension is created by forward stepping which generates extension moment at the contralateral hip. Energy requirement is similar to wheelchair mobility. If L3 is spared, the child may be able to use an AFO. Children with low lumbar lesions pull to stand and cruise near the expected age. They walk around 2 years of age with Trendelenburg lurch and gastrocnemius limp. Functional community ambulation is realistic. The mental age of 2 to 3 years is a prerequisite to learn crutch walking. Low thoracic lesion and upper lumbar lesions may achieve crutch walking by 4 to 5 years.

Low Lumbar and Sacral Lesions
Usually no braces, but may benefit from AFOs if plantar flexors are non-functional.

📖 Functional Community Ambulation

Thoracic lesions—0%–33%
High lumbar—31% achieve some degree of community ambulation.
Low lumbar—38% functional community ambulation less than 15 years of age. 95% functional community ambulation 15–31 years of age.
Sacral lesions—all able to achieve functional community ambulation.

Factors/Predictors for Ambulation

Sitting balance and motor level are early predictors of walking.
Deformities of the spine and lower extremities and obesity, are unfavorable factors for ambulation.
Wheelchair training: Training in wheelchair use can begin during the second year. An electric wheelchair is recommended at school age for a child with adequate cognitive function and emotional maturity.

Outcome

- Referral to preschool programs at age 3 years is legally mandated for children with disabilities. Most children with spina bifida complete high school with 50% continuing to further education. Independent living is achieved by 30%–60% in the United States
- The employment rate among those with spina bifida is 25%–50%
- Conception is possible in women, however, frequency of premature labor is increased
- Male sexual function is present in L5 lesions and sacral deficits, with reproductive potential related to lower and less severe lesions
- The incidence of spina bifida in offspring with one affected parent is 4%
- Urologic causes are responsible for around 40% of deaths between 5 to 30 years with survival during this period falling by 3% for every 5 years

NEUROMUSCULAR DISEASE IN CHILDREN

Neuromuscular diseases are disorders caused by an abnormality of any component of the lower motor neuron system: anterior horn cell, peripheral nerve, neuromuscular junction, or muscle. (Figure 10–19)

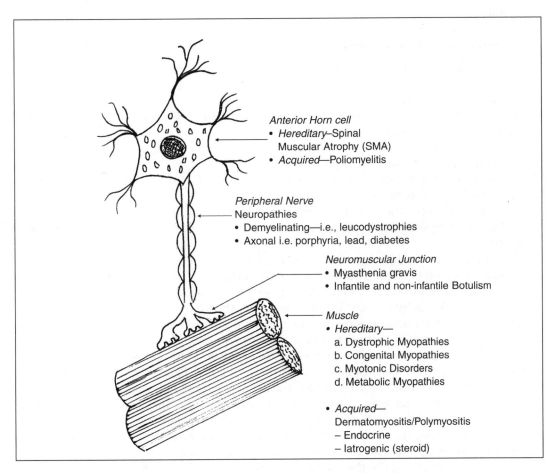

FIGURE 10–19. Anatomic Breakdown of Disorders of the Lower Motor Neuron.

- Neuromuscular disease may be acquired: poliomyelitis, Guillain-Barré syndrome, myasthenia gravis, polymyositis
- The most common are genetic: spinal muscular atrophy, hereditary motor sensory neuropathy, congenital myasthenia gravis and Duchenne's muscular dystrophy
- Molecular genetic advances have led to the discovery of specific genes for greater than 100 neuromuscular disorders
- Common symptoms of neuromuscular disease may include infantile floppiness or hypotonia, delay in motor milestones, feeding and respiratory difficulties, abnormal gait characteristics, frequent falls, difficulty with stairs or arising from the floor, and muscle cramps or stiffness

CHARACTERISTICS ON PHYSICAL EXAMINATION

1. 📖 Pseudohypertrophy seen in Duchenne's muscular dystrophy and Becker's muscular dystrophy. Increased gastrocnemius calf circumference caused by increase in fat and connective tissue, not true muscle
2. Stork leg appearance—focal atrophy of distal lower extremity muscles particularly seen in hereditary motor sensory neuropathy
3. Muscle fasciculations—seen in a variety of lower motor neuron disorders, especially common in spinal muscular atrophy
4. Hepatosplenomegaly—common in metabolic myopathy such as acid maltase deficiency and types 3 and 4 glycogenosis
5. Craniofacial changes and dental malocclusion—common in congenital myotonic muscular dystrophy, congenital myopathies, congenital muscular dystrophy and spinal muscular atrophy type II
6. 📖 Gowers' sign—results from proximal weakness of the pelvic girdle muscles causing patients to rise off the floor assuming a four-point stance on hands and knees, bridging the knees into extension while leaning the upper extremities forward, substituting for hip extension weakness by pushing off the knees with the upper extremities and sequentially moving the upper extremities up the thigh until an upright stance with full hip extension is achieved, not specific to any one neuromuscular disease
7. Toe walking/myopathic gait—weakness of hip extensors produces anterior pelvic tilt and tendency for trunk to be positioned anteriorly to the hip. Patients compensate by maintaining lumbar lordosis, which positions their center of gravity posterior to the hip, stabilizing the hip in extension. Weakness of hip extensors produces a tendency for knee instability and buckling. Patients compensate by decreased stance phase, knee flexion and posturing the ankle into plantar flexion. This produces a knee extension moment at foot contact, and plantar flexion of the ankle during mid to late stance helps to position the center of gravity anterior to the knee stabilizing the knee. Commonly seen in Duchenne's muscular dystrophy and Becker's muscular dystrophy
8. 📖 Trendelenburg gait/gluteus medius gait—weakness of hip abductors produces tendency toward lateral pelvic tilt and pelvic drop of swing phase side. Patient compensates by bending the trunk laterally over the stance hip joint
9. Steppage gait/foot slap—occurs secondary to distal weakness affecting ankle dorsiflexion and evertors. Steppage gait facilitates clearance of plantar flexed ankle

SPECIFIC NEUROMUSCULAR DISEASES

Myopathies: Dystrophic, Congenital, Myotonic

Dystrophic Myopathies

Duchenne's Muscular Dystrophy (DMD)
📖 Results from abnormality at the Xp21 gene loci and plasma membrane protein dystrophin deficiency. Chronic dystrophic myopathy is characterized by aggressive fibrotic replacement of the muscle and eventual failure of regeneration with muscle fiber death and fiber loss. Absent dystrophin or less than 3% normal is diagnostic of Duchenne's muscular dystrophy.

Definition: A steadily progressive, X-linked muscular dystrophy

Age of Onset: Within the first 5 years of life

Presenting Symptoms:
Delay in walking
Abnormal gait
Frequent falling
Difficulty climbing steps

Cardinal Clinical Signs:
Waddling gait, lordotic posture
Abnormal run
Difficulty rising from floor (Gowers' sign)
Inability to hop
Proximal muscle weakness, legs > arms
Prominence of calves

Associated features:
Cardiomyopathy (ECG abnormality)
Intellectual retardation (variable)
Deformities—equinovarus, scoliosis after loss of ambulation, fixed flexion contractures after loss of ambulation

Course and Prognosis:
Progressive loss of function
Loss of ambulation, usually by 8–12 years
Prone to respiratory infections in later stages
Life expectancy: late teens, early 20s

Investigations:
Creatinine Kinase (CK): grossly elevated
EMG: myopathic
Ultrasound: increased echo

Muscle Biopsy:
Progressive changes with time. Degeneration and regeneration, variation in fiber size, internal nuclei, proliferation of adipose and connective tissue

Genetics:
X-linked recessive; gene location Xp^{21}
Counseling for carrier status of female relative based on CK and application of new advances in recombinant DNA technology
Prenatal diagnosis, chorionic villous biopsy

Management:
Prevention of fixed deformities by passive stretching
Avoid immobilization with acute illnesses or injury
Promotion of ambulation with braces after loss of ability to walk
Prevention of scoliosis by attention to posture when chairbound, and provision of spinal supports
Operative treatment of progressive scoliosis
(Dubowitz, 1978)

- Incidence of Duchenne's muscular dystrophy is around 1 per 3500 male births. The majority of children are identified by 5–6 years old with symptoms most frequently of abnormal gait, frequent falls and difficulty climbing stairs
- Earliest weakness is seen in neck flexors during preschool years. Early on weakness is generalized, however, predominantly proximal. Pelvic girdle weakness precedes shoulder by several years. Ankle dorsiflexion is weaker than ankle plantar flexion. Ankle evertors are weaker than inverters. Knee extensors are weaker than flexors. Hip extensors are weaker than flexors. Hip abductors are weaker than adductors
- Greater than 40%–50% loss of muscle power occurs by age 6 years. The average age to wheelchair dependency is approximately 10 years with a range of 7–13 years. One study showed that all Duchenne's muscular dystrophy subjects who took ≥ 9 seconds to ambulate 30 feet lost ambulation within one year. Contractures are common in children greater than 13 years of age and mostly affect ankle plantar flexors, knee flexors, hip flexors, iliotibial band, elbow flexors and wrist flexors
- *Scoliosis*—Prevalence varies from 33%–100% and is related to age. 50% acquire scoliosis between ages 12–15 years. Scoliosis usually develops after 3–4 years in the wheelchair though no cause effect relationship has been established
- *Pulmonary*—Forced Vital Capacity (FVC) volumes increase during the first decade of life and plateau during early part of the second decade. There is a linear decline of FVC between age 10 and 20. Peak obtained FVC usually occurs in early part of the second decade and is an important prognostic indicator of severity of spinal deformity and severity of restrictive pulmonary compromise secondary to muscular weakness. FVC less than 40% is a contraindication to surgical spinal arthrodesis secondary to increased perioperative morbidity
- *Cardiac*—Dystrophin protein is present in myocardium and cardiac Purkinje fibers, therefore cardiac symptoms are part of the clinical picture. Nearly all patients greater than 13 years demonstrate abnormalities on EKG. These may include Q-waves in the lateral leads, elevated ST-segments, poor R-wave progression, increased R/S ratio, and resting tachycardia and conduction defects. Cardiomyopathy usually is first noticed at age greater than 10 years and is apparent in nearly all patients more than 18 years old. Cardiomyopathy and systolic dysfunction are poor prognostic indicators

Becker's Muscular Dystrophy

Definition:
An X-linked muscular dystrophy with similar clinical pattern to Duchenne type, but milder with slower progression

Age of Onset:
Variable: usually after 5 years of age and into adolescence or adult life

Presenting Symptoms:
Difficulty with running or climbing steps
Cramps on exercise

Cardinal Clinical Signs:
Mild functional disability
Proximal muscle weakness
Prominence of calves
Waddling gait, lordosis

Associated Features:
Cardiac involvement (mild, variable ECG changes)

Course and Prognosis:
Slowly progressive, variable course
Some cases practically static
Ambulation beyond 16 years
Life expectancy dependent on degree of progression and late respiratory deficit

Investigations:
CK: grossly elevated (similar levels to Duchenne's)
EMG: myopathic
Ultrasound: increased echo (variable)

Muscle Biopsy:
Variable dystrophic changes. Degeneration and regeneration
Variable loss of fibers and proliferation of adipose or connective tissue. Foci of atrophic fibers resembling denervation.

Genetics:
X-linked recessive
Allele of Duchenne's dystrophy, with same locus (Xp^{21})
Genetic counseling of heterozygote female carriers on basis of CK and in addition recombinant DNA technology

Management:
Promotion of activity
Prevention of fixed deformity (e.g., equinus) by passive stretching
Braces for promotion of ambulation if loss of ability to walk in late stages
Prevention and management of scoliosis if chairbound
(Dubowitz, 1978)

- Prevalence of Becker's muscular dystrophy (BMD) is 12–27 per one million, with a lower incidence than Duchenne's muscular dystrophy
- Becker's has a later onset, and a slower rate of progression
- Dystrophin is present at 20–80% normal levels or normal quantity and usually reduced or increased molecular weight of dystrophin resulting in abnormal function
- Becker's muscular dystrophy patients are able to walk into the late teenage years vs. Duchenne's muscular dystrophy where ambulation is arrested sooner
- Becker's muscular dystrophy and Duchenne's muscular dystrophy have similar distribution of weakness
- Around 75% of Becker's muscular dystrophy patients have EKG abnormalities

Congenital Muscular Dystrophy

Definition:
A heterogeneous group of cases presenting with clinical weakness or deformities in early infancy and having variable dystrophic changes in the muscle

Age of Onset:
At birth or in infancy or early childhood

Presenting Symptoms:
Hypotonia and weakness
Fixed deformities (arthrogryposis)
Variable sucking, swallowing, and respiratory difficulty
Delayed motor milestones in later onset cases

Cardinal Clinical Signs:
General hypotonia and weakness
Fixed deformities in relation to intrauterine posture
Variable weakness or contractures in later presenting cases

Associated Features:
Intellectual retardation (especially in Japan—Fukuyama type)
Dislocation of hips
Secondary deformities, e.g., scoliosis
Hydrocephalus and fundal changes (Santavuori type)

Course and Prognosis:
Variable
Many cases relatively static
May show functional improvement with time
May be fatal from respiratory deficit and risk of superadded infection

Investigations:
CK: variable from moderate elevation to normal levels
Ultrasonography: marked increase in muscle echo
EMG: myopathic pattern

Muscle Biopsy:
Variable. Some show extensive dystrophic changes with marked replacement of muscle by adipose tissue and variable connective tissue proliferation; some show mildly myopathic/dystrophic changes.

Genetics:
Autosomal recessive, (gene 9q 31–33; 6q)
Some cases probably sporadic
Some may be sequel to viral or other inflammatory process

Management:
Active physiotherapy to encourage mobility
Passive stretching of "fixed" deformities
Surgical correction of residual deformities at appropriate stage, e.g., equinovarus correction when able to stand
Avoid immobilization that promotes fixed deformity
Supportive treatment for respiratory problems
• Infants present with hypotonia, muscle weakness at birth or within the first few months of life, congenital contractures and a dystrophic pattern on muscle biopsy

- Children exhibit early contractures, equinovarus deformities, knee flexion contractures, hip flexion contractures and tightness of wrist flexors and long finger flexors

Facioscapulohumeral Dystrophy (FSH)

Definition:
Dominantly inherited dystrophy affecting primarily facial and shoulder girdle muscles

Age of Onset:
Variable, ranging from early childhood to adult life

Presenting Symptoms:
Disability relating to shoulder or facial muscles
Some cases have trunk and pelvic girdle weakness and difficulty with locomotion

Cardinal Clinical Signs:
📖 Facial weakness—patient cannot whistle
Shoulder girdle weakness
"Terracing" of shoulders on abduction
Lordosis and pelvic girdle weakness in some families

Associated features:
Deafness (variable)
Fundal changes (variable)

Course and Prognosis:
Very variable. Some may be mild and very slowly progressive, with normal lifespan, some have more marked progression of lower limb weakness and may lose ambulation in adult life
Variable degree of facial muscle weakness
Variable respiratory deficit in later stages

Investigations:
CK: may be normal or slightly elevated
EMG: normal or myopathic
Ultrasound: variable

Muscle biopsy:
Variable pathological change from focal atrophic fibers only to overtly dystrophic picture with variability in fiber size, splitting of fibers, internal nuclei and proliferation of connective and adipose tissue
Some cases have marked inflammatory response

Genetics:
Dominantly inherited, gene 4q35
Marked clinical variability within families. Subclinical cases may occur.
Genetic counseling needs careful clinical assessment of all family members to exclude subclinical.

Management:
Promotion of activity
Some cases benefit from surgical fixation of the scapulae to facilitate abduction of the arms
- Initial weakness affects facial muscles especially the orbicularis oculi, zygomaticus and orbicularis oris. The masseter, temporalis, extraocular, and pharyngeal muscles characteristically are spared. Sensory neural hearing deficit and impaired hearing function are more common than expected in FSH.

- Posterior and lateral scapular winging, high riding scapula and hyperlordosis are also seen. Hyperlordosis occurs in 20% of patients with FSH. FSH patients with scoliosis have mild and nonprogressive curves.
- Mild restrictive lung disease occurs in nearly 50% of patients with FSH with expiratory muscles more affected than inspiratory muscles. Cardiac complications in FSH are rare and patients generally have normal longevity.
- Usually there is no intellectual involvement.

(Dubowitz, 1978)

Emery-Dreifuss Muscular Dystrophy (EMD)

Definition:
An X-linked muscular dystrophy clinically distinct form Duchenne's and Becker's types

Age of Onset:
Late childhood, adolescence or adult life
Presenting Symptoms:
Difficulty with walking/running
Rigidity of neck or spine
Cardiac arrhythmia

Cardinal Clinical Signs:
Fixed deformities: equinus of feet, flexion deformity of elbows, rigidity of spine with limited neck and trunk flexion
Mild weakness
Focal wasting of muscles, especially upper arm (biceps and triceps) and lower leg (gastrocnemii, anterior group)

Associated Features:
Cardiac arrhythmia, may not be obvious clinically or on routine ECG, needs 24-hour Holter monitoring
Nocturnal hypoventilation, respiratory problems

Course and Prognosis:
Muscle weakness and functional disability very slowly progressive
Cardiac involvement may be life-threatening in early adult life

Investigations:
CK: slight to moderate elevation
EMG: myopathic
Ultrasound: focal involvement with increase in echo

Muscle Biopsy:
Mild dystrophic changes with variability in fiber size, internal nuclei, proliferation of connective tissue, degeneration or regeneration
Foci of atrophic fibers resembling denervation

Genetics:
X-linked recessive
Gene not near Duchenne and Becker dystrophy genes
Locus of gene Xq[28]
Counseling of heterozygote females on basis of CK elevation, minor changes on muscle biopsy and possible DNA polymorphisms in future

Management:
Promotion of ambulation
Prevention of deformities or their progression
Correction of fixed deformities of ankles if affecting ambulation
Close monitoring of cardiac status—may need cardiac pacemaker
Assessment of respiratory function
(Dubowitz, 1978)

- The muscle protein deficient in EMD is termed Emerin
- EMD usually presents in adolescence or early adulthood with atrophy in the upper arms and legs due to focal wasting of the calf muscles and biceps
- The hallmark of EMD clinically is early presence of contractures of the elbow flexors with limitation of full elbow extension. Heel cord tightness with ankle dorsiflexion weakness and toe walking may be present. Tightness of cervical and lumbar spinal extensor muscles resulting in limitation of neck and trunk flexion may occur

Limb Girdle Syndromes

Definition:
An autosomal recessive muscular dystrophy, of variable severity, resembling Becker's or Duchenne's muscular dystrophy

Age of Onset:
Wide, from early childhood to adolescence and adult life

Presenting Symptoms:
Difficulty with gait, running or climbing steps
Cramps on exercise

Cardinal Clinical Signs:
Abnormal gait, lordotic posture
Functional disability with hopping and rising from floor
Variable muscle weakness
Deformities after loss of ambulation, as in Duchenne's dystrophy
Prominence of calves in some

Associated features:
No consistent ones

Course and Prognosis:
Very variable
Progression usually slow but some cases severe and even more rapid than Duchenne type

Investigations:
CK: elevation variable—mild to moderate, sometimes gross
EMG: myopathic
Ultrasound: variable increase in echo; may show differential muscle involvement
Chromosome analysis in female cases to exclude translocation involving Xp^{21} site

Muscle Biopsy:
Dystrophic changes; variable
May be marked variability in fiber size and splitting of fibers
Degeneration and regeneration
Proliferation of adipose and connective tissue

Genetics:
Autosomal recessive; gene 15q

Management:
Promotion of ambulation
Prevention and treatment of deformities
(Dubowitz, 1978)

These are lower motor neuron disorders characterized by predominantly proximal weakness of shoulder and pelvic girdle muscles.

Congenital Myopathies

Central Core Myopathy
An autosomal dominant disorder with gene locus at 19q13.1. There is a high incidence of malignant hyperthermia with inhalation of anesthetic agents. There is a predominance of high-oxidative low-glycolytic type I fibers and relative paucity of type II fibers, resulting in relative deficiency of glycolytic enzymes. Patients demonstrate mild relatively nonprogressive weakness.

Minicore Disease
Autosomal recessive inheritance with predominance of type I fiber involvement. Present with hypotonia, delayed motor development, nonprogressive symmetric weakness of trunk and proximal limbs and diaphragmatic weakness with risk of nocturnal hypoventilation.

Nemaline Myopathy
(Rod-body myopathy)—Most typically occurs as autosomal recessive. Most cases present with a mild nonprogressive myopathy with hypotonia and proximal weakness. The autosomal dominant gene has been localized to chromosome 1q21-q23.

Myotubular Myopathy—recessive; Xq28
(Central nuclear myopathy)—This is present with early hypotonia, delay in motor milestones, generalized weakness proximal and distal musculature and ptosis with weakness of external ocular muscles and axial muscles.
Severe X-linked (congenital) Myotubular Myopathy—occurs with neonatal onset and severe respiratory insufficiency. The gene locus is at Xq28. Presents with severe generalized hypotonia, muscle weakness, dysphagia, and respiratory insufficiency. Children are often ventilator dependent at birth.

Congenital fiber type disproportion—recessive

Congenital type 1 fiber predominance—recessive

Mitochondrial myopathies (metabolic)—autosomal recessive; maternal inheritance

Miscellaneous subcellular organelles

Nonspecific congenital myopathies, Minimal-change myopathy
(Dubowitz, 1978)

This group of disorders usually presents with infantile hypotonia secondary to genetic defects causing primary myopathies without any structural abnormality of the central nervous system or peripheral nervous system.

Myotonic Myopathies

Myotonic Muscular Dystrophy (Steinert's disease)

Definition:
In addition to myotonia, this dominantly inherited syndrome comprises muscle weakness and wasting, cataracts, premature balding, cardiomyopathy with conduction deficits, gonadal atrophy and variable intellectual deficit and dementia. This adult type may start in childhood. In addition there is a distinct congenital type.

Age of Onset:
Usually adolescence/adult. May be present in at risk families, at an early age

Presenting Symptoms:
Weakness
Stiffness

Cardinal Clinical Signs:
Voluntary myotonia with sustained grip
Percussion myotonia of tongue or peripheral muscles
Facial weakness; inability to bury eyelashes
Ptosis, frontal balding, hatchet facies

Associated Features:
Cataracts
Delayed intellectual development

Course and Prognosis:
Affected children identified in at risk families are often symptom-free. They may later develop the full adult syndrome, but severity is extremely variable, even with a family,. Prognosis depends on associated cardiomyopathy and respiratory problems.

Investigations:
EMG: myotonia plus myopathy
ECG: Conduction defects; arrhythmia
Ultrasonography: increased muscle echogenicity

Muscle Biopsy:
In full blown adult type marked dystrophic changes plus internal nuclei and sarcoplasmic masses

Genetics:
Autosomal dominant with marked clinical heterogeneity
Gene, 19q13

Management:
Supportive treatment of dystrophy
Encourage activity
Myotonia not usually a problem
(Dubowitz, 1978)

- An autosomal dominant inherited disorder with incidence 1 per 8,000
- It affects skeletal muscle, smooth muscle, myocardium, brain and ocular structures. Associated findings include frontal baldness and gonadal atrophy, cataracts, and cardiac dysrhythmia.
- The characteristic facial features include long, thin face with temporal and masseter muscle wasting

- Myotonia, a state of delayed relaxation or sustained contraction of skeletal muscle, is seen with grip myotonia of the hand and percussion myotonia. Myotonic muscular dystrophy characteristically exhibits greater distal than proximal weakness with initial weakness often in the ankle dorsiflexors, evertors, inverters and hand muscles
- Cardiac involvement is common with EKG abnormalities in 70–75% with sudden death in less than 5% of patients
- Often IQ is significantly reduced

Myotonia Congenita (Thomsen's disease, Little Hercules)

Definition:
A disorder inherited as a dominant or recessive trait in which myotonia is the only or predominant feature

Age of Onset:
Any time from birth through infancy and childhood

Presenting Symptoms:
Stiffness after period of rest or sustained activity or posture
Stiffness and immobility on waking
Stiffness in cold weather
Difficulty releasing grip or object
Sustained eye-closure in crying infant

Cardinal Clinical Signs:
Myotonia following hand closure, eye closure, ocular deviation or other sustained movements
Percussion myotonia of tongue, thenar eminence or other muscles
Normal muscle power and function (usually)
Muscle hypertrophy

Associated features:
Myotonia following fright or sudden muscle tension
Persistent weakness in some cases
Overlap with hyperkalemic periodic paralysis in some families

Course and Prognosis:
Usually good. Patient can often control myotonia by activity
Tendency to improve with time

Investigations:
EMG: shows characteristic myotonic discharges, often on insertion of the needle

Muscle Biopsy:
Essentially normal
May be fiber hypertrophy

Genetics:
Recessive disorder probably more common than the dominant gene 7q35. Question as to whether paramyotonia congenita is a separate genetic entity or a variant of myotonia congenita.

Management:
Most patients manage without medication. When symptoms become disabling, therapeutic benefit may be obtained from quinine, procainamide, phenytoin, corticosteroids or tocainide.
(Dubowitz, 1978)

- Autosomal dominant inheritance. Symptoms usually present after birth. Symptoms are exacerbated by prolonged rest or inactivity and cold. Commonly, muscle hypertrophy is seen

Schwartz-Jampel Syndrome
- Autosomal recessive with symptoms of hypotonia, dwarfism, diffuse bone disease, narrow palpebral fissures and blepharospasm, micrognathia and flattened facies
- Symptoms are nonprogressive

Congenital Myotonic Dystrophy

Definition:
A syndrome peculiar to infants born to mothers with myotonic dystrophy. Characterized by severe hypotonia at birth, facial weakness and variable breathing and swallowing difficulties

Age of Onset:
In utero. Poor movements may be noted in second trimester. Always manifest at birth.

Presenting Symptoms:
Floppiness
Poor sucking and swallowing
Respiratory insufficiency

Cardinal Clinical Signs:
Marked hypotonia
Variable weaknesses; may have antigravity power in limbs
Facial weakness

Associated features:
Talipes equinovarus
Other deformities depending on in utero posture
Hydramnios; premature bladder
Thin ribs (x-ray)
Ventricular dilation, with or without periventricular hemorrhage
Delayed intellectual development

Course and Prognosis:
Respiratory insufficiency may be life-threatening, particularly if compounded by marked prematurity
If infant survives newborn period and swallowing difficulty resolves
(Hypotonia gradually resolves)
Marked delay in motor milestones
Variable delay in intellectual milestones
Speech difficulties

Investigations:
Examine mother for facial weakness and myotonia

Muscle Biopsy:
May be histologically normal
Delayed maturation on electron microscopy and immunocytochemistry

Genetics:
Dominant inheritance; mother always affected in congenital syndrome
Only infants with gene get hypotonic syndrome
Further affected children likely to have congenital syndrome
Prenatal diagnosis with DNA probes possible in some families

Management:
Respiratory support and tube feeding if appropriate to severity in infant
Passive stretching for equinovarus and other fixed deformities
Delay orthopaedic intervention for talipes until child standing
Speech therapist to advise on feeding difficulties and speech problems
Schooling appropriate to intellectual development
(Dubowitz, 1978)

Neuromuscular Junction Disorders

Transient neonatal myasthenia
- A transient disorder in a potentially normal infant of a myasthenic mother
- Occurs in 10–15% of infants born to myasthenic mothers and secondary to transplacental transfer of circulating acetylcholine receptor (AChR) antibodies from mother to fetus with symptoms appearing within the first few hours of birth
- Clinical signs include difficulty feeding, generalized weakness and hypotonia, respiratory difficulties, fetal cry, facial weakness and ptosis
- Usually self limiting with resolution in approximately two to three weeks

Congenital or infantile myasthenia
- This occurs in the infants of non-myasthenia mothers and may have an autosomal recessive inheritance. Antibodies to AChR are usually absent. There may be a number of different mechanisms involved

Juvenile myasthenia
- This is similar to the adult autoimmune type and has a high titre of AChR antibodies. It particularly affects adolescent girls and is often severe and labile

Clinical Features:
Ptosis and ophthalmoplegia are commonly present, together with weakness of other muscle groups including the face, the jaw, swallowing, speech, respiration, and also neck, trunk and limb muscles.

Investigations:
▫ Fatigability of muscle (surface electrodes) after stimulation of peripheral nerve(surface electrodes) at 4 or 10 Hz
Response to intravenous edrophonium (Tensilon)
Single fiber EMG, miniature endplate potentials (difficult in children)

Management:
Emergency intensive treatment for bulbar and respiratory paralysis
Neonatal—Prostigmine or pyridostigmine. Self-limiting
Congenital/Infantile—pyridostigmine
Juvenile (with Ab to AChR)—comprehensive regimen of Prostigmine, plasma exchange, thymectomy, alternate day steroid therapy, and azathioprine, carefully tailored to achieve and maintain full remission
(Dubowitz, 1978)

Autoimmune Myasthenia Gravis

- This presents with ophthalmoparesis, ptosis, facial weakness, dysphagia, speech problems, neck, trunk and limb weakness and often respiratory difficulties
- The proximal muscles are more affected than distal and upper limbs greater than lower limbs
- Relapse and remission are common
- Diagnosis is confirmed by response to an anticholinesterase drug such as edrophonium (Tensilon®)
- 📖 Repetitive nerve stimulation studies show a characteristic decrement in compound motor action potential (CMAP) with slow stimulation rates (2–5 Hz) over a train of 4–5 stimuli. Decrements of greater than 12%–15% are noted.
- Anticholinesterase receptors are detected in around 85%–90% of patients with generalized myasthenia gravis and around 50% with ocular myasthenia.

Infantile Botulism

- This usually presents between 10 days and 6 months with acute onset of hypotonia, dysphagia, constipation, weak cry and respiratory insufficiency
- Examination reveals weakness, ptosis, ophthalmoplegia with pupillary dilatation, decreased gag reflex and preservation of deep tendon reflexes
- Diagnosis is by EMG or measurement of Clostridium botulinum toxin in the stool

Non-infantile acquired botulism

- This occurs in older children and adults who acquire botulism through poorly cooked contaminated food with the toxin or through a wound contaminated with soil containing Clostridium botulinum
- Recovery may take months

Peripheral Nerve Disorders

Acute Inflammatory Demyelinating Polyradiculoneuropathy (Guillain-Barré syndrome) (AIDP)

📖 AIDP is a primarily demyelinating neuropathy with autoimmune causation. It often presents with a prodromal respiratory or gastrointestinal infection occurring within one month of onset. This often occurs with mycoplasma, cytomegalovirus, EBV (Epstein-Barr virus), Campylobacter jejuni, and various vaccinations. Weakness usually begins distally in the lower extremities with progressive ascending paralysis to involve the upper extremities. The most common cranial nerve abnormality is ipsilateral or bilateral lower motor neuron facial paralysis. Weakness generally peaks within two weeks of onset and time to maximum recovery is approximately seven plus or minus five months. Complete recovery occurs in most children. Treatment typically includes corticosteroids, plasma exchange, and IV immune globulin. Recovery is often good in children without treatment.

Chronic Inflammatory Demyelinating Polyradiculoneuropathy (CIDP)

This has a chronic relapsing course. Electrophysiologic studies show focal conduction block, temporal dispersion of CMAPs, prolongation of distal motor latencies, markedly slow conduction velocities, absent or prolonged H-wave and F-wave latencies.

Hereditary Motor Sensory Neuropathy (HMSN)

This is an inherited disease of peripheral nerves both motor and sensory with progressive neuromuscular impairment. The prevalence is 1 per 2,500 with onset usually in the first or second decade of life.

- Type 1 HMSN (Charcot Marie Tooth Type I—CMT Type I) occurs in 70%–80% of cases. It presents with a hypertrophic demyelinating neuropathy (onion bulbs) on nerve biopsy. The majority of CMT Type 1 patients demonstrate gene locus of chromosome at 17p11.2-12
- Type 2 HMSN (Charcot Marie Tooth Type II—CMT Type II) is an axonal neuropathy with normal or slightly decreased nerve conduction velocities. It presents at a later age with less involvement of small muscles of the hands. Wasting of calf and anterior compartment of the leg gives rise to "inverted champagne bottle" or "stork leg" appearance
- Type 3 HMSN (Dejerine-Sottas Disease)—a severe hypertrophic demyelinating polyneuropathy with onset in infancy or early childhood
- Type 4 HMSN (Refsum's Disease)—is an autosomal recessive disorder. Clinical features include distal muscle weakness, impaired sensation, and absent or diminished deep tendon reflexes. Weakness usually is present initially in the distal lower extremities and subsequently in the distal upper extremities. Slow progressive weakness, more proximally in the knees, elbows and pelvic and shoulder girdles may occur over decades

Toxic Neuropathies—These are rare in North American children and more common in other regions of the world.

Arsenic—This occurs as an axonal or demyelinating neuropathy. Diagnosis is from levels in the blood, urine, hair and nails.

Lead—This is most common secondary to ingestion of lead-based paint. Clinical findings of anorexia, nausea and vomiting, gastrointestinal disturbance, clumsiness, seizures, mental status changes, papilledema, and weakness predominantly in the lower extremities occur.

Mercury—This occurs from ingestion of mercuric salts, exposure to mercury vapor and/or use of topical ammonia and mercury ointments. Symptoms may include generalized encephalopathy, fatigue, predominantly distal motor axonal neuropathy, decreased or absent deep tendon reflexes, ataxic gait, and often distal sensory paresthesias.

Organophosphate poisoning—This occurs secondary to exposure to insecticides or lubricants from the plastic industry. Symptoms may include an encephalopathy (confusion and coma), sweating, abdominal cramps, diarrhea, and constricted pupils and motor polyneuropathy as a late effect.

N-hexane (Glue-sniffing) neuropathy—This occurs in teenaged recreational glue sniffers. It is predominantly a distal motor and sensory demyelinating polyneuropathy.

Chemotherapeutic agents, especially Vincristine—This often produces pure motor axonal polyneuropathy. Severity is dose related. Symptoms include a distal weakness, absent deep tendon reflexes, and often foot drop.

Metabolic neuropathy—This most often occurs with:
1. End stage renal disease—predominantly presents as a distal motor and sensory polyneuropathy with (glove and stocking) loss of sensation, loss of vibratory sense and distal weakness especially peroneal innervated musculature
2. Diabetic neuropathy—mixed motor and sensory polyneuropathy with both axonal changes and demyelination. It is less common in children than adults and may be related to degree of glucose control

Motor Neuron Disorders (Anterior Horn Cell)

Spinal Muscular Atrophy (SMA)—A group of inherited disorders characterized by weakness and muscle wasting, secondary to degeneration of both anterior horn cell of the spinal cord and brain stem motor nuclei without pyramidal tract involvement. There are three subtypes of autosomal recessive SMA described, all linked to chromosome 5q13.

SMA Type I (Werdnig-Hoffman Disease)—Severe SMA

Definition:
An autosomal recessive disorder of early infancy with severe axial and limb weakness due to degeneration of the anterior horn cell of the spinal cord

Age of Onset:
In utero or within the first few months of life

Presenting Symptoms:
Hypotonia and weakness
Sucking and swallowing difficulty
Respiratory problems

Cardinal Clinical Signs:
Severe limb and axial weakness; frog posture
Marked hypotonia
Poor head control
Diaphragmatic breathing, costal recession
Bell-shaped chest
Internal rotation of arms; jug-handle posture
Normal facial movements
Absent tendon reflexes
Weak cry

Course and Prognosis:
Despite severity, weakness usually non-progressive
Prone to respiratory infections
Prognosis poor; majority die of pneumonia in first year, most within 3 years

Investigations:
CK: normal
Motor nerve conduction velocity normal or reduced; poor motor action potential
Ultrasonography: normal or increased echo plus atrophy of muscle
EMG: features of denervation

Muscle Biopsy:
Large group atrophy plus isolated or clusters of large fibers (uniformly type I); early cases may show minimal changes—prepathological

Genetics:
Autosomal recessive; gene 5q11-q13

Management:
Pharyngeal suction if bulbar weakness present
Spinal brace in less severe cases to maintain sitting posture
Supportive treatment of pneumonia
(Dubowitz, 1978)

- The majority present within the first two months of life with generalized hypotonia and symmetrical weakness
- Symptoms include a weak suck, dysphagia, labored breathing during feeding, frequent aspiration, and a weak cry
- Examination reveals generalized hypotonia and symmetric weakness of the lower extremities more than upper extremities. Proximal muscles are more affected than distal muscles.

"Frog leg" position occurs when supine with lower extremities abducted and externally rotated.

- Diaphragmatic breathing occurs secondary to intercostal and abdominal muscle weakness and relatively preserved diaphragmatic function. Abdominal protrusion, paradoxical thoracic depression and intercostal retraction is seen. Facial weakness occurs in 50% with tongue fasciculation in 56–61%. Preservation of deep tendon reflexes does not exclude the diagnosis of SMA. ▢ Extraocular muscles and myocardium are spared.

SMA Type II—Intermediate SMA

Definition:
An autosomal recessive disorder characterized by weakness predominantly of the legs, with ability to sit unsupported but not to stand, due to degeneration of the anterior horn cells of the spinal cord

Age of Onset:
Usually between 6 and 12 months

Presenting Symptoms:
Weakness of legs
Inability to stand or walk

Cardinal Clinical Signs:
Symmetrical weakness of legs, predominantly proximal
Able to sit unsupported but unable to stand or take full weight on legs
Fasciculation of tongue (about 70%)
Tremor of hands
Tendon jerks absent or diminished
Facial muscles spared

Associated Features:
Scoliosis
Normal or advanced intellect
Variable intercostal weakness and respiratory problems
Hypotonia and excessive joint laxity, especially hands and feet

Course and Prognosis:
Muscle weakness usually static and non-progressive; may show functional improvement— some may have increasing weakness or disability over long period or during growth spurt or if putting on weight
Long-term prognosis dependent on respiratory function

Investigations:
CK: normal or moderately elevated
Ultrasonography: characteristic picture of increased echo in muscle atrophy and increased subcutaneous space
ECG: normal complexes – characteristic baseline tremor, especially in limb leads
EMG: evidence of denervation and re-innervation

Muscle Biopsy:
Characteristic pattern of large group atrophy plus variable clusters of enlarged fibers, uniformly or predominantly type I

Genetics:
Autosomal recessive, gene 5q11-q13, alleles of one gene to account for varying severities of SMA, or dual genes or separate genes

Management:
Prevention of scoliosis by early bracing
Treatment of scoliosis by spinal braces or surgery
Early achievement of standing posture in standing frame or calipers
Promotion of ambulation by appropriate orthoses
(Dubowitz, 1978)

- A progressive kyphoscoliosis and restrictive lung disease are seen in the late first decade of life
- The disease is slowly progressive with decline of less than one-half manual muscle testing unit per decade

SMA Type III (Kugelberg-Welander syndrome) – Mild SMA

Definition:
An autosomal recessive disorder characterized by proximal weakness, predominantly of the legs, due to degeneration of the anterior horn cells of the spinal cord

Age of Onset:
From the second year of life through childhood and adolescence into adulthood

Presenting Symptoms:
Difficulty with activities such as running, climbing steps, or jumping
Limitation in walking ability—quality or quantity

Cardinal Clinical Signs:
Abnormal gait; waddling, flat-footed, wide base
Difficulty rising from floor (Gowers' sign)
Proximal weakness; legs > arms
Hand tremor (variable)
Tongue fasciculation (variable)

Associated features:
Hypermobility of joints, especially hands and feet

Course and Prognosis:
Weakness usually relatively static; in some may be progressive
📖 Good long-term survival, depending on respiratory function

Investigations:
CK: normal or moderately elevated
Ultrasonography: characteristic picture of increased muscle echo plus loss of muscle bulk
EMG: evidence of denervation and re-innervation
Nerve conduction velocity normal

Muscle Biopsy:
Characteristic pattern of large group atrophy plus variable groups of normal or enlarged fibers, often uniformly type I; or retention of normal bundle architecture with fiber type grouping, and focal small group atrophy

Genetics:
Autosomal recessive, gene 5q11-q13
Less common dominant and X-linked forms

Management:
Encourage activity and ambulation
Rehabilitation in braces if ambulation lost
Vigorous treatment of respiratory infections
(Dubowitz, 1978)

- Weakness usually occurs between 18 months and the late teenage years. Proximal weakness occurs with pelvic girdle more affected than shoulder. Hip extensor weakness occurs with increased lumbar lordosis and anterior pelvic tilt. A waddling gait with pelvic drop and lateral trunk lean over stance phase side secondary to hip abductor weakness occurs.
- Fasciculations in the limb muscles and thoracic wall muscles are common.
- Scoliosis is frequent.
- Ventilatory failure secondary to restrictive lung disease is rare.

TABLE 10–31. Spinal Muscular Atrophy: Clinical Classification

Type	Onset	Course	Age at Death
1 (SEVERE)	Birth to 6 months	Never sit	Usually < 2 yrs
2 (INTERMEDIATE)	≤ 18 months	Never stand	> 2 yrs
3 (MILD)	≥ 18 months	Stand alone	adult

Munsat TL, Davies KE. International SMA consortium meeting. Neuromuscul Discord 1992; 2 (5–6): 423–428.

Spinocerebellar Degeneration Disease

Friedreich's Ataxia—A spinal cerebellar degeneration syndrome with onset before age 20 years. It is autosomal recessive and linked to chromosome 9q21. ▢ The protein found abnormal in Friedreich's ataxia is termed Frataxin. Symptoms include progressive ataxic gait, dysarthria, decreased proprioception or vibratory sense, weakness and absent DTRs. Prevalence of scoliosis approaches 100% with onset less than 10 years, usually presenting with more progressive severe scoliosis.

EXERCISE IN NEUROMUSCULAR DISEASE

- Eccentric or lengthening contractions produces more mechanical stress on muscle fibers than concentric or shortening contractions
- No systemic studies using Duchenne's muscular dystrophy populations have shown any deleterious effect of resistance exercise. Generally a submaximal strengthening program is prescribed
- Children with Duchenne's muscular dystrophy are demonstrated to have lower cardiovascular capacity and peripheral O_2 utilization with higher resting heart rate compared to controls
- Wheelchair reliance is imminent when knee extension strength becomes less than antigravity and time to ambulate 30 feet is greater than 12 seconds
- Duration of ambulation in Duchenne's muscular dystrophy has been successfully prolonged by 2 to 5 years by prompt surgery and bracing following loss of independent ambulation
- Little evidence supports the efficacy of early prophylactic lower extremity surgery in Duchenne's muscular dystrophy for independently producing prolonged ambulation

MANAGEMENT OF SCOLIOSIS IN NEUROMUSCULAR DISEASE

- A forced vital capacity of less than 30–40% of predicted may contraindicate scoliosis surgical correction secondary to increased perioperative morbidity.
- The management of spinal deformity with spinal orthotics is ineffective in Duchenne's muscular dystrophy and does not change the natural history of the curve.
- 📖 With neuromuscular disease beginning in the first decade of life, spinal bracing generally is used to improve sitting balance in patients unable to walk. Spinal arthrodesis is the most effective treatment of progressive scoliosis. Surgical intervention prior to a curvature of 35°, and prior to patient's vital capacity falling below 35%.
- Pulmonary complications are the number one cause in mortality in childhood neuromuscular disease.
- Respiratory insufficiency occurs from respiratory muscle weakness and fatigue, alteration of respiratory system mechanics and impairment of a central control of respiration.

RECOMMENDED READING

Behrman RE, Vaughan VC. *Nelson Textbook of Pediatrics*. Philadelphia: Williams & Wilkins; 1983.

Dubowitz V. *Color Atlas of Muscle Disorders in Childhood*. Chicago: Year Book Medical Publishers Inc.; 1989.

Dubowitz V. *Muscle Disorders in Childhood*. Philadelphia: W.B. Saunders; 1978.

Dubowitz V. *Muscle Disorders in Childhood* 2nd edition. Philadelphia: W.B. Saunders; 1995.

Menkes JH. *Textbook of Child Neurology* 5th edition. Baltimore: Williams & Wilkins; 1995.

Merenstein GB, Kaplan DW, Rosenberg AA. *Handbook of Pediatrics* 18th edition. Stamford: Appleton & Lange; 1997.

Molnar GE, Alexander MA. *Pediatric Rehabilitation* 3rd edition. Philadelphia: Hanley & Belfus; 1999.

Munsat TL, Davis KE. International SMA Consortium Meeting (26–28 June 1992, Bonn, Germany). *Neuromuscul Disord* 1992; 2 (5–6): 423–428.

O'Young B, Young MA, Stiens SA. *PM&R Secrets*. Philadelphia: Hanley & Belfus; 1997.

Stempien LM, Gaebler-Spira D. *Rehabilitation of Children and Adults with Cerebral Palsy*. In: Braddom RL. *Physical Medicine and Rehabilitation*. Philadelphia: W.B. Saunders; 1996.

Tolo VT, Wood B. *Pediatric Orthopaedics in Primary Care*. Baltimore: Williams & Wilkins; 1993.

11

ASSOCIATED TOPICS IN PHYSICAL MEDICINE AND REHABILITATION

SPASTICITY—Elie Elovic, M.D. and Edgardo Baerga, M.D.
MOVEMENT DISORDERS—Elie Elovic, M.D. and Edgardo Baerga, M.D.
WHEELCHAIRS—Steven Kirshblum, M.D. and Lisa Luciano, D.O.
MULTIPLE SCLEROSIS—David S. Rosenblum, M.D.
OSTEOPOROSIS—Barbara Hoffer, D.O. and Sara Cuccurullo, M.D.
BURNS—Alan Young, D.O. and Leslie Lazaroff, D.O.

■

SPASTICITY

DEFINITIONS

- **Muscle tone:** is the resistance of a muscle to passive stretch
- **Hypertonia:** is the subjective description of tone being greater than normal
- **Spasticity:** is a velocity-dependent resistance to movement felt by an examiner stretching a muscle group across a joint, resulting from the hyperexcitability of the stretch reflex. In spasticity, there is a catch and release, although the release may not be evident in severe cases
- **Rigidity:** is the resistance to stretch that is not velocity dependent—the examiner feels just about the same resistance to stretch irrespective of the velocity a muscle group is been stretched
- Spasticity results from the loss of the inhibitory and excitatory balance influencing the stretch reflex
- In spasticity, we commonly observe:
  1. Hypertonia
  2. ↑ Deep Tendon Reflexes (DTRs)
  3. Clonus
  4. Spread of reflexes beyond the muscle stimulated
- Spasticity is a component of the upper motor neuron syndrome (UMNS), which is also characterized by exaggerated phasic (tendon jerks) and tonic (spastic) stretch reflexes, released flexor reflexes in the lower extremities, and loss of movement dexterity

- **UMNS** characterized by positive and negative signs:

Positive signs	Negative signs
Spasticity	Weakness
Athetosis	Paralysis/paresis
Primitive reflexes	loss of dexterity
Rigidity	Fatigability
Dystonia	
↓ Cutaneous reflexes	
Loss of precise autonomic control	

METHODS TO QUANTIFY SPASTICITY

- There is no uniform way to quantify the severity of spasticity
- The Modified Ashworth Scale is a widely used qualitative scale for the assessment of spasticity; measures resistance to passive stretch. Clinical assessment of spasticity may also include muscle grading, Deep Tendon Reflexes (DTRs), and Range of Motion (ROM) measuring. (Table 11–1)

TABLE 11–1. Clinical Scale for Spastic Hypertonia (Modified Ashworth Scale)

0	No increase in tone
1	Slight increase in muscle tone, manifested by a catch and release or minimal resistance at the end of the ROM when the affected part(s) is moved in flexion or extension
1+	Slight increase in muscle tone, manifested by a catch, followed by minimal resistance throughout the remainder (less than half) of the ROM
2	More marked increase in muscle tone through most of the ROM, but affected part(s) easily moved
3	Considerable increase in muscle tone, passive movement difficult
4	Affected part(s) rigid in flexion or extension

From Katz RT. Spasticity. In: O'Young B, Young MA, Stiens SA. PM&R Secrets. Philadelphia; Hanley & Belfus, 1997, p. 487, with permission.

- Other methods for evaluating or assessing spasticity include the Bilateral Adductor Tone Score, the Visual Analog Scale, the Spasm Frequency Score, torque devices, and electrophysiologic studies (including dynamic multichannel EMG, tonic vibratory reflexes, and electrical tests related to the H reflex and F wave). Most of these methods are time consuming, involve expensive, specialized equipment, and/or used mainly in research

PROBLEMS-COMPLICATIONS THAT MAY RESULT DUE TO SPASTICITY

- Interferes with function
- Can cause extreme discomfort/pain in patients with intact sensation
- Disfigurement
- Interferes with nursing care
- Contractures
- Bone fractures
- Decubitus ulcers
- Interferes with hygiene
- In patients with fractures, malunion may occur
- Joint subluxation/dislocation
- ↑ risk of heterotopic ossification (HO)
- Acquired peripheral neuropathy

(Katz, 1997)

Benefits from spasticity

- May help some patients to ambulate, stand or transfer (e.g., stand pivot transfers)
- May assist in maintaining muscle bulk
- May assist in preventing Deep Vein Thrombosis (DVT)
- May assist in preventing osteoporosis
- ↓ pressure ulcer formation over bony prominences
- Can be used as "diagnostic tool" (spasticity can be a sign of exposure to a noxious stimuli—infection, bowel impaction, urinary retention, etc)

TREATMENT

Prevention

- Daily stretching ROM program
- Patient education
- Avoidance of noxious stimuli
  - Infection
  - Pain
  - DVT
  - HO
  - Pressure ulcers
  - Urinary retention

Patient and family/caretaker education

- Prevention can be achieved by emphasizing proper positioning, daily skin inspection, adequate bladder/bowel programs, etc.

Physical modalities and therapeutics

- Heat
- Cold
- Stretching
- Splinting
- Inhibitive casting (by application of serial casts)
- Proper positioning
- Functional electrical stimulation
- Vibration
- Relaxation techniques
- Motor re-education
- Biofeedback

Pharmacotherapy (Table 11–2)

TABLE 11–2. Antispasticity Medications

Medication	Mechanism of action	Side effects	Uses	Dose
Baclofen	• Analog of the inhibitory neurotransmitter **GABA**[1] • Binds to GABA-B receptors in the spinal cord inhibiting calcium influx into presynaptic terminals and suppressing the release of excitatory neurotransmitters	Generally mild • Sedation • Weakness • GI symptoms • Tremor • Insomnia • Confusion	Drug of choice for: – Spinal forms of spasticity – Multiple Sclerosis (MS)	• Start 5 mg bid or tid, ↑ dose by 5 mg q 3–5 days up to 80mg/day[2] • Sudden withdrawal of drug can cause seizures & hallucinations
Diazepam (Valium®)	• Acts centrally (on BS reticular formation system and spinal polysynaptic pathways) on GABA-A receptors, facilitating post-synaptic effects of GABA → inhibiting muscle contraction • Has no direct GABA-mimetic effect	• Sedation (most sedative) and memory impairment • Usually unsuitable in pts with TBI because of the deleterious effects on attention and memory	Useful in SCI spasticity	• Start 2 mg bid up to 60mg/day • Long half-life: 27 to 37 hrs
Dantrolene sodium (Dantrium®)	Acts peripherally in the striated muscle blocking Ca++ release from the sarcoplasmic reticulum, therefore, inhibiting muscle contractions (by ↓ the force produced by excitation-contraction coupling)	• Hepatotoxic—1% of pts [3] • Drowsiness/sedation (mild to moderate) • Weakness, fatigue, paresthesias, diarrhea, nausea, vomiting	Preferred drug spasticity of cerebral origin (stroke, CP, head injury)	• 25 mg/d up to 400 mg/d (100-200mg/d usually appropriate) • Liver Function Tests (LFTs) should be monitored
Clonidine (Catapres®)	Central alpha$_2$-adrenergic agonist	• Hypotension • Syncope • Nausea • Sedation • Depression • Dry mouth	• Largely studied in tx of SCI spasticity • Reported useful in tx of supraspinal (brainstem) spasticity	• 0.05 mg PO BID, ↑ up to 0.2 to 0.4mg/day • Transdermal Patch: Catapres®-TSS, begins with 0.1mg patch up to 0.3mg patch/wk
Tizanidine (Zanaflex®)	• Centrally acting alpha$_2$- adrenergic agonist, chemically related to clonidine • Presumably acts by ↑ presynaptic inhibition of motor neurons	• Drowsiness • Hypotension • Dry mouth • Bradycardia • Dizziness	Effective in spasticity to treat MS and stroke (comparable to diazepam and baclofen)	• May be started at 2–4 mg/day ↑ dose up to 8 mg tid (max 36mg/day) • LFTs monitoring suggested

[1]GABA = gamma-amino butyric acid

[2] 80 mg/day is the FDA's recommended max. dose; higher doses (100–120 mg/d), however, are frequently used and are usually well tolerated.

[3]Hepatotoxicity usually in females over 30 yrs, on high doses (> 300mg), for > 2 mo

Other oral agents

- Alpha agents
  - Phenothiazines
  - Thymoxamine
- GABA agonists
  - Progabide
  - Piracetam
- Phenytoin (Dilantin®)
- Gabapentin (Neurontin®)
- Chlorpromazine (Thorazine®)
- Glycine
- Threonine
- 📖 Cyclobenzaprine (Flexeril®)—acts primarily within the CNS at the brainstem as opposed to the spinal cord level, although its action in the latter may contribute to its overall skeletal muscle relaxant activity. Evidence suggests that the net effect of cyclobenzaprine is a reduction of tonic somatic motor activity, influencing both gamma and alpha motor systems. Skeletal muscle relaxants are generally not indicated for the treatment of spasticity
- Vincristine
- Cannabinoids
- Morphine

Chemical neurolysis/nerve blocks/motor point blocks

- Neurochemical agents can be used to reduce localized spasticity
- Local anesthetics, neurolytic agents, and neurotoxins can be applied to motor nerve branches, mixed nerves, or motor points to ↓ spasticity

1. **Local anesthetics**
   Local anesthetics block nerve conduction spasms for hours by interfering with the increase in permeability in Na^+ ions that normally occurs when the membrane is depolarized. It can be used to determine the potential efficacy of a longer-acting agent in treating spasticity
   Agents: lidocaine (Xylocaine®) or bupivacaine (Marcaine®)

2. **Chemical neurolytic agents**
   Chemical neurolytic agents can block spasticity for months to years. These agents induce demyelination and axonal destruction. They disrupt nerves by causing protein denaturation and axonal necrosis

   Agents:
   - Phenol (2% > 9%): anesthetic effect 1%–3% (producing demyelination with little axolysis); > 5% neurolytic (produce axonal destruction)
   - Ethyl alcohol (25%–100%)
   - These agents can be used to disrupt nerves within a trunk (mixed nerve or motor nerve block) or at the motor point where it attaches to the muscle
   - Complications/side effects of Phenol alcohol injections for spasticity:
     a) Dysesthesias (pain in the distribution of the sensory component of the blocked nerve) Incidence reported 10%–30%. Common when mixed nerves are injected; less frequent with motor nerve and motor point blocks)
     b) Muscle pain/tenderness
     c) Muscle weakness (might be "permanent", leading to deformity)
     d) Transient swelling
     e) Induration/nodule formation within the muscle
     f) DVT

g) Sprains

h) Phenol has a higher incidence of skin sloughs

i) Unlike alcohol, which has no systemic side effects when injected intravascularly, phenol can cause serious systemic reactions if injected intravascularly—causing convulsions, CNS depression, and cardiovascular collapse (usual doses of phenol are well below its lethal range). 8.5 gm of phenol can be lethal dose; should limit dose at single session to 20–30 cc of 5%

3. Neurotoxins/Botulinum toxin

- Botulinum toxin A—FDA approved for the treatment of blepharospasm, strabismus, torticollis, and hemifacial spasm
- Many off-label uses including spasticity as a result of UMNS
- Botulinum toxin produces denervation at the neuromuscular junction by blocking the release of acetylcholine, not the production of ACh
- Botulinum toxin is active at the peripheral cholinergic nerve terminals by inhibiting the release of acetylcholine and interfering with the uptake of cytoplasmic acetylcholine
- The toxin acts primarily at the neuromuscular junction but can act at other cholinergic sites including the pre- and post-ganglionic site of the autonomic nervous system

Contraindications

- Patients with known sensitivity to botulinum
- Patients receiving aminoglycoside or spectinomycin antibiotics
- Myasthenia gravis
- Lambert-Eaton syndrome
- Motor neuron disease
- Upper eyelid apraxia
- Safety during pregnancy and lactation has not been established yet

Administration and Dosing

- Can be given with or without EMG guidance (EMG is usually more helpful in localization of smaller muscles)
- Usual dosage 25–200 U per muscle—depends on size of muscle, size of patient and amount of spasticity
- Generally, maximum is 300–400 Units per session per 1–3 months
- In children, doses of 4–8 U/kg have been suggested
- As a general rule, sessions should be at least 3 months apart

Onset and duration of effects

- Onset of action occurs after 24–72 hrs after the procedure, but up to 7 days is not uncommon
- 📖 Peak effect: 4–6 weeks
- Effects last 2–6 mo

Side effects

- Unwanted weakness in injected or adjacent muscles (localized)
- Hematoma/bruising
- Flu-like syndrome (with headache, nausea, fatigue, general malaise)
- Dysphagia may occur from cervical injection (short-lived)
- Nerve trauma
- Local swelling
- Pain/soreness
- Localized erythema

- Antibody formation—to ↓ antibody formation, interval between injections should be as long as possible (at least 3 months) and doses should be as low as possible (use smallest effective dose). Antibody formation is often the source of secondary non-response

Intrathecal Baclofen Pump (ITB Pump)

- Intrathecal baclofen pump allows *direct delivery* of baclofen into the cerebrospinal fluid (CSF) (into the intrathecal space); it makes possible the administration of high doses of baclofen into the spinal cord, avoiding the untoward central system (CNS) effects associated with high oral doses of baclofen. Cervical: lumbar ratio is 1:3
- Components of the system include the pump and reservoir, which are implanted subcutaneously in the abdominal wall, and a catheter surgically implanted into the subarachnoid space
- ITB pump indicated for patients with generalized, diffuse spasticity with intolerance or lack of response to more conservative treatments (oral agents, nerve blocks, etc.)
- Originally used in patients with spinal forms of spasticity, Spinal Cord Injury (SCI), or Multiple Sclerosis (MS), and in Cerebral Palsy (CP) pts (when there is some preserved function below the level of the lesion)
- Intrathecal baclofen is delivered to the intrathecal space using the Medtronic SynchroMed infusion system; this pump is programmable. FDA has not approved it for cerebral origin >1 year.
- ITB pump are refilled on a 1-3 month basis via transcutaneous injections and lasts 5 years.
- Before implanting ITB pump, patients are generally given a trial run of baclofen administered either via an external pump with a catheter inserted percutaneously into the subarachnoid cord or via Lumbar Puncture (LP). If there is significant reduction of tone, frequency or severity of spasms, the patient is a good candidate for the pump (and is scheduled for ITB pump placement). Programmable aspect must be stressed as a critical feature. Adjustable via pump programmer. Dose can be continuous at various rates throughout the day

Side effects
- Drowsiness
- Headaches
- Dizziness
- Nausea
- Hypotension
- Weakness
  These are usually dose related and ↓ if dose is reduced by 10%–20%

Problems associated with pump itself
- Tube dysfunction (dislodging, kinking, disconnection, blockage)
- Pump failure
- Infection
- Errors in baclofen dosage

Signs/symptoms of baclofen overdose include
- Drowsiness
- Lightheadedness
- Nausea
- Bradycardia
- Weakness
- Seizures
- Resp. depression
- Loss of Consciousness (LOC) progressing to coma
  - The anticholinesterase, physostigmine, 2 mg IV, may be given to reverse the respiratory depression caused by baclofen overdose

- Seizures and hallucinations may occur due to sudden drug withdrawal. Greatest risk is when concentrations of solution changed

Other complications
- Skin breakdown
- Spinal headache (due to CSF leakage around the catheter)

Surgical Procedures

Orthopedic procedures
1. Tendon transfers
   - SPLATT—**split anterior tibial tendon transfer**—used for treatment of equinovarus deformity of the foot. In equinovarus deformity, the foot is plantar flexed (because of spastic gastrocnemius and soleus muscles) and the foot is inverted and supinated (because of spastic T. anterior). In the SPLATT procedure, the t. anterior muscle is split along its length (distally), and the distal end of the lateral half of the muscle is tunneled and attached into the cuboid and the third cuneiform bone. This creates an eversion force, which counteracts the in-turning, varus force at the ankle exerted by the remaining tibial portion of the t. anterior muscle. The SPLATT procedure is usually done in conjunction with tendo-Achilles lengthening (TAL), to the equinus (toe-pointing) deformity. The SPLATT makes the tibialis anterior a neutral inverter.
2. Tendon release
3. Tendon lengthening
4. Step-cut (Z-plasty) lengthening procedures
5. Tenotomy
6. Myotomy

Neurosurgical procedures
- ITB pump (mentioned above) and intrathecal morphine
- Dorsal rhizotomy—neurosurgical sectioning of selected dorsa; segmental roots to modulate afferent sensory input and reset muscle spindles so that there is less spasticity.
- Radiofrequency rhizotomy
- Peripheral neurectomy
- Neuroablative procedures
- Central electrical stimulators—including epidural (dorsal column) electrical stimulation and cerebellar stimulation
- Cordotomy (involves sectioning of portions of the spinal cord)
- Cordectomy (involves excision of portions of the spinal cord)
- Myelotomy (severing tracts of the spinal cord)

■

MOVEMENT DISORDERS

- Movement disorders includes a group of CNS neurodegenerative diseases associated with involuntary movements or abnormalities of skeletal muscle tone and posture
- The predominant area of involvement in movement disorders is the basal ganglia, but other pathways and structures can be affected. Basal ganglia are primarily inhibitory
- Typically, primary movement disorders are not associated with weakness or sensory loss

PARKINSON'S DISEASE

Parkinson's disease is by far the most common movement disorder, affecting 1% of the population > 50 years of age. (Table 11–3)

TABLE 11–3. Parkinson's Disease (PD)

Description	• Idiopathic Parkinson's disease is a basal ganglia disorder due to loss of cells in the substantia nigra (SN) and locus ceruleus (LC), where dopamine is produced, and degeneration of the nigrostriatal pathway (from SN to the corpus striatum); this results in a ↓ in dopamine content in the corpus striatum. • Microscopically, intracytoplasmic eosinophilic inclusions, called Lewy bodies, are found in damaged cells. • Dopamine depletion may produce a loss of inhibitory input to the cholinergic system (allowing excessive excitatory output). This leads to an imbalance of cholinergic input into the striatum. Dopaminergic input ↓ △ ↑ Cholinergic input
Epidemiology	• Male to female ratio = 3:2 • Prevalence: 160/100,000 • Incidence: 20/100,000 per year in the general population • 1% in persons > 50 years old

Signs/
Symptoms
	• Tremor at rest ("pill-rolling")—
	  – most common symptom, affecting 2/3 of patients
	  – On EMG, tremor seen as rhythmic alternating bursts in agonist and antagonist muscles
	• Bradykinesia/hypokinesia (slowness of movements)
	• Masked (expressionless) facies
	• Muscular rigidity ("cogwheel")
	• Festinating (shuffling) gait
	• Postural instability/ loss of postural reflexes (with tendency to fall to the side or backwards)
	• "Freezing" phenomena—transient inability to perform or restart certain task
	Also important:
	• Depression
	• Dementia (seen in up to 40% of Parkinson's patients)

Medical
Treatment
	Goal
	  1) ↑ dopamine action
	  2) ↓ cholinergic effect
	1. **L-Dopa:** metabolic precursor of dopamine given with Carbidopa®, a dopa-decarboxylase inhibitor that prevents systemic metabolism of L-dopa
	  L-Dopa + Carbidopa = Sinemet®
	2. **Dopamine agonists**
	  • Ergot derivatives—dopamine agonist agents that may produce symptomatic benefit by direct stimulation of dopamine receptors
	    – Bromocriptine = stimulates dopamine D_2 receptors
	    – Pergolide (Permax®) = stimulates dopamine D_1 and D_2 receptors
	  • Nonergot derivatives:
	    – Ropinirole (Requip®)
	    – Pramipexole (Mirapex®)
	3. **Amantadine (Symmetrel®):**
	  An antiviral agent; acts primarily by potentiating the release of endogenous dopamine. Also:
	  • Mild anticholinergic activity
	  • Somewhat inhibits dopamine re-uptake
	  • Glutamate receptors blocking

(continued)

TABLE 11–3. Parkinson's Disease (PD) *(Continued)*

Medical Treatment	4. **Anticholinergic agents** (muscarinic receptor antagonists) mostly useful in relieving tremor • Trihexyphenidyl (Artane®) • Benztropine (Cogentin®) • Procyclidine (Kemadrin®) • Orphenadrine (Disipal®) 5. **Inhibitors of dopamine metabolism** • Selegiline (Eldepryl®) Selective inhibitors of monoamine oxidase B (MAO B) such as selegiline (Eldepryl®) may reduce the oxidative damage in the Substantia nigra (antioxidant properties) and thus slow the disease progression; there is no evidence to support the earlier notion that this agent is neuroprotective and delays the natural progression of the disease.
	Note: The isoenzyme MAO B is the predominant form (compared to MAO A) in the striatum and is responsible for the majority of the oxidative metabolism of dopamine in the striatum.
	• Tolcapone (Tasmar®): catechol O-methyltransferase (COMT) inhibitor. COMT metabolizes dopamine and its precursor, levodopa, in the liver, GI tract and other organs. COMT inhibitors prevent dopamine metabolism and breakdown, the amount of levodopa that reaches the CNS. Tolcapone®, used as adjunct treatment to levodopa-carbidopa, may allow a reduction on the levodopa dosage.
Surgical Treatment	**Surgical treatment** • Surgical procedures are used to treat Parkinson's symptoms (rigidity, dyskinesias, tremor) in pts with advanced disease in whom antiparkinsonian meds are ineffective or poorly tolerated. • 📖 Techniques include destructive surgery or deep brain stimulation. – **Thalamotomy** (unilateral): technique in which there is surgical destruction of a specific group of cells in the thalamus, effectively reduces tremor (and sometimes rigidity) on the contralateral side. – **Pallidotomy** (unilateral posteroventral pallidotomy): procedure in which a portion of the globus pallidus is lesioned permanently. Compared to thalamic procedures, pallidotomy is more effective at improving dyskinesias, stiffness and "freezing" than in controlling tremors. – **Deep brain stimulation (DBS) of the thalamus:** Thalamic high-frequency stimulation (DBS) is done by placing an electrode into the ventral intermediate nucleus of the thalamus under electrophysiologic guidance. The electrode is connected to a pulse generator, which is activated and deactivated by passing a magnet over it. The procedure is associated with fewer complications than thalamotomy. Thalamic DBS effectively reduces tremor on the contralateral side (with less effect on bradykinesia and rigidity).
	Other treatments • Subthalamic nucleus (SN) stimulation: more effective in reducing rigidity and tremor than dyskinesias, bradykinesia. • Pallidal DBS • Tissue transplantation procedures (fetal SN cells to nigrostriate tracts; adrenal transplantation to caudate) are also been evaluated. • Botulinum toxin

(continued)

TABLE 11–3. *(Continued)*

Rehab Treatment	Rehab Treatment

	• Assessment of degree of rigidity, bradykinesia and decrease manual dexterity and how they affect ADLs. Adaptive equipment can be provided when deficits in upper extremity control limit efficient and safe function. Examples of adaptive equipment to improve feeding:
	  ▪ Plate-guards or specialized dishes
	  ▪ Weighted or large-handled cups and utensils
	  ▪ Swivel fork and spoons
	• Velcro® or zipper closures instead of buttons may improve dressing
	• Gait evaluation should be done, including speed and distance.
	• Assessment of fine motor tasks such as writing
	• Cognitive function (if clinically indicated)
	• Swallowing evaluation
	• Social isolation is common
	• Walking becomes impaired as the disease progresses

Differential Diagnoses

Differential diagnoses of PD include:
- Drug-induced parkinsonism: due to exposure to drugs such as neuroleptic agents (eg, haloperidol); metoclopramide (Reglan®), reserpine, amiodarone, lithium
- Toxin-induced parkinsonism (1-methyl-4-phenyl-1,2,3,6-tetrahydropyridine, manganese, carbon monoxide)
- Cerebrovascular accidents/Multiple lacunar strokes
- Brain tumors
- Dementia pugilistica (post-traumatic parkinsonism): parkinsonism associated with repeated trauma to the head.

Parkinson plus syndromes:
- Shy-Drager syndrome (progressive autonomic failure): parkinsonian features with dysautonomia (autonomic dysfunction)
- Olivopontocerebellar degeneration
- Multisystem atrophy: parkinsonian features with autonomic dysfunction
- Striatonigral degeneration: parkinsonian features with dystonia; tremor uncommon
- Progressive supranuclear palsy: gaze palsy (pt can't look downward), parkinsonian features with bradykinesia and rigidity (axial) >> tremor.

GENERAL DEFINITIONS OF MOVEMENT DISORDERS

Chorea

From the Greek = "to dance"; brief, rapid, forceful & dysrhythmic flinging of the limbs (or other body parts). In chorea there are nonstereotyped, unpredictable, jerky movements that interfere with purposeful motion. The most familiar, generalized form is Huntington's disease.

Athetosis

Slow, writhing, involuntary movements and inability to maintain the position of a limb or any other body part. Slower than choreiform movements and less sustained than dystonia; usually involves the face and distal upper extremities. Etiology = may be idiopathic, but can be related to another neurologic disease, such as stroke, tumor, or Wilson's disease.

Hemiballismus

Rare disorder characterized by sudden onset of violent, involuntary movements on one side of the body (unilateral and contralateral to the lesion), mainly of the arm. Usually associated with hemorrhage or infarction of the contralateral subthalamic nucleus.

HUNTINGTON CHOREA/HUNTINGTON'S DISEASE (HD) (Table 11–4)

TABLE 11–4. Huntington's Chorea

Description	• Hereditary disease (autosomal dominant) • Abnormal movements due to heightened sensitivity of striatal dopamine receptors • The disease predominantly strikes the striatum. Atrophy of the caudate nucleus can be seen on neuroimaging studies (CT, MRI) • Neurochemically, there is marked ↓ of GABA throughout the basal ganglia; there is also ↓ levels of substance P and enkephalins • Genetics: HD gene identified near the tip of the short arm of chromosome # 4 (4p16.3)
Epidemiology	• Prevalence in US and Europe: 4–8/100,000 in the general population • Usually begins at age 30–50

Signs/ Symptoms	Classic triad:
	1. Chorea/choreoathetosis (hyperkinetic, involuntary, jerky movements)
	2. Dementia and personality disorders
	3. Family history (dominant inheritance)
	   • Dysarthria
	   • Teeth grinding
	   • Facial grimacing
	   • Difficulty swallowing
	   • Depression
	Death occurs (on average) 15–20 years after the onset (usually from aspiration pneumonia)

Treatment	**Goal: ↓ dopamine action**
	At present, there is no known means of altering the progression of the disease or its fatal outcome
	
	Neuroleptics/dopamine receptor blockers
	1) Haloperidol (probably the most effective agent in suppressing the movement disorder)
	2) Phenothiazines:
	   a) Fluphenazine
	   b) Perphenazine
	Side effect: tardive dyskinesia
	
	Presynaptic dopamine depleters
	Reserpine and tetrabenazine: effective in treatment of chorea (side effect—hypotension)
	Agents for tx of depression, psychosis, irritability:
	• Clozapine
	• Fluoxetine
	• TCAs
	• Carbamazepine
	Attempts to replace the deficiency in GABA in HD by treating with GABA-mimetic agents have been unsuccessful

• In a small percentage of patients with HD, hypokinesia & rigidity are the presenting features (with similar presentation to PD). This is know as the *Westphal variant* and tends to have its onset at an earlier age.

MORE GENERAL DEFINITIONS OF MOVEMENT DISORDERS

Tremor

Rhythmic, oscillatory movements of a body part. Tremor may occur at rest (as in Parkinson's, see above) or during movement ("postural" tremor, "intention" tremor).

Movement Tremors

Essential Tremor
- Posture-maintaining tremor associated with sustained muscle contraction or stress
- Usually, early life-onset (in adolescence or early adult years); if tremor develops late in life it is often called senile tremor (which is a variant of essential tremor)
- Benign (pts should be reassured about this)
- May be familial (with autosomal dominant inheritance) or sporadic
- Tremor attenuates or disappears with intake of small amounts of alcohol
- Treatment: beta-blockers (eg, propanolol), primidone, anticholinergic drugs, surgery
- EMG: Simultaneous bursts produced from simultaneous contractures of agonist and antagonist muscles

Intention Tremor
- Intention tremor: Occurs with movement from point to point; it is evaluated with the "finger-to-nose" test. Cerebellar tremor is an example of intention tremor.

Tics

Sustained, nonrhythmic muscle contractions that are rapid and stereotyped, often occurring in the same extremity or body part during times of stress

Akathisia

Reversible motor restlessness accompanied by a sensation of unpleasant inner tension or anxiety; it is often confused with psychotic agitation. Can occur in 20%–40% of patients on antipsychotic drugs (thought to be an extrapyramidal reaction to dopamine blockade).

Myoclonus

Characterized by sudden, jerky, irregular, or periodic involuntary contractions of a muscle or group of muscles. It can be divided into reflex myoclonus, which is stimulus sensitive, occurring with volitional movements, muscle stretch, or superficial stimuli like touch; or nonspontaneous myoclonus, which is nonstimulus sensitive and occurs at rest.

Dystonia

Sustained muscle contraction that causes repetitive, twisting movements of variable speed and leads to abnormal posture. The most common focal dystonia is cervical dystonia—spasmodic torticollis with persistent contraction of the sternocleidomastoid muscle. Cervical dystonia including torticollis, is not the same as it includes lateracollis, anterior, and retrocollis. The SCM is just one of the muscles involved in cervical dystonia. Treatment is with botulinum toxin (Botox®).

Ataxia

Ataxia is the most important sign of cerebellar disease.

- *Cerebellar ataxia* is defined as lack of accuracy or coordination of movement that is not due to paresis, alteration in tone, loss of postural sense, or the presence of involuntary movements

- *Dysmetria* is a disturbance in the trajectory or placement of body part during active movement resulting either in hypometria where there is an undershooting of the target or hypermetria or overshooting of the target

- *Asynergia* or dyssynergia refers to difficulties within the sequence and speed of the components of movement

- *Dysdiadochokinesis* is difficulty with repetitive or fine movement

- *Kinetic tremor* is an oscillatory movement that occurs at the initiation of or during a movement. It has also be described as an intention tremor
- *Static tremor* occurs while a patient attempts to maintain a limb in a fixed position

Classification of Ataxias

In 1983 Harding introduced the now widely accepted classification system of ataxias. He divided them into two groups, hereditary and nonhereditary. The hereditary were further divided into autosomal dominant and autosomal recessive. (Tables 11–5, 11–6)

TABLE 11–5. Classification of Ataxia

Hereditary Ataxias
Autosomal recessive ataxias
Friedreich's ataxia
Congenital ataxia
Early-onset cerebellar ataxia
Ataxia-telangiectasia
Ataxia with isolated vitamin E deficiency
Autosomal dominant cerebellar ataxia (ADCA)
Without retinal degeneration
With additional non-cerebellar symptoms (ADCA I)
Spinocerebellar ataxia type (SCA 1)
SCA 2
SCA 3 (Machado-Joseph disease)
SCA 4
With a pure cerebellar syndrome (ADCA—III)
SCA 5
SCA 6
With a retinal degeneration (ADCA—II)
SCA 7
Dentatorubral-pallidoluysian atrophy
Episodic ataxias (EA)
EA—1
EA—2
Nonhereditary Ataxias
Idiopathic cerebellar ataxia (IDCA)
With additional noncerebellar symptoms or multiple system atrophy (IDCA-P/MSA)
Symptomatic ataxias
Alcoholism (alcoholic cerebellar degeneration)
Toxins (antiepileptics, lithium, solvents)
Malignancy (paraneoplastic cerebellar degeneration)
Malabsorption (acquired vitamin E deficiency)
Hypothyroidism
Physical causes (heat stroke, hyperthermia)

From Goetz CG, Pappert EJ. Textbook of Clinical Neurology. Philadelphia: W.B. Saunders, 1999: p. 680, table 35-1, with permission.

TABLE 11–6. Inherited Ataxias and Associated Chromosome and Genetic Mutations

Autosomal Recessive Ataxias		
Friedreich's ataxia	9q13-21	Intronic GAA repeat expansion
Ataxia-telangiectasia	11q22-23	Phosphatidyl inositol kinase
Ataxia with isolated vitamin E deficiency	8q	Alpha-tocopherol transport protein
Autosomal Dominant Cerebellar Ataxia		
Spinocerebellar ataxia type I (SCA 1)	6p21.3	CAG repeat expansion
SCA2	12q23-24.1	CAG repeat expansion
SCA3 (Machado-Joseph disease)	14q32.1	CAG repeat expansion
SCA4	16q24	
SCA5	11cen	
SCA6	19p13.1	Calcium channel (CAG repeat expansion)
SCA7	3p14-21.1	CAG repeat expansion
Denaturobral pallidoluysian atrophy (DRPLA)	12p12.3-13.1	CAG repeat expansion
Episodic ataxia (EA)		
EA-1	12p	Human potassium channel
EA-2	19p13.1	

From Goetz CG, Pappert EJ. Textbook of Clinical Neurology. Philadelphia: W.B. Saunders, 1999: p. 681, table 35-2, with permission.

Hereditary Autosomal Recessive Ataxias

Friedreich's Ataxia
- Caused by a problem with low production of messenger RNA from a gene X25
- Prevalence is 0.4 to 4.7/100,000
- Presents most commonly before age 25 and most likely between ages 10 and 15
- Patients present with progressive ataxia, areflexia of the lower limbs, impaired vibration or position sense
- Two-thirds of patients have extensor plantar reflexes. Progressive weakness of extremities, oculomotor abnormalities, rare nystagmus. Dysarthria, optic atrophy, reduced visual acuity, sensorineural hearing loss
- Nonneurologic signs; scoliosis, pes cavus, and hypertrophic obstructive cardiomyopathy

Easy-Onset Cerebellar Ataxia with Retained Tendon Reflexes
- Occurs before age 25 and is differentiated from Friedreich's ataxia by the presence of deep tendon reflexes. May be several different disorders with possible X linkage, as well as some noncongential sources
- Prevalence 0.5–2.3% per 100,000
- Starts by age 25, on average before age 17
- Presents with progressive ataxia of gait, stance and limb movements. Dysarthria, oculomotor disorders with half having impaired vibration or position sense

Hereditary Autosomal Dominant Disorders

Autosomal Dominant Disorders Without Retinal Degeneration.
- A group of disorders which are transmitted autosomally dominant with ataxia prominent presentation

Spinocerebellar Ataxia Type I
- Caused by abnormality at chromosome 6p
- Prevalence of 1.2 per 100,000
- Onset from adolescence to late adulthood with average of 35 years
- Progressive ataxia, dysarthria and cerebellar oculomotor abnormalities. Majority of patients have non-cerebellar symptoms including pyramidals signs, skeletal muscle atrophy and pale optic disks. Dysphagia is found late

Spinocerebellar Ataxia Type II
- Abnormality on chromosome 12q
- Unknown prevalence
- Onset from early childhood to late adulthood
- Progressive cerebellar syndrome with progressive ataxia, dysarthria and saccade slowing 50% have horizontal or vertical gaze palsy

Spinocerebellar Ataxia Type III—Machado-Joseph Disease
- Autosomal Dominant on chromosome 14q
- Prevalence 1.2 per 100,000 Presents early childhood to late adulthood with average around 40
- Different presentations however, all patients with progressive ataxia, dysarthria with many patients having gaze paralysis. Some patients have spasticity and hyperreflexia

Spinocerebellar Ataxia Type V
- Chromosome 11cen
- Presents from childhood to late adulthood. Primarily ataxia, dysarthria and cerebellar oculomotor disturbances

Autosomal Dominant Cerebellar Disorders with Retinal Degeneration
- Linked to chromosome 3p with unknown prevalence
- Onset between childhood to late adulthood with average 25
- When disease presents greater than 40 , majority present with ataxia with 50% progressive loss of vision. When onset before 40 all will have some visual disturbance with retinal degeneration and optic atrophy. With long disease can have gaze palsy, dysphagia, muscle weakness and hearing loss

Dentatorubral-Pallidoluysian Atrophy
- Found primarily in Japan with incidence there of 0.1 per 100,000. Average onset 30 years within range from infancy to late adulthood. Ataxia, dysarthria, and progressive dementia. When onset before 21 also have myoclonic epilepsy. Can have psychiatric disturbance, choreic or dystonic movements

Episodic Ataxia Type I
- Autosomal dominant disorder caused by potassium channel gene on chromosome 12p
- Unknown prevalence presents in early childhood with brief attacks of ataxia and dysarthria associated with interictal myokymia

Episodic Ataxia Type II
- Autosomal dominant disorder linked to chromosome 19p. Normally presents during childhood as early as 6 weeks to 30 years of age
- Different from type I because of long duration of attacks hours to greater than a day

Nonhereditary Idiopathic Cerebellar Ataxia
- Group of heterogeneous group of disorders beginning after age 25.
- Two major types:
  - Cerebellar type with degeneration of the cerebellar cortex
  - Plus type includes basal ganglia, pyramidal tract, and autonomic nervous system
- Starts around age 55 with ataxia, dysarthria, and cerebellar oculomotor abnormalities

■

WHEELCHAIRS

BASIC WHEELCHAIR PRESCRIPTION WRITING

There are many different wheelchairs to choose from, with many options. This section will cover basic principles to allow the clinician to prescribe the proper chair. Wheelchair prescriptions should maximize patient mobility and functional potential as well as prevent co-morbidity and restriction of remaining physiologic functional capabilities. Prior to wheelchair prescriptions, the clinician should complete a full medical history, assess the patient's strength, endurance, ROM, head and trunk control, skin integrity, sensation, sitting balance, as well as current functional status and future rehabilitation goals.

THE BASIC WHEELCHAIR

The configuration components and standard dimensions of the basic wheelchair manufactured in the United States are shown in the figure below. (Figure 11–1)

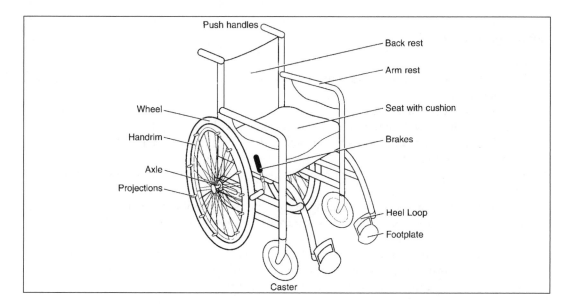

FIGURE 11–1. Manual Wheelchair. From Nesathurai S, ed. The Rehabilitation of People with Spinal Cord Injury: A House Officer's Guide. Boston: Arbuckle Academic Publishers, 1999, with permission.

In order to evaluate the specific needs of an individual wheelchair prescription the key items and proper patient measurements must be remembered. (Figure 11–2)

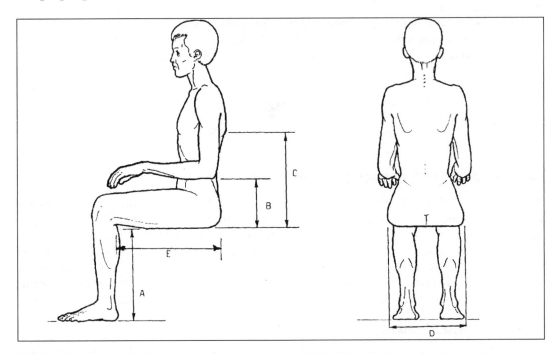

FIGURE 11–2. Critical body measures for wheelchairs (see text). From Wilson AB, Jr. Wheelchairs, A Prescription Guide, 2nd edition. New York: Demos Medical Publishing, 1992, with permision.

Seat (Figure 11–2)

Seat Width
- The selection of a proper seat is important for stability, comfort, ease of propulsion, and skin integrity
- There are two types of seats:
  - The vinyl sling seat—easy to fold, easy to clean, and lightweight
  - Solid Seat—firm, but provides better postural control. It is heavier and makes the chair more difficult to fold
- ⌨ Patients should not sit directly on either seat. All patients should receive some type of cushion
- Seat width is determined by measuring across the widest point of the hips (with clothing and any braces or orthosis). Once this distance is obtained, add one inch (1″) to this measurement. (Figure 11–2 D)
- ⌨ If the wheelchair is too narrow, transfers and access to the chair are difficult and pressure skin breakdown is more likely to develop. If the seat is too wide, truncal support is compromised, leading to scoliosis, back pain, and difficulty with wheelchair propulsion

Seat Depth
- This is determined by measuring from the dorsal buttocks to the popliteal fossa and subtracting 2–3″ from this measurement. If the backrest is cushioned, the thickness of the cushion must be added. (Figure 11–2 E)
- ⌨ If the seat depth is too shallow, ischial pressure is increased and stability of the chair is decreased

Seat Height
- This is determined by measuring from the bottom of the heel to the posterior thigh, then adding 2″ to compensate for leg rest clearance. (Figure 11–2 A) Consider the cushion thickness and its relative additional height. Foam cushions compress to 1/2 their normal size
- ⌨ Variations on seat height measurements occur in the foot drive, or hemiplegic chair, which is designed with the seat closer to the floor to allow the unaffected leg to propel the chair

Backrest
- Seat backs vary depending on the needs of the patient
- The backrest should be high enough to support the patient, but not inhibit movement
- The scapula should not hang over the chair. This is measured by the distance from the bottom of the buttocks to the level of the spine of the scapula. (Figure 11-2 C)
- If the backrest is too high, it may interfere with shoulder movement. If it is too low, it will not provide adequate trunk stability
- If the patient has good trunk control and can propel a wheelchair, 3″ is subtracted from this measurement
- If the patient has poor trunk muscles, but can still propel a wheelchair, 2″ is subtracted from this measurement
- If the patient has no upper extremity strength and poor trunk control, a full measurement is taken with the possible addition of a headrest and recliner mechanism

Recline and Tilt Backrest Mechanism
- These systems can be manually or power controlled and are for patients prone to skin pressure breakdown, patients who cannot sit fully erect, have poor sitting balance, poor endurance, orthostasis, respiratory needs, or otherwise need to be able to adjust the backrest. The most important reason is to perform adequate weight shifts and prevent skin breakdown. These systems add weight and bulk and require a longer wheel base to maintain adequate stability when the chair is reclined

A. Recliner Back
- Semirecliner can be adjusted to 30 degrees. The chair is 3″ longer and is more difficult to propel. Shear forces are increased when reclined
- Full recliner reclines to 90 degrees and is 6″ longer than the standard chair
- ⌨ There are low and zero shear recliners; however, no system will completely eliminate shear forces
- Power recliner advantages:
  Independent pressure relief
  Can assist in orthostatic episodes
  Allows for passive range of motion (PROM) of hip and knee
  Makes it easier to perform catheterization
  Can help mobilize secretion
- Power recliner disadvantages:
  May result in shear forces
  Can increase spasticity
  Increased turning radius

B. Tilt-in-Space (Fig. 11–3)
- This is an alternative to the recliner system

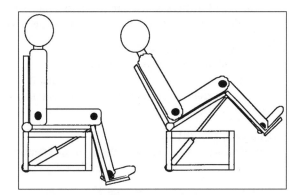

FIGURE 11–3 Schematic for tilt-in-space mechanism. The user remains in the same position but orientation changes. This allows pressure to be redistributed. From Cooper RA, Wheelchair Selection and Configuration. New York: Demos Medical Publishing, 1998, with permission.

- The entire seat and back are tilted as a single unit
- The angle of the seat and back itself does not change. The user remains in the same position but orientation changes. This allows pressure to be redistributed. This decreases shear forces to a minimum
- 📖 In order to redistribute skin pressure, the system must tilt at least 35–40 degrees. Most systems allow 45 degrees of tilt
- Tilt-in-space advantages:
    - Independent pressure relief
    - Can assist in orthostatic episodes
    - Alleviates shear
    - Diminishes effects of spasticity during position changes
    - Maintains seating position during weight shifts
    - Helps mobilize secretions
    - Tighter turning radius
- Tilt-in-space disadvantages:
    - No ROM benefits
    - May not offer as much pressure relief as a recliner
    - If using a leg bag, urine may run backwards in the tilted position
    - Difficult to maintain items on a lap tray when tilted
    - May require a raised door in van secondary to height of tilt-in-space wheelchair
    - More difficult to perform catheterization

Armrests

- Chair arms may be fixed, swing-away or fully removable; adjustable or fixed height, full length or desk arm; and made tubular or standard. Chair arms provide arm support, lateral support, and aid patients who must elevate their body at regular intervals to prevent pressure breakdown
- The arm height is measured from the buttocks to the bottom of the patient's bent elbow at 90 degrees. The measurement must be done with the cushion; 1" is added to this measurement

Fixed vs. Removable
- Fixed armrests are lighter, but not usually prescribed secondary to interference with transfers and activities of daily living. Fixed armrests do not add width to the chair
- Removable armrests are for patients that are close to being independent with transfers. The width is increased by 2". Weight is also increased

Full Length vs. Desk Arm
- Fixed and removable are available
- Full length offers more arm support and adjusts with sit to stand positioning. The disadvantage is that the patient will be unable to get close to any table
- Desk arm allows table access.

Adjustable Height Armrests
- Adjustable height is available as an alternative to ordering a fixed custom height
- Adjustable armrests are heavier than fixed

Tubular vs. Standard Armrests
- Tubular arms are more cosmetic, but not suited for heavier individuals (over 200 pounds)
- They are not used when upper extremity weight shifts are necessary.

Variations:
Wraparound armrests are removable and attach behind the seat. This feature does not increase the width of the wheelchair.

Swing-away or flip-up armrests are preferred by active SCI patients. Younger patients prefer no armrests if balance is not a concern. The removable desk arm is the most popular type prescribed

Wheels (Figure 11–4)

- The standard chair comes with 2–8" diameter front caster wheels and 2–24" diameter rear wheels. However, rear wheels with a diameter of 20–22" are available.
- Mag wheels are most common. They are one piece and are now cast with metal alloys or metal and plastic to weigh no more than the wire spoke wheel and are maintenance free
- Spoke wheels, similar to a bicycle wheel, are lighter and easier to propel and improve shock absorption. However, in the past, they required more maintenance secondary to bending and loosening

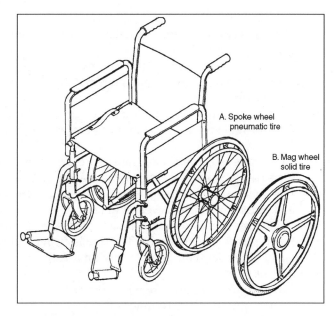

FIGURE 11–4. Wheels for wheelchairs. **A:** Spoke wheel, pneumatic tire. **B:** Mag wheel, solid tire. From Wilson, AB Jr. Wheelchairs, A Prescription Guide, 2nd ed. New York: Demos Medical Publishing, 1992, with permission

Adjusting Axle Position (Figure 11–5)

- 📖 The wheel axle can be moved forward to allow for easier "wheelies" in the SCI patient
- 📖 The axle can also be moved posteriorly to increase stability and compensate for the change in the location of the center of gravity in the absence of legs. This is a consideration in the bilateral amputee patient, or with a recliner or tilt system wheelchair
- 📖 The more posterior the rear wheels:
  The greater the rolling resistance
  The more energy required for propulsion
  The greater the turning radius
  The more stable the chair
- 📖 The more anterior the rear wheels:
  The less the rolling resistance
  Less energy is required to propel
  The smaller the turning radius
  The less stable the chair
  The more maneuverable the chair

Tires

There are several types of tires available for use with either the wire spoke or one-piece wheel.

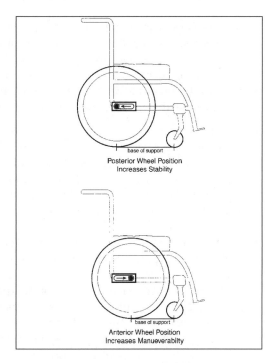

FIGURE 11–5. Adjusting Axle Position. From Nesathurai S. The Rehabilitation of People with Spinal Cord Injury: A House Officer's Guide. Boston: Arbuckle Academic Publishers, 1999, with permission

- *Solid rubber tires*
  - Have a very low rolling resistance on flat or smooth surfaces
  - Flat tires do not occur
  - Lack "cushioning" on rougher terrain.
  - Rubber tires are heavier than pneumatic.
- *Pneumatic tires*
  - Contain air inner tube and are lightweight
  - They provide the best ride on most surfaces, but not as good as rubber on smooth surfaces
  - 📖 If there is carpeting on most surfaces, pneumatic tires are best because carpeting increases the rolling resistance by a factor of 4
  - Pneumatic tires provide cushioning for outdoor use to allow a more comfortable ride and reduce wheelchair wear and tear
  - Pneumatic tires also come with an airless (flat-free) insert that is a soft rubber or *latex gel* that replaces the inner tube. The ride is cushioned and it does not go flat. However, it is slightly heavier than the basic pneumatic tire
- *All-terrain tires*
  - Have a wire tread and are wider overall
  - They require a standard inner tube
  - They are used for mobility on soft and sandy terrain and are up to 2-1/2" thick.
- *Kevlar® tires*
  - Made of Kevlar®
  - Can have air
  - Provide a durable and smooth ride

Camber
- Camber is the wheel angle against the vertical axis
- Camber makes the wheelchair easier to propel (especially at higher speeds), increases stability, and tightens the tuning radius
- An angle of 7 degrees maximizes lateral stability
- The disadvantages are increased overall width of the chair up to 6", increased tire wear, and lower seat height which may increase wear and tear of the shoulder joint

Handrims
- Handrims are attached to the driving wheels to allow propulsion and control safety without touching the tire directly to avoid soiling the hands
- The handrim is also smaller than the wheel making the chair easier to propel
- The larger the diameter of the handrim, the easier it is to grasp and propel, but it becomes heavier with increased thickness and requires an increased number of arm strokes to cover a given distance
- The standard handrim is the circular steel tube; however, for individuals who have difficulty with gripping the smooth surface vinyl, rubber or plastic coating is available with optional glove use
- There are also vertical, horizontal, or oblique projections to improve propulsion. However, horizontal and oblique projections increase the width of the chair
- Another variation is the one-hand drive chair for individuals with plexus injury, upper extremity amputee or hemiplegia. (Figure 11–6)
- The wheelchair can have interconnected driving wheels so that both wheels can be controlled from one side through a dual set of handrims
- When one handrim is moved independently of the other, only one wheel moves. When both rims are grasped together, both wheels are driven simultaneously

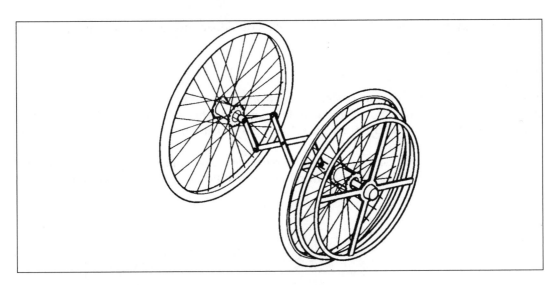

FIGURE 11–6. Mechanism for a one-hand drive chair. From Wilson AB, Jr. Wheelchairs, A Prescription Guide, 2nd ed. New York: Demos Medical Publishing, 1992, with permission.

Casters
- Casters allow steering of the wheelchair and are available in 8″, 5″, and 2″
- The smaller and narrower the caster, the lighter and more maneuverable the chair
- A smaller caster allows a shorter turning radius but performs poorly on outdoor surfaces and on carpets allowing the chair to wobble on uneven surfaces
- The 8″ diameter caster is standard on the basic chair. It is used on smooth surfaces and indoors. 8″ casters may also be ordered with pneumatic or semipneumatic tires to be used on rough surfaces or outdoors
- Larger diameter casters make it easier to maneuver curves, but may shake or flutter
- The 5″ model caster is used in many sports-chairs and on children's chairs
- Caster placement more posteriorly decreases the turning radius, decreases stability and increases maneuverability. (Refer to Figure 11–5)

Front Rigging
- The front rigging is the term used to describe the footrest and legrest collectively.
- Footrest consists of a support bracket with a foot plate
- Footrests are measured by taking the distance from the heel to the under surface of the thigh at the popliteal fossa. Footrests are usually adjustable and should have 2″ of clearance from the floor
- Footrests may be fixed or swing-away
- Swing-away footrests are the most common and allow for easier transfers. Swing-away removable rests help with portability of the chair. Swing-away rests are heavier than fixed
- Fixed footrests allow for a lighter chair, but interfere with transfers and portability
- Legrest consists of an elevating support bracket with swing-away mechanism, a foot plate and a calf pad to support the back of the leg when elevated
- Elevating legrests help with decreasing dependent edema and come with a calf support for the lower leg. Elevating legrests are essential in below the knee amputee patients, patients with knee extension contractures, or other joint abnormalities
- A footrest that is excessively long increases pressure over the lower posterior thigh or hit the floor on uneven surfaces. A footrest that is too short increases pressure over the ischial tuberosities by increasing knee elevation and shifting the patient within the seat. Foot- and

legrests may be ordered differently for each side depending on the patient's particular needs

Wheelchair Cushions (Figure 11–7)

Many different designs of seat cushions are available. Selection of seat cushions may be divided into 6 basic types shown in the table below. All wheelchairs should be used with a seat cushion. Patients should not sit directly on the constructed seat (sling or rigid) of the wheelchair.

Seating should provide proper pressure relief, enhance truncal and pelvic stability and provide comfort. Cushions should be durable and should not retain perspiration or unacceptable odors.

	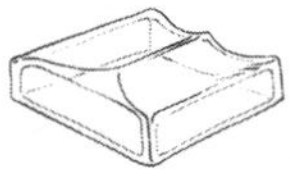 Contoured foam with gel insert	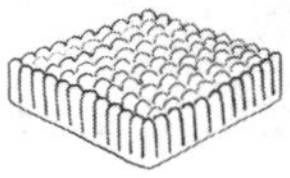 Air-filled villous	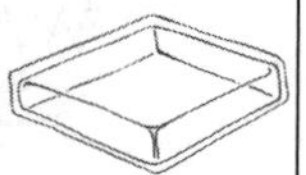 Gel-filled	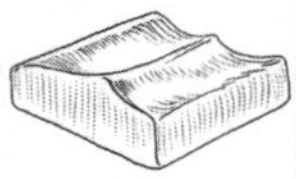 Coated contoured foam	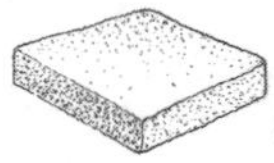 Foam	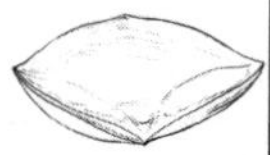 Air-filled
Pressure relief	GOOD	EXCELLENT	GOOD	FAIR TO GOOD	FAIR TO GOOD	FAIR
Seating stability	GOOD TO EXCELLENT	POOR TO FAIR	FAIR TO GOOD	EXCELLENT	GOOD	GOOD TO EXCELLENT
Heat dissipation	FAIR TO GOOD	GOOD TO EXCELLENT	EXCELLENT	FAIR TO POOR	FAIR	FAIR TO GOOD
Cleanability	EXCELLENT	EXCELLENT	EXCELLENT	EXCELLENT	POOR	EXCELLENT
Durability	GOOD TO EXCELLENT	FAIR TO GOOD	FAIR	EXCELLENT	FAIR TO GOOD	GOOD
Cost	HIGH	HIGH	MODERATE TO HIGH	MODERATE TO HIGH	LOW TO MODERATE	LOW

FIGURE 11–7. Wheelchair Cushions.

Safety Equipment

When ordering a wheelchair prescription, items should also include specific safety equipment.

Seat belt
- Seat belts should be worn for safety. The individual patient may be extremely cautious while seated in the chair, but unforeseen circumstances surrounding the individual may jar the chair enough to send a patient out of the chair. Seat belts are important not only for safety, but to maintain the pelvis in good position

Brakes or parking locks (Figure 11–8)
- Brakes or parking locks secure the wheels of the chair to avoid rolling away on uneven surfaces and to provide stability during transfers. Locks should not be used to slow a chair. The abrupt stop would result in overturning. Parking locks may be toggle or lever

Selection is based on available upper extremity and hand function. Locks may push or pull closed and can be mounted low or high. High mounted locks are easier but may interfere with transfers. Additional brake extensions are for patients who cannot reach form the ipsilateral side such as the hemiplegic patient.

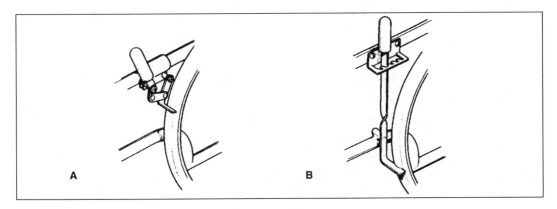

FIGURE 11–8. Two types of parking brakes. **A:** toggle type. **B:** lever type. Variations of these two types of brakes are available. From Wilson AB, Jr. Wheelchairs, A Prescription Guide 2nd ed. New York: Demos Medical Publishing, 1992, with permission.

Grade aides
- Grade aides prevent the chair from rolling backwards and are helpful for patients with limited strength and endurance where inclines prove challenging

Antitipping devices
- Antitipping devices can be fixed or removable and are extensions placed on the lower rail of the chair to prevent the chair from falling backwards. They are also available for attachment to the front-rigging to avoid forward tipping. Antitipping devices are mostly used in above-the-knee amputees and in spinal cord injury patients. However, antitipping devices may interfere with curb negotiation in patients independent in community wheelchair mobility.

Control mechanisms for power wheelchairs (Figure 11–9)

Joystick
The patient uses his hand to move the joystick for wheelchair control.

Head control
A specialized headrest allows the patient to drive the wheelchair.

Chin control
A mini joystick, which is used to steer the wheelchair, is mounted in front of the patient's chin.

Sip and puff
The patient pushes air through a straw allowing for control of the wheelchair, and, possibly an environment control unit

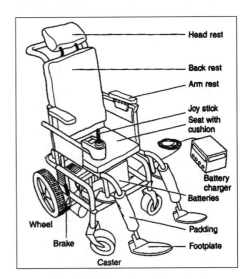

FIGURE 11–9. Typical Power Wheelchair. From Nesathurai S, ed. Rehabilitation of People with Spinal Cord Injury: A House Officer's Guide. Boston: Arbuckle Academic Publishers, 1999, with permission.

TABLE 11–7. Wheelchair Prescriptions for Spinal Cord Injury Patients Based on Motor Level

	Chair Type	Arms	Legs	Seat Belt/Tires	Seat Board	Cushion
High Tetraplegia C2–C4	• Power WC with power-tilt and/or recline • If ventilation dependent then ventilation tray • Control system: depending on functional capabilities (i.e. sip and puff, chin control, head control) • High seat back, head rest, trunk supports	• Upper extremity support such as lap board or arm trough • Removable desk top arms	• Legrests: elevating swing away, removable • Foot support loops	• Seat belt • Rubber tires: solid vs. pneumatic	Rigid Seat Board	• Can't weight shift • Requires excellent pressure relief seat cushion, i.e., air filled villous
C5 Tetraplegia	• Power WC with power tilt and/or recline • Modified joystick or head control to operate wheelchair • High seat back, headrest, trunk supports	• Upper extremity support such as lap board or arm trough • Removable desk top arms	• Legrests: elevating swing-away, removable • Foot support loops	• Seat belt • Rubber tires • (Can use manual WC with projections or lugs for indoor use)	Rigid Seat Board	• Requires excellent pressure relief seat cushion, i.e., air filled villous
C6 Tetraplegia POWER (can use either power or manual)	• Power WC, if independent in pressure relief, no need for power tilt or recline • Joystick controls • High back seat	• Removable desk top arms	• Legrests: elevating swing-away, removable • Foot support loops	• Seat belt • Rubber tires: solid vs. pneumatic	Rigid Seat Board	• Requires excellent pressure relief seat cushion, i.e., air filled villous
C6 Tetraplegia MANUAL (can use either power or manual)	• Manual WC: lightweight, adjustable chair with solid back • Adjustable wheel positioning • Brake extensions	• Removable desk top arms	• Legrests: elevating swing-away, removable • Foot support loops	• Seat belt • Rubber tires • Modified handrims i.e. lugs or plastic coated	Rigid Seat Board	• Requires excellent pressure relief seat cushion, i.e., air filled villous
C7–T1 Tetraplegia	• Manual WC: lightweight with solid back • Adjustable wheel position • Brake extension	• Removable desk top arms	• Legrests: elevating swing-away, removable • Foot support loops	• Seat belt • Rubber tires • Modified handrims i.e. lugs or plastic coated	Rigid Seat Board	• Requires excellent pressure relief seat cushion, i.e., air filled villous
T2 Paraplegia and Below	• Manual WC: lightweight • Adjustable wheel position • Back height may be lowered due to better truncal support	• Arm rests may not be necessary	• Legrests: elevating swing-away, removable • Foot support loops	• Seat belt • Rubber tires • Axle position can be placed anteriorly for improved maneuverability	Rigid Seat Board	• Good pressure relief seat cushion

768

TABLE 11-8. Wheelchair (WC) Prescriptions for Hypothetical Patients

	Chair Type	Arms	Legs	Seat Belt/Tires	Seat Board	Cushion
Orthopaedic Patient With BLE Edema	Standard WC–50 lbs.	Removable desk top arms	• Legrests elevating, swing-away, removable • Foot support are foot plates	• Seat belt • Rubber tires	Rigid Seat Board	Moderate pressure relief cushion
Orthopaedic Patient S/P MI	Light weight–37 lbs.	Removable desk top arms	• Legrests elevating, swing-away, removable • Foot support are foot plates	• Seat belt • Rubber tires	Rigid Seat Board	Moderate pressure relief cushion
Amputee	Standard amputee chair • Wheels set back further for center of gravity • Amputee board or legrest	Removable desk top arms or full length arms if patient has difficulty transferring	• *Amputated Side:* Amputee board • *Unaffected Side:* Legrests elevating, swing-away, removable Foot support are foot plates	• Seat belt • Rubber tires	Seat board with amputee extension	Moderate pressure relief cushion
Hemiplegic Patient	Standard or lightweight Hemiplegic chair: this chair is lower so the patient can self-propel with hand and foot (may need super low chair if 2″ cushion is ordered)	• Removable desk top arms or full length arms if patient has difficulty transferring • Arm board or lap board (clear if L. neglect present) • Brake extension on weak side	• *Hemiplegic Side:* Legrests elevating, swing-away, removable Foot support are foot plates • *Unaffected Side:* None	• Seat belt • Rubber tires • Seat board		Moderate pressure relief cushion
General Paraplegic Athlete (WC will vary significantly for different sports)	Standard lightweight WC 37 lbs. OR • Quickie WC 19 lbs. • Brakes set low for patients with large push stroke • Camber is adjusted according to sport • Anti-tippers are necessary in certain sports (front and/or rear) • Racing WC may have 3 or 4 wheels	Arm rests are usually not necessary	Footrests: plates or loops	Seat belt • Casters are smaller and narrower making the chair more maneuverable • Rubber tires are higher pressure making it easier to push	Seat Board	Good pressure relief seat cushion

In conclusion, the basic components of wheelchair prescriptions and measurement have been covered. However, there are many accessories available to assist with activities of daily living (ADLs) and everyday functional activities. There are special and custom seating systems available as well as externally powered wheelchairs and scooters, which have not been covered in this basic board review. For further reading and a more in-depth review please refer to the reading list at the end of this chapter.

■

MULTIPLE SCLEROSIS (MS)

DEFINITION

MS is a chronic progressive disease of the central nervous system. Brain and spinal cord are characterized by multiple areas of white matter demyelination (inflammation). These inflammatory sites lead to plaque formation that may recur and enlarge with subsequent exacerbations and remissions.

Older plaques may become sclerosed due to oligodendrocyte destruction, astrocyte proliferation and glial scarring. The oligodendrocyte makes up the myelin in the CNS and plaque formation results in a neuro-dysfunction of conduction (partial or complete) making impulse propagation of the action potential down the nerve impossible. In acute lesions, remyelination may occur which results in a "remission". The autoimmune response causes demyelination, axonal damage, and brain atrophy.

FACTS

- MS is the third leading cause of significant disability in the 20–50 age range
- The exact cause is unknown
- It affects F>M 2:1, Whites>>>>Blacks, Asians (Middle-aged adults)
- There is an increased incidence in the higher socioeconomic class
- (+) Family history involving siblings > parents (4–5%)
- Theories of pathogenesis
  - Genetic factors: Family history (siblings > children), Major histocompatability complex (MHC) on chromosome # 6 (noted more frequently in patients with MS than in controls).
  - Immunologic: T cells travels to the inflamed areas crossing the blood brain barrier
  - Viral: slow virus
- Geographic distribution: Prevalence rate is <1/100,000 in equatorial area compared to 4–6/100,00 in southern Europe and southern United States. In Canada, northern Europe and northern U.S., the rate is 30–80 cases/100,000. Approx. 350,000 people in the USA have MS
- Migration to temperate climate before age 15
- Pregnancy: decreases relapses, then increases after delivery. No change long term

SIX PATTERNS OF MS

1. Relapsing-Remitting

- ⌨ The most common pattern
- Early exacerbations followed by a complete remission. There are long periods of stability with an increase in disability after each remission period

2. Benign

- This results in mild symptoms, early exacerbations and complete remissions (resolution of inflammation, partial remyelination or rerouting of nerve transmission) with minimal or no disability seen after remission

3. Progressive-Relapsing

- Deterioration with relapses, with increasing degree of relapses and residual impairment

4. Primary Progressive

- An insidious onset with a steady progression of symptoms, few remissions and increasing disability. A progression to death can occur in weeks to months. It is more common in the older population

5. Secondary Progressive

- Relapsing, remitting, converting to steady deterioration

6. Malignant (> 5%)

- Rapid and severe (Kraft, 1981)

📖 PROGNOSTIC FACTORS (Table 11–9)

TABLE 11–9. Prognostic Factors of MS

Factors	Good Prognosis	Poorer Prognosis
Age of onset	< 35 years	Male, > 35 years
Symptoms	Monosymptomatic	Polysymptomatic
Onset	Sudden, good recovery with long remission	Rapidly progressive
Findings at onset	Sensory Optic neuritis	Motor (1st sign) Ataxia and tremor
Ambulation	Yes	No
Remission and Relapses	Longer, more complete remissions	Higher relapse rate
Disability	Low current disability	High disability

SIGNS AND SYMPTOMS

The signs and symptoms will depend on the location of the lesion in the central nervous system (CNS) white matter (spinal cord and brain). Onset of the disease may often present as an optic neuritis or transverse myelitis. In advanced stages, Charcot Triad, the combination of scanning speech, intention tremor, and nystagmus may be seen. Paresthesias and gait disturbances are commonly seen as an initial presentation, however, the most common clinical picture is a mixture of the abnormalities listed below.

Common symptoms

- Bladder and Bowel dysfunction
- Fatigue (📖 Central in nature)
- Pain
- Visual disturbances: Optic neuritis, diplopia, nystagmus
- Cerebellum and basal ganglia: ataxia, intention tremor
- Doral column: Sensory abnormalities (paresthesias), impairment of deep sensation, proprioception
- Corticospinal tract: Weakness and spasticity
- Frontal lobe dysfunction: Cognitive, memory, learning, and impaired emotional responses, depression
- Speech abnormalities: Dysarthria
- Brainstem abnormalities: Myokymia, deafness, tinnitus, vertigo, vomiting, transient facial anesthesia, dysphagia

> **Top 3 most prevalent symptoms**
> 1. Bladder and Bowel dysfunction
> 2. Fatigue (📖 Central in nature)
> 3. Pain
>
> (MS Society of Canada, 2003)

> **Top 3 problems affecting ADLs reported by patients:**
> 1. Fatigue
> 2. Balance difficulties
> 3. Weakness
>
> (Kraft, 1986)

📖 Common signs

Lhermitte's sign: Classic but not pathognomonic.
- Passive neck flexion causing an electric shock-like sensation radiating to the spine, shoulders as well as other areas. This sign is most likely a result of the increased sensitivity of the myelin to stretch or traction
- Upper motor neuron signs: Increased muscle stretch reflex (MSR) and plantar responses, spasticity
- Weakness
- Decreased sensation

Note: Not all new symptoms result from new MS lesion. Temporary aggravation of symptoms in old and previously silent lesions may be caused by fever, heat, stress, fatigue, or other medical problems, especially pulmonary or urinary tract infection, dehydration or medication side-effects. Aggravating factors and other medical problems must either be identified and treated, or ruled out.

DIAGNOSIS

Clinical Findings

- 📖 "Lesions scattered in time and space"; a lesion must occur in different locations in the CNS at different points of time.
- Neurologic deficits in 2 or more areas, reflecting white matter involvement, at 2 points in time for >24 hours separately by 1 month
- Age: 10–59 years, commonly 20–40 years
- Two separate attacks with the onset of symptoms at least 1 and up to 6 months apart or progression of the neurologic disease for greater than 6 months
- Two separate lesions in which the symptoms cannot be explained by a single lesion
- Objective deficits seen on exam
- Feature of typical signs and symptoms supported by diagnostic data

Diagnostic Data

📖 There is no pathognomonic test for MS. All labs are nonspecific and are to be interpreted within the clinical picture.

Cerebral Spinal Fluid (CSF) Examination
• Increased in Protein (myelin basic, 25%), Oligoclonal IgG bands (greatest sensitivity), IgG and WBCs

VEP (Visual Evoked Potentials) (high sensitivity along with MRI)
• P100 latency is abnormal (slowing secondary to plaques) in 75%

BAER (Brainstem Auditory Evoked Response)
• Investigates the pontine area displaying an absence or delay of wave formation secondary to the demyelinating process

SEP (Sensory Evoked Potentials)
• Prolongation of absolute peak or interpeak latency

EMG/NCS
• Sensory Nerve Action Potentials (SNAPs), Compound Motor Action Potentials (CMAPs), Conduction Velocity (CV) worsens as the myelin thins
• EMG may show Abnormal activity: Fibs, Positive Sharp Waves (PSW), Facial myokymia and a decrease Motor Unit Action Potentials (MUAP)
• Single Fiber Electromyography (SFEMG): jitter (Grana, 1994)
• Blink Reflex: May be abnormal

📖 MRI (Greatest sensitivity for the diagnosis of MS)
• Multifocal areas of increased intensity (plaques) on T2 weighted images are abnormal in 85% of the cases
• These ovoid-appearing plaques are located in the periventricular white matter (corpus callosum)
• Enhancement with gadolinium may precede the onset of deficits and identify active disease
• May visualize subclinical lesions

CT Scan
• Not effective in visualizing lesion of brainstem, cerebellum, and optic nerve.
• Cerebral atrophy is most common sign.

TREATMENT OF MS

During an acute exacerbation treatment should include a comprehensive rehabilitation program. Relative rest, hydration, bladder and bowel management, PT and OT speech (swallowing protection) and dietary (nutrition) are essential in the care of the patient.

Medications

Immunomodulator agents: Disease-modifying

Corticosteroids (Methylprednisolone)
• Used in short bursts for acute attacks secondary to its anti-inflammatory and anti-edema effects. Acute attacks = "exacerbation" which is new or worsening MS symptoms lasting > 24 hours and not related to metabolic factors (Urinary Tract Infection [UTI], etc.)
• Dose: ~1000mg/day Intravenous IV for 4–7days with a 2 week taper, switch to PO

- Risks: Gastrointestinal (GI) disturbance, fluid retention, mood swings, electrolyte imbalance, insomnia, acne, hyperglycemia, hypertension (HTN)
- Most responsive symptoms: Optic neuritis, brainstem, motor, acute pain, bowel and bladder
- Least responsive: Cerebellar, sensory
- Long-term use leads to increase increased risk of HTN, osteoporosis, diabetes, and cataracts
- Hastens recovery, but does not prevent further attacks or alter disease progression

Three Agents to Alter the Course of the Disease ("A, B, C's")

📖 *Interferon-A (Avonex®) A=Avonex*
- Dose: 6 million units IM Q week
- Side effects: flu-like symptoms, myalgia, fever, chills, asthenia
- 18% reduction in relapse rate

📖 *Interferon-B (Betaseron®) B=Betaseron*
- Dose: 8 million units Subcutaneous QOD.
- Side effects: Flu-like symptoms, increase liver function tests (LFTs), decreased WBC, myalgia, injection site reaction, injection site necrosis (5%)
- 30% reduction in relapse rate

📖 *Glatiramer acetate C=Copaxone*
- Dose: Subcutaneous Injection qd
- Side effects: Self-limited transient flushing, injection site reactions, post injection self-limiting chest tightness
- 32% reduction in relapse rate

📖 Serum neutralizing antibodies may form with Avonex® and Betaseron® (25%) decreasing efficacy

Immunosuppression agents are reserved for patients with unresponsive disabling MS. These are commonly used as second-line medications. The side effects need to be weighed when prescribing these medications and patients should be closely monitored.

Cyclosporin

Cyclophosphamide (Cytotoxin®)—modest improvement

Azathioprine—mixed results

Plasmapheresis

Methotrexate
   Side effects: mucosal ulceration, Bowel Movement (BM) abnormalities, GI.

Current Medications Under Review

Mitoxantrone—IV months, antineoplastic, for advanced MS—pending FDA review for this indication.

Intravenous Immunoglobulin (IVIG)—being studied.

REHABILITATION AND SYMPTOMATIC MANAGEMENT

"Rehab improves outcome in MS" (Greenspun, 1987)

Weakness and fatigue is seen in the Lower Extremity (LE) >> Upper Extremity (UE)

A goal of rehabilitation in MS patients is to prevent deconditioning, disuse atrophy, and muscle weakness to maximize functional potential.

Exercise improves conditioning not weakness.
- Aerobic training increases endurance. Light progressive resistive exercises prevent disuse atrophy allowing for multiple periods of rest. Do not exercise to the point of fatigue

Fatigue worsens with increased temperature, stress, and activity
- Swimming should be done at a cooler temperatures ~ < 84 degrees
- Heat worsens the condition, secondary to delaying impulse conduction. Only a slight increase in temperature is needed to result in a conduction block
- Recommendations: Medications (amantadine, Ritalin®) and avoid increases in temperature. Provigil shows promise as well. Selective Serotonin Reuptake Inhibitors (SSRIs) may help

Spasticity

Three categories of treatment
Physical: Remove noxious stimuli, ROM, positioning, casting and splinting and cryotherapy. Optimize bowel, bladder, and skin management.
Medications: Baclofen (PO or intrathecal) is the drug of choice, used in central spasticity. Other medications include tizanidine, dantrolene, diazepam, clonidine, and clonazepam. Motor point, blocks, nerve blocks and botulinum toxin injections are also used.
Surgery: Rhizotomies, tenotomies, and neurectomies.
An increase in spasticity may be an indication of a coexisting condition including infection, trauma, skin breakdown etc.

Incoordination, Ataxia, Tremor, Dysmetria

- Dysmetria is a lack of harmonious action between muscles during a voluntary movement in which the patient is unable to stop motion at a desired point
- The specific symptoms involved will depend on the specific location of the plaques in relation to the white matter tracts: spinocerebellar, cerebrum, and dorsal columns
- Rehabilitation includes: PT and OT for balance training, relaxation techniques; weighted ankle cuffs and utensils may assist ambulation and ADLs for the patients with proprioception abnormalities. Frenkel's exercises to treat ataxia
- Medications used with limited success: isoniazid (INH), primidone, clonazepam (Klonopin®), Depakote®, Inderal®, hydroxyzine

Sensory Disturbance Pain Syndrome

Therapeutic modalities (TENS, PT and OT), behavior modification and trials of various medications may be used to control the sensory dysesthesias that can be associated with MS. Medications include: Neurontin®, Tegretol®, TCA (Elavil®, Pamelor®), Dilantin®, capsaicin.

Fatigue—see above

Overwhelming exhaustion unique from normal fatigue
Better in morning
Impact motor, cognition, self-care, etc.
Worse with depression, heat intolerance, vigorous exercise, stress, spasticity
Rule out other causes (i.e., anemia, hypothyroidism, medication induced, depression, etc.)
Energy conservation, work simplification, economy of efforts, pacing, education

Visual Impairment/Eye Findings

Optic Neuritis
Acute (hours to days) inflammatory demyelination of the optic nerve. Seen in 1/4 of all MS patients

Clinical: Blurred vision, complete or partial loss of vision may be found in one eye. Vision loss may be preceded by pain around the eye. A central scotoma (area of blindness) is a common visual field defect. Residual decreased activity, photophobia, or pain possible.

Treatment: IV methylprednisolone is more effective than PO prednisone

📖 **Internuclear ophthalmoplegia**
- Demyelinating lesion of the medial longitudinal fasciculus (MLF)
- Paresis of the medial rectus muscle resulting in an inability to adduct the eye seen with voluntary lateral gaze. This lesion is usually accompanied by nystagmus
- Convergence, which does not run in the path of the MLF, involves a different pathway and is intact. Convergence runs from the retina to the midbrain nuclei via the pathway of the optic nerve, tract, chiasm and lateral geniculate terminating in the bilateral CN III nuclei
- Nystagmus, diplopia, blurred and decreased vision, patching and prisms

Bladder Dysfunction (Table 11–10)

(See Chapter 7: Spinal Cord Injury, for more in-depth discussion of bladder)

TABLE 11–10. Three Types of Bladders Seen in MS

	Failure to store (most common)	Failure to Empty	Combination/Bldder
Disorder	• Hyperactive bladder with a small capacity and weak sphincter (adrenergic)	• Big boggy bladder • Closed sphincter	• Detrusor sphincter dyssynergia (CDSD)
Problem	• Incontinence • Dribbling of urine	• Failure to void	• Bladder contracts • Sphincter closes • Backflow of urine to the kidney
Treatment	Smooth muscle relaxant (detrusor) • Ditropan® • Pro-Banthine® • Levsin® • Tolterodine (Detrol®)	Smooth muscle contractor • Urecholine External sphincter relaxant Alpha antagonist • Minipress®, Flomax®	• Intermittent cath • Anticholinergics for storing between cath. • Alpha-antagonists used by some. • Urethral stent or sphincterotomy
		• Self Intermittent Catheterization Placement	

Other Abnormalities

- **Bowel Dysfunction:** Constipation is commonly seen. An early bowel program is recommended
- **Dysphagia:** Impairment of cranial nerves (V, VII, IX, XII) may lead to swallowing abnormalities. Speech therapy to perform a swallowing evaluation is essential to prevent any complications such as aspiration. Delayed swallowing, pooling may be seen. Treatment includes exercise, positioning, and a change of food consistency
- **Dysarthria**
- **Sexual dysfunction**
- **Cognitive/affective impairments:** Euphoria may be caused by frontal lobe lesions or corticosteroids use. Depression is a common finding and should be addressed by rehab psych. 📖 The IQ of MS patients is usually intact, especially early on. Processing speed is often delayed. (Peterson, 1989)

- General intelligence in MS changes gradually over time, and verbal skills are affected less than performance skills
- 70% have neuropsychic abnormalities
- Suicide rate 7.5 × higher than normal population
- Decreased short-term memory, decreased reasoning, slow processing
- Depression

OUTCOME IN MS

In general, 85% of patients with MS will have a normal life expectancy, however, the unpredictable outcome of the disease and variable nature of its impairment make predicting it difficult.
- Seldom fatal
- 1/3 require ambulatory assistance within 10 years of diagnosis (2/3 don't)

Minimal Record of Disability (MRD)

This consists of different types of rating scales that profile the main dysfunctions of MS.
- The most common scale used is the Kurtzke Expanded Disability Status Scale (EDSS)
  - A 10-level rating scale used in MS examining 8 different neurologic systems
  - Rating scale:
        0 = normal
        4 = severe disability, but still ambulatory without aid
        8 = bedbound
        10 = death
  - Areas tested: pyramidal, cerebellar, brainstem, sensory, bowel and bladder, vision, mental status, and general.
- Other outcome scales used in MS include:
  - Kurtzke Functional Systems (FS)
  - Incapacity Status Scale (ISS)
  - Environmental Status Scale (ESS)

MRD = EDSS, ISS, and EES
FIM: Functional Independence Measure—assesses disability and the need for assistance. Does not assess vision. (Kurtzke, 1983) (See Figure 8–4)

▪

OSTEOPOROSIS

DEFINITION

Disease characterized by bone mass reduction and deterioration in the bone microarchitecture. It is caused by an imbalance between bone formation and bone resorption (ultimately leading to osteopenia).

Definition per World Health Organization (WHO)

1. **The young adult bone density mean** is the expected normal value of the patient's peak bone density at about age 20 compared to others of the same sex and ethnicity
2. **T score** is the standard deviation (SD) above or below the young adult mean

3. **Normal Bone Density:** Bone density within 1 standard deviation (SD) of the mean for young adults (T score > –1)
4. **Osteopenia:** Low bone mass with bone density between 1.0–2.5 standard deviation below the mean for young adults (T score between –1 and –2.5)
5. **Osteoporosis:** Bone density more than 2.5 SD below mean of normal young adult (T score ≤ 2.5)
6. **Z score:** Is the number of SD the patient's bone density is above or below the values expected for the patient's age, i.e., age-matched.
7. **Peak Bone Mass (PBM):** The highest level of bone mass achieved as a result of normal growth, generally occurs between adolescence and age 30 years, with variation at specific skeletal sites

T-score:	–2.5	–1	0	+1	2.5
	osteoporosis osteopenia		within normal range		

FACTS ABOUT OSTEOPOROSIS

- Most common metabolic bone disease
- In osteoporosis there is a normal ratio of organic and mineral components but less bone tissue, differs from osteomalacia (bone tissue is normal or increased, but reduced mineral content to organic component ratio).
- First clinical presentation is usually a fracture
- Major underlying cause of long bone fractures in the elderly is osteoporosis
- Diagnosis is not dependent on a fracture

EPIDEMIOLOGY

- There are >1.2 million fractures/year in the United States related to osteoporosis
- ~ 70% of fractures in people > 45 years old are related to osteoporosis
- 1/3 of females > 65 years old will have vertebral fracture
- In the greater population, > 75 years old, half the population affected, males and females equally
- Hip fracture is a significant cause of morbidity and mortality in Caucasian women aged 50 years and above, and to a lesser extent Caucasian men of similar age
  - 17.5% of these women will sustain a hip fracture compared to 6% of men
  - Fractures usually result in temporary disability, but approx. 50% of females with hip fractures admitted to nursing home, 14% of these patients in nursing home after 1 year
  - Morbidity: 50% of patients with hip fracture require assistance ADLs, 15%–25% long-term placement
  - Mortality: 10%–20% of patients die due to complications
- National Osteoporosis Foundation (NOF) uses the quality adjusted life year (QALY) of fractures to determine the impact of osteoporotic fractures on a person's life (Matkovic, 1996)

Living bone is never metabolically at rest, so it constantly remodels and reappropriates its matrix and mineral stores along lines of mechanical stress. The factors that control bone formation and resorption are not well understood, but in the adult skeleton under normal

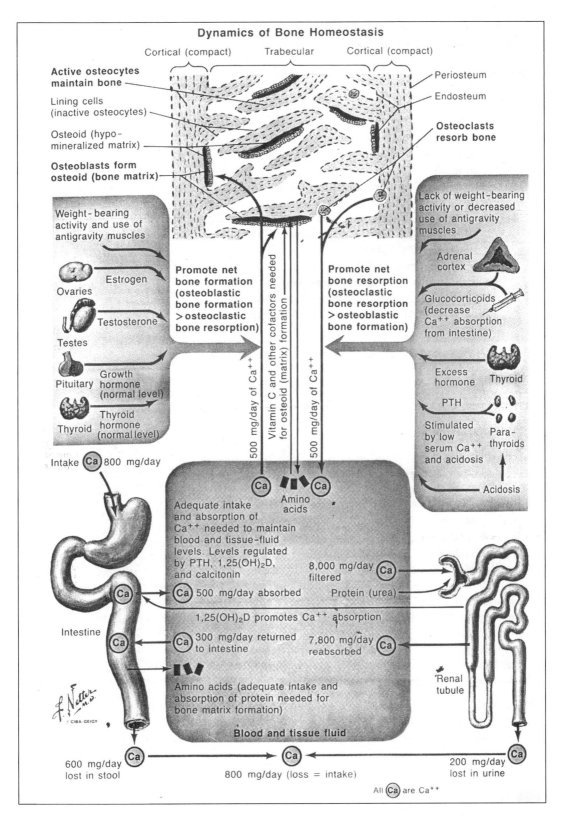

FIGURE 11–10. Calcium Cycle. From Kaplan FS. Prevention and Management of Osteoporosis. Clinical Symposia 1995; 47(1) Copyright Ciba-Geigy, with permission.

remodeling conditions, the two processes are exquisitely coupled so that net bone formation equals net bone resorption (Figure 11–10).

CLASSIFICATION

1. Generalized—affects different parts of whole skeleton

Primary
Basic etiology unknown
- Involutional—most common
  - Postmenopausal (Type I)
    Females 50–65 years old—affects women only within menopause, lasting 15–20 years
    Trabecular > cortical bone loss
    Most fractures in spine, hip, and wrist (Colles fracture) i.e., axial skeleton
  - Senile (Type II)—age-associated osteoporosis
    > 70 years old, 2 (F):1(M)
    Trabecular ≈ cortical bone loss
    Fractures: hip, spine, pelvis, humerus
- Juvenile—children and adolescents, self-limited
- Idiopathic—premenopausal females, middle-aged males

Secondary
Acquired or inherited diseases/medications (Type III)

Diseases:
- Hyperparathyroidism
- Hyperthyroidism
- Cushing's Disease
- Hypophosphatasia
- Hypogonadism
- Hypoestrogenism—anorexia, exercise induced amenorrhea
- Renal disease
- Chronic Obstructive Pulmonary Disease (COPD)
- Systemic Mastocytosis
- Rheumatoid Arthritis
- Diabetes Mellitus
- Idiopathic Hypercalciuria
- Gastrointestinal disease—malabsorption syndromes, liver disease, partial gastrectomy
- Alcoholism
- Nutrition—vitamin deficiency, calcium deficiency, high sodium, protein, phosphate, and caffeine intakes
- Malignancy—multiple myeloma, lymphoma, leukemia
- Immobility—paraplegia, hemiplegia, immobilization, prolonged bedrest
- Loss of ovarian function/estrogen depletion, testosterone deficiency

Medications:
- Corticosteroids—most common form of secondary osteoporosis, inhibits bone formation, mainly trabecular bone loss, compression deformities of the vertebrae and pelvis
- Heparin
- Anticonvulsants
- Excess Thyrosine
- Lithium
- Loop diuretics

2. Localized—discrete regions of reduced bone mass

Primary
- Transient regional—rare, migratory, predominantly involves hip, usually self-limited
- Reflex sympathetic dystrophy—radiographic changes may occur in first 3–4 weeks, showing patchy demineralization of affected area

Secondary
- Immobilization, inflammations, tumors, necrosis

RISK FACTORS FOR OSTEOPOROSIS:

Increased Risk
- Caucasian
- Female
- Advanced age
- Thin habitus
- Smoking
- Excess alcohol
- Excess caffeine intake
- Inactivity/Immobilization
- Diminished peak bone mass (PBM) at skeletal maturity
- History of fracture as adult
- Positive family history
- Loss of ovarian function/estrogen depletion, testosterone deficiency
- Exercise-induced amenorrhea

Decreased Risk
- Obesity

PATHOGENESIS

Multifactorial cause for reduced bone mass including genetic and environmental factors.

Main Determinants of Osteoporosis

Failure to achieve adequate peak bone mass (PBM) at skeletal maturity

Rate of bone loss

- After PBM is achieved, bone loss occurs gradually thereafter, with the most rapid bone loss in early post-menopausal period in females
- Rate of age related bone loss is approximately 0.25%–1.0% per year in males and females
- Immediate post-menopausal period: 3%–5% bone loss per year in females for approx. 5–7 years after onset of menopause
- Lifetime bone loss: 20%–30% in males, 45%–50% in females
- Greatest contributor to bone loss in mature adults is due to loss of gonadal function

Quality of bone microstructures and ability for bone tissue repair

- Normal bone turnover: There is an increase in bone resorption followed by increase in bone formation within 40–60 days = no net change (bone remodeling is coupled)
- Bone remodeling occurs throughout life and increases in older people
- Remodeling cycle takes approximately 3 months—osteoclasts resorb bone, then osteoblasts lay down new osteoid in cavity
- Major function of bone remodeling—repair of skeletal microfractures (trabecular perforation) and the release of Ca^+ into circulation

- The basic abnormality of osteoporosis is a disturbance of normal bone remodeling sequence at tissue level
- In osteoporosis: bone resorption increases without corresponding increase in bone formation = net loss on bone mass (negatively uncoupled)

PHYSIOLOGY

Cellular Components of Bone Remodeling

- **Osteoblasts**—bone forming cells form organic matrix which is mineralized to form normal lamellar bone
- **Osteoclasts**—bone resorption cells
- **Osteocytes**—osteoblasts incorporated in new bone matrix

Skeletal Mass Components

Cortical (compact) bone
- Dense outer shell of bone
- Concentric lamellae, Haversian systems
- 80% of skeleton, most in shafts (diaphysis) long bones
- Accounts for majority of skeletal mechanical strength

Trabecular bone (cancellous, spongy)
- Found in central medullary canal, encloses marrow space
- Irregular branching plates, circumferential lamellae
- 20% of total skeleton, found in vertebrae and flat bones (axial skeleton), ends of long bones
- Vertebral bodies 42%, whole vertebrae 25%
- More metabolically active than cortical bone
- Preferentially altered in osteoporosis type I

Minerals, Hormones, Vitamins
- Calcium phosphate—in the form of hydroxyapatite
  Major component of bone
  Regulated by Parathyroid Hormone (PTH), calcitonin, and vitamin D; 99% of a body's calcium is in bone
- PTH—regulated by Ca^+ concentration
  Effects:
      In bone—activates osteoclasts (bone resorption cells)
      In intestine—stimulates formation of vitamin D in kidneys (inactive form Vitamin D → active form Vitamin D), which results in increases Ca^+ uptake
      In kidneys—increased phosphate excretion increases calcium reabsorption
- Calcitonin
      Synthesized by C cells in thyroid glands
      Inhibits osteoclast activity and increases incorporation of Ca^+ into bone and decreases serum Ca^+ levels
- Vitamin D (1,25—Dihydroxyvitamin D_3)
      In intestine—enhances Ca^+ and phosphorus absorption in gut
      In kidneys—increases reabsorption of Ca^+, phosphorus

DIAGNOSIS

First clinical indication is usually a fracture
- Fracture of proximal femur, distal forearm
  Usually associated with minimal trauma

Pain usually present
- Fracture of vertebrae
Usually associated with minimal trauma
Pain or asymptomatic

EVALUATION

History/Physical Exam

Evaluate for presence of risk factors or medical conditions

Lab Studies

Lab studies performed mainly to exclude other diseases
Minimal work-up:
– serum Ca^+, phosphorus, total alkaline phosphatase
Maximum work-up:
– Ionized Ca^+, ESR, vitamin D, protein electrophoresis, thyroid function tests, simultaneous multiple analyzer 12 (SMA12), complete blood count (CBC), testosterone, serum and urine markers, urine Ca^+/Creatinine ratio
– Iliac crest bone biopsy with tetracycline labeling (osteoporosis—thin cortices and decreased number of trabeculae)

Markers of Bone Resorption

Elevated levels of calcium/creatinine ratio in fasting urine, hydroxyproline/creatinine ratio in fasting urine, collagen cross links (pyridinolines, telopeptides), TRAP (tartrate resistant acid phosphatase)

Markers for Bone Formation

Serum osteocalcin y-carboxyglutamic acid (GLA) protein
Serum total and bone specific alkaline phosphatase
Procollagen Propeptide

Bone Mass Measurement

X-ray
- Insensitive in assessment of quantifying bone mass; 30–35% bone mass loss occurs before demineralization detected
- *Findings:*
    Cortical thinning
    Trabecular pattern coarsened due to loss of small trabeculae
- *Findings in the spine:*
    Increased radiolucency
    Increased prominence of endplates
    Increased concavity of endplates if nucleus pulposus is not degenerated (codfish vertebrae)
    Anterior wedging
    Vertebral body height loss
    Compression fractures

Single Photon Absorptiometry (SPA)/ Single X-ray Absorptiometry (SXA)
- Inexpensive
- Low radiation dose
- Requires water bath or gel immersion

- Uses I^{125} (SPA, a radioactive isotope) or x-ray source (SXA)
- Site measured: Radius, calcaneus
- Limited to bone measurement of peripheral skeleton; unable to measure bone density of hip or spine

Dual Photon Absorptiometry (DPA)
- No water bath or immersion needed
- Uses AGD^{153} source, a radioactive isotope
- Less accurate and precise than dual energy x-ray absorptiometry (DXA)
- Increased scan time
- Sites measured: Proximal femur, lumbar spine

Dual Energy X-ray Absorptiometry (DXA)
- Preferred measurement technique "The Gold Standard" for bone density measurement
- Accurate, precise, fast
- Low radiation exposure (scan times are shorter than with DPA and radiation dose is very low)
- Uses x-ray source instead of an isotope source
- There is suspicion because the radiation source does not decay and the energy stays constant over time
- Allows assessment axial or peripheral skeleton or entire skeleton
- Sites measured: spine, hip radius
- Proximal femur density measurement useful for predicting hip fractures
- Lumbar spine density measurement useful for monitoring response to therapy
- Spinal osteophytes and aortic calcifications may contribute to false high readings

Quantitative Computed Tomography (QCT)
- Can localize an area of interest
- Allows measurement of trabecular bone alone of spine, apart from cortical bone
- High-dose radiation
- Expensive
- Sites measured: Spine, hip radius
- Accuracy compromised by increased fat content of bone marrow in elderly
- This technique is unique that it provides for true 3-dimensional imaging and reports bone density measurement as true volume density measurements.
- The advantage of QCT is its ability to isolate an area of interest from surrounding tissue.

Ultrasonography
- Inexpensive
- No radiation
- Not as precise as DXA
- Sites measured: Calcaneus, tibia, patella, fingers

Indications for Bone Mass Measurement
According to the National Osteoporosis Foundation's Scientific Advisory Board:
1. To aid in the diagnosis of significantly lowered bone mass in estrogen-deficient women as a guide for hormone replacement therapy.
2. To aid in therapeutic and diagnostic decision-making for those with apparent compression fracture or roentgenographic osteopenia. Even seemingly obvious vertebral compression fractures may actually represent old juvenile epiphysitis, positioning problems of the roentgenogram, or normal variations in vertebral body shape.
3. To diagnose low bone mass for those on long-term glucocorticoid steroids. Findings of significantly reduced bone mass may lead to reduction in dose.

4. To identify candidates for parathyroid surgery among those at risk for severe skeletal disease with asymptomatic primary hyperparathyroidism.

Other Indications Include
1. If risk factors present for fractures in peri-menopausal and post-menopausal women
2. Screen for bone loss in conditions in which osteopenia is a manifestation
3. Following response to treatment
4. Testosterone deficient men
5. Research—epidemiologic studies, clinical therapy trials

TREATMENT

Pharmacologic

- Preserve or improve bone mass
- Decrease bone resorption (anti-bone resorbers)

1. Calcium
- Mainstay for prevention and treatment of osteoporosis
- Optimal Calcium Requirements Recommended by the National Institutes of Health (NIH) Consensus Panel (Table 11–11)

TABLE 11–11. Calcium Requirements as Recommended by NIH

Age Group	Optimal Intake of Calcium (mg)
Birth–6 mos.	400
6 mos–1 year	600
1–5 yrs	800
6–10 yrs	800–1200
11–24 yrs	1200–1500
Men: 25–65 yrs	1000
Women: 25–65 yrs	1000
Postmenopausal women on estrogen: 50–65 yrs	1000
Postmenopausal women not on estrogen: 50–65 yrs	1500
Men and women > 65 yrs	1500
Pregnant and nursing women	1200–1500

- Immobilization + excess calcium intake predisposes patient to kidney stones; maintain urinary calcium excretion < 250 mg/24h in those without kidney stones

2. Vitamin D
   Increase calcium absorption in gut
   – Recommended doses:
      400–800 IU/day

3. Estrogen
- Mainstay for prevention and treatment for osteoporosis in females
- Mechanism of action:
      Suppresses interleukin 6 secretion with inhibition osteoclast recruitment
      Decreases bone resorption
      Increases calcium absorption in gut
- Dosing regimens:
      0.625mg/day conjugated estrogen cycled or continuous with progesterone 2.5 –10mg

Transdermal Estradiol: 0.05–0.10mg 2x/week
- Maintain therapy 10–20 yrs. after onset of post-menopausal symptoms
- Intact uterus: use progesterone to decrease buildup of endometrium
- If hysterectomy: may use estrogen only
- Benefits:
  Preserves bone mass at multiple skeletal sites
  Decreased incidence of fracture:
  ~ 50% risk reduction of spine fracture
  ~ 60% incidence reduction of hip/wrist fracture
  Prevents vasomotor symptoms
  Cardioprotective
- Side effects:
  Endometrial cancer: increased risk if estrogen given without progesterone
  Breast cancer: if prolonged use after menopause
  Thromboembolic disease
- Contraindications: Breast or uterine cancer, thrombophlebitis, hypercoagulable states, unexplained vaginal bleeding

4. Calcitonin (salmon)

Directly inhibits osteoclastic activity
- Benefits:
  Decreases pain in acute compression fractures through stimulation of beta endorphins
  Preserves bone mass
  ~ 36% incidence reduction of spine fractures
- Recommended doses:
  Nasal spray (Miacalcin®) 200 units/d
  Parenteral injection subcutaneously or intramuscularly (Calcimar®): prevention 100 IU QOD, treatment 100 IU QD
  Must have adequate concurrent intake of calcium and vitamin D
- Side effects: nasal irritation, facial flushing, local skin irritation, nausea

5. Bisphosphonates

- Alendronate (Fosamax®)
  More potent than Etidronate
  Recommended dosing: prevention 5 mg/d, treatment 10 mg/d
  Take 1/2 hour before food/drink/meds in morning, in upright position to avoid esophageal irritation
  ~ 49% risk reduction of spine fractures
  ~ 56% risk reduction of hip fractures
  Side effects: abdominal pain, nausea, dyspepsia, risk for esophageal ulceration
- Etidronate (Didronel®)
  Recommended dosing: 400 mg/d for 14 days every 3 months secondary to inhibition of normal mineralization
  Side effects: diarrhea

6. Selective Estrogen Receptor Modulators (SERMs)

- For prevention of osteoporosis in postmenopausal women unable to take estrogen due to side effects or risk of breast cancer
- Raloxifene (Evista®)
  Dosing: 60 mg/d
  Side effects: hot flashes, increased risk of DVT
- Increase bone formation (positive bone formers)
  Most considered experimental, not FDA approved

1. Sodium Fluoride: stimulates osteoblast formation; high dosage may increase risk of non-spinal fracture, bone fragility
2. Anabolic steroids: may have beneficial effect on bone mass but side effects prohibit their use; side effects: nausea, GI bleeding, joint pain
3. Testosterone: may benefit men with hypogonadism
4. Parathyroid hormone: may stimulate bone if given parenterally

Exercise (See Management)

Weight bearing (axial loading) and pull of functioning muscle preserves or increases bone mass

Avoidance of Risk Factors

MANAGEMENT

Depression

Most common psychological problem due to pain, functional decline
Treatment: psych support, antidepressants

Therapeutic Exercise

Tailored to fitness level and anticipated propensity to fracture or current fractures
Lessen bone loss, increase strength and balance to prevent falls and avoid fracture

Goals of Therapeutic Exercise
- Short Term—Education: proper posture, body mechanics, increasing strength and aerobic capacity
- Long Term—Prevention of falls and fractures: proper nutrition, strength, aerobic capacity with adequate spine support, pain management, psych support

Exercises
- Pectoral stretching, back extension
- Strengthening—back extension, isometric exercises to strengthen the abdomen, upper and lower extremities
- Deep breathing exercises
- Weight-bearing exercises—walking, low impact aerobics, jogging, stair-climbing (weight-bearing exercises improve bone density)
- Balance and transfer training
- Proper lifting techniques, body mechanics
- Posture correction—avoid kyphotic posture
- Avoid spine flexion exercises in spinal osteoporosis, which may predispose to vertebral compression fracture

TYPES OF FRACTURES AND SYNDROMES

Vertebral Fractures

Evaluation:
    History/Physical Exam
    Spine x-ray
    Bone scan: increased activity at sites of fractures indicate ongoing bone formation/healing
Acute vertebral fractures—may follow minor injury or physical activity
Most common osteoporotic fracture—vertebrae > hip > wrist

Compression Fractures
Most common site: lower thoracic, upper lumbar area
Involve anterior part of spine, vertebral body
Restrict flexion which loads anterior vertebral body

Microfractures–Trabeculae
Pain in the absence of fracture visible on x-ray
May be seen by bone-scan

Multiple Spine Fractures
Collapsed/anteriorly wedged vertebrae
    Kyphosis (Dowager's hump)
    Loss of height
    Abdominal proturbance, GI discomfort
    Pulmonary insufficiency
    Costal iliac impingement syndrome

Facet Joint Disease
Most prominent abnormality at vertebral collapse level with smaller lesions above and below level

Retropulsed Fragments
Back pain with neurologic symptoms in lower extremities

Costal Iliac Impingement Syndrome

Lower ribs impinge on iliac crest causing pain
Increased pain with lateral rotation and bending

Treatment
Relief with soft wide belt which sinks into pelvic cavity avoiding rib contact with iliac crest
Injection of sclerosing material into margins of iliac and lower ribs
Resection of lower ribs

PAIN MANAGEMENT

Pain caused by

- Recent compression fracture
- Mechanical derangement—paraspinal muscle spasm, kyphosis, arthritis, costal iliac impingement syndrome
- Differential diagnoses: neoplasm, herpes zoster, Polymyalgia Rheumatica, pancreatic disorders, abdominal aortic aneurysm

Acute Back Pain (Secondary to Acute Vertebral Fracture)
- Usually severe, most intense at fracture level
- Sharp pain increased with movement and alleviated with bedrest
- Severe pain lasting 2–3 weeks with decreased severity for 6–8 weeks
- May be asymptomatic

Treatment:
- Bedrest initially less than 1 week (1 day–1 week) graduating to bed activities and progressive ambulation
- Immobilization of fracture site, soft orthosis (corset)—rigid orthotic not used to prevent disuse osteoporosis

- Physical agents: local heat or cold
- Analgesics: to be given initially around the clock, narcotics initially, then within 1–2 weeks salicylates, NSAIDs and acetaminophen
- Avoid constipation and exertional exercises

Chronic Back Pain
- Pain less intense in acute fracture
- Mid-thoracic or lumbosacral
- Mechanical deformity, paraspinal muscle spasm
- Radiates laterally, associated with exertion

Treatment:
- Periods of bedrest 20–30 minutes BID
- Assess ADLs, use of devices to avoid aggravation of pain
- Orthosis
- Strengthening paravertebral, abdominal gluteal muscles, improve balance and flexibility, postural correction, proper body mechanics
- Avoid activities that increase vertebral compression forces
- Physical agents: heat or cold, TENS, acupuncture
- Analgesics: non-narcotic agents, Calcitonin
- Behavioral modifications: biofeedback, hypnosis, counseling

BACK SUPPORTS/BRACING

Orthoses

Indications for Using Bracing for Vertebral Fractures
- Pain relief: acute fracture—spine immobilization decreases paraspinal muscle spasm and overuse
- Stabilize spine
- Prevent further fracture
- Prevent soft tissue shortening
- Decrease flexion
- Compensate for weak erector spinal muscles

Contraindications to Back Bracing
- Hiatal hernia
- Inguinal hernia
- Orthopnea secondary to COPD
- Obesity
- Kyphoscoliosis

Risks of Prolonged Use of Orthosis
- Weakening/atrophy of trunk muscles
- Reduced spinal mobility
- Increased fracture risk due to weakening of supporting muscles—(this results in disuse osteoporosis)

Types of Orthoses (see also Chapter 6: Prosthetics and Orthotics)

1. Nonrigid Brace—used in stable fracture for pain management
- Abdominal Corset (elastic binder)
  Decrease pain: increase intra-abdominal pressure placing anteriorly directed force on vertebral bodies, also serves as a reminder to restrict motion

2. Rigid—(TL, TLSO, Jewett, CASH)—used in acute TL fractures
- Thoracolumbar support—assist spine extension via shoulder straps and paraspinal bars; increases intraabdominal pressure
- TLSO (Thoracolumbosacral Orthosis):
  Fixation from pelvis to shoulders
  Greatest immobility
  Increased noncompliance
- Jewett Brace
  Forces act to extend thoracolumbar region
- CASH (Cruciform Anterior Sternal Hyperextension)

Note: Orthotics that cause excessive hyperextension forces on the spine may induce posterior element type fractures in the osteoporotic patient, this therefore should be a consideration in this patient population.

Other Options:
- **Postural training supports** consist of small pouches containing weights up to 2 lbs. The pouch is suspended by loops from the shoulders, and is positioned just below the inferior angle of the scapula to counteract the tendency to bend forward and may be worn for 1-hour twice/day

FALLS AND FRACTURES

Hip Fractures: multifactorial causes with 2 major risk factors—osteoporosis and falls
Wrist fractures: most common fracture in females >75 years old.

Proximal Femur Fracture

- Muscle forces acting on hip are greater than the mechanical ability of femur to withstand these forces
- Direction of fall is a major risk factor for fracture
  Falls to side result in forces greater than muscle strength
  Elderly tend to fall sideways or drop in place

Risk Factors for Falling

- Decreased vision (poor depth perception)
- Sedative use
- Polypharmacy
- Cognitive impairment
- LE disability
- Foot problems
- Peripheral neuropathy
- Balance/gait abnormality
- Weakness (i.e., inability to rise form a chair without using one's arms)

Fall Prevention Program

- General conditioning exercises
- Assistive devices: canes, walkers, grab bars, tub benches
- Adequate shoe-wear, avoid high heels
- Modification of meds
- Improve balance

- Environmental modification: adequate lighting, removal of throw rugs, handrails for stairs, ramps

∎

REHABILITATION OF BURN INJURIES

BURNS—GENERAL INFORMATION

- A burn is the body's response to a thermal insult from an external agent such as heat , cold, chemicals, electricity, and radiation
- 85%–90% of burns are caused by heat
- 10%–15% of burns are from frostbite, chemical, and electrical damage
- 1.5 to 2.0 million people sustain burns each year in the U.S
- 60,000 to 80,000 of burn victims need hospitalization
- 5,000 people die each year from burns
- 35,000 to 50,000 people have temporary or permanent disability secondary to burns

Burns are the:
- Number 1 cause of accidental deaths in children under 2. The majority of burns in this age group occur as a result of abuse
- Number 2 in children under 4
- Number 3 in children under 19

Pathophysiology
- Normal skin figure (Table 11–12)

Cellular Response to Burns

Local reactions to burns include:
a) Exposed collagen causes platelet activation
b) Intense vasoconstriction secondary to epinephrine, prostaglandins, serotonin, and leukotrienes
c) Within a few hours—histamine release causing vasodilatation and increased capillary permeability allowing protein and albumin into the extravascular space followed by fluid causing severe edema
d) Late capillary permeability secondary to leukotrienes
e) Swelling and rupture of damaged cells
f) Platelet and leukocyte aggregation with clot formation from tissue thromboplastin, endotoxin, interleukin-1, and Hageman factor
g) Establishment of a hypermetabolic state

Systemic Response to Burns

- Loss of fluid into extravascular compartment resulting in hypovolemia and shock
- Hyperventilation with increased oxygen demand
- Inhalational injury causing decreased oxygenation and ARDS
- Initial decrease followed in several days by a significant increase in cardiac output
- Increase in blood viscosity
- Gastric dilation and ileus occurs in the first three days postburn
- Multi-organ system failure

CLASSIFICATION OF BURNS

Causative Agent

1. **Thermal**
   a) Heat—application creates a zone of coagulation, where tissue is destroyed and a zone of stasis, an area of decreased blood flow. This area may improve or get worse depending upon treatment
   b) Cold—damage occurs as a combination of actual freezing plus decreased blood flow and ischemia. Commonly, alcohol is involved in these injuries

2. **Electrical**—superficial damage may appear minimal; however, the deeper tissues (muscle and bone) may have severe injuries. The electrical current travels through the body following the path of least resistance. This turns out to be the nerves, arteries, veins, and bones. The current causes damage all along the course through the body. Because of its smaller cross-section area, there is a relatively greater resistance at the exit site, causing a greater build up of heat. This often leads to an explosive release of built up energy and significantly more extensive damage at the exit wound than entrance. Injury observed in conjunction with electrical burns includes:
   a) Radiculopathy from hyperextension caused by tonic/clonic contractions during electrocution.
   b) Peripheral neuropathy caused by direct injury from the current
   c) Cognitive impairment
   d) Spinal cord injury
   e) Formation of heterotropic bone around joints and in residual limbs
   f) Cardiopulmonary arrest
   g) Will be at risk of developing early onset of cataracts and hearing loss, both amenable to usual treatments

3. **Chemical burns**—from either acid or alkali exposure. These burns are typically underestimated and will frequently appear to be mild in severity. However, inappropriate or insufficient removal of the causative agent allows the injury to progress

4. **Radiation**—risk and severity of burn will depend upon duration and intensity of exposure. Response will vary from mild erythema to blistering and skin sloughing over a period of hours to days. If exposure is high enough, treatment can only be palliative

Depth of Burn (Table 11–12) (Figure 11–11)

Older Terminology
a) First degree; outer layers of epidermis injured, erythema, but no blistering
b) Second degree; involves epidermis into dermis but basal layer remains, blistering
c) Third degree; all epidermis and dermis destroyed; only white eschar remains
d) Fourth degree; muscle, nerve and bone damaged

Newer terminology
a) Superficial partial thickness; epidermis and upper part of dermis injured
b) Deep partial thickness; epidermis and large upper portion of dermis injured
c) Full thickness; all layers destroyed

TABLE 11–12. Degree of Burns

NORMAL SKIN	Epidermis and Dermis Intact	
FIRST DEGREE	Only the outer layers of epidermis are injured, sparing deeper layers. Erythematous, but no blistering.	
SECOND DEGREE Superficial partial thickness	Involves epidermis, but most of basal layer remains; blistering	
SECOND DEGREE Deep partial thickness	Involves the dermis; only the basal layer lining skin appendages remains; blistering.	
THIRD DEGREE Full thickness	Total destruction of epidermis and dermis.	

The degree of burn describes the depth of injury. Most injuries are of varying depths. (O'Young, 1997)

Size of burn

Rule of nines (Figure 11–12)
The Rule of 9's is an approximate way of estimating Adult Total Body Surface Area (BSA).
- Head = 9% BSA
- Each upper extremity = 9% BSA
- Each lower extremity = 18% BSA
- Anterior trunk = 18% BSA
- Posterior trunk = 18% BSA
- Perineum = 1% BSA

American Burn Association Classification

1. Minor
   a) < 15% BSA partial thickness (10% in child)
   b) < 2% BSA full thickness (not involving eyes, ears, face or perineum)
2. Moderate (most should be hospitalized)
   a) 15% to 20% BSA (10% to 20% in child)
   b) 2% to 10% BSA full thickness (not involving eyes, ears, face or perineum.)

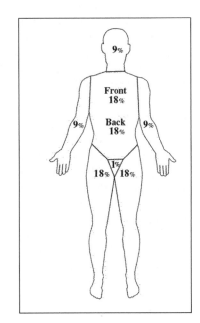

FIGURE 11–12. Rule of Nines.

3. Major (all should be hospitalized)
   a) > 25% BSA partial thickness (20% in child)
   b) ≥ 10% BSA full thickness
   c) All burns to eyes, ears, face or perineum.
   d) All electrical
   e) All inhalation
   f) All burns with fracture or major tissue trauma
   g) All with poor risk secondary to age or illness

FACTORS AFFECTING OUTCOME

1. **Age**—infants, children, and the elderly have a poorer rate of survival
2. **Total Body Surface Area**—the greater the area of involvement the worse the prognosis
3. **Depth of Burn**—as the total BSA that is full thickness increases the prognosis decreases
4. **Other Associated Injuries**—prognosis decreases as the number of concurrent injuries increases

PATIENT MANAGEMENT

Initial Treatment

Always begin any emergency assessment with an evaluation of the ABCs, airway , breathing, circulation. Special considerations include:
- Resuscitation with fluids, use Brooke, Evans, Baxter or Parkland formulas as a guide
- Parkland formula (4cc/kg body weight/% burned). One-half (1/2) of the total should be given in first 8 hours. The remaining amount is divided equally over the next 16 hours
- Escharotomy: an incision of burned tissue to relieve pressure from edema and hopefully avoid neurovascular compromise and amputation
- Nasogastric (NG) tube for abdominal decompression and foley catheter for volume management
- Tetanus toxoid
- Cleaning all wounds with sterile saline
- Application of topical antimicrobials. Systemic antibiotics should await specific indications and be culture driven
- Rapid and extensive debridement and grafting. The goal is to cover as much open area as possible in as short a period of time as possible. Nothing else will prevent complications, decrease pain, and promote rapid recovery as well as coverage of wounds

Wound Healing

Phases
1. Inflammatory Phase—response to injury with influx of neutrophils and macrophages
2. Proliferative Phase—with new matrix is laid with fibroblasts and in-growth of capillaries
3. Maturation Phase—resolution of inflammation in which collagen is laid down to form the scar.
4. Epithelialization—reestablishment of the basement membrane and epidermis
5. Wound Contraction—the open margins are brought together by fibroblasts
6. Wound Contracture—shrinkage of the scar through collagen remodeling. This causes functional restriction of motion

Treatment (Table 11–13)

Wounds are more likely to have hypertrophic scarring if they take longer than two weeks to heal. To reduce this, early debridement and skin grafting with good local wound care is required

- **Wound Dressings**—First use topical antibiotics (ie. Silvadene® or Bactroban®) then biological or synthetic dressings
- **Biological Dressings**—temporary cover for a burn wound to protect wound and decrease fluid loss from the site, decrease pain, and inhibits bacterial growth. May use autographs—split thickness (STSG) or full thickness (FTSG) skin grafts taken from donor sites on the patient; homographs—skin from the same species but not the patient (human cadavers or fetal membranes); and xenografts—skin from other species (pigs in the U.S. or frogs in Brazil). Homographs and xenografts are temporary coverings because the body will ultimately reject the foreign protein. They are utilized when too much BSA is involved and there is not enough uninjured skin to use for graphs, or until donor sites can be reharvested. Until then they provide the same benefits as STSG or FTSG.
- **Synthetic Dressings**—Much effort has gone into the development of synthetic membranes such as Biobrane®—a bi-laminate dressing that can be used temporarily to cover wounds until STSG are available
- **Cultured Epithelial Autocytes (CEA)**—CEA is skin that is cloned from a small 2.5 cm square piece of the patient's own skin. From that, literally yards of skin can be grown fairly rapidly. It is the patient's own skin so risk of rejection is minimized. Problems include: fragility (making application technically very difficult), lack of a basement membrane (it is only the epidermal layer meaning it cannot cover irregular surfaces well and easily slides off even after several days), and horrendous expense
- **Debridement**—removal of eschar to expose viable tissue and prepare the wound bed for coverage
  - **Mechanical**—wet to moist dressings, or hydro therapy to soften eschar
  - **Hydrotherapy**—consists of daily cleansing of wounds. Immersion tanks are not used secondary to the risk of cross contamination
  - **Enzymatic**—digest necrotic tissue without harming viable tissue. May be painful, increase body temperature, or cause bleeding. Can increase fluid loss therefore, should only be done 20% or less of BSA
- **Surgical debridement**
  - Tangential excision—1–10 days post burn, removing thin layers until normal viable tissue is exposed. May have significant bleeding. With early debridement and grafting, it has been shown to decrease hospital stay, mortality, and sepsis. (Helm, 1998).
- **Skin Grafting**—covering a wound with healthy skin
  - Used if wound is not expected to heal within 18–21 days
  - Allows early wound closure which reduces pain
  - Autologous
  - Full thickness. Utilizes all layers of epidermis and dermis. Will not contract as it matures. Obviously cannot be used to cover anything but small areas that are burned as available tissue is rapidly used up
  - Split thickness. Is meshed at the time of harvest giving largest possible area of coverage. Will contract as it heals
  - Homologous (cadaver) split skin (temporary)
  - Xenograft donor from another species (temporary)
  - Immobilize the joint above and below the graft for a minimum of 3 to 5 days to encourage healing
  - Minimize positional dependent edema to prevent graft loss

TABLE 11–13. Assessment and Treatment of Burn Injuries

Depth of Injury	Healing Time	Pain	Wound Outcome	Treatment Modalities
Superficial epidermis (First degree)	• 1–5 days	• Painful for 1–3 days, Ibuprofen or acetaminophen gives adequate analgesia	• No sequelae	• Elevation decreases pain of limb • Keep wound clean • Aloe or other moisturizer reduces dry skin and itching • If needed (usually in electrical injuries) therapy to prevent PTSD
Superficial dermis (Second degree/superficial partial thickness)	• 14 days	• Painful for 5–14 days • Acetaminophen with codeine or oxycodone gives adequate analgesia for wound care, exercise and sleep	• Possible pigment changes	• Wound care • Active exercise • Protective garments • Sunscreen • Therapy to prevent PTSD
Deep reticular dermis (Second degree/deep partial thickness)	• 21 days for spontaneous healing • If grafted after 10–14 days, less scar formation will be noted, with improved functional outcome; less pain, and shortened hospital stay	• Very painful until closure • Methadone or oral morphine continuously for baseline pain control • Parenteral or instant-release oral morphine and/or oxazepam and midazolam for dressing changes and stretching exercises	• Probable pigment changes • Reduced skin durability • Severe scarring • Sensory changes • Apocrine changes • Edema in dependent limbs	• Wound care • Anti-inflammatories, analgesics, antipruritics • Active exercise • Elevated positioning/orthotics • External vascular support garments • Moisturization and lubrication • Daily living skills • Psychological therapy • Therapy to prevent PTSD
Subcutaneous tissue (Third degree/full thickness)	• Graft needed, or if smaller, undermine to approximate with primary closure • Variable healing time	• Nonpainful initially due to destruction of nerve endings • Pain medication as above • Carbamazepine, phenytoin, or amitriptyline	• Same as above • Additional sweating loss • Possible loss of finger or toenails • Possible additional sensory loss • Alopecia over grafts • Areas of cultured epithelial autograft show permanent fragility, loss of temperature control, dry blistering skin with changed sensation	• Same as above • Post-op positioning/immobilization • Possible need for NSAIDs or other etidronate disodium to prevent heterotopic ossification (controversial early treatment) • Therapy to prevent PTSD • Very slow weaning from analgesics and anxiolytics • Vibration for pruritus
Muscle, tendon, bone (4th degree) (Old term in disfavor and rarely used)	• Amputation or reconstructive surgery, such as flaps, needed • Healing time variable	• Nonpainful initially due to destruction of nerve ending • Chronic pain treatment for neuromas and phantom limb pain and later bone spicules	• Variable • Early amputation with closure using non-injured tissue shortens hospital stay, decreases pain, and improves prosthesis fit	• Same as above • Deep tendon massage • Adapted equipment • Prosthetic fitting if indicated

Ibuprofen has the dual action of inflammation reduction at injury site and pain reception reduced at the CNS level.

PTSD = post traumatic stress disorder; NSAIDs = nonsteroidal antiinflammatory drugs

Rivers EA, Fisher SV. Burn Rehabilitation. In: O'Young B, Young, MA: Stiens, SA. PM&R Secrets. Philadelphia: Hanley & Belfus, 1997.

TABLE 11–14. Consequences of Burn Injury by Depth of Burn

	Absent or Impaired Morphology	Wound Consequences
Epidermis	Stratum basale Stratum spinosum Stratum granulosum Stratum lucidum Stratum corneum Melanocytes	Source for proliferating cells Decrease protection Increased water loss Water loss, microorganism growth, entry of noxious agents Repeated sunburn
Dermis (does not regenerate)	Altered collagen Increased collagen Aging collagen	Decreased tensile strength Scarring Altered surgical response
Nerves	Affected Absent	Pruritus/paresthesisas Decreased sensation, trauma, and burn risk
Vascular system	Impaired Absent Fragility	Impaired (especially venous return) No healing (depends on area) Re-injury risk
Basement membrane zone	Basal decidua and densa Rete pegs and dermal papillae	Blisters Blisters, fragility
Epidermal appendages	Sweat ducts Sebaceous glands Hair follicle	Impaired thermoregulation Loss of duct, sweat, and oil glands Loss of hair root, resultant alopecia
Fingernail bed	Basal cells for proliferation absent	Malformed or absent nail

Campbell MK, Covey MH, eds. Topics in Acute Care and Trauma Rehabilitation. Frederick, MD: Aspen, 1987.

REHAB ISSUES

Contractures

Scars will grow and contract. They will continue to contract until they mature in one to one and a half years or unless they are met by an opposing force. This contracture is particularly damaging over joints. Hypertropic scarring is cosmetically and psychologically devastating even in the absence of mechanical limitation. Need 25mm of pressure to counteract the contraction of a scar.

Positioning to prevent contracture (Fig 11–13)

- Position patient in extension and abduction. Patients tend to contract in flexion and adduction to reduce stretching in the injured skin.
- Position to prevent dependent edema.
- Use of special beds i.e., Kin Air® and ROHO to limit pressure, breakdown, and facilitate positioning.

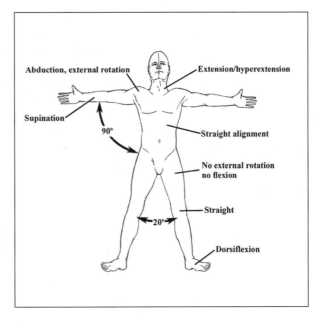

FIGURE 11–13. Anti-contracture Positioning—patient supine from ventral position.

Splinting

- Used with patients who are not compliant with positioning, or if there are exposed tendons or joints
- Splinting cannot be used without mobilization. A elbow that is frozen in full extension because it was splinted and never ranged is just as impaired as one that has contracted into full flexion because it was never splinted initially

Splints used:

Resting hand splint

1) For general hand burns to properly position patient
2) For hand burns with extensor tendons exposed

Dorsiflexion Lower Extremity

Knee-extension with foot dorsiflexion

Elbow extension

Transparent Face Mask—Made of silicon and used over healed grafts.

- Monitor skin easily
- Molded from the patient's own face for individual fit
- Protect contours of the face
- Prevents severe cosmetic deformities with even pressure across uneven surfaces, i.e., the nose
- Clear mask is more cosmetically and socially acceptable than a fabric mask
- Very hot, does not breathe and can cause maceration of the skin and even heat injury

Compression Garments

Used to help decrease hypertrophic scarring. It is thought that the pressure exerted on capillaries reduces blood flow; therefore, reducing the scar formation. These are worn 23 hours a day, only removed for washing. They are specifically measured to fit the burned areas: face masks, gloves, sleeves, jackets, or pants. They will need to be replaced frequently as they wear out and must be changed as the patient gains or loses weight.

Other Mechanisms to Control Hypertropic Scarring and Contractures

- Silastic gel has been found to reduce hypertrophic scar formation in the absence of pressure; however, the mechanism is not clear. It is used to line silicone masks and is applied over individual problem scar areas
- Steroids injected locally may reduce hypotrophic scarring
- Early mobilization is encouraged to maintain range of motion and prevent contractures. Balance splinting with mobilization
- Use assistive devices as needed for ambulation including Ankle Foot Orthosis (AFO)
- If torso is injured, maintain ROM with exercises
- Monitor for heterotopic ossification (HO)

Pain Control

Pain can be severe from burns, and adequate pain control is needed. Long-acting narcotics are used with short-acting for breakthrough pain. Dose may be high because metabolism of medications is higher in burn patients. Patient controlled analgesia (PCA) may be used to help the patient feel in more control. Consideration must be given to other causes of discomfort i.e. neuropathic pain, myofacial pain, pruritus, sleep deprivation and be treated aggressively and specifically. Mobilization must not be limited by pain.

Psychological Problems and Treatments for Burn Survivors

- Posttraumatic stress disorder (PTSD)
- Severe loss of personal identity with change in appearance. Little is more devastating than a change in our appearance
- Loss and change in position in the family and the community
- Financial and social stress
- Stress of constant pain
- Survivor guilt
- Depression
- Pre-existing psychological disorders
- Adjustment disorders
- Antidepressants
- Counseling
- Peer support of other burn survivors i.e., Phoenix Society
- Early reintegration into the community. Early and repeated emphasis upon return to vocational and avocational activity

Nutrition

Adequate calories must be given to maintain a positive nitrogen balance and promote muscle and skin repair. Healing will not take place without it, as the body is in a highly catabolic state. This may require as much as 2000 to 2200 calories and 15 gm of nitrogen per square meter of body surface per day. Additional vitamin C, vitamin A, zinc, copper, and manganese are important in wound care. The use of additional supplementation is essential. Once the acute phase has passed another problem may appear. Burned fat cells are not replaced. Overeating will cause weight gain into any area that has not lost cells and can lead to disfigurement secondary to relative obesity.

Exercise

- AROM (Active Range of Motion)
- Cardiovascular fitness
- Slow sustained stretching of the skin contractures:
  - Gentle application of superficial heat prior to stretch
  - Manual
  - Traction/weights
  - Serial casting/splinting
  - Paraffin
  - Massage/vibration

SPECIFIC PROBLEMS

Peripheral Neuropathy

- Present in 15–20% of burn patients with BSA of 20% or greater. (Helm, 1998)
- Etiology uncertain
- May have paresthesias, weakness
- Strength may recover well but usually easily fatigued

Multiple Mononeuropathy

Secondary to multiple crush syndrome caused by neurotoxins, metabolic or compression type injuries to nerves.

Bone and Joint Changes

- Decreased growth in children with burns near the epiphyseal plate
- Bone growth deformity after burn injury. Also must change the size of the compression garments frequently as children grow to prevent deformity. Particularly true with pressure to the mandible causing overbite

Osteophytes

- Found at the elbow and olecranon or coracoid process after burn injury

Heterotopic Ossification (HO)

- Ectopic bone deposition around joints and tendons
- Most common site of HO joint involvement in burns in elbow
- Reported in up to 23% of burn patients
- Recommend pain free active ROM

Scoliosis and Kyphosis

- Can be seen with burns of the chest or back
- May occur from protective posturing

Subluxations and Dislocations

- Seen with burns of the hands and feet, dorsal surface. During the healing process, skin pulls the joint into hyperextension, if chronic causes a subluxation
- Seen in MCP and MTP joints.
- Splint MCP in joint in flexion between 60 to 90 degrees, and exercise
- Use a surgical high-top shoe with a metatarsal bar 24 hours a day to prevent MTP subluxation

POSTACUTE PHASE

- Continue local wound care
- Prevention of new injury from mechanical irritants, the skin is now very sensitive.
- Lubricate skin several times a day
- Oral antihistamines and pressure garments (vascular support garments) for pruritus decrease edema, lessen hypertrophic scars, and speed wound healing. These garments should provide at least 25 mm Hg or more and be worn 23–24 hours per day to reduce hypertrophic scarring. (Helm, 1998)
- Provide protection from the sun as skin is susceptible to repeat burns. Use long sleeves, hats and sunscreen
- The skin will also be susceptible to topical irritants such as oil and gas and these should be avoided
- Extremes of heat should be avoided in full thickness burns as sweat glands are lost and the ability to cool the body through sweating is lost

SPASTICITY AND MOVEMENT DISORDERS
RECOMMENDED READING

Adams RD, Victor M, Ropper AH. *Principles of Neurology* 6th ed. New York: McGraw-Hill; 1997.

Goetz CG, Pappert EJ. *Textbook of Clinical Neurology.* Philadelphia: W.B. Saunders; 1999.

Katz RT. Spasticity. In: O'Young B, Young MA, Stiens SA (eds.). *PM&R Secrets.* Philadelphia: Hanley & Belfus; 1997.

Katz RT. Management of Spasticity. In: Braddom RL (ed.). *Physical Medicine and Rehabilitation.* Philadelphia: W.B. Saunders; 1996: 580–604.

Physician's Desk Reference 53rd ed. Montvale, NJ: Medical Economics; 1999.

Rosenthal M, Griffith ER, Bond MR, Miller JD. *Rehabilitation of the Adult and Child with Traumatic Brain Injury.* 3rd ed. Philadelphia: F.A. Davis; 1999.

Rowland LP. *Merritt's Textbook of Neurology* 8th ed. Philadelphia: Lea & Febiger; 1989.

Sliwa JA. Neuromuscular rehabilitation and electrodiagnosis. 1. Central neurologic disorders. *Arch Phys Med Rehabil* 2000; 81: S8–S10.

WHEELCHAIRS
RECOMMENDED READING

Buschbacher RM, Adkins J, Lay B, Braddom RL. Prescriptions of Wheelchairs and Seating Systems. In: Braddom RL (ed.). *Physical Medicine and Rehabilitation.* Philadelphia: W.B. Saunders; 1996: 381–400.

Cooper RA. *Wheelchair Selection and Configuration.* New York: Demos Medical Publishing; 1998.

Currie DM, Hardwick K, Marburger RA. Wheelchair Prescription and Adaptive Seating. In: DeLisa JA, Gans BM (eds.). *Rehabilitation Medicine: Practices and Principles* 3rd ed. Philadelphia: Lippincott-Raven; 1998: 763–788.

O'Young B, Young MA, Stiens SA. *PM&R Secrets.* Philadelphia; Hanley and Belfus; 1997.

Nesathruai S (ed.). *Rehabilitation of People with Spinal Cord Injury: A House Officer's Guide.* Boston: Arbuckle Academic Publishers; 1999.

Wilson AB Jr. *Wheelchairs: A Prescription Guide* 2nd ed. New York: Demos Medical Publishing; 1992.

MULTIPLE SCLEROSIS
REFERENCES

Grana EA, Kraft GH. Electrodiagnostic abnormalities in patients with multiple sclerosis. *Arch Phys Med Rehabil* 1994; 75: 778–782.

Greenspun B, Stineman M, Agri R: Multiple scleroses and rehabilitation outcome. *Arch Phys Med Rehabil* 1987; 68: 434–437.

Kraft GH, Freal JE, Coryell JK. Disability, disease duration, and rehabilitation service needs in multiple sclerosis: Patient perspectives. *Arch Phys Med Rehabil* 1986; 67: 164–168.

Kraft GH, Freal JE, Coryell JK, Hanan CL, Chitnis N. Multiple sclerosis: Early prognostic guidelines. *Arch Phys Med Rehabil* 1981; 62(2): 54–58.

Kurtzke, JF. Rating neurologic impairment in multiple sclerosis: An expanded disability status scale (EDSS). *Neurology* 1983; 33(11): 1444–152.

Multiple Sclerosis Society of Canada. MS Information. Multiple Sclerosis: Its Effect on You and Those You Love. www.mssociety.ca (accessed 8/30/02).

MULTIPLE SCLEROSIS
RECOMMENDED READING

Adams RD, Victor M, Ropper AH. *Principles of Neurology* 6th ed. New York: McGraw-Hill; 1997: 902–25.

Darley FL, Aronson AE, Brown JR. *Motor Speech Disorders.* Philadelphia: W.B. Saunders; 1975.

Kurland LT. Trauma and multiple sclerosis. *Ann Neurol* 1994; 36: S33–S77.

Peterson RC, Kokmen E. Cognitive and psychiatric abnormalities in multiple sclerosis. *Mayo Clin Proc* 1989; 64(6): 657–663.

Rolak LA. *Neurology Secrets: Questions You Will Be Asked—On Rounds, in the Clinic, at the Bedside* 2nd ed. Philadelphia: Hanley & Belfus; 1998: 191–198.

Rosenblum D, Saffir M. Multiple Sclerosis. In: Grabois M, Garrison S, Hart L, Lehmkuhl D (eds.). *Physical Medicine and Rehabilitation—The Complete Approach.* Malden, MA: Blackwell Scientific; 2000: 1370–1400.

Sliwa JA, Cohen BA. Multiple Sclerosis. In: DeLisa JA, Gans BM (eds.). *Rehabilitation Medicine: Principles and Practice* 3rd ed. Philadelphia: Lippincott-Raven; 1998: 1242–1257.

OSTEOPOROSIS
RECOMMENDED READING

American Academy of Orthopaedic Surgeons, American Association of Orthopaedic Surgeons Bulletin, 1999; 47(4): 33–36.

Bonner FJ Jr, Fitzsimmons A, Chestnut CD III, Lindsay R. Osteoporosis. In: DeLisa JA, Gans BM (eds.). *Rehabilitation Medicine: Practices and Principles* 3rd ed. Philadelphia: Lippincott-Raven; 1998: 1453–1476.

Kaplan FS. Prevention and management of osteoporosis. *Clin Symp* 1995; 47(1): 2–32.

Kaplan FS. Osteoporosis. *Clin Symp* 1983; 35(5): 1–32.

Matkovic V, Colachis SC III, Ilich JZ. Osteoporosis: Its Prevention and Treatment. In: Braddon RL (ed.). *Physical Medicine and Rehabilitation.* Philadelphia: W.B. Saunders; 1996: 851–75.

O'Young B, Young MA, Stiens SA. *PM&R Secrets.* Philadelphia: Hanley & Belfus; 1997.

Physical Medicine and Rehabilitation Clinics of North America, *Osteoporosis.* Philadelphia: W.B. Saunders; August 1995; 6(3).

Springer. Osteoporosis review of the evidence for prevention, diagnosis and treatment and cost-effective analysis. *Osteoporosis Internl* 1998; 8(S4).

BURNS
RECOMMENDED READING

American Burn Association. *Proceedings from the Annual Meeting.* 1992, 1993.

Artz CP, Moncrief JA, Pruitt BA Jr. *Burns: A Team Approach.* Philadelphia: W.B. Saunders; 1979.

Campbell MK, Covey MH (eds.). *Topics in Acute Care and Trauma Rehabilitation.* Frederick, MD: Aspen Publishers, 1987.

Helm PA, Fisher SV, Cromes GF Jr. Burn Injury Rehabilitation. In: DeLisa JA, Gans BM (eds.). *Rehabilitation Medicine: Practices and Principles* 3rd ed. Philadelphia: Lippincott-Raven; 1998: 1575–98.

Martyn JAJ. *Acute Management of the Burned Patient.* Philadelphia: W.B. Saunders; 1990.

Richard RL, Staley MJ. Burn Care and Rehabilitation Principles and Practice. Philadelphia: F.A. Davis; 1994.

Rivers EA, Fisher SV. Burn Rehabilitation. In: O'Young B, Young MA, Stiens SA (eds.). *PM&R Secrets.* Philadelphia: Hanley & Belfus, 1997.

■
EPILOGUE

I hope you enjoyed this textbook and it has helped crystallize the facts needed to pass boards and practice the field of physical medicine and rehabilitation. It was not meant to be the final text but a complete factual outline to enable both the seasoned and the neophyte to gain a vast amount of knowledge and background pathophysiology of diseases that cause disabling conditions. It will serve as an excellent quick reference to you for years to come. One must always remember, "we see what we are looking for, we look for what we know and what we do not know, we never see". Learning is a lifelong experience. Enjoy the experience and continue looking for the unseen.

Thomas E. Strax, M.D.

INDEX

Boldface numbers indicate illustrations and tables.